Comprehensive Healthcare Simulation

Series Editors

Adam I. Levine

Samuel DeMaria Jr.

More information about this series at http://www.springer.com/series/13029

Ali Alaraj
Editor

Comprehensive Healthcare Simulation: Neurosurgery

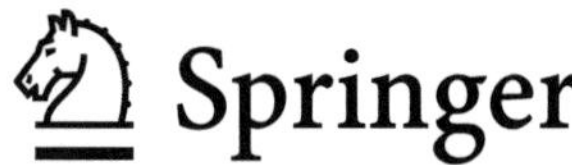

Editor
Ali Alaraj
Department of Neurosurgery
University of Illinois Hospital & Health Sciences System
Chicago, IL, USA

ISSN 2366-4479   ISSN 2366-4487   (electronic)
Comprehensive Healthcare Simulation
ISBN 978-3-319-75582-3   ISBN 978-3-319-75583-0   (eBook)
https://doi.org/10.1007/978-3-319-75583-0

Library of Congress Control Number: 2018941465

This Springer imprint is published by the registered company Springer International Publishing AG part of Springer Nature.
The registered company address is: Gewerbestrasse 11, 6330 Cham, Switzerland

Preface

The art of science of neurosurgery has been taught through past and recent history from one generation to another. The past history has relied on some forms of *simulation* to train the upcoming physicians. Initially that includes simulation of surgical procedures mostly on cadavers. Recently, with new technological advances, there has been an expansion of the simulation tools that are available for us for training. Different medical and surgical specialties have developed different modules for the training; the implementation of such training modules varies from one medical/surgical specialty to others. Within the medical specialties, the simulation modules focus more on physical examinations and analysis of emergent scenarios, while the surgical specialties had to come up with different ways to teach surgical skills. That created a huge obstacle to have simulation modules that can realistically mimic the human anatomy, its hemodynamics, and hemostasis as well as the physical properties of the human organs. Neurosurgery field like other surgical specialties have its own unique challenges. Neurosurgical trainees face great challenges in learning to plan and perform increasingly complex procedures in which there is little room for error. The brain is anatomically the most challenging organ in the body. Any surgical training module has to take into consideration the relationship of the skin, bone, brain tissue, and the ventricular system, thus expanding the complexity of any simulation module. The neurosurgical community has embarked on a very complex challenge of creating alternative surgical skill tools that would introduce the technical skills to the new residents, without putting patients at an increased risk.

In this textbook *Comprehensive Healthcare Simulation: Neurosurgery*, we tried to shed the light on the previous, current, and possible futuristic simulation methods that would enhance our ability to train future neurosurgeons. The textbook divides training tools into *physical*, *biological*, and *virtual reality* models. In each chapter, the corresponding authors go into details describing the nature of these models, their current application, and the current evidence of their value in the training. The choice of these models should take into consideration validity, cost-effectiveness, and ease of access.

Modes of simulation include detailed descriptions of cadaveric simulation, lifelike cadaveric simulation, fidelity manikin simulation, and microsurgical skills training in animal models and present on various currently available computer-based augmented reality simulators. The use of physical simulators has a promising role because of its low cost. The advantage of segmented reality simulation includes training on task-specific simulators, including simple ventriculostomy procedures, expanding into spinal instrumentation, and ultimately including the most complex aneurysm clipping procedures. The textbook also presents the role and future of 3D printing and 3D visualization of medical imaging. This field is only expected to expand which will revolutionize how we interpret medical imaging, how we would teach basic anatomy to medical students, and how to have a rehearsal of surgical anatomy and approaches prior to the surgical procedure using patient-specific data.

The role of such simulation modalities has been very essential in focused level-specific courses; this has been embraced in neurosurgical societies in the United States and internationally. These courses will prove to be helpful as they bring simulation material and faculty in one form. This textbook's aim is to provide a platform where residents in training, practicing neurosurgeons, and organized neurosurgery can go to review the best evidence for the role of simulation in neurosurgical training. I hope that the readers will find the material in this textbook helpful and useful in this rapidly changing field. I would certainly love to get feedback that can be used to enhance the second edition of this textbook.

Chicago, IL, USA   Ali Alaraj

Contents

Contributors

Aviva Abosch, MD, PhD Department of Neurosurgery, University of Colorado, Denver, CO, USA

Emad Aboud, MD, IFAANS Department of Neurosurgery, Arkansas Neuroscience Institute, Little Rock, AR, USA

Talal Aboud Department of Neurosurgery, Arkansas Neuroscience Institute, Little Rock, AR, USA

Ghaith Aboud, MD Department of Neurosurgery, Arkansas Neuroscience Institute, Little Rock, AR, USA

Ali Alaraj, MD Department of Neurosurgery, University of Illinois at Chicago, Chicago, IL, USA

Wafa Alduais Alshafai Neurosurgical Academy A.N.A, Toronto, ON, Canada

Kaith K. Almefty, MD Department of Neurosurgery, Barrow Neurological Institute, St. Joseph's Hospital and Medical Center, Phoenix, AZ, USA

Nabeel Saud Alshafai Alshafai Neurosurgical Academy A.N.A, Toronto, ON, Canada

Rami James N. Aoun, MD, MPH Department of Neurosurgery, Mayo Clinic, Phoenix, AZ, USA

Precision Neurotherapeutics Lab, Mayo Clinic, Phoenix, AZ, USA

Neurosurgery Simulation and Innovation Lab, Mayo Clinic, Phoenix, AZ, USA

Gregory Arnone, MD Department of Neurosurgery, University of Illinois at Chicago, Chicago, IL, USA

Adam Arthur University of Tennessee Health Sciences Center and Semmes-Murphey Neurologic and Spine Institute, Memphis, TN, USA

Nicholas C. Bambakidis Department of Neurological Surgery, University Hospitals Case Medical Center, Cleveland, OH, USA

Jaafar Basma Department of Neurosurgery, University of Tennessee Health Science Center, Memphis, TN, USA

Evgenii Belykh, MD Department of Neurosurgery, Barrow Neurological

Institute, St. Joseph's Hospital and Medical Center, Phoenix, AZ, USA

Department of Neurosurgery, Irkutsk State Medical University, Irkutsk, Russia

Bernard R. Bendok, MD, MSCI Department of Neurological Surgery, Otolaryngology, and Radiology, Mayo Clinic, Phoenix, AZ, USA

Precision Neurotherapeutics Lab, Mayo Clinic, Phoenix, AZ, USA

Neurosurgery Simulation and Innovation Lab, Mayo Clinic, Phoenix, AZ, USA

Antonio Bernardo Weill Cornell Medicine, Neurological Surgery, New York, NY, USA

Michael A. Bohl, MD Department of Neurosurgery, Barrow Neurological Institute, St. Joseph's Hospital and Medical Center, Phoenix, AZ, USA

Denise Brunozzi Department of Neurosurgery, University of Illinois at Chicago, Chicago, IL, USA

Roukoz Chamoun, MD Department of Neurosurgery, University of Kansas Medical Center, Kansas City, KS, USA

Fady T. Charbel, MD Department of Neurosurgery, University of Illinois at Chicago, Chicago, IL, USA

Alexander I. Evins Weill Cornell Medicine, Neurological Surgery, New York, NY, USA

Kyle M. Fargen Department of Neurological Surgery, Wake Forest University, Winston-Salem, NC, USA

Mark B. Frenkel Department of Neurosurgery, Wake Forest Baptist Medical Center, Winston Salem, NC, USA

Aman Gupta, MBBS Department of Neurosurgery, Mayo Clinic, Phoenix, AZ, USA

Precision Neurotherapeutics Lab, Mayo Clinic, Phoenix, AZ, USA

Neurosurgery Simulation and Innovation Lab, Mayo Clinic, Phoenix, AZ, USA

Rahim Ismail Department of Neurosurgery, University of Illinois at Chicago, Chicago, IL, USA

Department of Neurosurgery, University of Rochester Medical Center, Rochester, NY, USA

Connie Ju Department of Neurological Surgery, Case Western Reserve University, Cleveland, OH, USA

Teddy E. Kim Department of Neurological Surgery, Wake Forest University, Winston-Salem, NC, USA

Ralf A. Kockro Department of Neurosurgery, Hirslanden Hospital, Zurich, Switzerland

Sabine E. M. Kreilinger Department of Anesthesiology (MC 515), University of Illinois Health and Sciences System, Chicago, IL, USA

Chandan Krishna, MD Department of Neurosurgery, Mayo Clinic, Phoenix, AZ, USA

Precision Neurotherapeutics Lab, Mayo Clinic, Phoenix, AZ, USA

Neurosurgery Simulation and Innovation Lab, Mayo Clinic, Phoenix, AZ, USA

Ali Krisht Department of Neurosurgery, Arkansas Neuroscience Institute, Little Rock, AR, USA

Amanda Kwasnicki Department of Neurosurgery, University of Illinois at Chicago, Chicago, IL, USA

Michael Lawton Barrow Neurologic Institute, Phoenix, AZ, USA

Baruch B. Lieber Department of Neurological Surgery, Cerebrovascular Research Center, Stony Brook University Medical Center, Stony Brook, NY, USA

Cristian Javier Luciano Bioengineering, Biomedical and Health Information Sciences, University of Illinois at Chicago, Chicago, IL, USA

Laura Stone McGuire Department of Neurosurgery, University of Illinois at Chicago, Chicago, IL, USA

J. Mocco Department of Neurological Surgery, Mount Sinai Hospital, New York, NY, USA

Peter Nakaji, MD Department of Neurosurgery, Barrow Neurological Institute, St. Joseph's Hospital and Medical Center, Phoenix, AZ, USA

Steven Ojemann Department of Neurosurgery, University of Colorado, Denver, CO, USA

Edwing Isaac Mejia Orozco Department of Research and Development, Holo Surgical S.A., Warsaw, Poland

Jonathan R. Pace Department of Neurological Surgery, University Hospitals Case Medical Center, Cleveland, OH, USA

Jeremy C. Peterson, MD Department of Neurosurgery, University of Kansas Medical Center, Kansas City, KS, USA

Mark C. Preul, MD Department of Neurosurgery, Barrow Neurological Institute, St. Joseph's Hospital and Medical Center, Phoenix, AZ, USA

Rudy J. Rahme, MD Department of Neurosurgery, Northwestern Feinberg School and Medicine and McGaw Medical Center, Chicago, IL, USA

Shivani Rangwala, BS Department of Neurosurgery, University of Illinois at Chicago, Chicago, IL, USA

Ben Roitberg Department of Neurological Surgery, Case Western Reserve University School of Medicine, MetroHealth Campus, Cleveland, OH, USA

Hassan Saad Department of Neurosurgery, Arkansas Neuroscience Institute, Little Rock, AR, USA

Chander Sadasivan Department of Neurological Surgery, Cerebrovascular Research Center, Stony Brook University Medical Center, Stony Brook, NY, USA

Mithun G. Sattur, MBBS Department of Neurosurgery, Mayo Clinic, Phoenix, AZ, USA

Precision Neurotherapeutics Lab, Mayo Clinic, Phoenix, AZ, USA

Neurosurgery Simulation and Innovation Lab, Mayo Clinic, Phoenix, AZ, USA

Luis Serra Galgo Medical SL, Barcelona, Spain

Kushal J. Shah, MD Department of Neurosurgery, University of Kansas Medical Center, Kansas City, KS, USA

Sophia F. Shakur Department of Neurosurgery, University of Illinois at Chicago, Chicago, IL, USA

John H. Shin, MD Department of Neurosurgery, Massachusetts General Hospital, Harvard Medical School, Boston, MA, USA

Konstantin V. Slavin, MD Department of Neurosurgery, University of Illinois at Chicago, Chicago, IL, USA

Maksim Son Alshafai Neurosurgical Academy A.N.A, Toronto, ON, Canada

Theodosios Stamatopoulos, MD Department of Neurosurgery, Massachusetts General Hospital, Harvard Medical School, Boston, MA, USA

CORE-Center for Orthopedic Research at CIRI-AUTh, Aristotle University Medical School, Thessaloniki, Hellas, Greece

Barbara Stanley Department of Anaesthetics, Brighton and Sussex University Hospitals NHS Trust, Brighton, UK

Jay Vachhani University of Tennessee Health Sciences Center and Semmes-Murphey Neurologic and Spine Institute, Memphis, TN, USA

Erol Veznedaroglu Drexel Neurosciences Institute, Philadelphia, PA, USA

Talia Weiss College of Applied Health Sciences, University of Illinois at Chicago, Chicago, IL, USA

Matthew E. Welz, MS Department of Neurosurgery, Mayo Clinic, Phoenix, AZ, USA

Precision Neurotherapeutics Lab, Mayo Clinic, Phoenix, AZ, USA

Neurosurgery Simulation and Innovation Lab, Mayo Clinic, Phoenix, AZ, USA

Stacey Q. Wolfe Department of Neurological Surgery, Wake Forest University, Winston-Salem, NC, USA

Henry H. Woo Department of Neurological Surgery, Cerebrovascular Research Center, Stony Brook University Medical Center, Stony Brook, NY, USA

Vijay Yanamadala, MD Department of Neurosurgery, Massachusetts General Hospital, Harvard Medical School, Boston, MA, USA

Wei Hsun Yang Department of Neurosurgery, Arkansas Neuroscience Institute, Little Rock, AR, USA

Dali Yin Department of Neurosurgery, University of Illinois at Chicago, Chicago, IL, USA

Part I

Introduction to Simulation in Neurosurgery

History of Simulation

Nabeel Saud Alshafai and Wafa Alduais

Introduction

As we believe in the statement of the philosopher Confucius "Study the past, if we would divine the future," this chapter is dedicated to addressing the history of neurosurgical simulation. The objective of this chapter is to highlight the important historical background of simulation development over the years from the nonmedical era till it became one of the essential tools in neurosurgical training.

Early Use of Simulation in Military

Looking back at ancient history, simulation was first used by European military leaders for practicing decision-making and operational strategies. Petteia (Fig. 1.1) was used by the Greek as a war game in 500 BC, and it was a board game resembling war to plan military tactics [1]. Chess is recognized as another form of simulation used during the sixth century by Indians [2] and likewise for Kriegsspiel (German word for "wargame") which was developed by Prussian army in the nineteenth century [3].

History of Simulation Using Cadavers

Simulation was also used as an educational tool in medicine. Cadaveric dissections have historically been considered the ultimate anatomic simulators and continue to play an indispensable role in current neurosurgical training [4]. The earliest simulation attempt in medicine via cadaveric dissection was first performed during the era of Alcmaeon of Croton, a Greek philosopher in the sixth century BC (Fig. 1.2) [5]. In the latter half of the sixth century BC, most of the famous medical schools in Magna Graecia were found in Croton. Unlike what was practiced during that time to treat patients using the supernatural powers and magic, diseases of the human body were examined in a scientific and experimental way in these medical schools. Alcmaeon was one of the most active physicians interested in human physiology, devoted to science, and was a skillful experimentalist in the medical tradition of Croton [6].

In 275 BC, Herophilus of Chalcedon (Turkey 335–280 BC) is considered the founder of the first school of anatomy in Alexandria. He encouraged the human cadaveric dissection studies which have led to significant advances in the medical knowledge [7, 8]. These advances included recognizing the difference between arteries and nerves as well as between motor and sensory nerves, distinguishing the ventricles of

N. S. Alshafai (✉) · W. Alduais
Alshafai Neurosurgical Academy A.N.A,
Toronto, ON, Canada

© Springer International Publishing AG, part of Springer Nature 2018
A. Alaraj (ed.), *Comprehensive Healthcare Simulation: Neurosurgery*,
Comprehensive Healthcare Simulation, https://doi.org/10.1007/978-3-319-75583-0_1

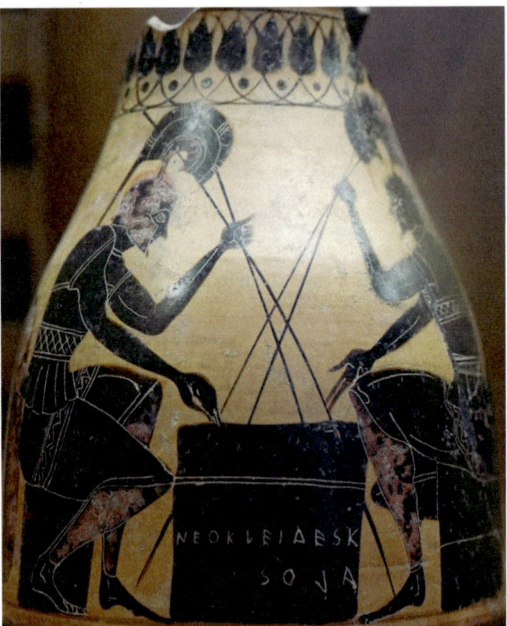

Fig. 1.1 Achilles and Ajax playing the board game Petteia [16]

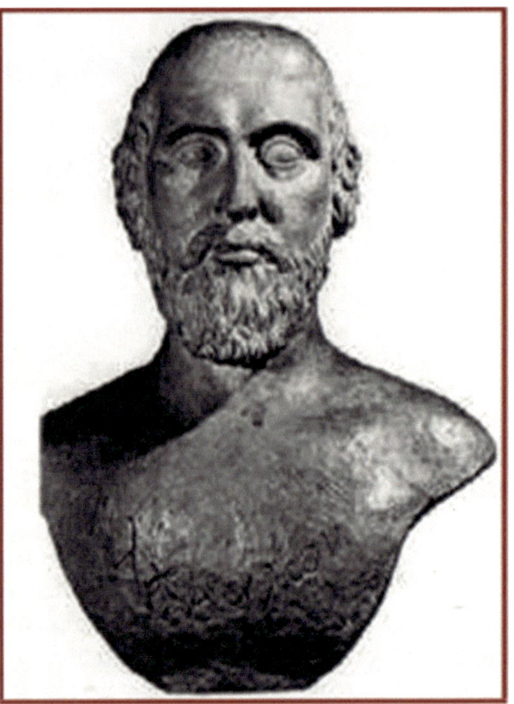

Fig. 1.2 Sculpture of Alcmaeon of Medicine Museum, University of Rome (Italy), donation by G. Arcieri [89]

the brain, differentiating between cranial and spinal nerves, and discovering and naming the confluence of dural sinuses near the internal occipital protuberance, which was named after him (torcular herophili) [9, 10].

Galen (AD 129–c.200/c.216) was considered the second most famous physician in history after Hippocrates [11]. His work provided further clarification of the human body [12, 13]. Because Roman law had prohibited the dissection of human cadavers since about 150 BC, Galen performed anatomical dissections on living and dead animals (Fig. 1.3). This work was useful because Galen believed that the anatomical structures of these animals closely mirrored those of humans [14]. For around 1500 years after Galen's death, to study medicine was to study Galen [13]. However, although his anatomical experiments on animal models led him to a more complete understanding of the circulatory system, nervous system, respiratory system, and other structures, his work contained scientific errors which was later shown by Ibn al-Nafis (Arab physician) mainly describing accurately the respiratory and circulatory systems [16]. There is some debate about whether or not Ibn al-Nafis participated in dissection to come to his conclusions about pulmonary circulation as some scholars believe that he must have participated or seen a human heart to describe the circulation this accurately [17].

Leonardo da Vinci (1452–1519) started his study in the anatomy of the human body under the apprenticeship of Andrea del Verrocchio. As an artist, he quickly became master of topographic anatomy, drawing many studies of muscles, tendons, and other visible anatomical features [18] (Fig. 1.4). As a successful artist, Leonardo was given permission to dissect human corpses. Leonardo made over 240 detailed drawings and wrote about 13,000 words toward a treatise on anatomy [18]. He created models of the cerebral ventricles with the use of melted wax [19].

Andreas Vesalius (1514–1564; whose meticulous monographs formed the basis of modern human anatomic studies) (Fig. 1.5) contributed to the new Giunta edition of Galen's collected works and began to write his own anatomical text

Fig. 1.3 Galen dissecting a monkey, as imagined by Veloso Salgado (pt) in 1906 [15]

based on his own research [21]. In 1543, Vesalius took residence in Basel to help Johannes Oporinus publish the seven-volume De humani corporis fabrica (On the fabric of the human body), a groundbreaking work of human anatomy [22].

History of Simulation Using Synthetic Physical Models

The first medical simulators were simple models of human patients. Since antiquity, these representations in clay and stone were used to demonstrate clinical features of disease states and their effects on humans. Models have been found from many cultures and continents. These models have been used in some cultures (e.g., Chinese culture) as a "diagnostic" instrument, allowing women to consult male physicians while maintaining social laws of modesty. Models are used today to help students learn the anatomy of the musculoskeletal system and organ systems [24].

The development of plastic physical model that can reproduce human responses was encouraged to overcome the limitations of cadaveric models in the medical training. "Resusci Anne" was a cardiopulmonary resuscitation manikin which was developed by Åsmund Lærdal (Fig. 1.6), a Norwegian

publisher and toy manufacturer in the 1950s [25]. Resusci Anne is considered as one of the first significant events in the history of medical simulation. She was initially designed for the practice of mouth-to-mouth breathing, and her face was based on the death mask of the Girl from the River Seine, a famous French drowning victim [26].

In the late 1960s, Abrahamson and Denson at the University of Southern California created the first anesthesia simulator (Sim One) which is a computer-controlled manikin [27]. The manikin had sophisticated features as it was able to breathe; has a heartbeat, temporal and carotid pulse (synchronized), and blood pressure; opens and closes its mouth; blinks its eyes; and responds to four intravenously administered drugs and two gases (oxygen and nitrous oxide) administered through mask or tube. The physiologic responses to what is done to it are in real time and occur "automatically" as part of a computer program [28]. However, due to its high cost, Sim One did not get much acceptance back then.

In 1968, Dr. Michael Gordon of the University of Miami Medical School demonstrated Harvey cardiology mannequin (Fig. 1.7) for the first time at the American Heart Association Scientific Sessions under the title of a Cardiology Patient Simulator. It is a full-sized mannequin that

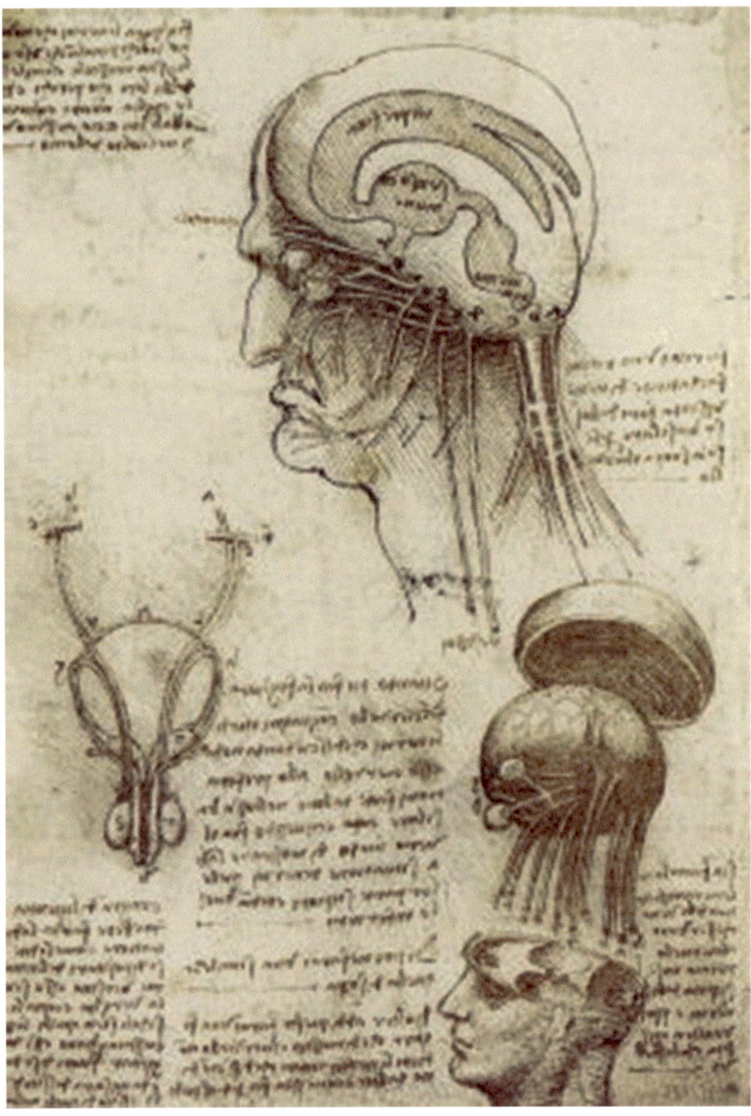

Fig. 1.4 Leonardo's physiological sketch of the human brain and skull (1510) [20]

simulates 27 cardiac conditions. The simulator displays various physical findings, including blood pressure by auscultation, bilateral jugular venous pulse wave forms and arterial pulses, precordial impulses, and auscultatory events in the four classic areas; these are synchronized with the pulse and vary with respiration. Harvey is capable of simulating a spectrum of cardiac diseases by varying blood pressure, breathing, pulses, normal heart sounds, and murmurs [29].

In the late 1980s, comprehensive anesthesia simulation environment (CASE 1.2) was developed by Dr. David Gaba and colleagues at Stanford Medical School as the first prototype of a mannequin simulator for investigating human performance in anesthesia [31]. Simultaneously, a multidisciplinary team at the University of Florida led by Dr. Michael Good and mentored by Dr. J S Gravenstein developed the Gainesville Anesthesia Simulator (GAS). The idea started from an interest in training anesthesia residents in basic clinical skills [32]. Many other different simulator mannequins were developed since that time in different countries, e.g., ACCESS (Anesthesia Computer Controlled Emergency Situation Simulator) was developed in the UK as a part-task trainer for anesthesia skills [33].

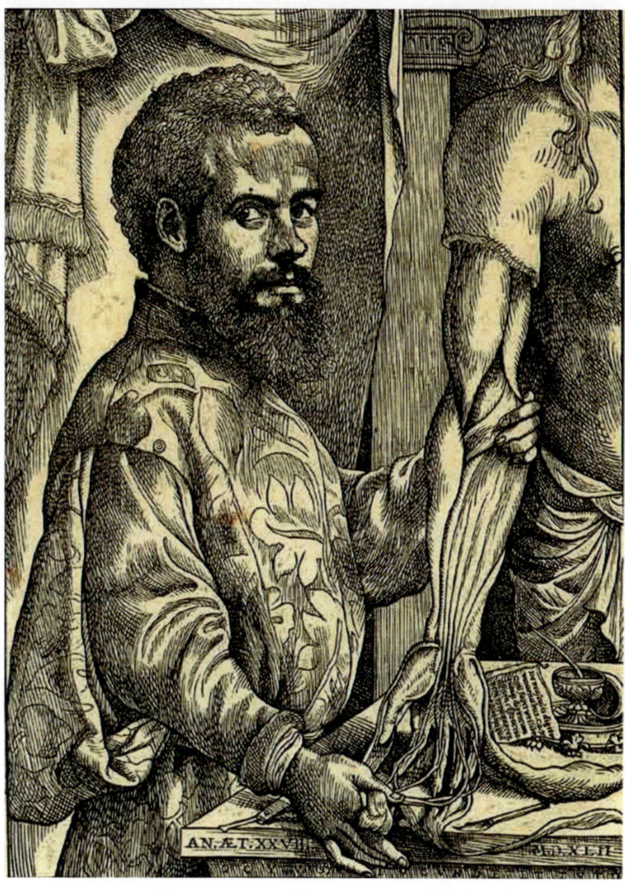

Fig. 1.5 Andreas Vesalius (1514–1564), the founder of modern human anatomy, provided further knowledge of anatomy-based systematic cadaveric dissection [23]

In 2012, Rowena (Realistic Operative Workstation for Educating Neurosurgical Apprentices) was designed with high fidelity features. She consists of a complete head with all the external features and surface landmarks. It consists of realistic layers to simulate the scalp, bone, and dura; the latter two include all sutures and appropriate vascular markings. A lot of research has gone into making these layers behave as realistically as possible, and, in particular, they are "bonded" together in a way that enables them to be dissected apart in a most realistic fashion. Rowena has no ferrous metal components and can therefore be scanned easily with MRI. First adult model was used, and then later, a pediatric model was developed [34].

History of Procedural Simulation

The earliest publication of a procedure simulation was reported in 1987 by Gillies and Williams for fiber-endoscopic training [35]. Baillie et al. described a computer simulation for teaching basic ERCP techniques in 1988 [36]. A large number of procedural simulators have been developed in different medical domains, including neurosurgery. One of the earliest neurosurgical simulation procedure planning was reported in the year 2000 by Phillips NI et al. for simulating ventricular catheterization [37]. Procedural simulation has evolved in different subspecialties of neurosurgery over the years (Table 1.1).

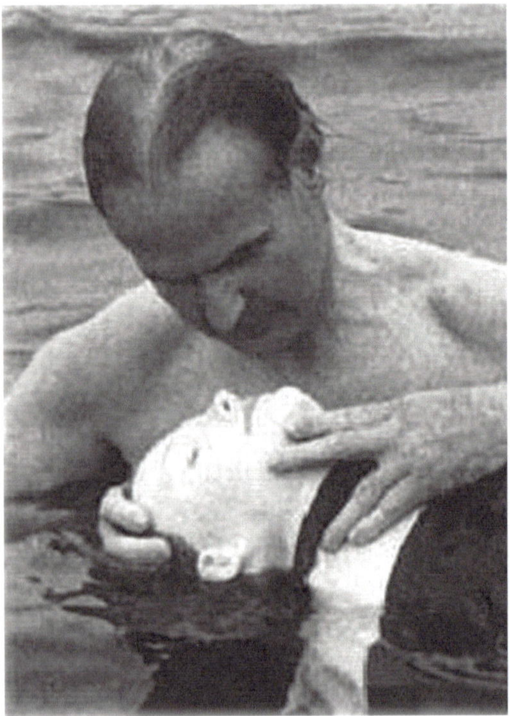

Fig. 1.6 Åsmund Lærdal with Resusci Anne, in about 1970 [26]

History of the Use of Human Simulator

In 1963 the idea of patient actor was first introduced by a neurologist from the University of Southern California to teach medical students during neurology clerkship. Initially designated as simulated patients, these were actors taught to portray different patient conditions [69]. In the 1970s, a patient instructor (patient with chronic stable findings) was used to teach physical examination and diagnostic skills to medical students. In 1993, the Association of American Medical Colleges sponsored a survey of medical schools regarding the use of standardized patient simulation which showed that this method was used largely by the medical schools in the USA. The Medical Council of Canada was the first to incorporate the standardized patient examination into licensure in 1993 [70].

In 2010, Musacchio et al. presented a critical care training program using Human Patient Simulator for neurosurgical trainees. Topics included spinal shock, closed head injury, and

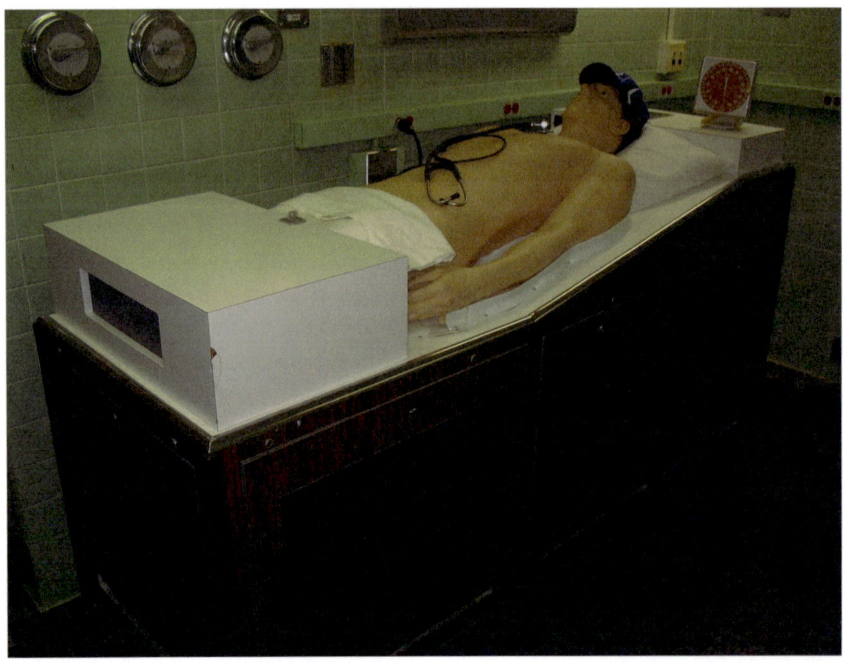

Fig. 1.7 Older version of Harvey Cardiovascular Patient Simulator [30]

Table 1.1 Procedural simulation in different neurosurgical subspecialties

Subspecialty	Procedure simulation
General and Emergency Neurosurgery	General skills include operative techniques and emergency procedures simulator [38] Neurosurgical critical care simulator [39] VR simulator for hemostasis [40] Burr hole and trauma craniotomy simulators have been developed by the National Capital Area Simulation Center (Uniformed Services University, Bethesda, Maryland) to teach residents as well as military surgeons who are being deployed to manage neurotrauma cases [41] Emergency neurosurgical procedures, including ventriculostomy and decompressive craniectomy [42] Ventriculostomy simulators, including VR models with haptic feedback and mixed-reality simulator [43–45]
Spine Neurosurgery	Immmersive Touch (Immersive Touch, Inc., Chicago, Illinois, USA), a VR platform combined with haptic technology called Sensimmer, has developed a lumbar pedicle screw model [90] Patient-specific mixed-reality simulator for spine procedures [46] A percutaneous VR simulator for vertebroplasty [47]
Vascular Neurosurgery	Cadaveric model with colored fluid under pulsating pressure for arteries simulating live surgery [48] Human placenta for vascular training simulating aneurysm models for clipping and endovascular treatment [49, 50] Bypass simulators [51] Simulator-based angiography [52] Complex aneurysm simulators [53–55]
Pediatric Neurosurgery	Computer-assisted 3D visualization and simulation system for fronto-orbital advancement in children with trigonocephaly [91] Anatomical Simulator for Pediatric Neurosurgery (ASPEN; Pro Delphus, São Paulo, Brazil) [55] Synthetic simulator for pediatric lumbar pathologies [56]
Tumor resection and skull base	Dextroscope simulator for vascular pathologies, cranial nerve decompression, tumor resection, and epilepsy procedures [57] Neuro Touch Cranio (VR simulator for brain tumor resection) [58] Voxel-Man Group (Hamburg, Germany) developed VR temporal bone simulators [59]
Minimally invasive Neurosurgery	ROBO-SIM (manipulator-assisted virtual procedure in minimally invasive neurosurgery) [60] Virtual neuroendoscopy system for surgical planning known as VIVENDI [61] NeuroTouch Endo. The VR platform is a simulator for endoscopic transsphenoidal surgery that integrates haptic feedback via tactile tool manipulators [62]
Stereotactic Neurosurgery	Monte Carlo simulations are 3D dosimetry tools suitable for adequate SRS therapy [63] Robotic radiosurgery systems [64] Hamamoto et al. introduced a tractography simulator to estimate dose tolerance of the optic radiation [65] Patient-specific mixed-reality simulator for percutaneous stereotactic lesion procedure for trigeminal neuralgia [46]
Functional Neurosurgery	Nowinski et al. introduced a DBS simulator system based on a reconstruction of a 3D stereotactic atlas of brain structure and vasculature using MR studies [66] Intracranial electrode implantation for epilepsy [67, 68]

cerebral vasospasm. Based on their experience, the neurosurgical critical care simulator helped residents and students to enhance their critical care education and the benefit for learning in a fail-safe scenario [71].

Historical Prospective of How Aviation Contributed to Current Advances in Neurosurgical Simulation

Medical simulation as we know it today was modeled primarily on those simulators initially implemented in the aviation industry in the early twentieth century. Up to our knowledge, the first reported aviation simulator was the Antoinette biplane in 1909 which was produced by a French manufacturer [72, 73].

In 1928, Edwin Link (Fig. 1.8) invented the first flight simulator, a prototype "blue box" flight trainer, believing that there must be an easier, safer, and less expensive way to learn how to fly [74]. Link opened his own flying school in 1930 to demonstrate the educational value of his trainer.

In 1934, after several catastrophic and fatal accidents, the Army purchased six Link Trainers to improve training. In World War II, military needs increased for the trainer throughout the world and led to other Link inventions: the Celestial Navigation Trainer, a bomber crew trainer, and the first airplane-specific model [76]. In 1955, civil aviation embraced simulation technology; and the Federal Aviation Administration required simulation recertification to maintain commercial pilots' licenses. The birth of analog computers in the 1950s increased the complexity

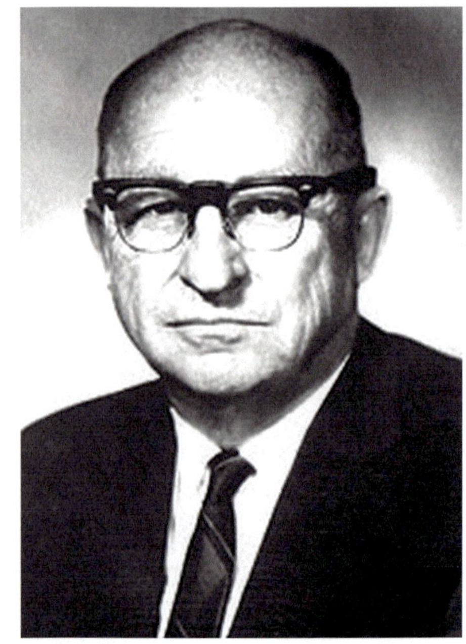

Fig. 1.8 Edwin Link [75]

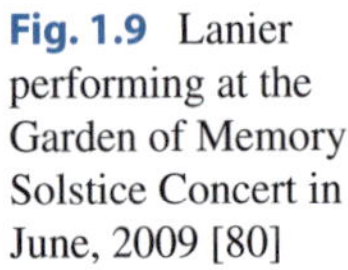

Fig. 1.9 Lanier performing at the Garden of Memory Solstice Concert in June, 2009 [80]

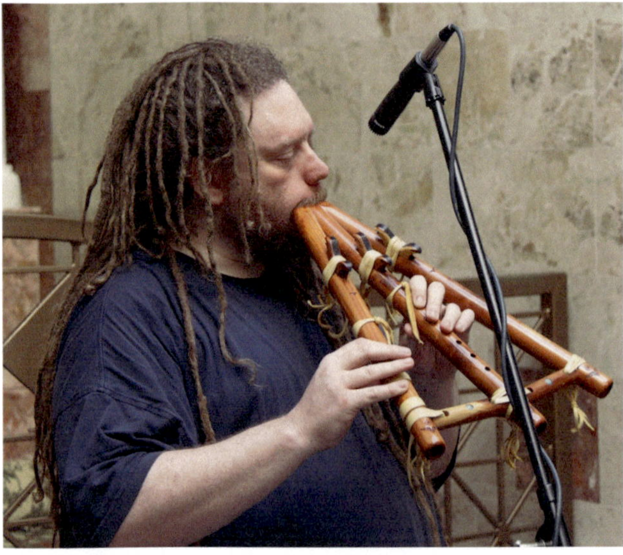

and realism of flight simulation [77]. It took us almost a century to arrive at the sophisticated flight simulators in use today.

The same principle used in flight simulation has been applied to assist surgeons. Computer-based surgical simulation was initially limited to presenting case scenarios using text and static images to be answered in branching-tree Bayesian methodology [78]. However, the first interactive and image-based computer simulation, virtual reality, was introduced in 1987 by Jaron Lanier (Fig. 1.9) (a computer philosophy writer, computer scientist, visual artist, and composer of classical music) [79, 80].

One of the first VR simulators in medical field was a leg simulator developed by Scott Delph and Joseph Rosen and was used to practice Achilles' tendon repair and then show the effect the procedure on gait [81]. At approximately the same time, Lanier and Satava developed the first VR simulator for general surgery, and although they looked at it as primitive initial step, they believed that it will represent the foundation for an educational base that is as important to surgery as the flight simulator is to aviation [82].

The first commercially successful surgical simulator was the MIST-VR (minimally invasive surgery trainer-virtual reality) by Seymour et al. [83]. ENT Sinus Surgery Simulator was one of the most sophisticated early simulators and was developed by the company that began by making aviation simulators" Lockheed Martin Corporation" [84].

Vascular Intervention Simulation Trainer (VIST), by Immersion Medical, is considered as the most sophisticated form of hybrid simulators. The initial hybrid simulators were created by HT Medical; however, the most successful has been a suite of gastrointestinal (GI) endoscopy simulators by Simbionix, Inc., in 2000 [78].

Motion tracking simulators were first developed at the Imperial College in London. Darzi et al. (2001) have developed the Imperial College Surgical Assessment Device (ICSAD) and have demonstrated that it is possible to quantitatively track the motion of the hands (see below) with the result in a measurable "motion signature" [85]. Eye trackers were also developed by Mylonas and Darzi and their colleagues in 2004 at the Imperial College [86].

In 2007, another area of simulation emerged, incorporating the simulation directly into the surgical work station of a robotic surgery system, such as the da Vinci of Intuitive Surgical, Inc. [87]. The modeling of simulator's dynamics problem has been extensively addressed in other paradigms, such as the modeling of rocket engines and nuclear detonations, and many of the algorithms developed in these fields were simplified for use in a real-time environment and proved to be useful in the solution of the dynamic haptic problem as well [88].

References

1. Smith R. The long history of gaming in military training. Simul Gaming. 2009;41:6–19.
2. Murray HJR. A history of chess: the original. 1913th ed. New York: Skyhorse Pub; 2012.
3. Robison RA, Liu CY, Apuzzo ML. Man, mind, and machine: the past and future of virtual reality simulation in neurologic surgery. World Neurosurg. 2011;76(5):419–30.
4. Moore KL. A history of anatomy: The post-Vesalian era. Clinical Anatomy. 1998;11(4):284–284.
5. Debernardi A, Sala E, D'aliberti G, Talamonti G, Franchini AF, Collice M. Alcmaeon of Croton. Neurosurgery. 2010;66(2):247–52.
6. Bradley P. The history of simulation in medical education and possible future directions. Med Educ. 2006;40(3):254–62.
7. Ghasemzadeh N, Zafari AM. A brief journey into the history of the arterial pulse. Cardiol Res Pract. 2011;28:2011.
8. Potter P. Herophilus of Chalcedon: an assessment of his place in the history of anatomy. Bull Hist Med. 1976;50(1):45.
9. Wiltse LL, Pait TG. Herophilus of Alexandria (325–255 BC): the father of anatomy. Spine. 1998;23(17):1904–14.
10. King LS. Doctors: the biography of medicine. JAMA. 1988;260(18):2729–30.
11. Kunkler K. The role of medical simulation: an overview. Int J Med Rob Comput Assisted Surg. 2006;2(3):203–10.
12. Limbrick DD Jr, Dacey RG Jr. Simulation in neurosurgery: possibilities and practicalities: foreword. Neurosurgery. 2013;73:S1–3.
13. Aufderheide AC. The scientific study of mummies. Cambridge: Cambridge University Press; 2003.
14. By Veloso Salgado – NOVA Medical School I Faculdade de Ciências Médicas da Universidade

Nova de Lisboa, Public Domain. https://commons.wikimedia.org/w/index.php?curid=59771497.

15. https://commons.wikimedia.org/wiki/File:Claudius_Galenus_(1906)_-_Veloso_Salgado.pnghttps://en.wikipedia.org/wiki/Achilles#Achilles.2C_Ajax_and_a_game_of_petteia.

16. Rocca J. Galen on the brain: anatomical knowledge and physiological speculation in the second century AD. Studies in ancient medicine. 2003;26:1.

17. Le Floch-Prigent P, Delaval D. The discovery of the pulmonary circulation by Ibn al Nafis during the 13th century: an anatomical approach (543.9). FASEB J. 2014;28(1 Supplement):543–9.

18. Da Vinci L. The notebooks of Leonardo da Vinci. Courier Corporation; 2012.

19. Jones R. Leonardo da Vinci: anatomist. Br J Gen Pract. 2012;62(599):319-319.

20. By Leonardo da Vinci., http://www2.warwick.ac.uk/fac/med/study/ugr/mbchb/societies/surgical/events/invited_lecture_-/, Public Domain, https://commons.wikimedia.org/w/index.php?curid=52376553 .

21. Rehder R, Abd-El-Barr M, Hooten K, Weinstock P, Madsen JR, Cohen AR. The role of simulation in neurosurgery. Childs Nerv Syst. 2016;32(1):43–54.

22. Catani M, Sandrone S. Brain renaissance: from Vesalius to modern neuroscience. Oxford: Oxford University Press; 2015.

23. By Attributed to Jan van Calcar – Page xii of De humani corporis fabrica (1534 edition), showing portrait of Andreas Vesalius. Original scan of page cropped to show portrait alone, contrasted slightly to 70 in Microsoft Photo Editor. The original book from which the scan arises is a copy of the 1543 edition stored in the collection of the U.S. National Library of Medicine, a division of the National Institutes of Health (NIH)., Public Domain. https://commons.wikimedia.org/w/index.php?curid=425785

24. Meller G. A typology of simulators for medical education. J Digit Imaging. 1997;10:194–6.

25. Rosen KR. The history of medical simulation. J Crit Care. 2008;23(2):157–66.

26. Cooper JB, Taqueti V. A brief history of the development of mannequin simulators for clinical education and training. Qual Saf Health Care. 2004;13(suppl 1):i11–8.

27. Denson JS, Abrahamson S. A computer-controlled patient simulator. JAMA. 1969;208(3):504–8.

28. Abrahamson S, Denson JS, Wolf RM. Effectiveness of a simulator in training anesthesiology residents. Qual Saf Health Care. 2004;13(5):395–7.

29. Cooper JB, Taqueti V. A brief history of the development of mannequin simulators for clinical education and training. Postgrad Med J. 2008;84(997):563–70.

30. By Gene Hobbs – Own work, CC BY-SA 3.0. https://commons.wikimedia.org/w/index.php?curid=15302566 .

31. Gaba DM, DeAnda A. A comprehensive anesthesia simulation environment: re-creating the operating room for research and training. Anesthesiology. 1988;69(3):387–94.

32. Good ML, Lampotang S, Gibby G, Gravenstein JS. Critical events simulation for training in anesthesiology. J Clin Monit Comput. 1988;4:140.

33. Byrne AJ, Hilton PJ, Lunn JN. Basic simulations for anaesthetists a pilot study of the ACCESS system. Anaesthesia. 1994;49(5):376–81.

34. Ashpole RD. Introducing Rowena: a simulator for neurosurgical training. Bull R Coll Surg Engl. 2015;97(7):299–301.

35. Gillies DF, Williams CB. An interactive graphic simulator for the teaching of fibrendoscopic techniques. In: Marechal G, editor. EUROGRAPHICS 1987. Amsterdam: North Holland; 1987. p. 127–38.

36. Baillie J, Gillies DF, Cotton PB, Williams CB. Computer-simulation for basic ERCP training-a working model. In Gastrointestinal endoscopy; 1989 Mar 1 (Vol. 35, No. 2, pp. 177–177). 11830 Westline Industrial Dr, St Louis, Mo 63146–3318: Mosby-Year Book INC.

37. Phillips NI, John NW. Web-based surgical simulation for ventricular catheterization. Neurosurgery. 2000;46(4):933–7.

38. Sharpe R, Koval V, Ronco JJ, Dodek P, Wong H, Shepherd J, FitzGerald JM, Ayas NT. The impact of prolonged continuous wakefulness on resident clinical performance in the intensive care unit: a patient simulator study. Crit Care Med. 2010;38(3):766–70.

39. Musacchio MJ, Smith AP, McNeal CA, Munoz L, Rothenberg DM, von Roenn KA, Byrne RW. Neuro-critical care skills training using a human patient simulator. Neurocrit Care. 2010;13(2):169–75.

40. Gasco J, Patel A, Ortega-Barnett J, Branch D, Desai S, Kuo YF, Luciano C, Rizzi S, Kania P, Matuyauskas M, Banerjee P. Virtual reality spine surgery simulation: an empirical study of its usefulness. Neurol Res. 2014;36(11):968–73.

41. Acosta E, Liu A, Armonda R, Fiorill M, Haluck R, Lake C, Muniz G, Bowyer M. Burrhole simulation for an intracranial hematoma simulator. Stud Health Technol Inform. 2006;125:1.

42. Lobel DA, Elder JB, Schirmer CM, Bowyer MW, Rezai AR. A novel craniotomy simulator provides a validated method to enhance education in the management of traumatic brain injury. Neurosurgery. 2013;73:S57–65.

43. Banerjee PP, Luciano CJ, Lemole Jr GM, Charbel FT, Oh MY. Accuracy of ventriculostomy catheter placement using a head-and hand-tracked high-resolution virtual reality simulator with haptic feedback. Journal of Neurosurgery. 2007;107(3):515–21.

44. Hooten KG, Lister JR, Lombard G, Lizdas DE, Lampotang S, Rajon DA, Bova F, Murad GJ. Mixed reality ventriculostomy simulation: experience in neurosurgical residency. Oper Neurosurg. 2014;10(4):565–76.

45. Lemole GM Jr, Banerjee PP, Luciano C, Neckrysh S, Charbel FT. Virtual reality in neurosurgical education: part-task ventriculostomy simulation with

dynamic visual and haptic feedback. Neurosurgery. 2007;61(1):142–9.

46. Bova FJ, Rajon DA, Friedman WA, Murad GJ, Hoh DJ, Jacob RP, Lampotang S, Lizdas DE, Lombard G, Lister JR. Mixed-reality simulation for neurosurgical procedures. Neurosurgery. 2013;73(suppl_1):S138–45.

47. Ng TP, Hui KP, Tan WC. Integrative haptic and visual interaction for simulation of PMMA injection during vertebroplasty. Stud Health Technol Inform. 2006;119:96–8.

48. Aboud E, Al-Mefty O, Yaşargil MG. New laboratory model for neurosurgical training that simulates live surgery. J Neurosurg. 2002;97(6):1367–72.

49. Oliveira Magaldi M, Nicolato A, Godinho JV, Santos M, Prosdocimi A, Malheiros JA, Lei T, Belykh E, Almefty RO, Almefty KK, Preul MC. Human placenta aneurysm model for training neurosurgeons in vascular microsurgery. Oper Neurosurg. 2014;10(4):592–601.

50. Kwok JC, Huang W, Leung WC, Chan SK, Chan KY, Leung KM, Chu AC, Lam AK. Human placenta as an ex vivo vascular model for neurointerventional research. J Neurointerv Surg. 2013:neurintsurg-2013.

51. Higurashi M, Qian Y, Zecca M, Park YK, Umezu M, Morgan MK. Surgical training technology for cerebrovascular anastomosis. J Clin Neurosci. 2014;21(4):554–8.

52. Fargen KM, Arthur AS, Bendok BR, Levy EI, Ringer A, Siddiqui AH, Veznedaroglu E, Mocco J. Experience with a simulator-based angiography course for neurosurgical residents: beyond a pilot program. Neurosurgery. 2013;73(suppl_1):S46–50.

53. Mashiko T, Otani K, Kawano R, Konno T, Kaneko N, Ito Y, Watanabe E. Development of three-dimensional hollow elastic model for cerebral aneurysm clipping simulation enabling rapid and low cost prototyping. World Neurosurg. 2015;83(3):351–61.

54. Wurm G, Lehner M, Tomancok B, Kleiser R, Nussbaumer K. Cerebrovascular biomodeling for aneurysm surgery: simulation-based training by means of rapid prototyping technologies. Surg Innov. 2011;18(3):294–306.

55. Coelho G, Warf B, Lyra M, Zanon N. Anatomical pediatric model for craniosynostosis surgical training. Childs Nerv Syst. 2014;30(12):2009–14.

56. Mattei TA, Frank C, Bailey J, Lesle E, Macuk A, Lesniak M, Patel A, Morris MJ, Nair K, Lin JJ. Design of a synthetic simulator for pediatric lumbar spine pathologies. J Neurosurg Pediatr. 2013;12(2):192–201.

57. Anil SM, Kato Y, Hayakawa M, Yoshida K, Nagahisha S, Kanno T. Virtual 3-dimensional preoperative planning with the dextroscope for excision of a 4th ventricular ependymoma. min-Minimally Invasive Neurosurgery. 2007;50(02):65–70.

58. Delorme S, Laroche D, DiRaddo R, Del Maestro RF. NeuroTouch: a physics-based virtual simulator for cranial microneurosurgery training. Oper Neurosurg. 2012;71(suppl_1):ons32–42.

59. Nash R, Sykes R, Majithia A, Arora A, Singh A, Khemani S. Objective assessment of learning curves for the Voxel-Man TempoSurg temporal bone surgery computer simulator. J Laryngol Otol. 2012;126(7):663–9.

60. Radetzky A, Rudolph M, Starkie S, Davies B, Auer LM. ROBO-SIM: a simulator for minimally invasive neurosurgery using an active manipulator. Stud Health Technol Inform. 2000;77:1165–9.

61. Freudenstein D, Bartz D, Skalej M, Duffner F. New virtual system for planning of neuroendoscopic interventions. Comput Aided Surg. 2001;6(2):77–84.

62. Delorme S, Laroche D, DiRaddo R, Del Maestro RF. NeuroTouch: a physics-based virtual simulator for cranial microneurosurgery training. Oper Neurosurg. 2012;71(suppl_1):ons32–42.

63. Boudou C, Balosso J, Estève F, Elleaume H. Monte Carlo dosimetry for synchrotron stereotactic radiotherapy of brain tumours. Phys Med Biol. 2005;50(20):4841.

64. Dieterich S, Cavedon C, Chuang CF, Cohen AB, Garrett JA, Lee CL, Lowenstein JR, Taylor DD, Wu X, Yu C. Report of AAPM TG 135: quality assurance for robotic radiosurgery. Med Phys. 2011;38(6):2914–36.

65. Hamamoto Y, Manabe T, Nishizaki O, Takahashi T, Isshiki N, Murayama S, Nishina K, Umeda M. Influence of collimator size on three-dimensional conformal radiotherapy of the cyberknife. Radiat Med. 2004;22(6):442–8.

66. Nowinski WL, Chua BC, Volkau I, Puspitasari F, Marchenko Y, Runge VM, Knopp MV. Simulation and assessment of cerebrovascular damage in deep brain stimulation using a stereotactic atlas of vasculature and structure derived from multiple 3-and 7-tesla scans. J Neurosurg. 2010;113(6):1234–41.

67. Noordmans HJ, Van Rijen PC, Van Veelen CW, Viergever MA, Hoekema R. Localization of implanted EEG electrodes in a virtual-reality environment. Comput Aided Surg. 2001;6(5):241–58.

68. Pieters TA, Conner CR, Tandon N. Recursive grid partitioning on a cortical surface model: an optimized technique for the localization of implanted subdural electrodes. J Neurosurg. 2013;118(5):1086–97.

69. Barrows HS, Abrahamson S. The programmed patient: a technique for appraising student performance in clinical neurology. Acad Med. 1964;39(8):802–5.

70. Wallace P. Following the threads of an innovation: the history of standardized patients in medical education. Caduceus (Springfield, Ill). 1997;13(2):5.

71. Musacchio MJ, Smith AP, McNeal CA, Munoz L, Rothenberg DM, von Roenn KA, Byrne RW. Neuro-critical care skills training using a human patient simulator. Neurocrit Care. 2010;13(2):169–75.

72. Ullrich WF. A history of simulation: part II-early days. Military Simulation & Training. 2008. p. 27–30.

73. Singh H, Kalani M, Acosta-Torres S, El Ahmadieh TY, Loya J, Ganju A. History of simulation in medicine: from Resusci Annie to the Ann Myers Medical Center. Neurosurgery. 2013;73:S9–14.

74. The Link Trainer. Stark Ravings Web site. http://www.starksravings.com/linktrainer/linktrainer.htm.
75. https://en.wikipedia.org/w/index.php?curid=32934125.
76. A brief history and lineage of our CAE-Link Silver Spring operation. http://lifeafterlink.org/brochure.shtml.
77. Setting the Standard in Simulation and Training for 80+ Years. https://www.link.com/about/pages/history.aspx.
78. Satava RM. Historical review of surgical simulation—a personal perspective. World J Surg. 2008;32(2):141–8.
79. Lanier J. Virtual reality: the promise of the future. Interact Learn Int. 1992;8(4):275–9.
80. By Canticle at en.wikipedia, CC BY-SA 3.0. https://commons.wikimedia.org/w/index.php?curid=9074729
81. Delp SL, Loan JP, Hoy MG, Zajac FE, Topp EL, Rosen JM. An interactive graphics-based model of the lower extremity to study orthopaedic surgical procedures. IEEE Trans Biomed Eng. 1990;37(8):757–67.
82. Satava RM. Virtual reality surgical simulator. Surg Endosc. 1993;7(3):203–5.
83. Seymour NE, Gallagher AG, Roman SA, O'brien MK, Bansal VK, Andersen DK, Satava RM. Virtual reality training improves operating room performance: results of a randomized, double-blinded study. Ann Surg. 2002;236(4):458.
84. Edmond CV, Wiet GJ, Bolger LB. Virtual environments: surgical simulation in otolaryngology. Otolaryngol Clin N Am. 1998;31(2):369–81.
85. Datta V, Mackay S, Mandalia M, Darzi A. The use of electromagnetic motion tracking analysis to objectively measure open surgical skill in the laboratory-based model. J Am Coll Surg. 2001;193(5):479–85.
86. Mylonas G, Darzi A, Yang GZ. Gaze contingent depth recovery and motion stabilization for minimally invasive robotic surgery. Medical Imaging and Augmented Reality. 2004. p. 311–9.
87. Albani JM, Lee DI. Virtual reality-assisted robotic surgery simulation. J Endourol. 2007;21(3):285–7.
88. Spicer MA, Van Velsen M, Caffrey JP, Apuzzo ML. Virtual reality neurosurgery: a simulator blueprint. Neurosurgery. 2004;54(4):783–98.
89. https://neurosurgerycns.wordpress.com/2010/02/08/free-article-alcmaeon-of-croton/.
90. Alaraj A, Charbel FT, Birk D, Tobin M, Luciano C, Banerjee PP, Rizzi S, Sorenson J, Foley K, Slavin K, Roitberg B. Role of cranial and spinal virtual and augmented reality simulation using immersive touch modules in neurosurgical training. Neurosurgery. 2013;72(suppl_1):A115–23.
91. Rodt T, Schlesinger A, Schramm A, Diensthuber M, Rittierodt M, Krauss JK. 3D visualization and simulation of frontoorbital advancement in metopic synostosis. Childs Nerv Syst. 2007;23(11):1313–7.

Part II

Physcial Models Simulation

2

Shivani Rangwala, Gregory Arnone,
Fady T. Charbel, and Ali Alaraj

Introduction

External ventricular drainage (EVD) is a therapeutic measure implemented in cases of trauma, hemorrhage, and hydrocephalus in neurosurgical patients. Placement of an EVD provides the feature of intracranial pressure (ICP) measurement and subsequent release of excess cerebrospinal fluid from the ventricles in cases of raised ICP. A ventriculostomy involves puncturing the cerebral ventricles to access the cerebrospinal fluid contents and is a skill taught early in neurosurgical training. Simulation in neurosurgery can augment resident expertise in core procedural competencies, with no additional risk to patient care—making ventriculostomy simulation an essential feature for neurosurgical resident training.

Electronic supplementary material: The online version of this chapter https://doi.org/10.1007/978-3-319-75583-0_2 contains supplementary material, which is available to authorized users.

S. Rangwala · G. Arnone · F. T. Charbel · A. Alaraj (✉)
Department of Neurosurgery, University of Illinois at Chicago, Chicago, IL, USA
e-mail: Alaraj@uic.edu

History of Ventriculostomy

Ventricular catheter placement is a key skill set all neurosurgeons master early in their training. Further, external ventricular drainage (EVD) is one of the most commonly performed neurosurgical procedures and allows excess cerebrospinal fluid in the ventricles to be externally drained. The first documented EVD was performed by Claude-Nicolas Le Cat in 1744 [1]. Carl Wernicke performed the first sterile placement of an external ventricular device in 1881 [1–3]. External diversion of excess cerebrospinal fluid continued to gain popularity into the late 1800s [1, 2]. Eventually, the technology advanced catheter material and internalization of shunts, paving way for modern ventricular shunts. Our current design for ventricular shunts first appeared in 1950 and continues to be improved upon [2]. Aside from the impressive evolution of ventricular catheters, the technique of placement remains consistent over the last century.

Early comments on ventricular puncture technique were published in 1850, sharing the poor results of puncturing the lateral ventricles of a hydrocephalic infant through the fontanelle [1]. Through trial and error, the technique further evolved as neurosurgeons investigated ideal anatomical locations and theorized benefits and consequences of CSF drainage. W.W. Keens was the first to report on EVD technique and later will be credited for one of the optimal points for EVD placement. Keen's point is defined as "3 cm superior and 3 cm posterior to the pinna" and will provide a lateral entry point to the lateral ventricle [1]. In collaboration with Harvey Cushing, Theodore Kocher described a point for ventricular access that was "in the midpupillary line, 10 cm posterior to the nasion," which would famously be called Kocher's point [1, 4]. Other points of entry have been explained in the literature, such as von Bergmann's frontal approach or Dandy's point, but what is most closely associated with the current approach is described by H. Tillman in 1908 [5, 6]. Tillman suggested use of Kocher's point for EVD placement, which continues to be a famous reference point in modern neurosurgery [1]. Ventriculostomy procedures are not only applicable in cases of hydrocephalus but have expanded in relevance to cases of trauma and hemorrhage, with approximately 25,000 ventriculostomies performed annually [7]. As a consequence, EVD placement is one of the first skills taught to young neurosurgical residents and should be mastered early in training to minimize risk to patients [1, 8–10].

Simulation in Surgery

The concept of using simulation to prepare individuals for highly skills tasks originated in military and aviation industries, where simulation was an essential component of training. Simulation has since been introduced into training surgical residents, a highly technical specialty with minimal room for error [11]. The purpose of an effective simulator, as outlined by Kahol et al., is to develop both cognitive and psychomotor skills, two key tenets required in developing surgical expertise [10, 12]. There is an expanding literature of support for the use of simulation in surgical training—ensuring residents have access to various procedural scenarios without the high-stakes environment of an operating room. Studies have found that general surgery residents with virtual reality simulation training outperform their colleagues who lack simulation training when compared in operating room tasks [11,

13, 14]. Within surgical subspecialties, neurosurgery demands a high level of technical expertise, and there is a growing need to expand simulation opportunities to strengthen resident training.

General Neurosurgical Training

Neurosurgical residency is a demanding and high-intensity training environment. Recent policy changes in resident duty hour restrictions and physician evaluations demand an efficient training modality at no increased risk to patient care. Simulation serves this purpose and allows residents to strengthen basic neurosurgical skills before working on patients. In a systematic review of simulation in neurosurgery performed by Kirkman and colleagues, ventriculostomy was the most common procedure simulated [15, 16]. EVD placement is considered a low-risk procedure which is taught early on in neurosurgical training and is typically performed by first and second year residents [1, 17]. Junior residents often struggle with the procedural elements of EVD placement, requiring multiple passes before a successful ventricular puncture [18]. To avoid potential risks (hemorrhage, infection, malpositioned catheter, even possibly death) and to accurately assess competency, simulation (primarily virtual reality modalities) is recommended to train neurosurgical residents in basic procedural tasks [17, 19, 20].

Ventriculostomy Simulation

Several classes of simulation technologies are available within neurosurgery, but few provide specific simulation for ventriculostomy [21]. Simulation can be nonvirtual in nature, where a physical construct allows learners to attempt basic procedural skills. Alternatively, virtual reality haptic simulation uses diverse sensory modalities to accurately reproduce a holistic procedural experience. Each simulation type has its benefits and drawbacks.

Physical Simulation Training

Traditionally, simulation in resident training has involved cadaveric dissections, mannequins, and synthetic models that allow residents to practice basic procedural skills [15]. Cadaveric dissections do not provide accurate simulation of a ventriculostomy procedure due to lack of intact ventricular pressures. Innovations in 3D printing now allow realistic printing of anatomically correct cranial models. Physical models offer the benefit of allowing residents to identify and feel anatomic landmarks to determine entry point, such as Kocher's point, closely simulating actual ventriculostomy procedures.

Ryan and colleagues [10] describe a cost-effective physical simulator developed using 3D printing to practice EVD placement. The simulator contains a gel-based brain mold encased with a partial solid cranial mold and a gravity-driven pressure system to control ventricular pressures This gel-based 3D-printed simulator showed positive potential in neurosurgical training of ventriculostomy procedures when qualitatively assessed by residents and medical students [10].

Tai and colleagues developed a 3D-printed physical simulator from Stealth head CT scans to practice EVD placement. The construct consists of a skull frame, skull cap, replaceable skin insert, and phantom brain model containing pressure-controlled ventricles to mimic real-life ventricle pressures (Fig. 2.1a, b). The prototype was tested out by 17 neurosurgeons across 3 different training sites, ranging from resident to attending level training, and was determined to be a promising early model, with room for improvement before it can be implemented in resident training [22].

Mixed Simulation Training

Mixed simulation strikes a balance between physical models and virtual reality with haptic feedback. This platform allows trainees to practice on anatomically accurate physical constructs and make decisions based on real-time sensory feedback, optimizing development of procedural knowledge [23–25]. Bova and colleagues [23] have developed a patient-specific 3D-printed physical model which links to a virtual reality system. This system will simulate ventriculostomy procedures, percutaneous stereotactic lesion procedures, and spinal instrumentation [23]. For ventriculostomy simulation, the trainee identifies where to make the burr hole based on surface landmarks on the physical simulator, drills a hole with a handheld drill (stopping before breaching the inner table), and then prepares for ventriculostomy catheter. The physical head model is linked via an electromagnetic tracking system to a virtual head, allowing the trainee to analyze their catheter trajectory and see the final catheter tip location [23, 24] (Fig. 2.2).

Hooten et al. [24] tested accuracy of this mixed simulation for ventriculostomy on 263 residents, who agreed the simulation was realistic and beneficial to training. Senior residents were found to perform the simulation faster and more accurately than junior residents, further supporting how real-life clinical skills translate to simulation proficiency [24]. Mixed simulation improves upon the physical simulation model, providing better feedback for training purposes.

Virtual Reality Simulation Training

More advanced technology utilizes a virtual reality platform combined with a haptic system to completely immerse the user in the full neurosurgical procedure experience. The user is presented with a virtual 3D head, which was developed from real patient data sets to depict normal anatomy. Haptic systems provide real-time sensory feedback to parallel different tissue types and resistance encountered during different procedural steps [26–29]. Two neurosurgical simulators exist—ImmersiveTouch and NeuroTouch. Between these two, however, only ImmersiveTouch offers specific modules to recreate ventriculostomy procedures [19, 26, 27, 29].

ImmersiveTouch is one of the leading simulation platforms that combines a haptic device with high-resolution stereoscopic display to illustrate

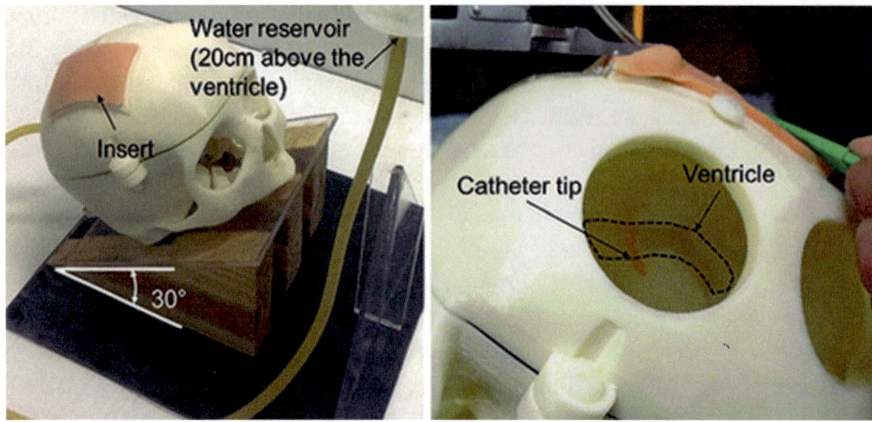

Fig. 2.1 A physical model of the skull including the ventricular system used for training for placement of frontal ventriculostomy. (With permission, Tai et al. [22])

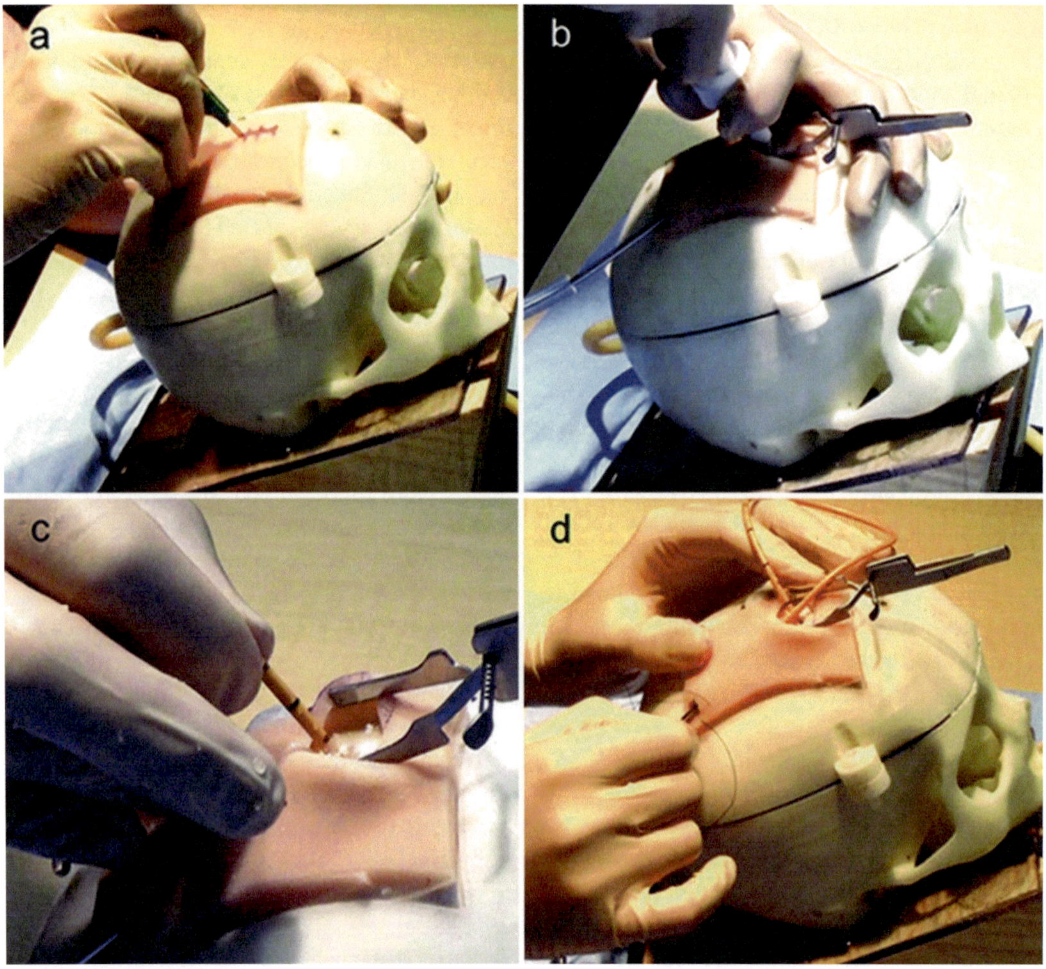

Fig. 2.2 Images from a representative physical model EVD simulator evaluation showing scalp incision (**a**), bone drilling (**b**), catheter placement (**c**), and tunneling and suturing (**d**). (With permission, Tai et al. [22])

various neurosurgical procedures [19, 29]. Developed through a joint effort between neurosurgery and engineering at the University of Illinois and University of Chicago, ImmersiveTouch offers several different modules, including ventriculostomy simulation. The system gives real-time feedback on the location of the catheter during insertion and grades the user based on predetermined performance measures (including burr hole location, overall catheter trajectory, length of catheter inserted into the ventricles, and final distance between the tip of the catheter and foramen of Monro) [19, 30]. To simulate a ventriculostomy procedure, the user sits at a console and is given stereoscopic goggles which track their head position with respect to the virtual 3D head to constantly reorient their point of view (Fig. 2.3). In their hands, the user is given a stylus to mimic a virtual catheter, which is equipped with haptic feedback, and a toggle which adjusts light and 3D anatomical planes of the virtual head [9, 31]. The training modules start by identification of the surgical landmarks, creating the burr hole, and then introducing the virtual ventricular catheter into the burr hole and later into the ventricular space (Fig. 2.4, Video 2.1). As the ventricular catheter is advanced, there is a change in the tactile feedback once the catheter enters the CSF space. The module does identify if the cannulation is successful when the catheter changes its color to green (Fig. 2.4f); the module also allows the operator to virtually cut through the brain to identify the exact location of the catheter (Fig. 2.4g, h, i). The module also identify when the catheter is outside the ventricular system, where the catheter color turns red (Fig. 2.5). There is also another module for occipital ventriculostomy (Fig. 2.6). After trying the module with normal anatomy, Lemole et al. expanded the application of ImmersiveTouch to abnormal ventricle anatomy. Residents were able to successfully cannulate "shifted ventricles" after multiple attempts, emphasizing the learning curve with procedures that ImmersiveTouch accurately creates [32] (Figs. 2.7 and 2.8).

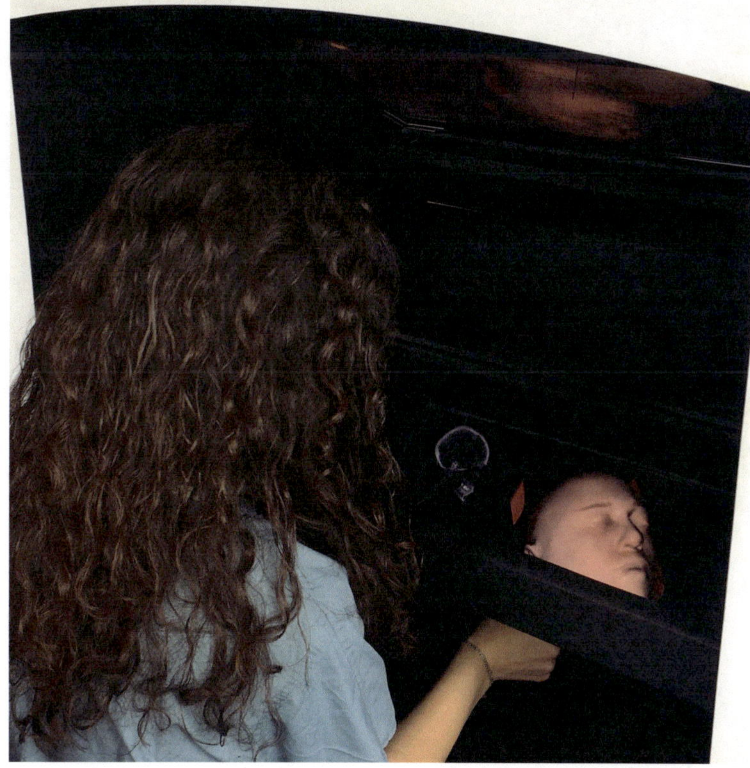

Fig. 2.3 The ImmersiveTouch simulator setup, the virtual model is seen through a reflected mirror. (Courtesy of ImmersiveTouch, with permission)

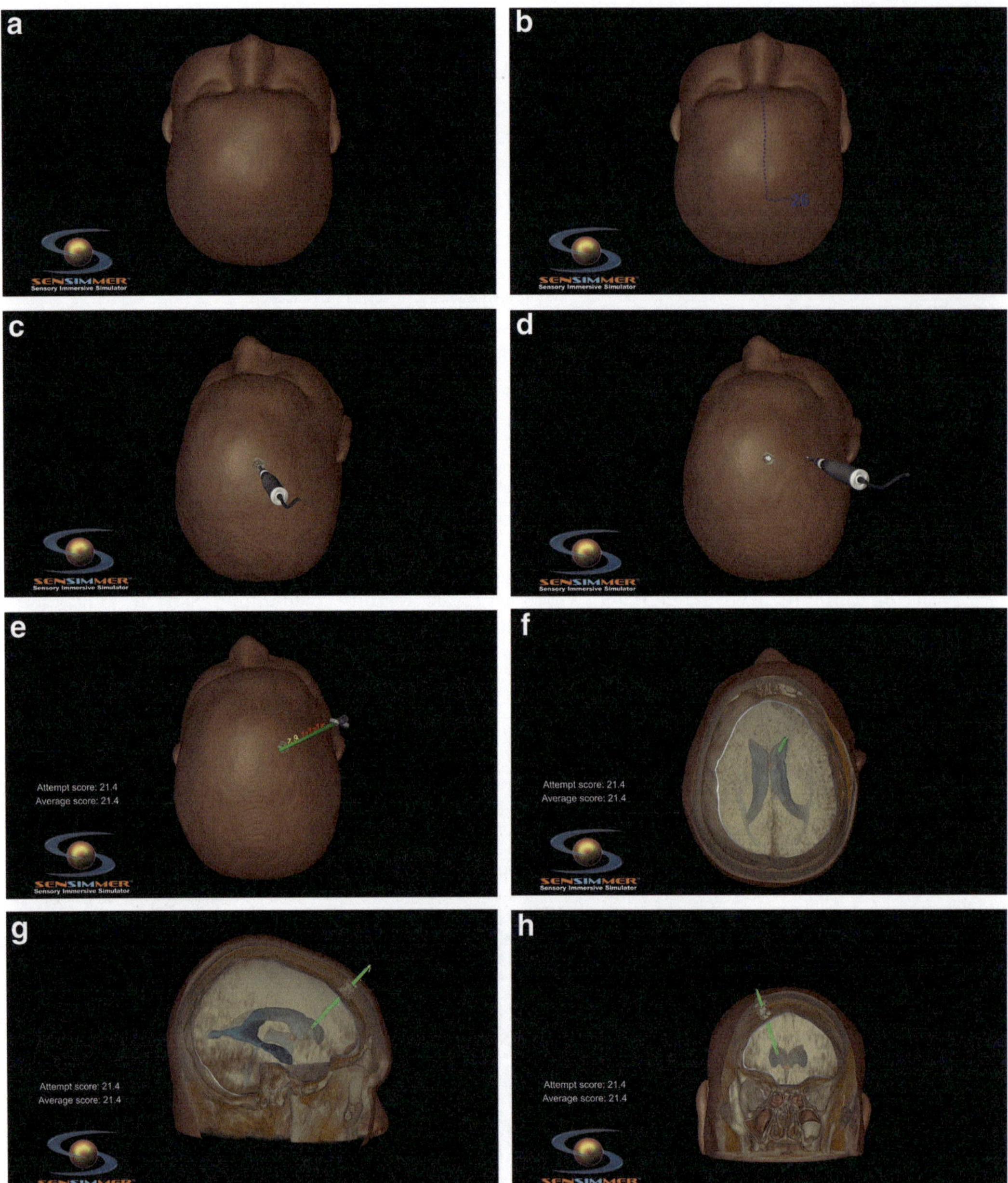

Fig. 2.4 ImmersiveTouch simulator steps including head positioning (**a**), skin landmarks identification (**b**), burr hole drilling (**c**, **d**), ventricular catheter placement (**e**), virtual cutting in the axial plane (**f**), sagittal plane (**g**), and coronal place (**h**). (Courtesy of ImmersiveTouch, with permission)

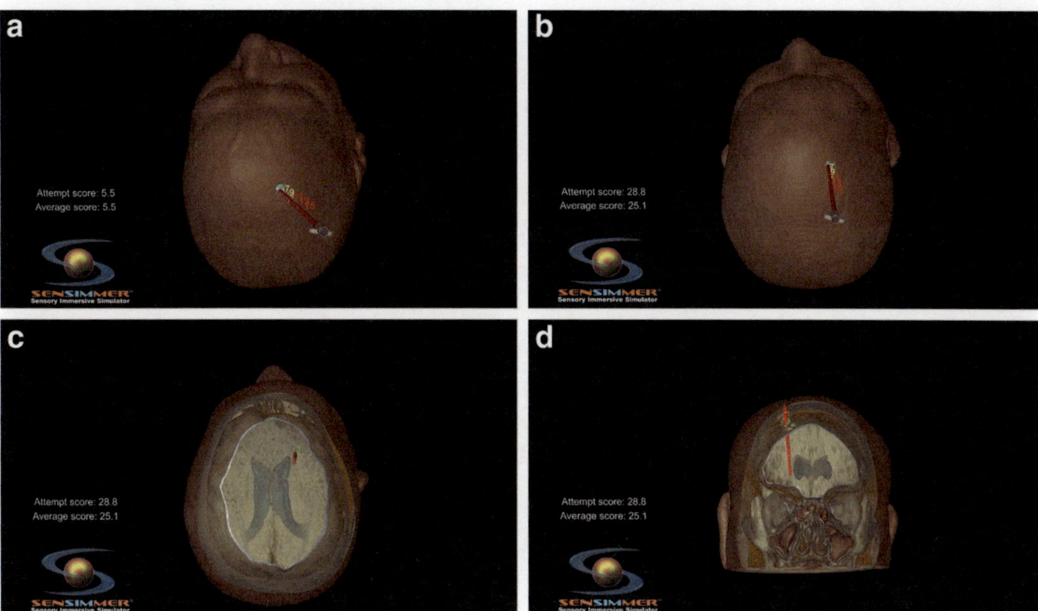

Fig. 2.5 ImmersiveTouch ventricular catheter misplaced outside the ventricular system identified as red color (**a**), different angle misplaced catheter (**b**), virtual cut through the brain in axial (**c**), coronal (**d**) sectioning identifying the location of the catheter outside the frontal horn. (Courtesy of ImmersiveTouch, with permission)

Benefits of Current Technology

The implications of simulation in neurosurgery are an ongoing investigation, but early results are promising. Ventriculostomy is a standard procedure which all residents learn early in their training. Schirmer et al. used ImmersiveTouch to simulate the ventriculostomy procedure in a trauma module developed for CNS Resident Simulation Symposium with positive results. Residents who practiced with ImmersiveTouch modules showed improved ventriculostomy results, with junior residents benefiting more than senior residents from the simulation [20, 30]. When testing residents and fellows at the 2006 AANS meeting, Banerjee et al. found that ImmersiveTouch ventriculostomy module simulated accurate catheter placement, with comparable results to a retrospective study of freehand pass catheter placement on 97 patients, supporting reproducibility of the real procedure by this module [18, 19, 29, 31]. Neurosurgical residents and fellows commented that the sensory and visual information provided in ventriculostomy simulation was realistic and helped develop relevant procedural skills [9, 19, 20, 29]. Further, ImmersiveTouch contains normal and abnormal anatomy modules, challenging residents to practice with a variety ventriculostomy scenarios to improve their skills for the bedside [20, 32].

Limitations of Existing Technology

The limitations of physical simulators depend on our 3D printing technology. The challenge lies within choosing appropriate materials to print out the simulator, such that it best models the biomechanical properties of brain tissue and ventricles. Tai et al. used a gelatin-like material with a realistic simulation experience [22, 33]. Another downside of physical simulators is the long-time wear and tear of the product, requiring frequent replacement of parts after use, such as the one-time-use skull insert developed by Tai et al. [22] The limitations of physical systems also hold true for the physical component of mixed simulators. Despite the long-term cost of replacement, physical simulators (with manufacturing costs of approximately $1000) do not compare to the high cost of VR systems [22].

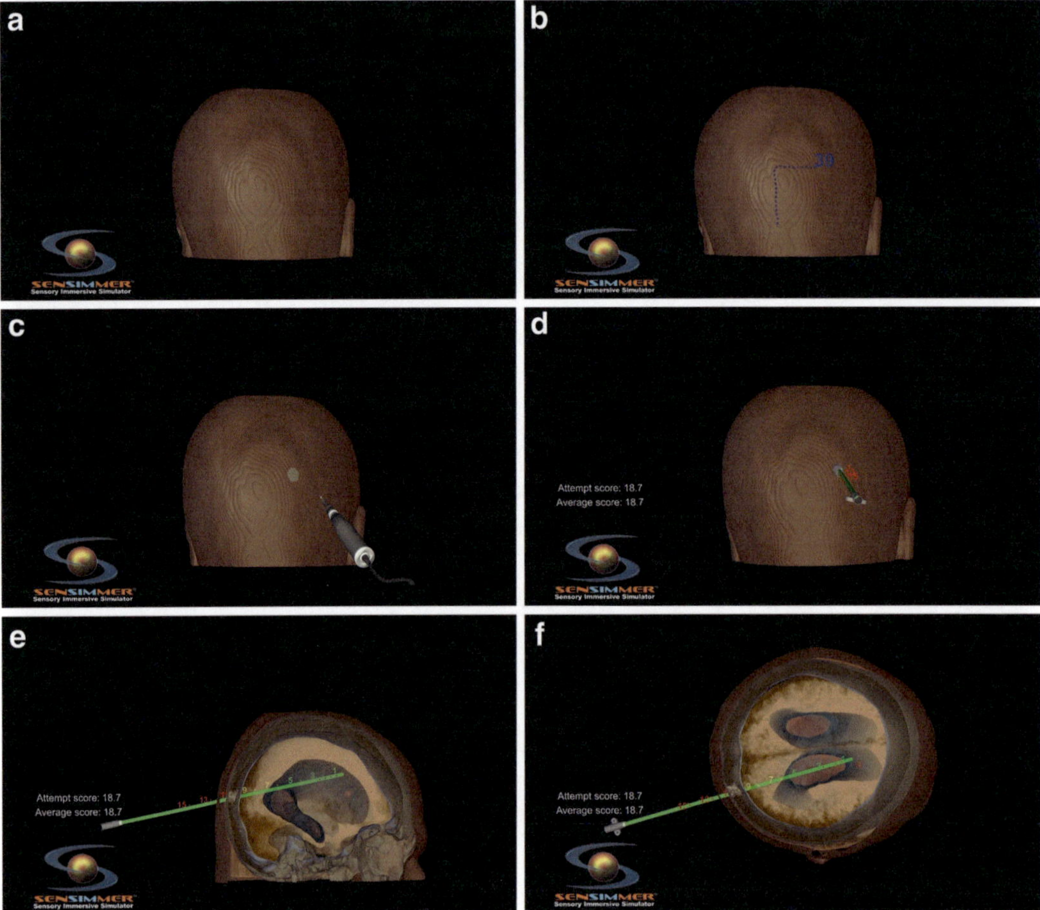

Fig. 2.6 ImmersiveTouch occipital ventriculostomy planning including head positioning (**a**), skin landmark identification (**b**), burr hole (**c**), ventricular catheter placement (**d**), virtual cutting of the brain in sagittal plane (**e**), and axial planes (**f**) identifying the location of the catheter within the ventricular system. (Courtesy of ImmersiveTouch, with permission)

One drawback to VR systems is the high financial cost, limiting its access to most neurosurgical residency programs. The estimated cost upfront is variable, with lease options starting at $20,000 and purchase options starting at $75,000. Not included in these estimations are time and resources for initial setup and future maintenance once the system starts to be used for resident training [30].

Further, the VR systems are bulky and demand a workspace for setup. Depending on the structure of a residency program, accessibility may be limited for residents to practice on these systems away from their daily routine on the wards [26]. All simulation systems should augment, not replace, hands-on training residents receive. Haptic feedback and processing continues to be modified, and while current technology is effective, it does not perfectly mimic the complexity of the actual placement of an EVD and real-time complications residents may encounter.

Conclusions

The recent advancement in technology did bring new training modules for the training of ventriculostomy. These modules include the physical models and the virtual reality-based modules. Those modules have been widely used in the training of neurosurgical residents.

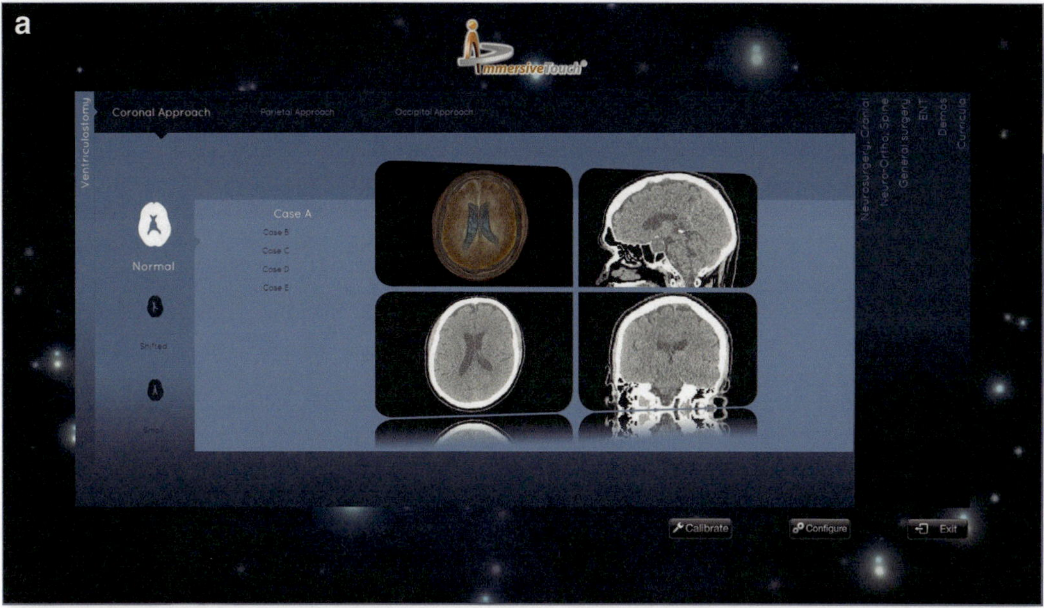

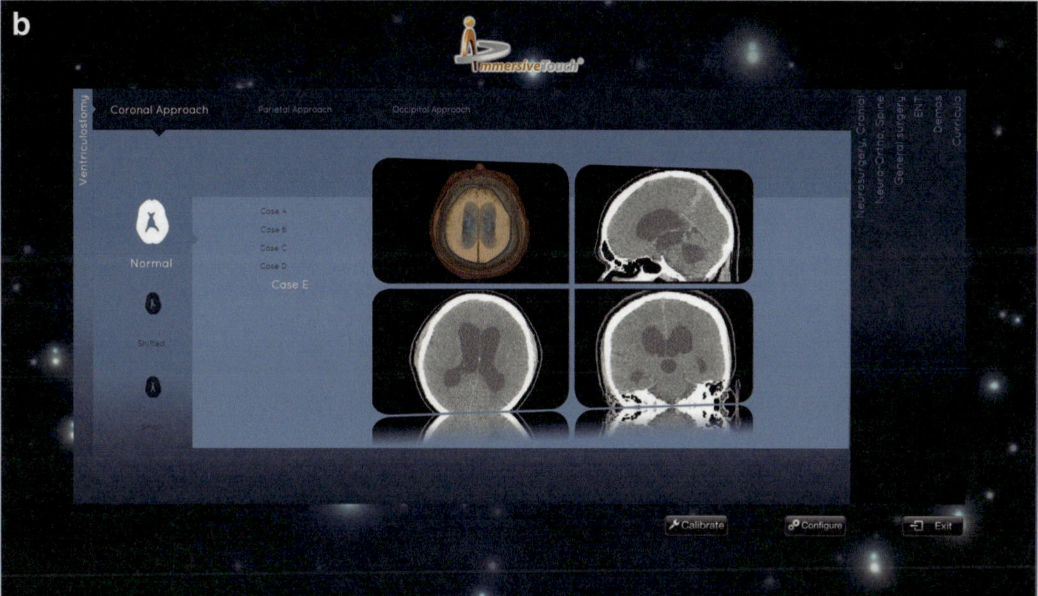

Fig. 2.7 ImmersiveTouch ventriculostomy modules in normal ventricular anatomy (**a**) hydrocephalus (**b**) shifted ventricle (**c**) and very small ventricles (**d**). (Courtesy of ImmersiveTouch, with permission)

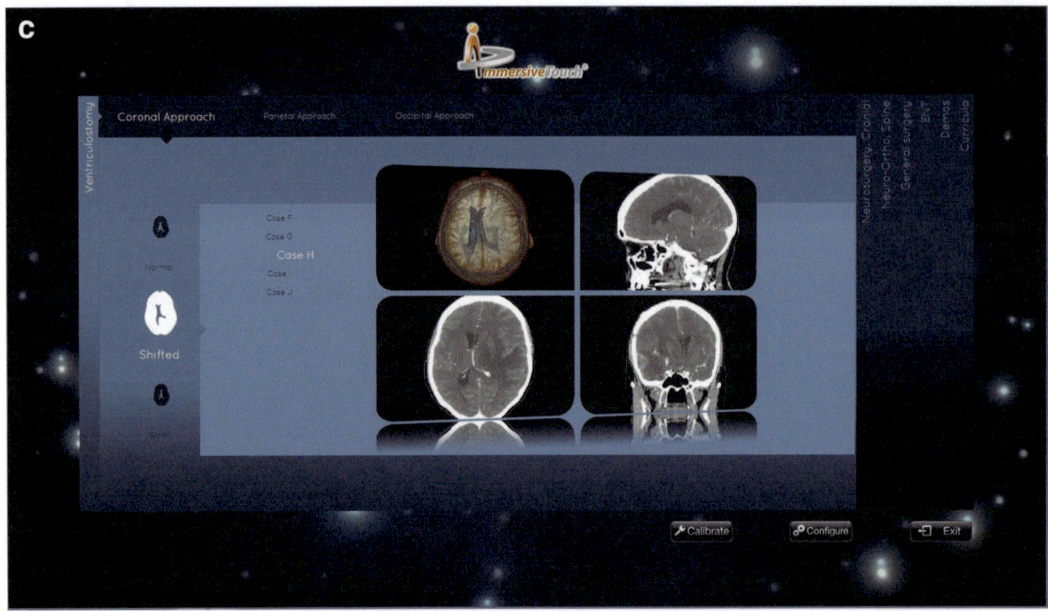

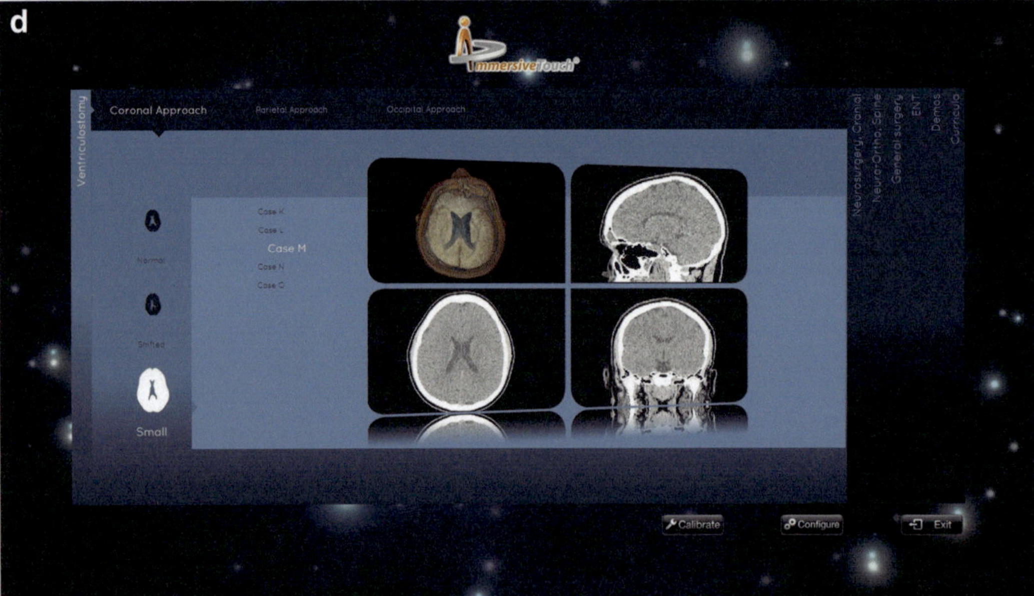

Fig. 2.7 (continued)

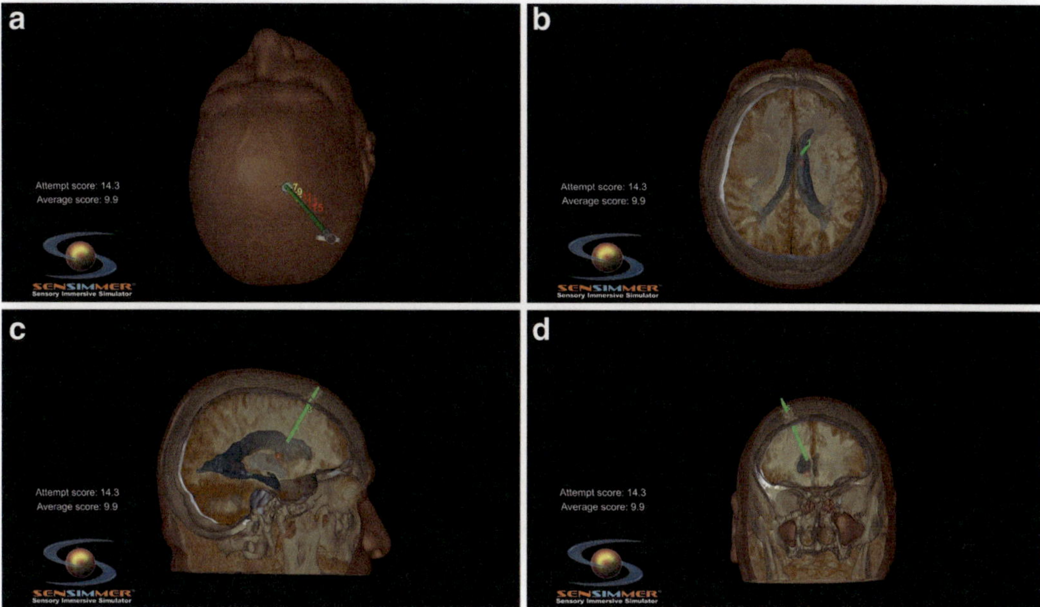

Fig. 2.8 ImmersiveTouch ventriculostomy training in a shifted ventricle with catheter placed in the ventricle (**a**), axial (**a**), sagittal (**b**), and coronal (**c**) cuts showing the location of the catheter within the ventricular system. (Courtesy of ImmersiveTouch, with permission)

References

1. Srinivasan VM, O'Neill BR, Jho D, Whiting DM, Oh MY. The history of external ventricular drainage. J Neurosurg. 2014;120(1):228–36.
2. Weisenberg SH, TerMaath SC, Seaver CE, Killeffer JA. Ventricular catheter development: past, present, and future. J Neurosurg. 2016;125(6):1504–12.
3. Keen WW. Surgery of the lateral ventricles of the brain. Lancet. 136(3498):553–5.
4. Schültke E. Theodor Kocher's craniometer. Neurosurgery. 2009;64(5):1001–4; discussion 4–5.
5. Kaufmann GE, Clark K. Emergency frontal twist drill ventriculostomy. Technical note. J Neurosurg. 1970;33(2):226–7.
6. Dandy WE. An operative procedure for hydrocephalus. Bull Johns Hopkins Hosp. 1922;33:189–90.
7. Sekula RF, Cohen DB, Patek PM, Jannetta PJ, Oh MY. Epidemiology of ventriculostomy in the United States from 1997 to 2001. Br J Neurosurg. 2008;22(2):213–8.
8. Kakarla UK, Kim LJ, Chang SW, Theodore N, Spetzler RF. Safety and accuracy of bedside external ventricular drain placement. Neurosurgery. 2008;63(1 Suppl 1):ONS162–6; discussion ONS6–7.
9. Lemole GM, Banerjee PP, Luciano C, Neckrysh S, Charbel FT. Virtual reality in neurosurgical education: part-task ventriculostomy simulation with dynamic visual and haptic feedback. Neurosurgery. 2007;61(1):142–8; discussion 8–9.
10. Ryan JR, Chen T, Nakaji P, Frakes DH, Gonzalez LF. Ventriculostomy simulation using patient-specific ventricular anatomy, 3D printing, and hydrogel casting. World Neurosurg. 2015;84(5):1333–9.
11. Grantcharov TP. Is virtual reality simulation an effective training method in surgery? Nat Clin Pract Gastroenterol Hepatol. 2008;5(5):232–3.
12. Kahol K, Vankipuram M, Smith ML. Cognitive simulators for medical education and training. J Biomed Inform. 2009;42(4):593–604.
13. Grantcharov TP, Kristiansen VB, Bendix J, Bardram L, Rosenberg J, Funch-Jensen P. Randomized clinical trial of virtual reality simulation for laparoscopic skills training. Br J Surg. 2004;91(2):146–50.
14. Seymour NE, Gallagher AG, Roman SA, O'Brien MK, Bansal VK, Andersen DK, et al. Virtual reality training improves operating room performance: results of a randomized, double-blinded study. Ann Surg. 2002;236(4):458–63; discussion 63–4.
15. Suri A, Patra DP, Meena RK. Simulation in neurosurgery: past, present, and future. Neurol India. 2016;64(3):387–95.
16. Kirkman MA, Ahmed M, Albert AF, Wilson MH, Nandi D, Sevdalis N. The use of simulation in neurosurgical education and training. A systematic review. J Neurosurg. 2014;121(2):228–46.
17. Fried HI, Nathan BR, Rowe AS, Zabramski JM, Andaluz N, Bhimraj A, et al. The insertion and Management of External Ventricular Drains: an evidence-based consensus statement : a statement for healthcare professionals from the Neurocritical Care Society. Neurocrit Care. 2016;24(1):61–81.

18. Huyette DR, Turnbow BJ, Kaufman C, Vaslow DF, Whiting BB, Oh MY. Accuracy of the freehand pass technique for ventriculostomy catheter placement: retrospective assessment using computed tomography scans. J Neurosurg. 2008;108(1):88–91.

19. Alaraj A, Charbel FT, Birk D, Tobin M, Luciano C, Banerjee PP, et al. Role of cranial and spinal virtual and augmented reality simulation using immersive touch modules in neurosurgical training. Neurosurgery. 2013;72(Suppl 1):115–23.

20. Yudkowsky R, Luciano C, Banerjee P, Schwartz A, Alaraj A, Lemole GM, et al. Practice on an augmented reality/haptic simulator and library of virtual brains improves residents' ability to perform a ventriculostomy. Simul Healthc. 2013;8(1):25–31.

21. Chan S, Conti F, Salisbury K, Blevins NH. Virtual reality simulation in neurosurgery: technologies and evolution. Neurosurgery. 2013;72(Suppl 1):154–64.

22. Tai BL, Rooney D, Stephenson F, Liao PS, Sagher O, Shih AJ, et al. Development of a 3D-printed external ventricular drain placement simulator: technical note. J Neurosurg. 2015;123(4):1070–6.

23. Bova FJ, Rajon DA, Friedman WA, Murad GJ, Hoh DJ, Jacob RP, et al. Mixed-reality simulation for neurosurgical procedures. Neurosurgery. 2013;73(Suppl 1):138–45.

24. Hooten KG, Lister JR, Lombard G, Lizdas DE, Lampotang S, Rajon DA, et al. Mixed reality ventriculostomy simulation: experience in neurosurgical residency. Neurosurgery. 2014;10(Suppl 4):576–81; discussion 81.

25. Lampotang S, Lizdas D, Rajon D, Luria I, Gravenstein N, Bisht Y, et al. Mixed simulators: augmented physical simulators with virtual underlays. IEEE Virtual Reality. Orlando. 2013.

26. Cobb MI-PH, Taekman JM, Zomorodi AR, Gonzalez LF, Turner DA. Simulation in neurosurgery: a brief review and commentary. World Neurosurg. 2016; 89:583–6.

27. Delorme S, Laroche D, DiRaddo R, Del Maestro RF. NeuroTouch: a physics-based virtual simulator for cranial microneurosurgery training. Neurosurgery. 2012;71(1 Suppl Operative):32–42.

28. Escobar-Castillejos D, Noguez J, Neri L, Magana A, Benes B. A review of simulators with haptic devices for medical training. J Med Syst. 2016;40(4):104.

29. Alaraj A, Lemole MG, Finkle JH, Yudkowsky R, Wallace A, Luciano C, et al. Virtual reality training in neurosurgery: review of current status and future applications. Surg Neurol Int. 2011;2:52.

30. Schirmer CM, Elder JB, Roitberg B, Lobel DA. Virtual reality-based simulation training for ventriculostomy: an evidence-based approach. Neurosurgery. 2013;73(Suppl 1):66–73.

31. Banerjee PP, Luciano CJ, Lemole GM, Charbel FT, Oh MY. Accuracy of ventriculostomy catheter placement using a head- and hand-tracked high-resolution virtual reality simulator with haptic feedback. J Neurosurg. 2007;107(3):515–21.

32. Lemole M, Banerjee PP, Luciano C, Charbel F, Oh M. Virtual ventriculostomy with 'shifted ventricle': neurosurgery resident surgical skill assessment using a high-fidelity haptic/graphic virtual reality simulator. Neurol Res. 2009;31(4):430–1.

33. Chen RK, Shih AJ. Multi-modality gellan gum-based tissue-mimicking phantom with targeted mechanical, electrical, and thermal properties. Phys Med Biol. 2013;58(16):5511–25.

Physical Simulators and Replicators in Endovascular Neurosurgery Training

3

Chander Sadasivan, Baruch B. Lieber, and Henry H. Woo

Medical Simulation

Simulated medical training has evolved from simple models derived from sheep lungs and livers used by temple priests in Mesopotamia, through the complex models of human anatomy produced by Galen, Vesalius, and Da Vinci and the Resusci Anne and Harvey simulators developed half a century ago [1, 2] to the current array of sophisticated machines simulating procedures ranging from childbirth to battlefield trauma. Due to this technological maturity, the use of medical simulation has rapidly widened over the past decade as physicians and physician-trainees appreciate the ability to learn new skills in a controlled environment instead of in patients. Simulators offer an optimal avenue for the development of skill levels for trainees under work-hour restrictions and for the maintenance of skill levels for physicians at low-volume centers [3, 4]. Traditional vascular surgery is gradually being replaced by endovascular (interventional) surgery for the treatment of various vascular diseases, and endovascular medical devices are being brought to market at a rapid rate requiring interventional physicians to continually learn the use of these new devices. The traditional use of animal models for training is also declining because both endovascular device technology and medical simulation technology have moved past the relatively simplistic scenarios that can be replicated in animals (simple geometries, smaller vessel sizes, etc. [4]) at a relatively high cost (ethical as well as financial). Further, the use of simulators in medicine, and in particular, endovascular surgery, allows for the potential fulfilment of the fundamental principle of doing no harm in an era in which technological complexity and the current medical education system contribute to about 200,000 deaths from preventable adverse events in hospitalized patients in the United States [5].

The positive results of simulator training have been borne out by numerous studies that have demonstrated benefits in reduced costs, increased interest and confidence among students and trainees, reduced training times, increased teamwork among operative team members, as well as improved procedure efficiencies (reduced volume of injected contrast, shorter fluoroscopy and procedure times, etc.) with fewer complications [1, 4, 6–17]. High-fidelity simulators facilitate greater improvements in surgical skills, especially for experienced practitioners performing sophisticated procedures [9, 11, 18–20]. Simulators also allow for treatment planning where the optimal choice and sequence of devices such as stents, coils, or embolics can be evaluated

C. Sadasivan (✉) · B. B. Lieber · H. H. Woo
Department of Neurological Surgery, Cerebrovascular Research Center, Stony Brook University Medical Center, Stony Brook, NY, USA
e-mail: csadasivan@sbumed.org; blieber@sbumed.org; henry.woo@stonybrookmedicine.edu

© Springer International Publishing AG, part of Springer Nature 2018
A. Alaraj (ed.), *Comprehensive Healthcare Simulation: Neurosurgery*,
Comprehensive Healthcare Simulation, https://doi.org/10.1007/978-3-319-75583-0_3

prior to treatment [21]. Medical simulators thus facilitate numerous benefits to treatment outcome and patient care, and the inherent error associated with the "see one, do one, teach one" paradigm can be mitigated via experience gained with simulation training.

Other Simulation Models

It should be noted that several physical head phantoms have been developed using various tissue simulants to suit various requirements of imaging, surgical planning, or surgical simulation with increasing utilization of 3D printing over the past decade [22–24]. These include agar gel-bound ferric oxide and hydroxyapatite to model hemorrhage and calcification, respectively [25]; paraffin wax as extracranial soft tissue and manganese chloride solution as brain matter for magnetic resonance imaging [26]; 3D printing of calcium sulfate [27] and polyamide nylon with glass beads [28] as temporal bone substitute for ear surgery training (nylon powder- and photopolymer-based 3D-printed bone structures have also been used for operative assessment of acetabular fracture patterns [29, 30]); 3D-printed epoxy resin chambers filled with dipotassium phosphate solution and agarose gel to mimic bone and brain tissue, respectively [31]; and mixtures of paraffin, Teflon, and calcium carbonate based on elemental compositions to duplicate atomic numbers and physical and electron densities of bone and soft tissue [32]. Combined skull and cerebrovascular models have been made with nylon and glass beads powder or rigid photopolymers to mimic skull, and silicone rubbers and flexible photopolymers to represent vasculature [33, 34]; the nylon and glass powder was found to qualitatively equal surgical drilling and rongeuring of human bone [33, 34]. Various media (paraffin wax, polyurethane, epoxy resin) have been permeated into skull structures printed with a specific powder/binder printer (ProJet, 3D Systems) to help mimic acoustic attenuation properties of neonatal skulls and fracture forces of human sinuses [35, 36].

Several virtual endovascular simulators are also available [20]; these rely on haptic feedback from software that attempts to encode the behavior of the medical devices being simulated. Virtual systems have several advantages such as portability, short "setup" times, no radiation, no physical device expense, and automatic performance feedback. On the other hand, they can suffer from relatively poor haptic feedback, training under a simplistic environment can lead to learned complacency in novice trainers, device tracking and deployment behavior is only as effective as the software code, and new devices cannot be simulated until their behavior is encoded. This chapter will focus on high-fidelity physical simulators, or replicators, for endovascular neurosurgery training.

Replicators (High-Fidelity Physical Endovascular Simulators)

The term "simulator" has become synonymous with virtual systems, and thus, a different descriptor is needed to describe physical systems. Additionally, standalone physical components such as vascular models and pumps have generally been available for research, device testing, as well as training purposes in either a commercial (Table 3.1, Fig. 3.1) or laboratory setting [37–39] for several years. We have chosen the term "replicator" here in order to distinguish

Table 3.1 List of commercial companies selling pulsatile pumps and vascular replicas for physical neuroendovascular simulation; it should be noted that this list is not exhaustive

Component	Company
Pulsatile pumps	Shelley Medical Imaging Technologies
	Medical Implant Testing Lab
	Vivitro Labs
	Harvard Apparatus
	Vascular Simulations
Vascular replicas	Elastrat Sarl
	United Biologics
	DialAct
	BDC Laboratories
	FAIN Biomedical
	Vascular Simulations

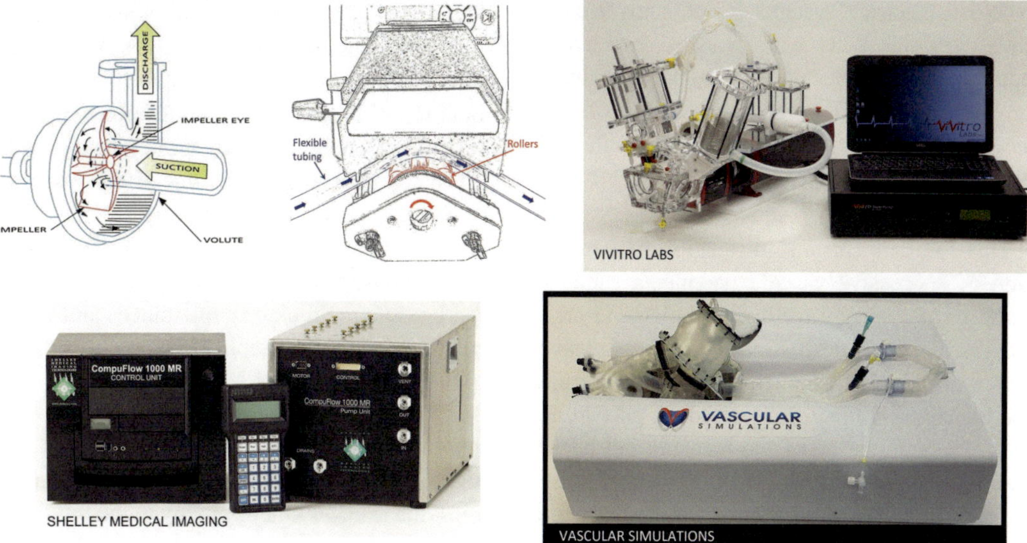

Fig. 3.1 Images or schematics of different types of pumps. Clockwise from top left: a centrifugal pump, a peristaltic pump, and three commercially available pulsatile flow pumps – ViVitro Labs SuperPump, Vascular Simulations Replicator, and Shelley Medical Imaging Technologies CompuFlow. Centrifugal pump schematic from pumpfundamentals.com. (all images used with permission)

comprehensive, high-fidelity physical simulators from both virtual systems and standalone physical components. A neuroendovascular replicator, then, must comprise certain components such as anatomically accurate vascular replicas, physiological pulsatile flow, and proper X-ray attenuation parameters along with other physical considerations of the endovascular compartment such as blood-matched fluid viscosity, physiological luminal friction against catheters, and parenchyma-equivalent suspension of the vessels. Additional details on the requirements for replicators are listed below.

Flow Pumps

Physiological Pulsatile Flow   The hemodynamics of the cardiovascular system are extremely complex due not only to the time-dependent ejection of the stroke volume by the left ventricle every cardiac cycle but also the structure and properties of the arterial network through which blood traverses [40–42]. As the ventricular pressure rises above the aortic pressure during ventricular contraction, the aortic valve opens, causing a rapid ejection of fluid into the aorta, which, by being compliant, also substantially distends. At the end of systole, when the ventricular pressure drops below the aortic pressure and the aortic valve snaps shut, the fluid "rebounding" into the compliant vessel causes a signature increase in the aortic pressure waveform called the dicrotic notch. The ventricle relaxes and, as the mitral valve opens, it fills with blood from the atrium during diastole. The increased pressure in the ascending aorta during the systolic ejection of fluid sets up a pressure gradient (pressure gradients drive flow, not pressures) relative to the downstream vascular segment causing the fluid to successively course through the vascular system overcoming several forms of resistance such as viscous resistance of the fluid, frictional resistance against the walls, and geometric resistance stemming from the curvatures and bifurcations as well as structural narrowing through to the capillary bed. During diastole, the aorta relaxes or recoils and pushes fluid into the next downstream segment resulting in a more gradual decay of pressures (diastolic periods are about twice as long as systolic periods). This compliant behavior of the vasculature led to the Windkessel (air chamber) theory, which, in analogy to electrical systems, is frequently used to model vascular beds with physical resistance, capacitance, and inductance (in sum, impedance) components [43, 44]. Pressure gradient, flow, and impedance are related as voltage, current, and electrical impedance, respectively.

This fluid mechanical distension and relaxation of successive vascular segments sends a pressure pulse wave traveling through the arterial tree. As it travels downstream, this pulse wave reflects off of arterial branch points and a portion of it travels back upstream toward the ascending aorta. The summation of the forward and backward traveling waves results in increasing pulse pressures in the large arteries as compared to the aorta [41, 45](Fig. 3.2, the mean arterial pressure continually decreases); both the mean and pulse pressure significantly reduce in the smaller arteries through to the capillaries where there is essentially no pulsatility. The dampening mechanism of the compliant vessels results in a continual decrease in flow pulsatility through the entire arterial tree to steady flow in the capillaries (Fig. 3.2).

This brief summary of the pressures and flows in the cardiovascular tree underlines the importance of a few points with regard to high-fidelity simulation of blood flow dynamics: the temporal nature of pressures and flows at the vascular inlet must match physiology; the large artery vasculature wherein endovascular training is conducted must be complete, in the correct anatomical location, and possess physiological compliances; and distal bed/microcirculatory resistances and compliances must be replicated with proper Windkessel components.

Pumps Mechanical pumps have a variety of designs, but two general categories are dynamic pumps that transfer kinetic energy to the fluid and positive displacement pumps where a volume of fluid is periodically trapped and forced out of the pump [46, 47]. The main goal of pumps is to supply what is traditionally called "hydraulic head" in the system in order to overcome the system pressures, gravitational, and frictional forces and drive the working fluid at requisite flow rates. A common steady-flow, or continuous-flow, pump that could be used in physical simulators is the

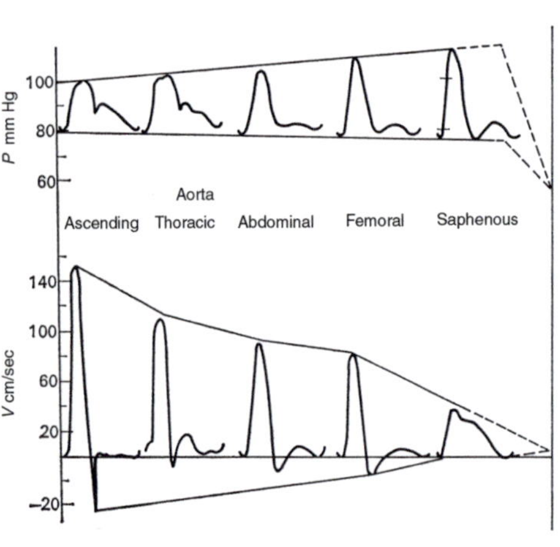

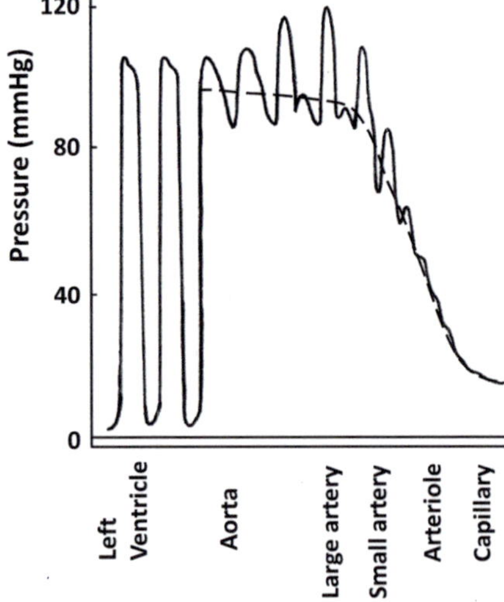

Fig. 3.2 Pressure (left top and right) and flow (left bottom) pulsatility in the cardiovascular system. The pulse pressure increases in the large arteries downstream of the aorta due to reflected pressure waves, but the mean arterial pressure reduces (right dashed line) to maintain a pressure gradient for forward flow. The amplitude of flow pulsa- tions continually decreases, and both pressure and flow pulsatility reduce drastically from the small arteries (tail end of right panel and broken lines on left panel) to achieve steady flow in the capillaries. Left panel from McDonald 1974, Fig. 13.4 [41](right panel modified from O'Rourke and Hashimoto 2007 [45], with permission)

centrifugal pump (a dynamic pump). The basic design of a centrifugal pump consists of a motor that is able to achieve very high rotational speeds connected to a shaft with impeller blades housed inside a pump casing (Fig. 3.1). Dynamic pumps operate with Bernoulli's principles where the fluid is accelerated to a high kinetic energy from spinning the blades. The high kinetic energy fluid is converted into potential energy to generate the discharge pressures required to drive flow through the flow circuit. Centrifugal pumps generate steady flow because, as long as the motor driving the flow rotates at a constant speed, the output is maintained at a constant pressure and flow (Fig. 3.3). Axial flow or propeller pumps are another common form of dynamic pumps that work on similar principles; both these pump types are used in circulatory support devices [48].

The majority of other pump designs have transient flow output and are positive displacement pumps. There are a large variety of positive displacement pumps, from diaphragm pumps to sliding vane pumps, but the two more common ones are piston pumps and peristaltic pumps [46, 47]. Piston pumps have a simple design with a piston centered inside a cylindrical pump housing. Mechanical motion of the piston fills the housing by creating a suction pressure at the inlet and discharges the fluid by creating a positive pressure at the outlet; unidirectional check valves at the inlet and outlet ensure flow is maintained in a single direction. Peristaltic pumps are widely used small scale pumps because of their low cost and versatility of operation and have a similar driving mechanism as the peristaltic motion of intestines. These pumps have a motor connected to a shaft, at end of which multiple rollers (or an eccentric cam) are attached. The rollers lie within a disc-shaped housing. A flexible tubing continuous with the inlet and outlet ports of the pump runs along the inner periphery of the housing such that the tube is pinched in between the rollers and the housing. Rotation of the motor and thus the rollers traps a set volume of fluid in the tube between the rollers that is then displaced and discharged through the outlet (Fig. 3.1). An advantage of peristaltic pumps is that the fluid remains within the flexible tubing and does not come into contact with any other pump parts; fatigue wear usually occurs in the flexible tubing that can be easily replaced. These pumps are considered transient flow because they essentially output fluid boluses in a cyclic pattern (Fig. 3.3). While this is pulsatile in the sense that it is non-steady and cyclical, such flows must be distinguished from physiological pulsatile flow. Pulsatile flow pumps require far more sophisticated control systems and feedback mechanisms.

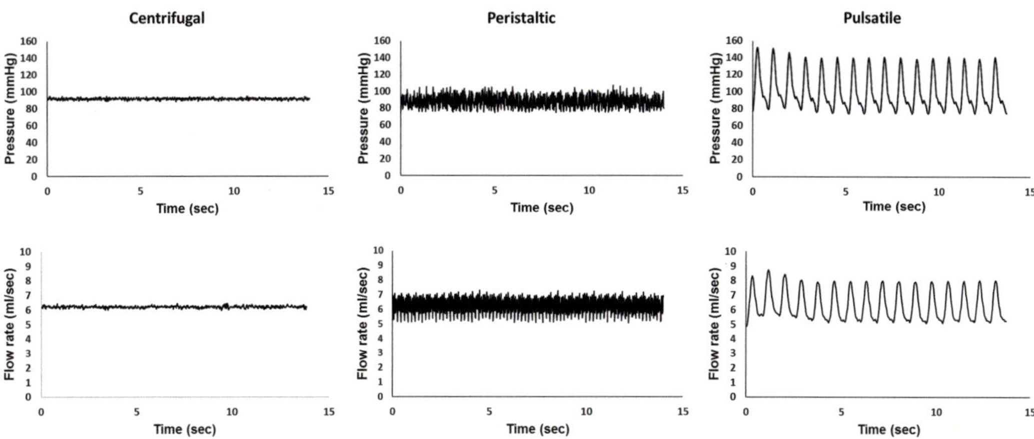

Fig. 3.3 Pressure (top) and flow (bottom) profiles in a 5 mm diameter tube with a centrifugal, peristaltic, and pulsatile pump. All pumps have a mean flow rate of 6.3 cc/s

Pulsatile Flow Pumps Commercial (Table 3.1, Fig. 3.1) and academic pumps that are electromechanically controlled to produce physiological pulsatile flow for benchtop (simulator) use have been developed. It should be noted that numerous ventricular-assist, bridge-to-transplant, or heart replacement devices exist that utilize similar pumping mechanisms (centrifugal, propeller, diaphragm) to produce continuous, or by modulating the driving mechanisms, pulsatile flow [49–53]; these pumps are not discussed here. Programmable piston pumps for simulator use can take any desired flow waveform as input and use software to control the voltages applied to adjust the torque and rotation speed of motors that drive a piston to accurately output the desired waveform. Other systems use actuation (contraction) of compliant chambers simulating the left ventricle by hydraulic or pneumatic mechanisms (by pressuring air or liquid outside the chamber to "squeeze" it) to output physiologically realistic ventricular outputs; different heart valve structures can usually be inserted in these machines to improve physiological accuracy. As mentioned above, the physiological flow output from such pumps needs to be matched with replicas of arterial trees having physiological compliance in order to replicate the hemodynamics with high fidelity. Distal arterial bed resistances and compliances of the flow circuit usually need to be manually adjusted by the user to achieve proper transmission of pressures and flows, but feedback systems can also be built into the hydraulic and electronic circuits to automatically control these parameters and maintain homeostatic pressures and flows. In order to replicate the Windkessel phenomenon, distal compliance or capacitance is usually simulated by adjusting the height of an air column, while resistances can be simulated with resistance valves or narrow channels in the flow circuit [44]. Control feedback can be built in by acquiring and interpreting digital signals from appropriately positioned pressure and flow sensors in the circulation to adjust pump performance in real time.

Working Fluid In order to maintain hemodynamic fidelity, the working fluid that is pumped by pulsatile pumps must mimic blood in terms of its primary mechanical properties – density (1.06 g/cc) and viscosity (~0.04 g/cm.s). This can be accomplished with aqueous solutions of various thickening agents such as glycerin or sorbitol. Blood behaves as a non-Newtonian fluid (its viscosity increases at low shear rates), but this effect is only significant in the small vessels and the microcirculation and can be overlooked for the large vessels in which most endovascular training is conducted. If precise blood flow behavior is required in sluggish flow regimes, for example, in large cavernous aneurysms, the working fluid composition can be altered to mimic non-Newtonian behavior by adding different ingredients such as polyvinyl alcohol, borax, or xanthan gum [54, 55]. Depending on the training scenario, the optical clarity of the vessel can be improved by matching the refractive indices of the vessel replica and fluid [56]. Finally, for endovascular devices that are made of shape-memory materials, the temperature of the blood mimicking fluid must be physiological or near physiological for the devices to deploy properly.

Vascular Replicas

Vascular replicas of cerebrovascular pathologies have been manufactured for research and device testing for nearly three decades by numerous groups using a variety of methods ranging from vascular casts of cadaver heads to direct 3D printing [38, 57–69]. Figure 3.4 shows several common paths to manufacture cerebrovascular replicas. The design phase usually involves volume reconstruction and image segmentation of patient imaging scans (rotational angiography, computerized tomography, magnetic resonance) or construction of idealized/simplified geometries in computer-aided design (CAD) software. A mold is then created from the design by 3D printing or machining; an acrylic/epoxy cast of the vasculature from a cadaver head can also serve as a mold. The oldest casting technique is

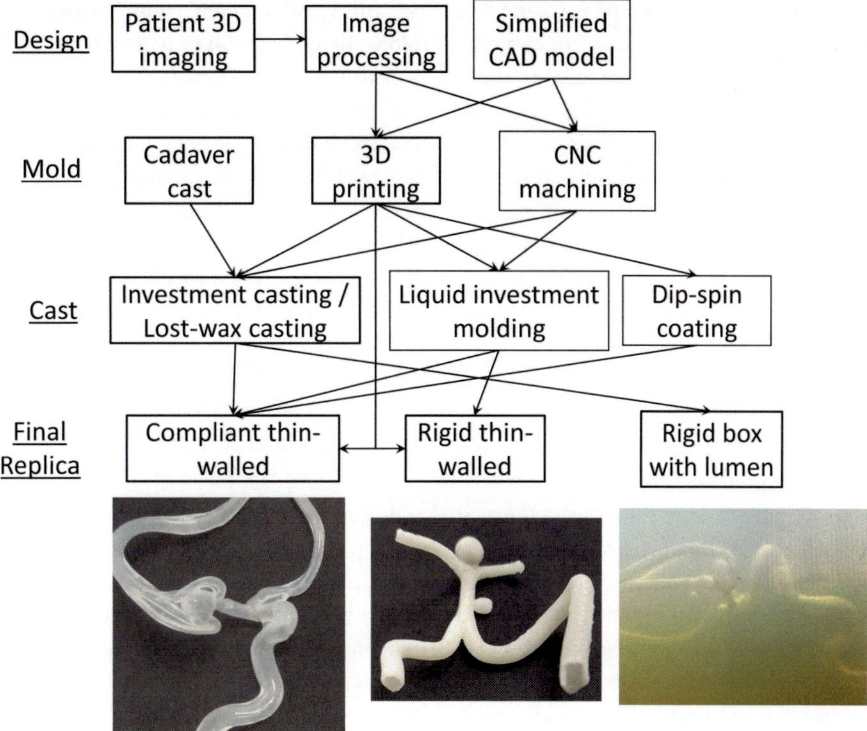

Fig. 3.4 Common methods of manufacturing cerebro-vascular replicas; several paths can be taken to obtain a vascular replica depending on requirements, and several tools and techniques can be used to accomplish each process. Bottom left to right: a compliant thin-walled silicone replica, a rigid 3D-printed replica with 500 micron wall thickness, and a rigid silicone box replica with vascular lumen. CAD computer aided design, CNC computer numeric control

lost-wax casting or investment casting, which uses a negative mold to create a wax replica onto (or into) which a compliant polymer or rigid resin can be casted and the required geometry obtained after melting out the wax. Alternately, liquid polymers can be injected or infused into a mold using liquid investment molding or coated onto the mold using dip-spin coating (processes are described with more detail below). Many of these paths can also be used to cast a block of material within which the vessel geometry is cored out. Advances in 3D printing have made it possible to essentially skip the molding and casting stages and directly print rigid as well as soft vascular replicas. However, control over the material properties of the soft prints in order to match physiological vascular wall properties is still in the incipient stages. In general, the material chosen for manufacturing the replicas must be a

durable material with appropriate fatigue resistance that can be formed into complex geometries that has (or can be coated for) physiological luminal friction coefficients against catheters and wires and matches the distensibility of arteries. The primary material used thus far has been silicone due to its versatility (availability, storage, wide range of material properties based on composition, durability, etc.).

Liquid Investment Molding Investment casting usually involves creating a metal pattern tool or die that is a negative of the outer surface of the desired part, injecting molten wax into this die to form a wax replica of the desired part, coating the wax replica with ceramic to form a ceramic shell, melting out the wax, pouring molten metal into the ceramic shell, and then destroying the ceramic shell (with water jets, vibration, etc.) to obtain the final cast part, which can then be polished and finished. As can be imagined, these steps can produce intricate outer shapes or surfaces. If inner surfaces are also required (e.g., so as to make complex lumen shapes), then additional steps – building a core die, pouring ceramic into the die to form a ceramic core, and assembling the ceramic core into the previous pattern die – are required to obtain the wax replica that can then be coated with a ceramic shell and cast to obtain parts that have both inner and outer surfaces.

Liquid injection molding usually involves injecting low-temperature liquid silicone (two separate liquid components mix to form the final silicone) under high pressure into a heated metal mold within which the silicone cures; the mold is then opened to release the silicone part. The benefits of using 3D printing to reduce the time and cost of these traditional molding/casting methods by, for example, printing the pattern dies or wax replicas or integral core and shell molds, have been noted over the past two decades [70–72]. A combination of these techniques has been utilized to manufacture cerebrovascular replicas by 3D printing integral core and shell molds, injecting or infusing liquid silicone under relatively low pressures into the mold at room temperatures, allowing the silicone to cure, and destroying the mold to obtain the final silicone replica [38]; an example of the process is shown in Fig. 3.5 to manufacture an aortic bifurcation with femoral port access.

Dip-Spin Coating Dip coating is a traditional manufacturing process where molds (or mandrels or substrates) are dipped (immersed and extracted) into a coating solution after which the coating material is allowed to cure and either the coated material is peeled off the mold to obtain the final part or the substrate with the coated material forms the final part. Spin coating involves the deposition of a coating solution at the center of a rotating substrate, which allows the coating material to evenly cover the substrate via centrifugal force. Dip-spin coating combines these two processes where thin films are formed on parts by placing the parts in a rotating cham-

ber, filling the chamber with coating solution to allow for coating films to form on the parts by centrifugal force, extracting the parts from solution, and letting the solution cure. An amalgam of these techniques has been used to develop a dip-spin coating method to manufacture vascular replicas where 3D-printed molds/mandrels are dipped into a coating solution, rotated to obtain even coating thicknesses, curing the coating material, and removing the mold to obtain the final replica [37, 57, 73]. Several parameters of the process such as solution viscosity, number of coats, immersion, extraction, and rotation times and speeds are important to the process [37, 74].

Figure 3.6 shows one version of the dip-spin coating process to manufacture a carotid cavernous silicone replica. The rotational angiogram (any three-dimensional imaging such as computed tomography or magnetic resonance angiography could also be used) from patient imaging is imported into a medical image processing software (Mimics, Materialise, Leuven, Belgium), and the three-dimensional structure is pruned to maintain the relevant vasculature. Inlet and outlet segments are then added so to be able to assemble the replica into the circulatory flow system. The design is converted to stereolithography (STL) format and 3D printed with a rapid prototyper (Dimension Elite, Stratasys, Eden Prairie, MN) that prints the structure with ABS (acrylonitrile butadiene styrene) plastic at a resolution of 180 μm. The plastic core is then smoothed with a solvent in order to reduce surface roughness. The smoothed core is dipped in a silicone solution and spun using a multi-axis spinner so as to obtain an even coating thickness. Additional coats are applied depending on the required thickness. The core with coated silicone is placed in a convection oven at 75 °C for 36 h to cure the silicone, and the core is then destroyed to obtain a compliant thin-walled luminal replica of the patient geometry. Nearly each step of this process from design to mold processing to the silicone used is critical and needs to be controlled to maintain geometric accuracy of the anatomical lumen. Various commercial entities (Table 3.1) have manufactured such cerebral aneurysm replicas using the different

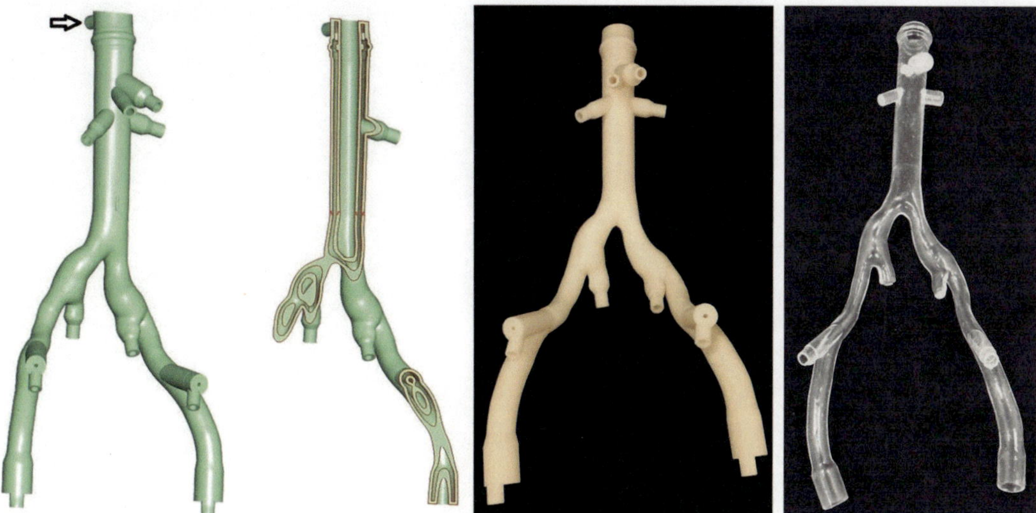

Fig. 3.5 Left to right: design of an abdominal aortic bifurcation mold; the arrow points to the silicone injection port, cross-section view showing the integral core, and shell structure with a lumen into which liquid silicone flows, 3D-printed mold, final silicone part after mold removal

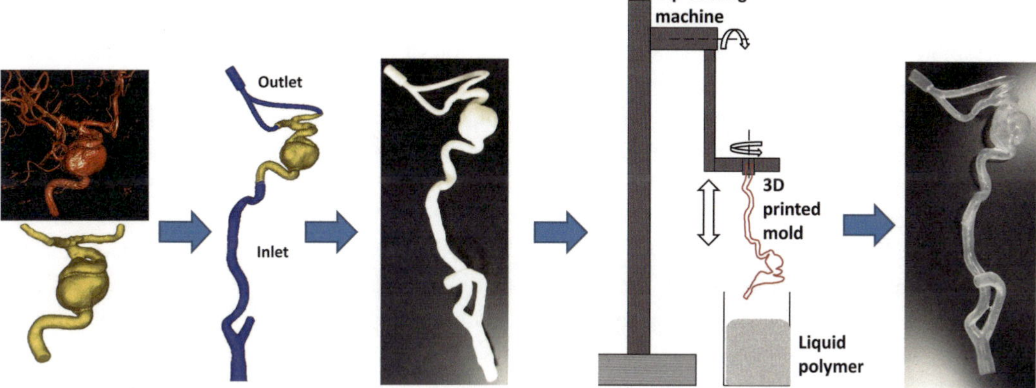

Fig. 3.6 The general process of manufacturing a vascular replica by dip coating. Left to right: the original patient 3D imaging is pruned to retain regions of interest, inlet and outlet segments are added to fit the vasculature into the circulatory system, the geometry is 3D printed to obtain a mold, the mold is coated with a liquid polymer, the polymer is cured, and then the mold is destroyed to result in a replica of the vascular lumen. Multi-axis translations and rotations of the dip-coating machine are usually required to obtain even coats of the polymer

processes mentioned above for training and treatment planning with coils, flow diverters, stents, or intra-aneurysmal devices. Vascular replicas can also be manufactured with clot ports for introduction of thrombus into preferred arterial sites to simulate mechanical thrombectomy procedures, or replicas of arteriovenous malformations can be manufactured for simulating embolization procedures (Fig. 3.7).

Vasculature in a replicator that produces physiological pressure waveforms must also possess distensibility that is equivalent to that of human arteries. Numerous definitions of dynamic distensibility or compliance exist, but all of them are iterations of the ratio of percentage change in vascular volume to change in pressure (systolic volume – diastolic volume)/(diastolic volume*pulse pressure). The mechanical properties of human

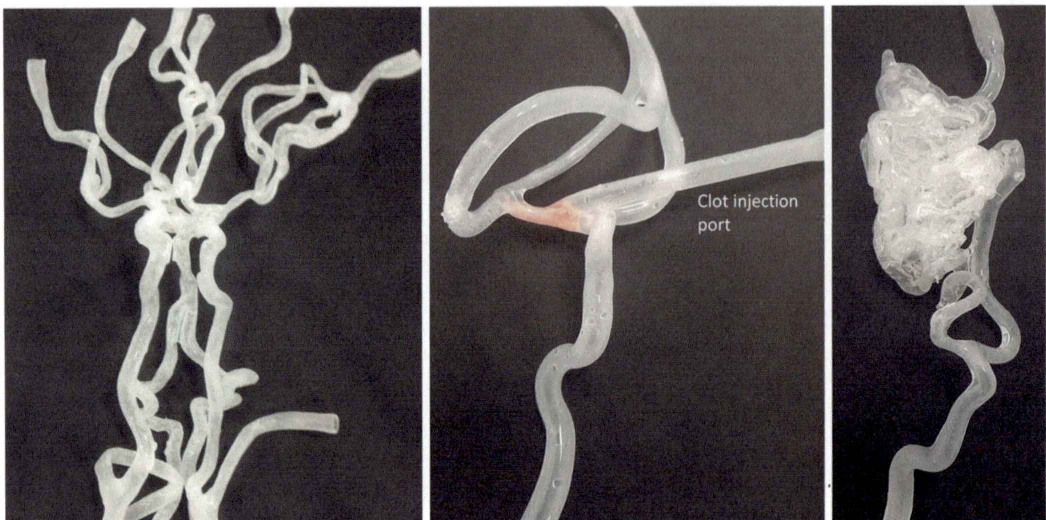

Fig. 3.7 Images of compliant silicone replicas of (left to right) a circle of Willis, a middle cerebral artery occlusion with synthetic thrombus injected through a "clot port," and an arteriovenous malformation

arteries have been evaluated by several groups [75–89]. Wall thicknesses are about 0.75–1.0 mm extracranially and ~0.5 mm intracranially [77–80, 84], the dynamic compliance can be about 8–12% per 100 mmHg (ISO 7198 definition of dynamic compliance) at 60 years of age (most studies measure the common carotid) [75–77, 82, 83, 87], and the circumferential elastic modulus is about 0.5–1.0 megapascals (MPa) [38, 77, 78, 80, 85, 86, 89]. The dynamic compliance is essentially related to the arterial diameter, elastic modulus, and wall thickness (compliance = diameter/(modulus*thickness)). Other arterial properties include a burst strength of 2000–5000 mmHg [87, 88, 90] and suture retention strength of ~200 gram-force [87, 88]. The stiffness of rubbers is measured on the Shore hardness scale and a silicone composition with hardness of 25 Shore A will approximately have an elastic modulus of 0.5 MPa. Thus, if a mold of a cerebral vessel that is anatomically accurate can be coated with this silicone to have a wall thickness varying from 1 mm extracranially to 0.5 mm intracranially, the silicone replica should have a dynamic compliance that is matched to physiology.

The endovascular behavior of wires, catheters, and device delivery systems such as pushability, trackability, and torquability is crucially dependent on the luminal coefficient of friction of the vascular replicas. The sliding coefficient of friction of porcine aorta against catheters varies from 0.04 (low-density polyethylene) to 0.1 (siliconized latex) depending on catheter material [91, 92]. In contrast, the coefficient of friction of raw silicone can be extremely high and ranges from about 0.6 to far greater than 1 [91, 93, 94] depending on the opposing surface material. The luminal friction of silicone vascular replicas thus has to be reduced by at least an order of magnitude for endovascular use. This is usually accomplished by coating the lumen with a friction-reducing agent, using the silicone replica with a working fluid that induces slip, or both. Apart from silicone, polyvinyl alcohol (PVA) has been mentioned as a superior tissue substitute, and it also possesses intrinsically low-friction coefficients, making it suitable for interventional surgery; cerebrovascular replicas have previously been manufactured from PVA [68, 93, 95–100].

Finally, as intracranial vessels lie within the subarachnoid space against the brain parenchyma, they are not free-floating and are subject to a certain degree of flexion as catheters and devices are tracked through them. As a first-order approximation of the physiological extravascular space, vascular replicas can be suspended in a gelatinous medium that simulates this flexion. Material properties of brain tissue have been characterized previously [101–103]; dynamic viscosities, for example, range from 60 to 180 poise.

X-ray Attenuation

Although most neurointerventional procedures are conducted under digital subtraction angiography or fluoroscopic roadmap visualization, a skull structure with physiological attenuation is required in order to simulate bony landmarks or subtraction artifacts or to learn the amount and rate of contrast injection required to properly visualize arterial opacification, especially for novice trainees. A skull phantom is also required to simulate the demand placed on the angiographic imaging chain for visualization of the increasingly fine and complex structures of newer-generation endovascular devices.

Mechanical and X-ray attenuation properties of bone have been studied [104–125]. The total thickness of the skull varies from 5 to 10 mm overall, with the inner and outer cortical tables constituting 20–25% each and the trabecular diploe constituting the remaining 50–60%; average skull thickness can be assumed to be 7–8 mm

[107, 114–119]. The density of cortical bone is around 1.6–1.85 g/cc [114, 121, 123, 124]. Cortical bone is generally orthotropic (isotropic in transverse and radial directions) and possesses longitudinal elastic modulus of 16–21 gigapascals (GPa), transverse elastic modulus of ~11 GPa, shear modulus of 3.5–6 GPa, and Poisson's ratio of 0.2–0.5 [114, 120–125]; the tensile and compressive strengths in the longitudinal and transverse directions are 0.135 GPa and 0.05 GPa and 0.2 GPa and 0.13 GPa, respectively [124, 125]. Corresponding properties of trabecular bone may be about one-half to one-tenth of these values [124]. The X-ray attenuation of trabecular bone is around 200–300 HU [106, 108, 112], while that of cortical bone is around 1500–1700 HU [106, 109, 111, 113] such that a value of around 700–800 HU [110] can be assumed for average bone. The attenuation of brain parenchyma, which is around 30 HU [126], also needs to be simulated to increase the accuracy of the radio-density. Cortical bone and brain parenchyma X-ray attenuation profiles are available from the National Institute of Standards and Technology (http://physics.nist. gov/PhysRefData/XrayMassCoef/tab4.html).

If the parenchyma is simulated by a gel, then numerous media such as barium sulfate, iodinated agents, or titanium dioxide can be added to the gel to increase the radio-opacity. Radiographic

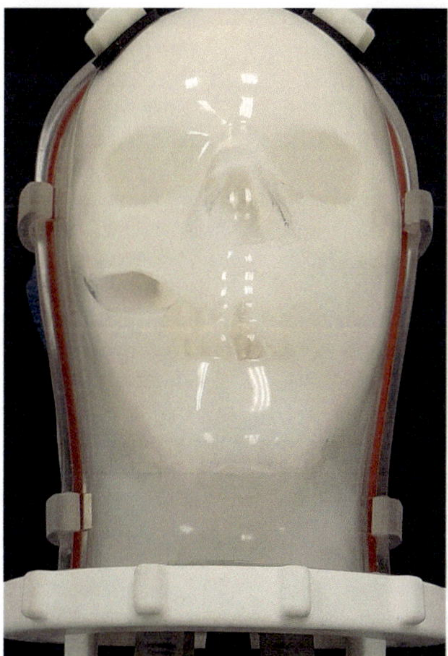
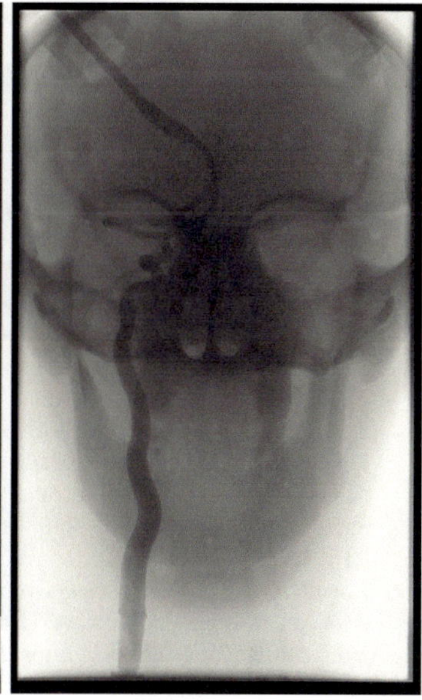

Fig. 3.8 (left) Image of a skull phantom embedded with vascular replicas suspended in a gel. Both the gel (~35 HU) and the skull (800–1000 HU) have physiological X-ray attenuations. (right) Native angiogram of right common carotid vascular replica within the skull

skull phantoms are usually manufactured by casting plastic modified to the requisite Hounsfield attenuation into a mold. Although not yet implemented, 3D printing can potentially be used to manufacture patient-specific skulls with matched radio-opacity; for example, the infiltrant postprocessing techniques associated with the powder/binder 3D printing technology mentioned previously [35, 36] could be used to permeate attenuation-modifying materials into the porous printed structure.

A native angiogram of contrast injection into pulsatile flow through the major intracranial arteries suspended in a gel and embedded within a skull with physiological X-ray attenuations is shown in Fig. 3.8. Further increases in fidelity – inclusion of parenchymal blush, delineation of cortical and trabecular bone, venous sinuses, and a scalp/skin substitute – can be accomplished with current know-how.

Acknowledgment We thank Brandon Kovarovic for his assistance in writing portions of the Flow Pumps section.

Conflict of Interest All authors have a significant financial interest in Vascular Simulations, LLC.

References

1. Kunkler K. The role of medical simulation: an overview. Int J Med Rob Comput Assisted Surg. 2006;2(3):203–10. https://doi.org/10.1002/rcs.101.
2. Rosen KR. The history of medical simulation. J Crit Care. 2008;23(2):157–66. https://doi.org/10.1016/j.jcrc.2007.12.004.
3. Bath J, Lawrence P. Why we need open simulation to train surgeons in an era of work-hour restrictions. Vascular. 2011;19(4):175–7. https://doi.org/10.1258/vasc.2011.oa0284.
4. Nesbitt CI, Birdi N, Mafeld S, Stansby G. The role of simulation in the development of endovascular surgical skills. Perspect Med Educ. 2016;5(1):8–14. https://doi.org/10.1007/s40037-015-0250-4.
5. James JT. A new, evidence-based estimate of patient harms associated with hospital care. J Patient Saf. 2013;9(3):122–8. https://doi.org/10.1097/PTS.0b013e3182948a69.
6. Roguin A, Beyar R. Real case virtual reality training prior to carotid artery stenting. Catheter Cardiovasc Interv. 2010;75(2):279–82. https://doi.org/10.1002/ccd.22211.
7. Dawson DL. Training in carotid artery stenting: do carotid simulation systems really help? Vascular. 2006;14(5):256–63.
8. Tedesco MM, Pak JJ, Harris EJ, Jr., Krummel TM, Dalman RL, Lee JT. Simulation-based endovascular skills assessment: the future of credentialing? J Vasc Surg. 2008;47(5):1008–1; discussion 14. https://doi.org/10.1016/j.jvs.2008.01.007.
9. Lee JT, Qiu M, Teshome M, Raghavan SS, Tedesco MM, Dalman RL. The utility of endovascular simulation to improve technical performance and stimulate continued interest of preclinical medical students in vascular surgery. J Surg Educ. 2009;66(6):367–73. https://doi.org/10.1016/j.jsurg.2009.06.002.
10. Nestel D, Van Herzeele I, Aggarwal R, Odonoghue K, Choong A, Clough R, et al. Evaluating training for a simulated team in complex whole procedure simulations in the endovascular suite. Med Teach. 2009;31(1):e18–23. https://doi.org/10.1080/01421590802337104.
11. Aggarwal R, Mytton OT, Derbrew M, Hananel D, Heydenburg M, Issenberg B, et al. Training and simulation for patient safety. Qual Saf Health Care. 2010;19(Suppl 2):i34–43. https://doi.org/10.1136/qshc.2009.038562.
12. Boyle E, O'Keeffe DA, Naughton PA, Hill AD, McDonnell CO, Moneley D. The importance of expert feedback during endovascular simulator training. J Vasc Surg. 2011;54(1):240–8 e1. https://doi.org/10.1016/j.jvs.2011.01.058.
13. Willaert WI, Aggarwal R, Van Herzeele I, O'Donoghue K, Gaines PA, Darzi AW, et al. Patient-specific endovascular simulation influences interventionalists performing carotid artery stenting procedures. Eur J Vasc Endovasc Surg. 2011;41(4):492–500. https://doi.org/10.1016/j.ejvs.2010.12.013.
14. Eidt JF. The aviation model of vascular surgery education. J Vasc Surg. 2012;55(6):1801–9. https://doi.org/10.1016/j.jvs.2012.01.080.
15. Hseino H, Nugent E, Lee MJ, Hill AD, Neary P, Tierney S, et al. Skills transfer after proficiency-based simulation training in superficial femoral artery angioplasty. Simul Healthc. 2012;7(5):274–81. https://doi.org/10.1097/SIH.0b013e31825b6308.
16. Markovic J, Peyser C, Cavoores T, Fletcher E, Peterson D, Shortell C. Impact of endovascular simulator training on vascular surgery as a career choice in medical students. J Vasc Surg. 2012;55(5):1515–21. https://doi.org/10.1016/j.jvs.2011.11.060.
17. Duran C, Bismuth J, Mitchell E. A nationwide survey of vascular surgery trainees reveals trends in operative experience, confidence, and attitudes about simulation. J Vasc Surg. 2013;58(2):524–8. https://doi.org/10.1016/j.jvs.2012.12.072.
18. Robinson WP, 3rd, Schanzer A, Cutler BS, Baril DT, Larkin AC, Eslami MH, et al. A randomized comparison of a 3-week and 6-week vascular surgery simulation course on junior surgical residents' performance of an end-to-side anastomosis. J Vasc

Surg. 2012;56(6):1771–80; discussion 80–1. https://doi.org/10.1016/j.jvs.2012.06.105.

19. Lonn L, Edmond JJ, Marco J, Kearney PP, Gallagher AG. Virtual reality simulation training in a high-fidelity procedure suite: operator appraisal. J Vasc Interv Radiol. 2012;23(10):1361–6 e2. https://doi.org/10.1016/j.jvir.2012.06.002.

20. Eslahpazir BA, Goldstone J, Allemang MT, Wang JC, Kashyap VS. Principal considerations for the contemporary high-fidelity endovascular simulator design used in training and evaluation. J Vasc Surg. 2014;59(4):1154–62. https://doi.org/10.1016/j.jvs.2013.11.074.

21. Fargen KM, Siddiqui AH, Veznedaroglu E, Turner RD, Ringer AJ, Mocco J. Simulator based angiography education in neurosurgery: results of a pilot educational program. J Neurointerv Surg. 2012;4(6):438–41. https://doi.org/10.1136/neurintsurg-2011-010128.

22. Klein GT, Lu Y, Wang MY. 3D printing and neurosurgery – ready for prime time? World Neurosurg. 2013;80(3–4):233–5. https://doi.org/10.1016/j.wneu.2013.07.009.

23. Rengier F, Mehndiratta A, von Tengg-Kobligk H, Zechmann CM, Unterhinninghofen R, Kauczor HU, et al. 3D printing based on imaging data: review of medical applications. Int J Comput Assist Radiol Surg. 2010;5(4):335–41. https://doi.org/10.1007/s11548-010-0476-x.

24. Ventola CL. Medical applications for 3D printing: current and projected uses. P T. 2014;39(10):704–11.

25. Nute JL, Le Roux L, Chandler AG, Baladandayuthapani V, Schellingerhout D, Cody DD. Differentiation of low-attenuation intracranial hemorrhage and calcification using dual-energy computed tomography in a phantom system. Investig Radiol. 2015;50(1):9–16. https://doi.org/10.1097/rli.0000000000000089.

26. Shmueli K, Thomas DL, Ordidge RJ. Design, construction and evaluation of an anthropomorphic head phantom with realistic susceptibility artifacts. J Magn Reson Imaging. 2007;26(1):202–7. https://doi.org/10.1002/jmri.20993.

27. Schwager K, Gilyoma JM. Ceramic model for temporal bone exercises – an alternative for human temporal bones? Laryngorhinootologie. 2003;82(10):683–6. https://doi.org/10.1055/s-2003-43242.

28. Suzuki M, Ogawa Y, Kawano A, Hagiwara A, Yamaguchi H, Ono H. Rapid prototyping of temporal bone for surgical training and medical education. Acta Otolaryngol. 2004;124(4):400–2.

29. Hurson C, Tansey A, O'Donnchadha B, Nicholson P, Rice J, McElwain J. Rapid prototyping in the assessment, classification and preoperative planning of acetabular fractures. Injury. 2007;38(10):1158–62. https://doi.org/10.1016/j.injury.2007.05.020.

30. Niikura T, Sugimoto M, Lee SY, Sakai Y, Nishida K, Kuroda R, et al. Tactile surgical navigation system for complex acetabular fracture surgery.

Orthopedics. 2014;37(4):237–42. https://doi.org/10.3928/01477447-20140401-05.

31. Gallas RR, Hunemohr N, Runz A, Niebuhr NI, Jakel O, Greilich S. An anthropomorphic multimodality (CT/MRI) head phantom prototype for end-to-end tests in ion radiotherapy. Zeitschrift fur medizinische Physik. 2015;25:391–9. https://doi.org/10.1016/j.zemedi.2015.05.003.

32. Shikhaliev PM. Dedicated phantom materials for spectral radiography and CT. Phys Med Biol. 2012;57(6):1575–93. https://doi.org/10.1088/0031-9155/57/6/1575.

33. Mori K, Yamamoto T, Oyama K, Ueno H, Nakao Y, Honma K. Modified three-dimensional skull base model with artificial dura mater, cranial nerves, and venous sinuses for training in skull base surgery: technical note. Neurol Med Chir. 2008;48(12):582–7; discussion 7–8.

34. Wurm G, Lehner M, Tomancok B, Kleiser R, Nussbaumer K. Cerebrovascular biomodeling for aneurysm surgery: simulation-based training by means of rapid prototyping technologies. Surg Innov. 2011;18(3):294–306. https://doi.org/10.1177/1553350610395031.

35. Gatto M, Harris RA, Sama A, Watson J, editors. Investigating the effectiveness of three-dimensional-printing for producing realistic physical surgical training phantoms. Annals of DAAAM for 2010 and 21st International DAAAM Symposium "Intelligent Manufacturing and Automation: Focus on Interdisciplinary Solutions", October 20, 2010 – October 23, 2010; 2010; Zadar: Danube Adria Association for Automation and Manufacturing, DAAAM.

36. Gatto M, Memoli G, Shaw A, Sadhoo N, Gelat P, Harris RA. Three-dimensional printing (3DP) of neonatal head phantom for ultrasound: thermocouple embedding and simulation of bone. Med Eng Phys. 2012;34(7):929–37. https://doi.org/10.1016/j.medengphy.2011.10.012.

37. Arcaute K, Wicker RB. Patient-specific compliant vessel manufacturing using dip-spin coating of rapid prototyped molds. J Manuf Sci E T ASME. 2008;130(5):0510081–05100813. https://doi.org/10.1115/1.2898839.

38. Chueh JY, Wakhloo AK, Gounis MJ. Neurovascular modeling: small-batch manufacturing of silicone vascular replicas. AJNR Am J Neuroradiol. 2009;30(6):1159–64. https://doi.org/10.3174/ajnr.A1543.

39. Chaudhury RA, Atlasman V, Pathangey G, Pracht N, Adrian RJ, Frakes DH. A high performance pulsatile pump for aortic flow experiments in 3-dimensional models. Cardiovasc Eng Technol. 2016;7(2):148–58. https://doi.org/10.1007/s13239-016-0260-3.

40. Fung YC. Biomechanics : circulation. 2nd ed. New York: Springer; 1997.

41. McDonald DA. Blood flow in arteries. 2nd ed. Baltimore: The Williams & Wilkins Company; 1974.

42. Lieber BB, Sadasivan C. Hemodynamics, Macro circulatory. Encyclopedia of biomaterials and biomedical engineering. 2nd ed (Online Version). CRC Press; 2008. p. 1356–1367.

43. Segers P, Rietzschel ER, De Buyzere ML, Stergiopulos N, Westerhof N, Van Bortel LM, et al. Three- and four-element Windkessel models: assessment of their fitting performance in a large cohort of healthy middle-aged individuals. Proc Inst Mech Eng H J Eng Med. 2008;222(4):417–28.

44. Kung EO, Taylor CA. Development of a physical windkessel module to re-create in-vivo vascular flow impedance for in-vitro experiments. Cardiovasc Eng Technol. 2011;2(1):2–14. https://doi.org/10.1007/s13239-010-0030-6.

45. O'Rourke MF, Hashimoto J. Mechanical factors in arterial aging: a clinical perspective. J Am Coll Cardiol. 2007;50(1):1–13. https://doi.org/10.1016/j.jacc.2006.12.050.

46. Volk MW. Pump characteristics and applications. Mechanical engineering, vol. 103. New York: M. Dekker; 1996.

47. Armignacco P, Garzotto F, Bellini C, Neri M, Lorenzin A, Sartori M, et al. Pumps in wearable ultrafiltration devices: pumps in wuf devices. Blood Purif. 2015;39(1–3):115–24. https://doi.org/10.1159/000368943.

48. Moazami N, Fukamachi K, Kobayashi M, Smedira NG, Hoercher KJ, Massiello A, et al. Axial and centrifugal continuous-flow rotary pumps: a translation from pump mechanics to clinical practice. J Heart Lung transplant. 2013;32(1):1–11. https://doi.org/10.1016/j.healun.2012.10.001.

49. Jahren SE, Ochsner G, Shu F, Amacher R, Antaki JF, Vandenberghe S. Analysis of pressure head-flow loops of pulsatile rotodynamic blood pumps. Artif Organs. 2014;38(4):316–26. https://doi.org/10.1111/aor.12139.

50. Pirbodaghi T, Axiak S, Weber A, Gempp T, Vandenberghe S. Pulsatile control of rotary blood pumps: does the modulation waveform matter? J Thorac Cardiovasc Surg. 2012;144(4):970–7. https://doi.org/10.1016/j.jtcvs.2012.02.015.

51. Cuenca-Navalon E, Laumen M, Finocchiaro T, Steinseifer U. Estimation of filling and afterload conditions by pump intrinsic parameters in a pulsatile total artificial heart. Artif Organs. 2016;40(7):638–44. https://doi.org/10.1111/aor.12636.

52. Gu YJ, van Oeveren W, Mungroop HE, Epema AH, den Hamer IJ, Keizer JJ, et al. Clinical effectiveness of centrifugal pump to produce pulsatile flow during cardiopulmonary bypass in patients undergoing cardiac surgery. Artif Organs. 2011;35(2):E18–26. https://doi.org/10.1111/j.1525-1594.2010.01152.x.

53. Sajgalik P, Grupper A, Edwards BS, Kushwaha SS, Stulak JM, Joyce DL, et al. Current status of left ventricular assist device therapy. Mayo Clin Proc. 2016;91(7):927–40. https://doi.org/10.1016/j.mayocp.2016.05.002.

54. Jungreis CA, Kerber CW. A solution that simulates whole blood in a model of the cerebral circulation. AJNR Am J Neuroradiol. 1991;12(2):329–30.

55. Anastasiou AD, Spyrogianni AS, Koskinas KC, Giannoglou GD, Paras SV. Experimental investigation of the flow of a blood analogue fluid in a replica of a bifurcated small artery. Med Eng Phys. 2012;34(2):211–8. https://doi.org/10.1016/j.medengphy.2011.07.012.

56. Yousif MY, Holdsworth DW, Poepping TL. Deriving a blood-mimicking fluid for particle image velocimetry in Sylgard-184 vascular models. Conf Proc IEEE Eng Med Biol Soc. 2009;2009:1412–5. https://doi.org/10.1109/iembs.2009.5334175.

57. Seong J, Sadasivan C, Onizuka M, Gounis MJ, Christian F, Miskolczi L, et al. Morphology of elastase-induced cerebral aneurysm model in rabbit and rapid prototyping of elastomeric transparent replicas. Biorheology. 2005;42(5):345–61.

58. Santore J, Sadasivan C, Fiorella DJ, Lieber BB, Woo HH, editors. Creation of patient-specific silicone vascular replicas of aneurysm-parent vessel complexes. AANS/CNS Cerebrovascular Section Annual Meeting; 2012. Hilton New Orleans Riverside, New Orleans.

59. Kerber CW, Heilman CB. Flow dynamics in the human carotid artery: I. Preliminary observations using a transparent elastic model. AJNR Am J Neuroradiol. 1992;13(1):173–80.

60. Knox K, Kerber CW, Singel SA, Bailey MJ, Imbesi SG. Stereolithographic vascular replicas from CT scans: choosing treatment strategies, teaching, and research from live patient scan data. AJNR Am J Neuroradiol. 2005;26(6):1428–31.

61. Yagi T, Sato A, Shinke M, Takahashi S, Tobe Y, Takao H, et al. Experimental insights into flow impingement in cerebral aneurysm by stereoscopic particle image velocimetry: transition from a laminar regime. J R Soc Interface / R Soc. 2013;10(82):20121031. https://doi.org/10.1098/rsif.2012.1031.

62. Anderson JR, Diaz O, Klucznik R, Zhang YJ, Britz GW, Grossman RG, et al. Validation of computational fluid dynamics methods with anatomically exact, 3D printed MRI phantoms and 4D pcMRI. Conf Proc IEEE Eng Med Biol Soc. 2014;2014:6699–701. https://doi.org/10.1109/embc.2014.6945165.

63. Khan IS, Kelly PD, Singer RJ. Prototyping of cerebral vasculature physical models. Surg Neurol Int. 2014;5:11. https://doi.org/10.4103/2152-7806.125858.

64. Russ M, O'Hara R, Setlur Nagesh SV, Mokin M, Jimenez C, Siddiqui A, et al. Treatment planning for image-guided neuro-vascular interventions using patient-specific 3D printed phantoms. Proceedings of SPIE – the International Society for Optical Engineering. 2015;9417. https://doi.org/10.1117/12.2081997.

65. Ikeda S, Arai F, Fukuda T, Negoro M, Irie K. An in vitro patient-specific biological model of the cerebral artery reproduced with a membranous configuration for simulating endovascular intervention. J Rob Mechatronics. 2005;17(3):327–34.

66. Mashiko T, Otani K, Kawano R, Konno T, Kaneko N, Ito Y, et al. Development of three-dimensional hollow elastic model for cerebral aneurysm clipping simulation enabling rapid and low cost prototyping. World Neurosurg. 2015;83(3):351–61. https://doi.org/10.1016/j.wneu.2013.10.032.

67. Wetzel SG, Ohta M, Handa A, Auer JM, Lylyk P, Lovblad KO, et al. From patient to model: stereolithographic modeling of the cerebral vasculature based on rotational angiography. AJNR Am J Neuroradiol. 2005;26(6):1425–7.

68. Yu CH, Ohta M, Kwon TK. Study of parameters for evaluating the pushability of interventional devices using box-shaped blood vessel biomodels made of PVA-H or silicone. Biomed Mater Eng. 2014;24(1):961–8. https://doi.org/10.3233/bme-130891.

69. Benet A, Plata-Bello J, Abla AA, Acevedo-Bolton G, Saloner D, Lawton MT. Implantation of 3D-printed patient-specific aneurysm models into cadaveric specimens: a new training paradigm to allow for improvements in cerebrovascular surgery and research. Biomed Res Int. 2015;2015:939387. https://doi.org/10.1155/2015/939387.

70. Bassoli E, Gatto A, Iuliano L, Violante MG. 3D printing technique applied to rapid casting. Rapid Prototyp J. 2007;13(3):148–55. https://doi.org/10.1108/13552540710750898.

71. Cheah CM, Chua CK, Lee CW, Feng C, Totong K. Rapid prototyping and tooling techniques: a review of applications for rapid investment casting. Int J Adv Manuf Technol. 2005;25(3–4):308–20. https://doi.org/10.1007/s00170-003-1840-6.

72. Sachs E, Cima M, Williams P, Brancazio D, Cornie J. Three dimensional printing: rapid tooling and prototypes directly from a CAD model. J Eng Ind. 1992;114(4):481–8. https://doi.org/10.1115/1.2900701.

73. Wicker R, Cortez M, Medina F, Palafox G, Elkins C, editors. Manufacturing of complex compliant cardiovascular system models for in-vitro hemodynamic experimentation using CT and MRI data and rapid prototyping technologies. ASME Summer Bioengineering Conference; 2001 Jun 27–Jul 1; Snowbird: ASME.

74. Arcaute K, Palafox GN, Medina F, Wicker RB, editors. Complex silicone aorta models manufactured using a dip-spin coating technique and water-soluble molds. 2003 Summer Bioengineering Conference; 2003 June 25–29; Key Biscayne.

75. Van Merode T, Hick PJ, Hoeks AP, Rahn KH, Reneman RS. Carotid artery wall properties in normotensive and borderline hypertensive subjects of various ages. Ultrasound Med Biol. 1988;14(7):563–9.

76. Hirai T, Sasayama S, Kawasaki T, Yagi S. Stiffness of systemic arteries in patients with myocardial infarction. A noninvasive method to predict severity of coronary atherosclerosis. Circulation. 1989;80(1):78–86.

77. Luc M, Polonsky T, Lammertin G, Spencer K. Automated border detection for assessing the mechanical properties of the carotid arteries: comparison with carotid intima-media thickness. J Am Soc Echocardiogr. 2010;23(5):567–72. https://doi.org/10.1016/j.echo.2010.01.024.

78. Kamenskiy AV, Dzenis YA, MacTaggart JN, Lynch TG, Jaffar Kazmi SA, Pipinos II. Nonlinear mechanical behavior of the human common, external, and internal carotid arteries in vivo. J Surg Res. 2012;176(1):329–36. https://doi.org/10.1016/j.jss.2011.09.058.

79. Hayashi K, Handa H, Nagasawa S, Okumura A, Moritake K. Stiffness and elastic behavior of human intracranial and extracranial arteries. J Biomech. 1980;13(2):175–84.

80. Franquet A, Avril S, Le Riche R, Badel P, Schneider FC, Boissier C, et al. Identification of the in vivo elastic properties of common carotid arteries from MRI: a study on subjects with and without atherosclerosis. J Mech Behav Biomed Mater. 2013;27:184–203. https://doi.org/10.1016/j.jmbbm.2013.03.016.

81. Tanaka H, Dinenno FA, Monahan KD, Clevenger CM, DeSouza CA, Seals DR. Aging, habitual exercise, and dynamic arterial compliance. Circulation. 2000;102(11):1270–5.

82. Hansen F, Mangell P, Sonesson B, Lanne T. Diameter and compliance in the human common carotid artery – variations with age and sex. Ultrasound Med Biol. 1995;21(1):1–9.

83. Lenard Z, Fulop D, Visontai Z, Jokkel G, Reneman R, Kollai M. Static versus dynamic distensibility of the carotid artery in humans. J Vasc Res. 2000;37(2):103–11. https://doi.org/10.1159/000025721.

84. Sato T, Sasaki T, Suzuki K, Matsumoto M, Kodama N, Hiraiwa K. Histological study of the normal vertebral artery – etiology of dissecting aneurysms. Neurol Med Chir. 2004;44(12):629–35; discussion 36.

85. Drangova M, Holdsworth DW, Boyd CJ, Dunmore PJ, Roach MR, Fenster A. Elasticity and geometry measurements of vascular specimens using a high-resolution laboratory CT scanner. Physiol Meas. 1993;14(3):277–90.

86. Dobrin PB. Mechanical properties of arteries. Physiol Rev. 1978;58(2):397–460.

87. Konig G, McAllister TN, Dusserre N, Garrido SA, Iyican C, Marini A, et al. Mechanical properties of completely autologous human tissue engineered blood vessels compared to human saphenous vein and mammary artery. Biomaterials. 2009;30(8):1542–50. https://doi.org/10.1016/j.biomaterials.2008.11.011.

88. L'Heureux N, Dusserre N, Konig G, Victor B, Keire P, Wight TN, et al. Human tissue-engineered blood

vessels for adult arterial revascularization. Nat Med. 2006;12(3):361–5. https://doi.org/10.1038/nm1364.

89. Monson KL, Goldsmith W, Barbaro NM, Manley GT. Axial mechanical properties of fresh human cerebral blood vessels. J Biomech Eng. 2003;125(2):288–94.

90. Sarkar S, Salacinski HJ, Hamilton G, Seifalian AM. The mechanical properties of infrainguinal vascular bypass grafts: their role in influencing patency. Eur J Vasc Endovasc Surg. 2006;31(6):627–36. https://doi.org/10.1016/j.ejvs.2006.01.006.

91. Kazmierska K, Szwast M, Ciach T. Determination of urethral catheter surface lubricity. J Mater Sci Mater Med. 2008;19(6):2301–6. https://doi.org/10.1007/s10856-007-3339-4.

92. Caldwell RA, Woodell JE, Ho SP, Shalaby SW, Boland T, Langan EM, et al. In vitro evaluation of phosphonylated low-density polyethylene for vascular applications. J Biomed Mater Res. 2002;62(4):514–24. https://doi.org/10.1002/jbm.10249.

93. Ohta M, Handa A, Iwata H, Rufenacht DA, Tsutsumi S. Poly-vinyl alcohol hydrogel vascular models for in vitro aneurysm simulations: the key to low friction surfaces. Technol Health Care. 2004;12(3):225–33.

94. Persson BNJ. Silicone rubber adhesion and sliding friction. Tribol Lett. 2016;62(2). https://doi.org/10.1007/s11249-016-0680-0.

95. Kosukegawa H, Mamada K, Kuroki K, Liu L, Inoue K, Hayase T, et al. Measurements of dynamic viscoelasticity of poly (vinyl alcohol) hydrogel for the development of blood vessel biomodeling. J Fluid Sci Tech. 2008;3(4):533–43. https://doi.org/10.1299/jfst.3.533.

96. Kosukegawa H, Shida S, Hashida Y, Ohta M, editors. Mechanical properties of tube-shaped poly (vinyl alcohol) hydrogel blood vessel biomodel. ASME 2010 3rd Joint US-European Fluids Engineering Summer Meeting; 2010. Montreal: Fluids Engineering Division.

97. Yu C, Kosukegawa H, Mamada K, Kuroki K, Takashima K, Yoshinaka K, et al. Development of an in vitro tracking system with poly (vinyl alcohol) hydrogel for catheter motion. J Biomech Sci Eng. 2010;5(1):11–7. https://doi.org/10.1299/jbse.5.11.

98. Kosukegawa H, Kiyomitsu C, Ohta M, editors. Control of wall thickness of blood vessel biomodel made of poly (vinyl alcohol) hydrogel by a three-dimensional-rotating spin dip-coating method. ASME 2011 International Mechanical Engineering Congress and Exposition; 2011. Denver: ASME.

99. Mutoh T, Ishikawa T, Ono H, Yasui N. A new polyvinyl alcohol hydrogel vascular model (KEZLEX) for microvascular anastomosis training. Surg Neurol Int. 2010;1:74. https://doi.org/10.4103/2152-7806.72626.

100. Spetzger U, von Schilling A, Brombach T, Winkler G. Training models for vascular microneurosurgery. Acta Neurochir Suppl. 2011;112:115–9. https://doi.org/10.1007/978-3-7091-0661-7_21.

101. Saboori P, Sadegh A. Material modeling of the head's subarachnoid space. Sci Iran. 2011;18(6):1492–9.

102. Fallenstein GT, Hulce VD, Melvin JW. Dynamic mechanical properties of human brain tissue. J Biomech. 1969;2(3):217–26.

103. Cotter CS, Smolarkiewicz PK, Szczyrba IN. A viscoelastic fluid model for brain injuries. Int J Numer Methods Fluids. 2002;40(1–2):303–11. https://doi.org/10.1002/fld.287.

104. Chen X, Lam YM. Technical note: CT determination of the mineral density of dry bone specimens using the dipotassium phosphate phantom. Am J Phys Anthropol. 1997;103(4):557–60. https://doi.org/10.1002/(sici)1096-8644(199708)103:4<557::aid-ajpa10>3.0.co;2-#.

105. Giambini H, Dragomir-Daescu D, Huddleston PM, Camp JJ, An KN, Nassr A. The effect of quantitative computed tomography acquisition protocols on bone mineral density estimation. J Biomech Eng. 2015;137(11). https://doi.org/10.1115/1.4031572.

106. Mah P, Reeves TE, McDavid WD. Deriving Hounsfield units using grey levels in cone beam computed tomography. Dentomaxillofac Radiol. 2010;39(6):323–35. https://doi.org/10.1259/dmfr/19603304.

107. Delye H, Clijmans T, Mommaerts MY, Sloten JV, Goffin J. Creating a normative database of age-specific 3D geometrical data, bone density, and bone thickness of the developing skull: a pilot study. J Neurosurg Pediatr. 2015;16(6):687–702. https://doi.org/10.3171/2015.4.peds1493.

108. Lee S, Chung CK, Oh SH, Park SB. Correlation between bone mineral density measured by dual-energy X-ray absorptiometry and Hounsfield units measured by diagnostic CT in lumbar spine. J Korean Neurosurg Soc. 2013;54(5):384–9. https://doi.org/10.3340/jkns.2013.54.5.384.

109. Kowalczyk M, Wall A, Turek T, Kulej M, Scigala K, Kawecki J. Computerized tomography evaluation of cortical bone properties in the tibia. Ortop Traumatol Rehabil. 2007;9(2):187–97.

110. Turkyilmaz I, Ozan O, Yilmaz B, Ersoy AE. Determination of bone quality of 372 implant recipient sites using Hounsfield unit from computerized tomography: a clinical study. Clin Implant Dent Relat Res. 2008;10(4):238–44. https://doi.org/10.1111/j.1708-8208.2008.00085.x.

111. Lim Fat D, Kennedy J, Galvin R, O'Brien F, Mc Grath F, Mullett H. The Hounsfield value for cortical bone geometry in the proximal humerus – an in vitro study. Skelet Radiol. 2012;41(5):557–68. https://doi.org/10.1007/s00256-011-1255-7.

112. Schreiber JJ, Anderson PA, Hsu WK. Use of computed tomography for assessing bone mineral density. Neurosurg Focus. 2014;37(1):E4. https://doi.org/10.3171/2014.5.focus1483.

113. Cassetta M, Stefanelli LV, Pacifici A, Pacifici L, Barbato E. How accurate is CBCT in measuring bone density? A comparative CBCT-CT in vitro

study. Clin Implant Dent Relat Res. 2014;16(4):471–8. https://doi.org/10.1111/cid.12027.

114. Peterson J, Dechow PC. Material properties of the human cranial vault and zygoma. Anat Rec A Discov Mol Cell Evol Biol. 2003;274(1):785–97. https://doi.org/10.1002/ar.a.10096.

115. Delye H, Verschueren P, Depreitere B, Verpoest I, Berckmans D, Vander Sloten J, et al. Biomechanics of frontal skull fracture. J Neurotrauma. 2007;24(10):1576–86. https://doi.org/10.1089/neu.2007.0283.

116. Adeloye A, Kattan KR, Silverman FN. Thickness of the normal skull in the American blacks and whites. Am J Phys Anthropol. 1975;43(1):23–30. https://doi.org/10.1002/ajpa.1330430105.

117. Lynnerup N, Astrup JG, Sejrsen B. Thickness of the human cranial diploe in relation to age, sex and general body build. Head Face Med. 2005;1:13. https://doi.org/10.1186/1746-160x-1-13.

118. Lynnerup N. Cranial thickness in relation to age, sex and general body build in a Danish forensic sample. Forensic Sci Int. 2001;117(1–2):45–51.

119. Sabanciogullari V, Salk I, Cimen M. The relationship between total calvarial thickness and diploe in the elderly. Int J Morphol. 2013;31(1):38–44.

120. Kobler JP, Prielozny L, Lexow GJ, Rau TS, Majdani O, Ortmaier T. Mechanical characterization of bone anchors used with a bone-attached, parallel robot for skull surgery. Med Eng Phys. 2015;37(5):460–8. https://doi.org/10.1016/j.medengphy.2015.02.012.

121. Park HK, Dujovny M, Agner C, Diaz FG. Biomechanical properties of calvarium prosthesis. Neurol Res. 2001;23(2–3):267–76. https://doi.org/10.1179/016164101101198424.

122. Zysset PK, Guo XE, Hoffler CE, Moore KE, Goldstein SA. Elastic modulus and hardness of cortical and trabecular bone lamellae measured by nanoindentation in the human femur. J Biomech. 1999;32(10):1005–12.

123. Dechow PC, Nail GA, Schwartz-Dabney CL, Ashman RB. Elastic properties of human supraorbital and mandibular bone. Am J Phys Anthropol. 1993;90(3):291–306. https://doi.org/10.1002/ajpa.1330900304.

124. Keaveny TM, Hayes WC. Mechanical properties of cortical and trabecular bone. In: Hall BK, editor. Bone: Bone growth – B. Boca Raton: CRC Press; 1993. p. 285–344.

125. Reilly DT, Burstein AH. The elastic and ultimate properties of compact bone tissue. J Biomech. 1975;8(6):393–405.

126. Camargo ECS, González G, González RG, Lev MH. Unenhanced computed tomography. In: González RG, Hirsch JA, Koroshetz WJ, Lev MH, Schaefer PW, editors. Acute ischemic stroke: imaging and intervention. Berlin, Heidelberg: Springer Berlin Heidelberg; 2006. p. 41–56.

Kushal J. Shah, Jeremy C. Peterson,
and Roukoz Chamoun

Introduction

Neurosurgical training has evolved with technological advances. Traditionally, neurosurgery was taught on real people in the operating room. The conventional dictum of "see one, do one, teach one" has been long-standing. The changes in the work hour restrictions and other cultural changes have led to the need to develop other training tools.

Education has also transpired on cadavers. Cadavers are an excellent method for teaching anatomy. However, they tend to be expensive, and the preservation techniques do affect the dissection planes. Additionally, they usually lack pathology.

As technology has advanced, neurosurgeons are using navigation systems as a method of training. More recently, simulators have been used. Simulators are an excellent teaching tool but are not quite realistic enough for higher-level procedural practice.

3D printed models have the benefit of providing patient-specific tools to teaching various approaches and techniques. "Stereolithography is a method and apparatus for making solid objects by successively 'printing' thin layers of the curable material, one on top of the other" [1].

This technique allows the creation of complex 3D models of the skull, brain, spine, and other anatomical parts of the body. The more advanced 3D printers allow multiple colors and materials, giving the tissues a more realistic appearance and feel. Not surprisingly, the costs of the advanced 3D printers are much higher than more basic printers.

At our institution, we utilize the uPrint SE Plus 3D printer made by Stratasys.

This chapter will outline the various ways that 3D printed models are a valuable teaching tool in neurosurgical training.

Cranial

Aneurysm Clipping

Microsurgical dissection and clipping of cerebral aneurysms are one of the highest skill dependent procedures performed in neurosurgery. Classically, these skills have been developed while working on cadavers and observing more senior neurosurgeons. With the increased use of endovascular techniques, the number of aneurysms being clipped has declined worldwide. The cases that are clipped are, in general, the more difficult and challenging cases that are not amiable to endovascular treatment. This has greatly decreased the opportunities for training

K. J. Shah · J. C. Peterson · R. Chamoun (✉)
Department of Neurosurgery, University of Kansas
Medical Center, Kansas City, KS, USA
e-mail: kjs5wf@mail.umkc.edu; jpeterson6@kumc.edu;
rchamoun@kumc.edu

© Springer International Publishing AG, part of Springer Nature 2018
A. Alaraj (ed.), *Comprehensive Healthcare Simulation: Neurosurgery*,
Comprehensive Healthcare Simulation, https://doi.org/10.1007/978-3-319-75583-0_4

neurosurgeons to employ skills learned in cadaver courses to less complex aneurysms. Cadavers containing pathology specific to aneurysm surgery are not common. 3D printing has started to answer the call for a better training environment as related to aneurysm surgery (Fig. 4.1).

3D printing of cerebrovasculature, especially aneurysms, was one of the first uses of 3D printing in neurosurgery. D'Uso et al. [2] were the first to use three-dimensional data from computed tomographic angiography (CTA) and magnetic resonance angiography (MRA) to fabricate intracranial vasculature biomodels with stereolithography in 1999. They conducted a prospective 16-patient study to evaluate the accuracy and functionality of the process that uses a laser beam to solidify layers of a photosensitive liquid resin. This process was described as producing vasculature that accurately represented the intraoperative findings in all but one aneurysm which contained an intraluminal thrombus. The data obtained only included intraluminal data. CTA was found to include both arterial and venous structures which had to be determined based on anatomical knowledge. Perforating vessels with a diameter less than 1 mm were windowed out and not provided in the models. Comparison between the biomodeling and a postmortem specimen was demonstrated within the paper. The study showed that the surgeons found the biomodels to be helpful when educating patients, positioning the patient, and during the surgical procedure. The accuracy allowed measurements to be taken and transferred to the operative suite to clarify anatomical relationships. Limitations to the study included the difficulty of portraying small vessels and removing the support material without removing pertinent anatomy. Another challenge was determining the amount of thresholding for segmentation which was operator dependent which may have introduced error. The build time for their models was an average of 3 days and cost $300 per model.

Wurm et al. [3] conducted a prospective study of 13 aneurysms from 1999–2003. The first three cases were performed using CTA and an SLA 250 (3D Systems, Valencia CA) which had a build layer thickness of 0.25 mm. The CTA imag-

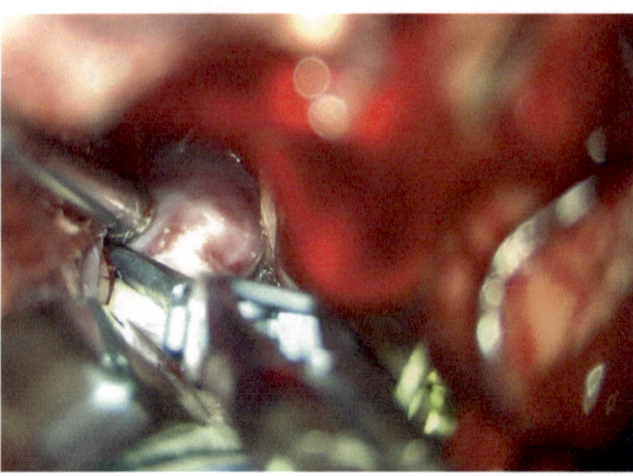

Fig. 4.1 Cerebral aneurysm clipping of anterior communicating artery aneurysm

ing was found to have poor resolution in comparison to the rapid prototyping machine. 3D rotational angiography data was then used in the rest of the patients. The last model was created with an SLA 3500 (3D Systems, Valencia CA) which had a build layer thickness of 0.0625 mm. The improvement in imaging data, postprocessing techniques, and stereolithography technology helped increase the accuracy throughout this study. The model accuracy was compared to intraoperative videos. These models were felt to be valuable in improving 3D anatomy understanding and relationships of the aneurysm to branching vessels. Due to the rigidity of the models, they did not provide help with the evaluation of the geometry of the aneurysm neck and simulation of clipping or provide an opportunity for dissecting exercises. They had an approximately 50-h delay from the time of imaging to obtaining the model within their study (Fig. 4.2).

Wurm et al. [4] continued to refine their methods to make the models more functional for dissection and clip application. They first were able to use 3D rotational angiography to obtain data of the relevant vasculature in relation to the bone. They first attempted to fabricate a model using their previous work with stereolithography to create a model of the bone and vasculature as well as a mold to create a less rigid silicone aneurysm to better simulate actual clipping. In order to improve the functionality of the model, they were the first to move to PolyJet Matrix 3D printing. This process involves jetting a liquid

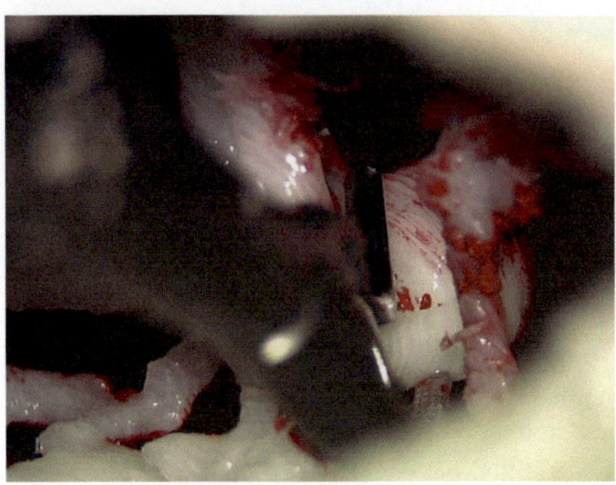

Fig. 4.2 After trialing multiple clips and directions, the best clip and position have been tested on a 3D model

photopolymer then immediately curing the liquid with a high-intensity ultraviolet light source. This technology offers the ability to print objects made of multiple model materials of any mix of rigid and flexible properties within a single build. The builds had to contain three parts: solid skull, vessels of a different color, and an aneurysm that was flexible. The vessels and bone were opaque rigid polymers, and the aneurysm was an amber translucent, rubberlike, flexible photopolymer material. Due to the print size, the skull and vessels had to be printed in two parts, and the aneurysm was a separate third part. The aneurysm and parent vessels were hollowed out to allow for placement over the rigid vasculature of the model and allowed replacement of the aneurysm section for multiple clippings. Data transfer and production took 1.5 weeks and cost approximately 2000 Euro. They concluded that this model provided an avenue for simulation-based training that offered an opportunity for improvement of surgical skills and allowed good haptic feedback of aneurysm clipping. These models still were unable to provide feedback about the intrinsic factors of the vessel walls. They also did not include information about the structures directly around the aneurysm that are important in approaching the aneurysm, such as the sylvian fissure anatomy and surrounding brain tissue.

Kimura et al. [5] reported a different technique of creating a hollow, elastic aneurysm and vessels based on CTA information. The elastic, rubberlike polymer vessels were created by a PolyJet printer. After the vessels were printed, they were placed under a UV light which cured the outer surface of the material. The inner uncured portion of the vessels was cleared by curetting, thus making the model hollow. They then created a hard bone model that contained resin and talc that hardened after irradiation. The hollow vessel model was attached to the skull by flexible wires or plastic clay in the orientation expected during surgery. They performed this process on three retrospective and eight prospective patients. For the prospective cases, surgical planning was conducted prior to surgery, and five out of the eight cases used the same number of clips in the same orientation as planned. These models were then used for training of novice neurosurgeons, and the lumen of the aneurysm was observed pre- and post-clipping with the use of a flexible vascular endoscope. The models took around 3–7 days for production and cost 300–400 US dollars. Limitations were the need to affix the vascular model to the hollow model, time to create the model, and inability to represent surrounding tissues.

The vascular detail obtained from CTA has greatly improved over the years, and a group out of Brazil looked at the accuracy of creating anatomical models of aneurysms based off of CTA data [6]. They used a PolyJet printer to create small segments of the aneurysm and surrounding vessels and compared measurements of the aneurysm model as compared to measurements taken from a digital subtracted angiogram (gold standard). All three prototypes accurately represented the angioarchitecture measurements obtained from the angiogram. The process took on average 20 h per print and cost $130. They present that the process was quicker and cost less in their paper, but the degree of anatomy displayed was less than previous papers. The main fallbacks to this paper are that the aneurysms were not hollow and did not include surrounding tissue data. They did demonstrate the need for advanced anatomical knowledge when creating the model, especially when determining the correct level of windowing of CTA data to include relevant small vasculature without introducing artifact to the print.

The paper by Mashiko et al. [7] used a different technique to create models of 20 patients, 12 of which underwent clipping; 3 cases showing endovascular methods to be preferred; 1 patient who died prior to treatment; and 4 remaining in the planning stage at that time. The 3D data was obtained from CTA. The aneurysm and parent vessels were printed in acrylonitrile-butadiene-styrene (ABS) plastic. The base material and excess material were removed manually, and the vessels were smoothed with putty created from ABS mixed with small amounts of xylene. Molding silicone was then painted over the ABS vessel model and allowed to harden. After the silicone had hardened, the vessels were then placed in a xylene bath which melted the ABS into gel that could be squeezed and washed out of the hollow silicone model. The hollow elastic models were placed into the orientation of the hard plastic model for visualization of the field of view when approaching the aneurysm. Aneurysm clips could be placed in the presumed intraoperative orientation and compared to the actual procedure. The models provided good anatomical representation, but four cases had slight modification at the time of surgery. Three cases required booster clips as the aneurysm neck was thicker than portrayed, and one aneurysm had an adherent vessel to the aneurysm neck which was not detailed preoperatively. The data presented was subjective in nature by questionnaire which was a cited weakness of the paper. The aneurysms were durable and could withstand 25–80 clip applications. The time required for creating the models was around 14–24 h depending on the size of the print. The system setup was around $66,500, but the material cost per aneurysm print was about JPY 200–600 or $2–6 and approximately $150 for full skull print. They demonstrate that with in-house printing, the initial cost is the most prohibitive factor. They were able to present a cost saving as compared to the proceeding 20 aneurysm clipping cases at their institution. The previous 20 cases required eight wasted clips compared to zero during the study with 3D modeling.

The hollow vascular 3D models were used by Benet [8] and placed within cadavers to simulate dissection and clipping of aneurysms. They used two 3D printed aneurysm models from two preoperative patients and then placed these aneurysms in their anatomical location bilaterally on two cadavers [8]. The aneurysm data was obtained from an MRA and printed with a rubberlike material. The models were implanted into the cadavers using minimal dissection of the arachnoid cisterns and attached to the cadaveric vasculature using cyanoacrylate or anastomosed using 8-0 suture, depending on training versus research model, creating a vascular model similar to the actual patient (Fig. 4.3, Table 4.1).

Dissection was then performed and simulation of clip application was carried out. They cite that the models had similar flexibility and allowed manipulation comparable to surrounding cadaveric vessels. The aneurysms were also sturdy enough to cause mass effect on surrounding tissue without abnormal deformation. One limitation of this technique is that bony anatomy varied between the real aneurysm patient and the cadaver (Fig. 4.4).

Lan et al. [10] created multicolor 3D craniocerebral models demonstrating the aneurysm and select surrounding tissue like the optic nerve. CT, MRI, and CTA data were used as available. A newer generation printer was used that is capable of printing multiple material hardness, color, or transparency in a single print. The aneurysm model could be printed down to vessels 1 mm in diameter. The model provided aneurysm anatomical information in relation to the optic nerve, parasellar area, and clinoid process during clipping. The detail of the prints was at a resolution of 0.016 mm, and the aneurysm model took 2 h to print and 20 h for the remaining craniocerebral model. The material costs were around $20–200 per print depending on the size.

Andereggen et al. [11] created six models of complex cerebral aneurysms to facilitate better understanding of treatment and the possible need for bypass and occlusion of the lesions. They used CTA and 3D angiography data to construct accurate anatomical relationships for complex aneurysms. Improvement in 3D registration software based on neuroimaging has improved the ability to augment manual segmentation with semiautomatic segmentation of objects which

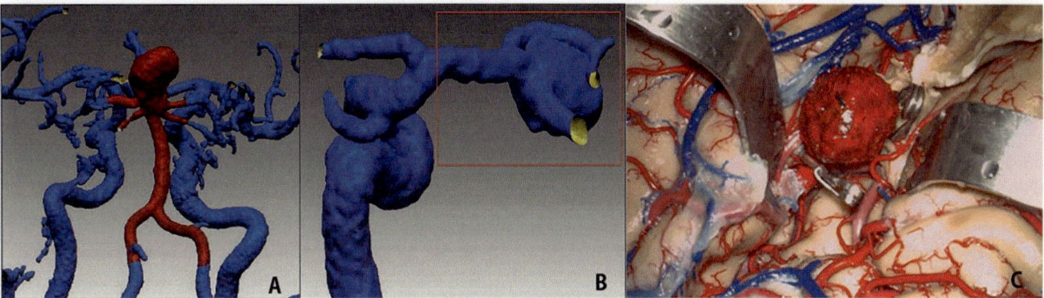

Fig. 4.3 (**a**) MRA-generated model of basilar apex aneurysm, (**b**) MRA-generated model of middle cerebral artery aneurysm, (**c**) implanted 3D printed aneurysm into cadaver [8]

Table 4.1 Surgical simulation experiments for aneurysm clipping in cadaver [8]

3D model	Approach for implantation	Side of implantation	Approach for clipping
Basilar tip	Orbitozygomatic	Left	Right orbitozygomatic
	Orbitozygomatic	Right	Left orbitozygomatic
	Orbitozygomatic	Left	Right orbitozygomatic
	Orbitozygomatic	Right	Left orbitozygomatic
Middle cerebral artery	Pterional	Left	Left pterional
	Minipterional	Right	Right minipterional
	Pterional	Left	Left pterional
	Pterional	Right	Right minipterional

was used in this study. They could delineate bony anatomy, intra-aneurysmal anatomy, extracranial vasculature, and previous aneurysm coils based on multimodality imaging. These objects were then oriented in relation to each other using surface-based registration software. This facilitated the training on determining the best area for craniotomy and area for protection of the extracranial vasculature for bypass. Their study was limited by the fact that all materials were printed in rigid material and that small perforating vessels could not be visualized on the printed model.

Mahiko et al. [12] created a 3D model of an MCA aneurysm and hollow brain to measure and simulate force encountered when retracting brain tissue for fissure dissection and applied this to training. The skull and silicone vasculature were created with a similar process as the already reviewed articles. The brain was created by printing a negative mold of the brain surface that was used to fabricate a 4 mm wall of soft polyurethane. The open side of the brain was covered with an acrylic plate with a tube attachment to fill the lumen with water. A force sensing brain spatula was constructed, and pressure on the spatula and the column of water in the lumen and tubing were tracked during sylvian fissure opening. The models were created in approximately 96 h and materials cost approximately $17. These models did incorporate brain tissue in relation to the aneurysm but, for the purpose of the study, did not provide details of nerves, cisterns, or dura/arachnoid for detailed dissection.

Ryan et al. [13] further developed this model to increase functionality of simulation for cerebral aneurysm clipping. CT, CTA, and MRI were used to create a model that optimized reproducibility and adaptability to patient-specific pathology. The vascular model was created from nine patient datasets. Each aneurysm and parent vessel were segmented into an individual aneurysm and then recombined into a single Circle of Willis. Each segment was able to be printed individually for future replacement of each aneurysm. The process allowed for the hollow aneurysm sleeves (shore value A27) to slip over the hard non-aneurysmal vascular tree. The vessels were dyed red. The brain was created using

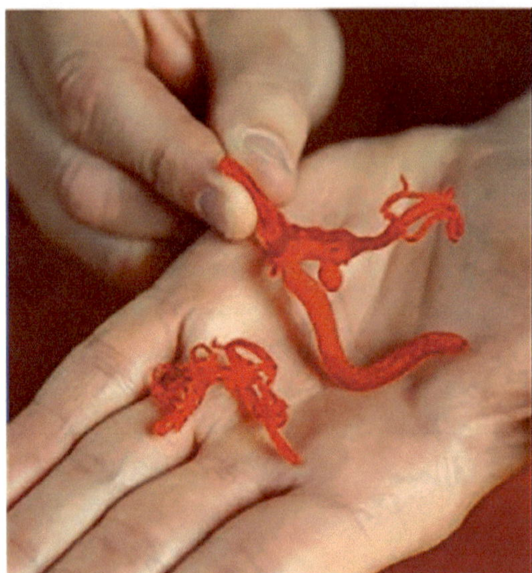

Fig. 4.4 Vessel only models demonstrating the aneurysm and associated vessels [9]

a normal MRI to create separate parts of the left frontal and parietal lobes, the right frontal and parietal lobes, the left temporal and occipital lobes, the right temporal and occipital lobes, the cerebellum, and the brainstem including the optic nerve. These segments were each printed in ABS and the surfaces were smoothed. A mold was created around each section using casting silicone. The final brain was created with a lower elastic modulus silicone to better simulate the turgor of a normal brain. The skull was printed from a normal patient dataset as described above with material similar to bone in hardness. The skull was printed with a longitudinal split to allow for easier replacement of the brain and vascular models. The model effectively integrated the brain and cranium into the training, thus providing an accurate representation of the operative corridor for various aneurysms and allowed for adequate simulation of aneurysm clipping with appropriate equipment. The modular form of the model proposes to decrease future cost from the initial price of just under $1000 by having the individual modular parts costing less than $10. This feature may also provide a generalized model with increased speed of printing and incorporating patient-specific aneurysms into the model, therefore making it possible to

plan for surgery in ruptured aneurysm cases. One limitation of the model is that only a truncated optic nerve was allowed, while the other cranial nerves were unable to be included. Another limitation, related to current 3D printers, is that small perforating vessels are unable to be captured. There was no ability to include material to simulate arachnoid dissection in this model. 3D printers at this time were unable to create vascular walls less than 0.45 mm making the aneurysm clipping characteristics different than real tissue parameters (Fig. 4.5).

To demonstrate the process used in creating three-dimensional models, we offer an illustrative case of an elective 7 mm right anterior communicating artery aneurysm clipping. The case was planned to be done from a left pterional approach based on imaging review until intraoperative planning on a 3D model demonstrated the best avenue to be a right orbitozygomatic approach (Fig. 4.5). The case was rehearsed by using clip and clip appliers from several angles (Fig. 4.2). After drilling out the bone for an orbitozygomatic approach, it was also noted that the surgical route would require transgression of the frontal sinus, which allowed operative planning for this portion of the case. The model was brought into the operating room to guide positioning of the patient. Our experience with this case demonstrated how this technique helps surgeons find the optimal surgical corridor as well as clip selection (Fig. 4.6).

Skull Base/Tumor

Another area of neurosurgery that requires extensive training is tumor surgery, especially at the skull base. As radiation and chemotherapy options continue to evolve, the number of surgical cases decline. One avenue for continued development of skills and anatomical relationships is to use 3D printed models to replace cadaver lab training.

The anatomical accuracy required for these models to provide relevant operative experience was validated by using a neuronavigation system in a paper by Waran et al. [14] The neuronavigation

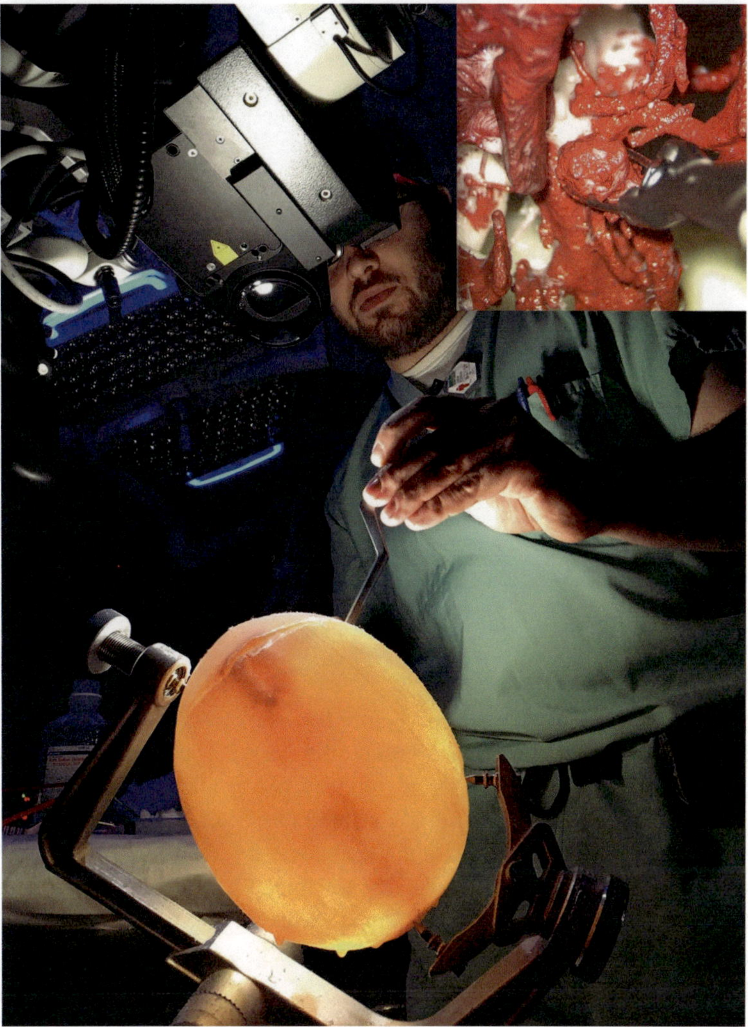

Fig. 4.5 Residents rehearse clip application under the microscope on a 3D model

technology has advanced greatly to the point that they are reliably used more frequently in operative cases. They used fine cut 1 mm CT scan data to produce the five skulls. The skulls were each registered to a surface registration neuronavigation system. One model was created with accurate representation of the overlying facial contours. All models were easily registered. Ten small surface area landmarks were tested on each skull and verified on the navigation system. All ten points on each model correlated with the imaging.

This level of accuracy is important when dealing with skull base anatomy, especially in the temporal bone. Three articles discuss their experience with using 3D printed models for temporal bone skills labs. The first paper by Cruz and Francis [15] attempted to assess the validity of such a model based on previous cadaveric and operative experiences. The data was from CT scans of normal human cadaveric temporal bone with 12 micron resolution. The material was a cast powder and bonding agent which produces physical characteristics similar to temporal bone. Color was added to differentiate various structures. The cast powder could be removed from hollow structures such as mastoid air cells and the cochlea. The facial nerve, carotid artery, and sigmoid sinus were initially printed as hollow structures with appropriately

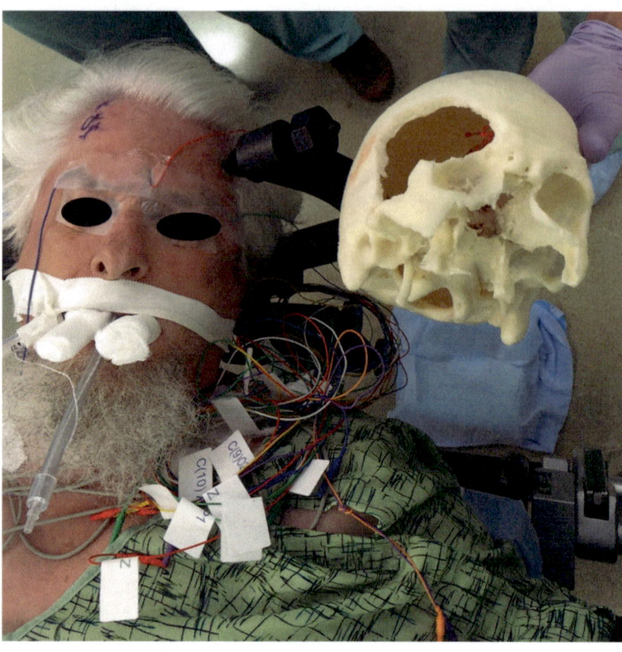

Fig. 4.6 Patient positioned based on 3D model to allow optimal exposure for aneurysm clipping

colored edges and filled with colored wires. Silicone sheets were used to simulate the dura and tympanic membranes. Nine trainees performed specific tasks on three 3D printed temporal bones. Afterward, questionnaires to assess the experience were conducted. They concluded that the models provided anatomical realism and provided a good replacement to cadaveric temporal bone.

The second paper, by Hochman et al. [16], was conducted in a similar matter with comparable conclusions. The main difference is that trainees performed a dissection on a cadaveric specimen and a 3D printed model of that same specimen. The models were printed in slices with segmented pieces for relevant anatomy like the dura, carotid artery, otic capsule, facial nerve, and others. These segments were then placed into the correct orientation with the printed bone. Subsequently, they were bound together based on predefined fiducials by a cyanoacrylate and hydroquinone mixture. Interestingly, this allowed the model to have features like a urethane facial nerve with a bronze inner core which could signify injury to the structure during dissection.

The final paper, by Wanibuchi et al. [17], used a synthetic resin and inorganic filler to create a model with a selective laser sintering technique. The temporal bone was made in two pieces thus allowing dye to be placed within the semicircular canals and facial canal. The sigmoid sinus was then filled with blue silicone. The major advantage of using this technique is the thermal stability of the material which could withstand high-speed drilling. This technique also allows for inclusion of precise anatomical structures with bone-like properties and feel.

Another area requiring extensive training and understanding of complex anatomy is the resection of skull base tumors. We have found three articles dedicated to this area of interest. The first study performed by D'Urso et al. [18] included a prospective evaluation of 11 stereolithographic printed skull base tumors. The cases included three acoustic schwannomas, five meningiomas, one sphenoidal lytic dermoid cyst, one retro-orbital melanoma extending into the middle fossa, and one giant pituitary macroadenoma. The system used at this time was a first-generation 3D printer and thus lacked the ability to include multiple objects. Each part (i.e., tumor, skull, vessels) had to be painted individually which made it difficult to determine the true transition zone of normal and abnormal tissues.

Kondo et al. [19] used newer technology and were able to print four cases of skull base tumors with multiple materials and colors to represent the internal carotid artery, basilar artery, brainstem, bone, and tumors. The purpose of the study was to print the models with either no tumor, solid tumor, or a variable degree of mesh representing the tumor to determine visibility of deep structures at the time of surgery. The printing technique used was binder jetting. They concluded that printing skull base tumors as a hollow core with a mesh outline provide a significant improvement in evaluation of deep structures while maintaining the three-dimensional relationship of the tumor to pertinent tissue at high risk for injury during surgery.

The last article was from the work conducted at our institution [20]. We described a method of using high-resolution skull base CT and MRI in three patients with petroclival tumors to determine the area of view afforded by a middle cranial fossa approach or retrosigmoid approach [20]. We used our institution's neuronavigation system to fuse the image datasets to segment the bone and tumor. These files were converted to STL files and processed on computer aided drafting software. The printer used fused deposition modeling to create the solid 3D model. The area of tumor was painted after performing each craniotomy. The neuronavigation software was then used to define the amount of surface area visible through each operative corridor. Our printer costs around $50,000, and cost for each skull was approximately $150. In this study we were unable to include the surrounding structures like the brain and brainstem, cranial nerves, and vasculature to determine the influence of this anatomy on the operative view (Fig. 4.7, Table 4.2).

Pituitary/Endoscopic

Traditional neurosurgical techniques have included large incisions and craniotomies for various skull base approaches. As technology has evolved, endoscopic techniques have as well. The use of the endoscope has become a common tool for the treatment of various neurosurgical pathologies including pituitary tumors, intraventricular tumors, and hydrocephalus.

New technologies are exciting but can take time for adoption. Training clinicians on the use of new equipment is traditionally done through cadaver courses and mentorship by working with someone who is more comfortable and experienced with the equipment. 3D printed models are another avenue to learn the use of a new technique without placing a real patient at risk.

Endoscopic third ventriculostomy (ETV) and biopsy are common neurosurgical procedures. Waran et al. [21] describe how they created a cranial model with a pineal tumor and hydrocephalus. Three surgeons performed the various steps of an ETV with pineal biopsy and scored each step on a scale of 1–5 on realism. Their overall score was 4.5 out of 5, leading to a realistic and natural experience. They were also able to use neuronavigation successfully. They noted that these models were able to mimic certain tactile responses seen in actual surgery.

Pituitary tumors account for one of the most common primary brain tumors. Therefore, transsphenoidal surgery is a very common procedure for many neurosurgical departments [22]. At our institution, we performed a study using a 3D model to teach skull base anatomy through a transsphenoidal approach for neurosurgery residents [23]. All the residents were brought to the operating room prior to any formalized teaching and were asked to identify critical structures which included the sella turcica, cavernous sinus, optic nerve, and the paraclinoid carotid artery. The residents were then split into two groups. Group A residents were taught about the anatomy through a didactic lecture which included 2D images. Group B residents were taught in this same didactic lecture but also learned through neurosurgical simulation using the 3D printed model. The residents were tested in the operating room again to identify the same critical structures. Group A residents were then taught with the 3D printed model and tested for a third time. The results demonstrated improvement in the identification of important anatomic landmarks after training using the 3D model (Table 4.3).

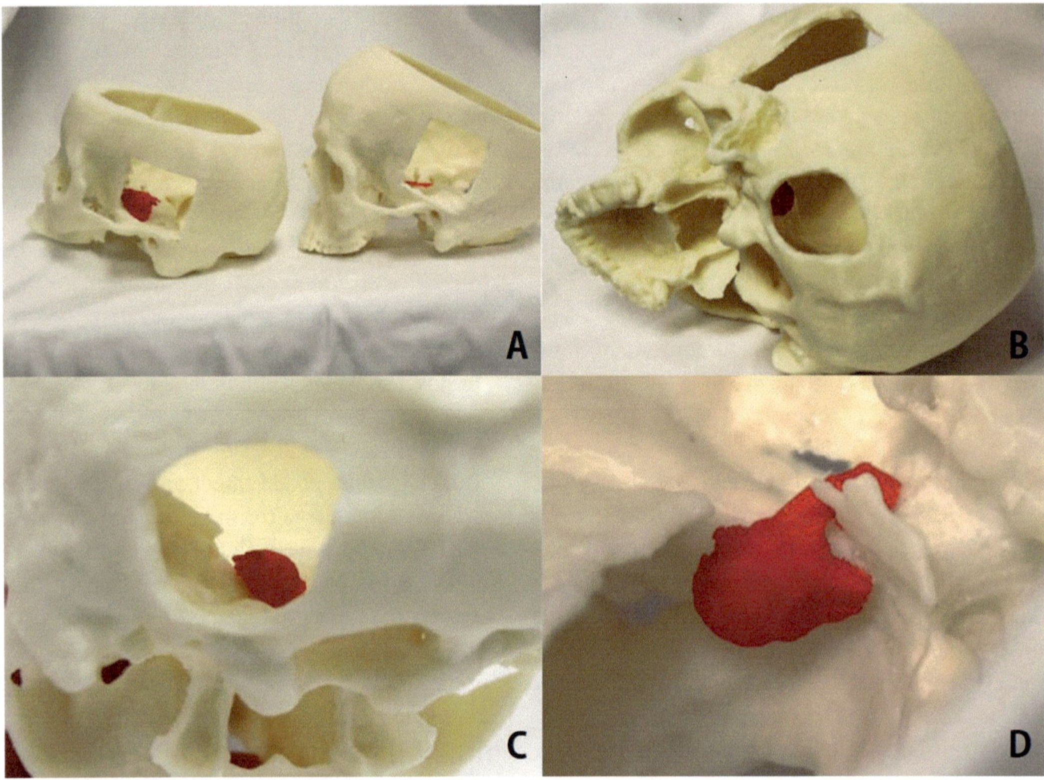

Fig. 4.7 (**a**) Middle cranial fossa approach to petroclival tumor, (**b**) retrosigmoid approach to tumor, (**c**) view of tumor through foramen magnum, (**d**) zoomed in view of petroclival tumor

Table 4.2 Surface area of petroclival tumors accessible from two skull base approaches [20]

Skull base approach	Middle fossa approach	Retrosigmoid approach
Patient 1	52 mm²	148 mm²
Patient 2	103 mm²	188 mm²
Patient 3	378 mm²	75 mm²

This article objectively illustrates improvement in anatomical knowledge after practicing using this 3D model [23] (Fig. 4.8).

Endoscopic endonasal anatomy and the drilling of the appropriate anatomy are one of the challenges a surgeon faces when performing endoscopic skull base procedures. Performing this skill is different than other neurosurgical procedures given that the surgeon is working through a narrow corridor with limited visualization and many critical structures surrounding the bony landmarks. The surgeons surveyed support the use of this 3D model for training in endoscopic endonasal anatomy [24] (Fig. 4.9).

Basilar invagination is a difficult pathology to treat that requires extensive training. Traditionally, this was performed via a transoral approach. However, newer endoscopic techniques describe this via a transnasal approach. Narayanan et al. [26] reveal how this procedure can be performed on a 3D model with basilar invagination. Fifteen ENT surgeons with various levels of experience were involved in the study showing the utility of this model in simulating this technique. They noted limitations with anterior nasal anatomy and transnasal access; however the remaining portions of the procedure were well simulated. 3D models have a clear advantage over cadavers in that cadavers rarely have pathology (Fig. 4.10).

Table 4.3 Results of testing of anatomical landmarks [23]

	Group A					Group B	
	No teaching	Lecture alone	Lecture +3D simulation			No teaching	Lecture +3D simulation
R1	3	6	8		R5	3	7
R2	2	4	6		R6	2	7
R3	4	6	6		R7	4	8
R4	2	4	8		R8	2	8
Average	**2.75**	**5**	**7**		**Average**	**2.75**	**7.5**

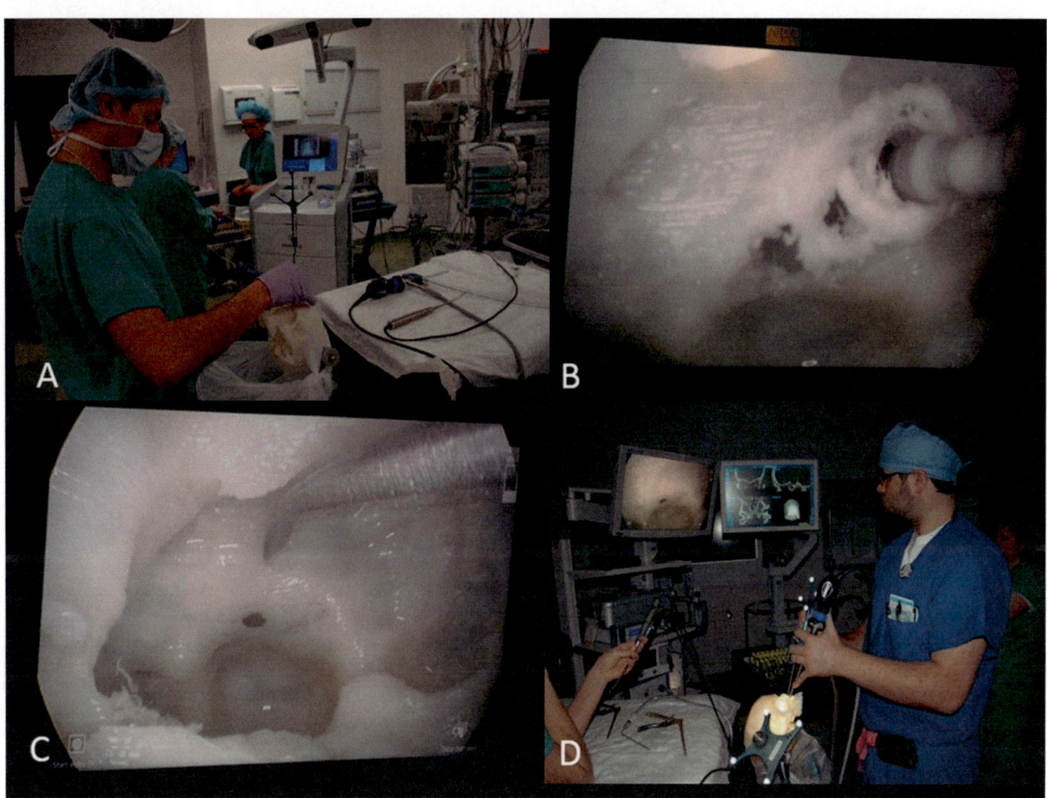

Fig. 4.8 (**a**) Registration of 3D printed model, (**b**) drilling of the sphenoid sinus through the endoscope, (**c**) identification of various anatomic structures through the endoscope, (**d**) residents practicing endoscopic navigation

Minor Procedure/EVD

Bedside procedures are common in neurosurgery and often lifesaving. These include external ventricular drains (EVDs), lumbar punctures and drains, central lines, intubations, etc. Bedside procedures are often performed by junior residents with appropriate supervision.

EVDs are commonly performed procedures for the treatment of hydrocephalus, intraven- tricular hemorrhage, cerebrospinal fluid leak, and other diagnoses. These procedures are often taught on live patients under close super- vision. Cadavers are not great teaching tools due to preservation techniques affecting the ventricular system [28]. Simulators have also been explored as a method for teaching EVD placement. Luciano et al. have developed a vir- tual reality-based simulator for this purpose [29].

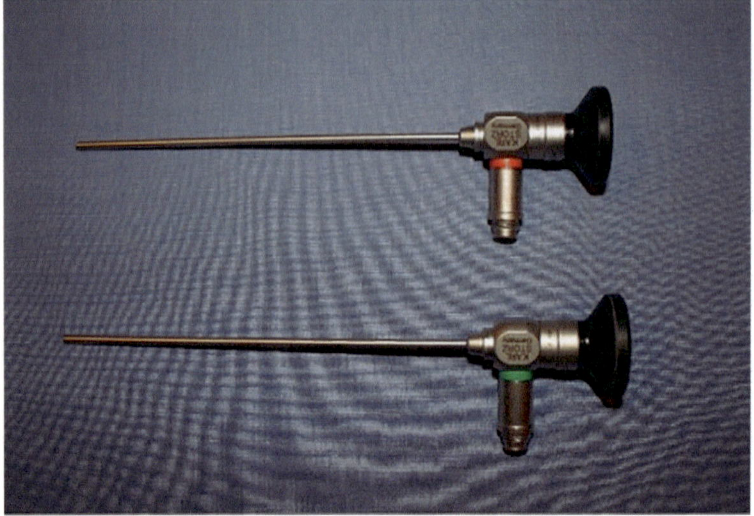

Fig. 4.9 Hopkins rod rigid endoscopes, 2.7 mm diameter, zero and 30° angled, length 14 cm [25]

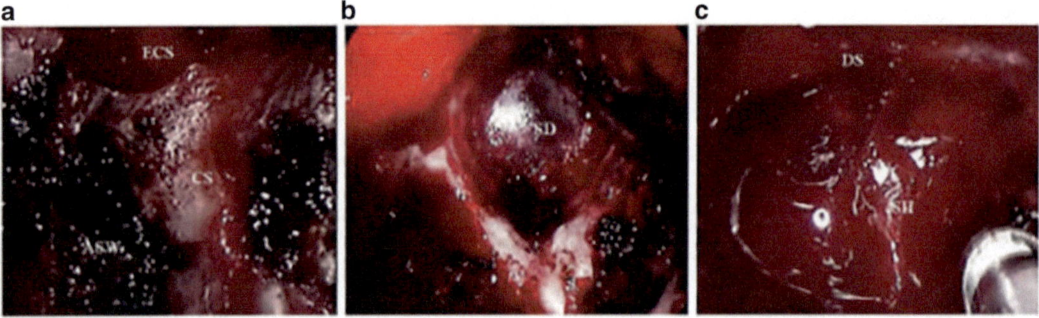

Fig. 4.10 Intraoperative endoscopic view of endoscopic transsphenoidal excision of the sellar tumor. (**a**) Anterior wall of sphenoid sinus, (**b**) exposure of the sella dura, (**c**) sella region after tumor resection [27]

3D models have also been developed as instructional tools for the placement of EVDs. Tai et al. [28] have developed a 3D model with a disposable insert for EVD placement. The insert is an artificial scalp for which the user can mimic placement of the EVD through similar tissues. The ventricle is filled with water and controlled by the water reservoir (Fig. 4.11).

Tai et al. studied their 3D model with a total of 17 surgeons. They gave the highest score to the "value of simulator as a training tool for novice neurosurgeons." Users performed skin incision, skin retraction, burr hole drilling, sharp opening of dura, catheter passage into the brain, tunneling, and skin closure.

Ryan et al. [31] also describe a 3D model they created for the purpose of neurosurgical training. Ten individuals (residents and students) were involved in the study where they counted number of passes into the ventricular system prior to successful cannulization. Their study displayed how these models could be created for an affordable price of $4 per brain model. This is much less than other models.

3D printing technology has advanced sufficiently to replicate the various layers of the body. Waran et al. [32] describe creating a model with skin, bone, dura, and tumor varying in consistency for the appropriate layers. A drawback to their model is the expense: $2000 for the reusable base and $600 for the disposable surgical insert.

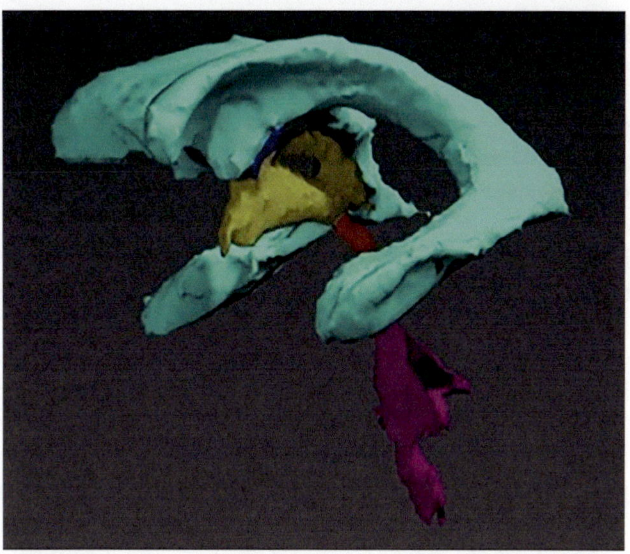

Fig. 4.11 The ventricular system of the brain [30]

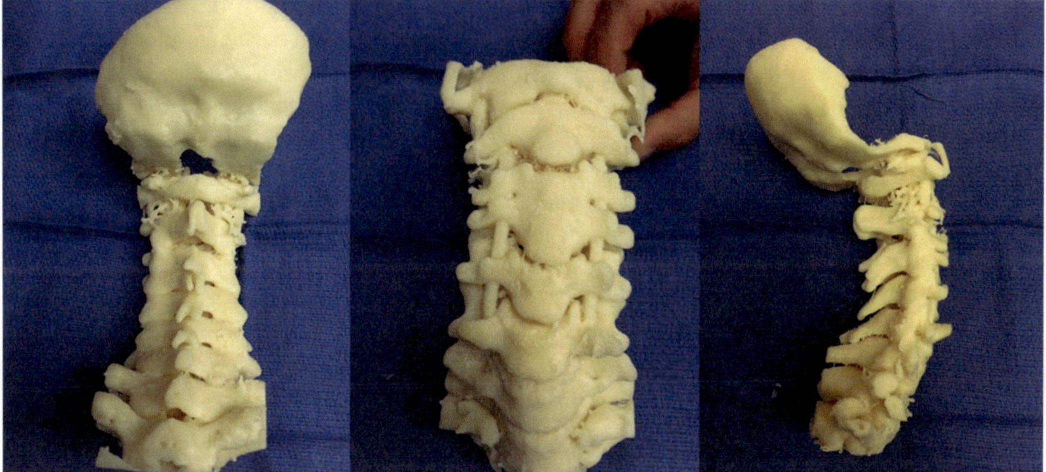

Fig. 4.12   3D printed model of the cervical spine created from CTA cervical spine

This same group has developed a method of 3D printing to test registration skills in neuronavigation platforms. They successfully registered and navigated accurately all models in their study [14].

External ventricular drain placement training can be augmented by the use of 3D models. Technology has made these 3D models more realistic allowing them to be registered in neuronavigation systems as well as allowing for the various layers of the human head to be replicated.

Spine

Spinal surgery accounts for a high percentage of neurosurgical procedures. Understanding the anatomy of the various aspects of the spine is critical to performing safe spinal surgery. 3D printed models can also be used to aide in the understanding of this anatomy (Fig. 4.12).

Neurosurgeons commonly encounter unique and challenging cases. Revision spine surgery with deformity can be one of these situations. Selecting the appropriate approach is critical, but not always easily chosen when only reviewing imaging. The creation of a custom patient model is one method of deciphering the optimal surgical approach. Physicians at NYU printed a patient-specific 3D model of an 11-year-old boy with multiple congenital abnormalities who previously underwent C1-C2 laminectomy and instrumentation. Their model of the cranioverte-bral junction included bone and vessels. They reviewed the various possible approaches and finally decided on a posterior approach with the aid of the 3D model [33].

A group of authors from India describe the use of craniovertebral junction models for surgical planning. They printed 3D models of 11 cases. They used these models to study the facet joints, size of the pedicles, the course of the vertebral arteries, and other important anatomic land-marks. They concluded that the information and ability to study the models were invaluable for surgical planning [34].

The thoracic spine has its own set of chal-lenges. Thoracic pedicle screw placement can be problematic due to the small size of the pedicles. Hu et al. have shown a rapidly prototyped drill template to assist in the placement of these pedi-cle screws [35] (Fig. 4.13).

Otsuki et al. [37] demonstrated that in revision spine surgery, 3D printed guides for pedicle screw placement could be created on a 3D printer. They are small, but with multiple arms that fit the bone surface precisely to align the guide. These guides were able to accurately place pedicle screws.

Revision lumbar surgery for discectomy is more challenging than the first operation. Scar tissue formation and bony removal from the first surgery are a couple of the complicating factors. Li et al. [38] published an article in which they printed 3D models of the spine where one cohort of patients underwent revision lumbar discectomies. The other cohort had routine care. They demonstrated a statistically significant decrease in operating time and blood loss when using the 3D model. However, there was no dif-ference in outcomes.

The world of custom implants has been grow-ing in medicine with spine surgery being no exception. Spetzger et al. [39] demonstrated that an implant for an anterior cervical discectomy and fusion (ACDF) could be created. On preop-erative planning, osteophytes were identified, which were subsequently drilled. The custom implant that had been created resulted in a highly accurate fit. The cage self-located into the correct position. This cage didn't move in any direction once the distraction was released. Their implant was created from EIT cellular titanium™ (Fig. 4.14).

Continuing the topic of custom implants, Xu et al. [41] describe a very interesting case of Ewing's sarcoma. After posterior resection and fixation, they approached the tumor anteriorly performing a C2 vertebral body resection. They created an anterior cervical spine implant made of porous metal, which was created by 3D printing. This was inserted in surgery and secured in place.

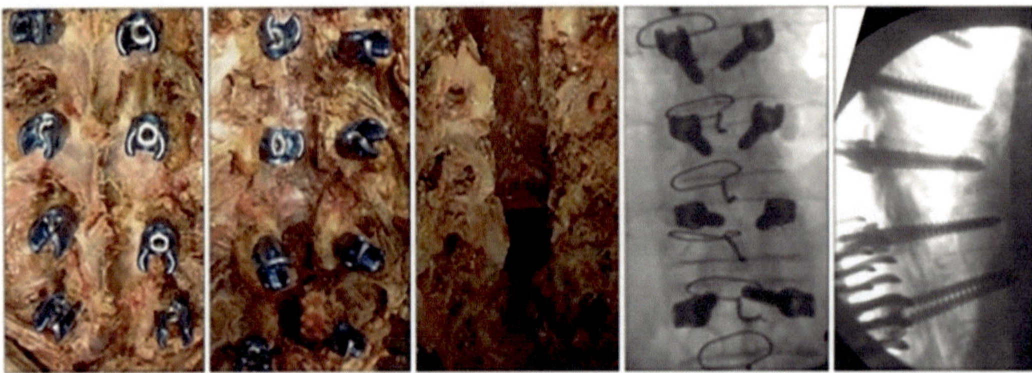

Fig. 4.13 Transpedicular screws inserted into the thoracic spine [36]

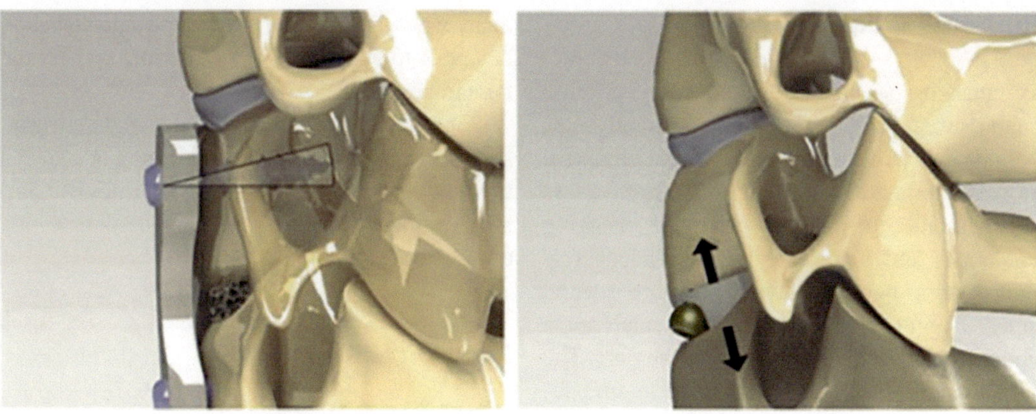

Fig. 4.14 Anterior plate with graft in place [40]

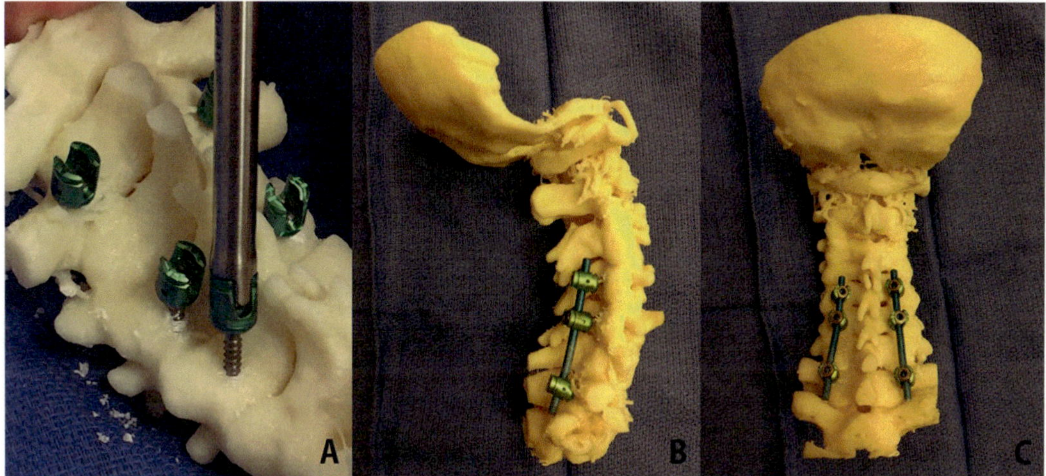

Fig. 4.15 (**a**) Placement of lateral mass screws into 3D printed model, (**b**) lateral view and (**c**) posterior view of 3D printed model after performing cervicothoracic instrumentation

3D printed models are an excellent tool to teach spinal anatomy. Li et al. [42] used 3D printed models to test spinal anatomy knowledge in medical students. They were studying spinal fractures. They randomized the students into three groups: CT only, 3D image, and 3D printed model. They found that students in the 3D printed model group performed significantly better than those in the CT only group. This study reinforces the idea that 3D models can be used as an effective teaching tool (Fig. 4.15).

It is obvious why surgeons find 3D models helpful. Interestingly, radiologists also find them valuable. A cervical spine model was generated from CT data that worked as a phantom in both CT and MR. The authors propose that such models could be used to simulate MRI-guided interventions such as cryosurgeries [43].

Future Direction

As imaging technology and 3D printing techniques and equipment continue to advance, these models will have a greater impact on neurosurgical training that ever before. These advances and measures are required given the changing regulations and requirements to be adequately trained as a neurosurgeon. There are several papers coming out in the endovascular arena which is a growing area within neurosurgery. The largest requirements at this point are to have models that can be printed at one time without required assembly, represent anatomy at a high resolution, and have tissue characteristics approaching the level seen clinically. We feel that once you can adequately represent brain tissue with similar physical properties to actual brain, this avenue will greatly excel. A trainee will be able to conduct a practice session with real-life equipment without the possibility of harm that is inherent to a surgical cause.

Conclusion

3D models in neurosurgery are a valuable resource in neurosurgical training. This chapter has displayed its various applications in cranial and spinal neurosurgery. The ability to print an actual patient model prior to performing a neurosurgical procedure allows the trainee to rehearse the procedure without causing harm.

Various authors have contributed to the literature on the numerous ways they have used 3D printed models in neurosurgery. The selection of 3D printers available is astounding with the most complex and advanced printers that have the ability to print multiple different colors and consistencies. These attributes allow for printing a hard bony skull and soft, flexible vessels.

As technology continues to advance, so will the models we can create in neurosurgery. The more realistic the models become, the more applicable to training they will be. In the current era of training in the 80-hr work week, exposure to accurate 3D printed models will help supplement training in the operating room. In many ways, it is safer to practice on a precise replica prior to performing the procedure on a living human being.

3D models will likely be a mainstay in neurosurgical training. Their aide in learning is unquestionable. The future remains bright for neurosurgical training using 3D models as an excellent teaching tool.

References

1. Hull CW, inventor; Google Patents, assignee. Method and apparatus for production of three-dimensional objects by stereolithography1996.
2. D'Urso PS, Thompson RG, Atkinson RL, Weidmann MJ, Redmond MJ, Hall BI, et al. Cerebrovascular biomodelling: a technical note. Surg Neurol. 1999;52(5):490–500.
3. Wurm G, Tomancok B, Pogady P, Holl K, Trenkler J. Cerebrovascular stereolithographic biomodeling for aneurysm surgery. Technical note. J Neurosurg. 2004;100(1):139–45.
4. Wurm G, Lehner M, Tomancok B, Kleiser R, Nussbaumer K. Cerebrovascular biomodeling for aneurysm surgery: simulation-based training by means of rapid prototyping technologies. Surg Innov. 2011;18(3):294–306.
5. Kimura T, Morita A, Nishimura K, Aiyama H, Itoh H, Fukaya S, et al. Simulation of and training for cerebral aneurysm clipping with 3-dimensional models. Neurosurgery. 2009;65(4):719–25; discussion 25–6.
6. Erbano BO, Opolski AC, Olandoski M, Foggiatto JA, Kubrusly LF, Dietz UA, Zini C, et al. Rapid prototyping of three-dimensional biomodels as an adjuvant in the surgical planning for intracranial aneurysms. (1678–2674 (Electronic)).
7. Mashiko T, Otani K, Kawano R, Konno T, Kaneko N, Ito Y, et al. Development of three-dimensional hollow elastic model for cerebral aneurysm clipping simulation enabling rapid and low cost prototyping. LID – S1878–8750(13)01357–0 [pii] LID – https://doi.org/10.1016/j.wneu.2013.10.032 [doi]. (1878–8750 (Electronic)).
8. Benet A, Plata-Bello J, Abla AA, Acevedo-Bolton G, Saloner D, Lawton MT. Implantation of 3D-printed patient-specific aneurysm models into cadaveric specimens: a new training paradigm to allow for improvements in cerebrovascular surgery and research. Biomed Res Int. 2015;2015:939387.
9. Khan IS, Kelly PD, Singer RJ. Prototyping of cerebral vasculature physical models. Surg Neurol Int. 2014;5(2229–5097 (Print)):11.
10. Lan Q, Chen A, Zhang T, Li G, Zhu Q, Fan X, et al. Development of three-dimensional printed Craniocerebral models for simulated neurosurgery. World Neurosurg. 2016;91:434–42.

11. Andereggen L, Gralla J, Andres RH, Weber S, Schroth G, Beck J, et al. Stereolithographic models in the interdisciplinary planning of treatment for complex intracranial aneurysms. Acta Neurochir. 2016;158(9):1711–20.

12. Mashiko T, Konno T, Kaneko N, Watanabe E. Training in brain retraction using a self-made three-dimensional model. World Neurosurg. 2015;84(2):585–90.

13. Ryan JR, Almefty KK, Nakaji P, Frakes DH. Cerebral aneurysm clipping surgery simulation using patient-specific 3D printing and silicone casting. World Neurosurg. 2016;88:175–81.

14. Waran V, Devaraj P, Hari Chandran T, Muthusamy KA, Rathinam AK, Balakrishnan YK, et al. Three-dimensional anatomical accuracy of cranial models created by rapid prototyping techniques validated using a neuronavigation station. J Clin Neurosci. 2012;19(4):574–7.

15. Da Cruz MJ, Face FHW. Content validation of a novel three-dimensional printed temporal bone for surgical skills development. J Laryngol Otol. 2015;129(Suppl 3):S23–9.

16. Hochman JB, Rhodes C, Wong D, Kraut J, Pisa J, Unger B. Comparison of cadaveric and isomorphic three-dimensional printed models in temporal bone education. Laryngoscope. 2015;125(10):2353–7.

17. Wanibuchi M, Noshiro S, Sugino T, Akiyama Y, Mikami T, Iihoshi S, et al. Training for Skull Base surgery with a colored temporal bone model created by three-dimensional printing technology. World Neurosurg. 2016;91:66–72.

18. D'Urso PS, Anderson RL, Weidmann MJ, Redmond MJ, Hall BI, Earwaker WJ, et al. Biomodelling of skull base tumours. J Clin Neurosci. 1999;6(1):31–5.

19. Kondo K, Harada N, Masuda H, Sugo N, Terazono S, Okonogi S, et al. A neurosurgical simulation of skull base tumors using a 3D printed rapid prototyping model containing mesh structures. Acta Neurochir. 2016;158(6):1213–9.

20. Muelleman TJ, Peterson J, Chowdhury NI, Gorup J, Camarata P, Lin J. Individualized surgical approach planning for petroclival tumors using a 3d printer. J Neurol Surg B Skull Base. 2016;77(3):243–8.

21. Waran V, Narayanan V, Karuppiah R, Thambynayagam HC, Muthusamy KA, Rahman ZA, et al. Neurosurgical endoscopic training via a realistic 3-dimensional model with pathology. Simul Healthc. 2015;10(1):43–8.

22. Jane JA Jr, Sulton LD, Laws ER Jr. Surgery for primary brain tumors at United States academic training centers: results from the Residency Review Committee for neurological surgery. J Neurosurg. 2005;103(5):789–93.

23. Shah KJ, Peterson JC, Beahm DD, Camarata PJ, Chamoun RB. Three-dimensional printed model used to teach skull base anatomy through a transsphenoidal approach for neurosurgery residents. Oper Neurosurg [Internet]. 2016;12:326–9.

24. Tai BL, Wang AC, Joseph JR, Wang PI, Sullivan SE, McKean EL, et al. A physical simulator for endo-scopic endonasal drilling techniques: technical note. J Neurosurg. 2016;124(3):811–6.

25. Pollak N, Azadarmaki R, Ahmad S. Feasibility of endoscopic treatment of middle ear myoclonus: a cadaveric study. ISRN Otolaryngol. 2014;2014:175268.

26. Narayanan V, Narayanan P, Rajagopalan R, Karuppiah R, Rahman ZAA, Wormald PJ, et al. Endoscopic skull base training using 3D printed models with pre-existing pathology. Eur Arch OtorinoLaryngol. 2015;272(3):753–7.

27. Song Y, Wang T, Chen J, Tan G. Endoscopic transsphenoidal resection of sellar tumors with conchal sphenoid sinus: a report of two cases. Oncol Lett. 2015;9(2):713–6.

28. Tai BL, Rooney D, Stephenson F, Liao PS, Sagher O, Shih AJ, et al. Development of a 3D-printed external ventricular drain placement simulator: technical note. J Neurosurg. 2015;123(4):1070–6.

29. Luciano C, Banerjee P, Lemole GM Jr, Charbel F. Second generation haptic ventriculostomy simulator using the ImmersiveTouch system. Stud Health Technol Inform. 2006;119:343–8.

30. Manson A, Poyade M, Rea PA. Recommended workflow methodology in the creation of an educational and training application incorporating a digital reconstruction of the cerebral ventricular system and cerebrospinal fluid circulation to aid anatomical understanding. BMC Med Imaging. 2015;15:44.

31. Ryan JR, Chen T, Nakaji P, Frakes DH, Gonzalez LF. Ventriculostomy simulation using patient-specific ventricular anatomy, 3D printing, and hydrogel casting. World Neurosurg. 2015;84(5):1333–9.

32. Waran V, Narayanan V, Karuppiah R, Owen SL, Aziz T. Utility of multimaterial 3D printers in creating models with pathological entities to enhance the training experience of neurosurgeons. J Neurosurg. 2014;120(2):489–92.

33. Pacione D, Tanweer O, Berman P, Harter DH. The utility of a multimaterial 3D printed model for surgical planning of complex deformity of the skull base and craniovertebral junction. J Neurosurg. 2016;125:1–4.

34. Goel A, Jankharia B, Shah A, Sathe P. Three-dimensional models: an emerging investigational revolution for craniovertebral junction surgery. J Neurosurg Spine. 2016(1547–5646 (Electronic)):1–5.

35. Hu Y, Yuan ZS, Spiker WR, Dong WX, Sun XY, Yuan JB, et al. A comparative study on the accuracy of pedicle screw placement assisted by personalized rapid prototyping template between pre- and post-operation in patients with relatively normal mid-upper thoracic spine. Eur Spine J. 2016;25(6):1706–15.

36. Hyun SJ, Kim YJ, Cheh G, Yoon SH, Rhim SC. Free hand pedicle screw placement in the thoracic spine without any radiographic guidance : technical note, a cadaveric study. J Korean Neurosurg Soc. 2012;51(1):66–70.

37. Otsuki B, Takemoto M, Fujibayashi S, Kimura H, Masamoto K, Matsuda S. Utility of a custom screw insertion guide and a full-scale, color-coded 3D

plaster model for guiding safe surgical exposure and screw insertion during spine revision surgery. J Neurosurg Spine. 2016;25(1):94–102.

38. Li C, Yang M, Xie Y, Chen Z, Wang C, Bai Y, et al. Application of the polystyrene model made by 3-D printing rapid prototyping technology for operation planning in revision lumbar discectomy. J Orthop Sci. 2015;20(3):475–80.

39. Spetzger U, Frasca M, Konig SA. Surgical planning, manufacturing and implantation of an individualized cervical fusion titanium cage using patient-specific data. Eur Spine J. 2016;25(7):2239–46.

40. Palepu V, Kiapour A, Goel VK, Moran JM. A unique modular implant system enhances load sharing in anterior cervical interbody fusion: a finite element study. Biomed Eng Online. 2014;13(1):26.

41. Xu N, Wei F, Liu X, Jiang L, Cai H, Li Z, et al. Reconstruction of the upper cervical spine using a personalized 3D-printed vertebral body in an adolescent with Ewing Sarcoma. Spine. 2016;41(1):E50–4.

42. Li Z, Li Z, Xu R, Li M, Li J, Liu Y, et al. Three-dimensional printing models improve understanding of spinal fracture – a randomized controlled study in China. Sci Rep. 2015;5:11570.

43. Mitsouras D, Lee TC, Liacouras P, Ionita CN, Pietilla T, Maier SE, et al. Three-dimensional printing of MRI-visible phantoms and MR image-guided therapy simulation. Magn Reson Med. 2016;77(2):613–22

Synthetic Replica for Training in Microsurgical Anastomosis: An Important Frontier in Neurosurgical Education

5

Rudy J. Rahme, Chandan Krishna, Mithun G. Sattur, Rami James N. Aoun, Matthew E. Welz, Aman Gupta, and Bernard R. Bendok

Introduction

"See one, do one, teach one"; The Halstedian apprenticeship model established over a century ago has been the norm in surgical education until the mid-1980s [1, 2]. In 1984, the unfortunate and well-publicized death of a young woman, Libby Zion, at the New York Hospital, led to a series of events – political, legal, and otherwise – that eventually led to the remodeling of this educational paradigm. This culminated in a set of rulings and recommendations for significant changes in graduate medical education focused on curbing resident fatigue, which was assumed (but never proven) to be a major factor behind medical errors [2]. Following suite, the Accreditation Council for Graduate Medical Education (ACGME) convened and published a set of guidelines for resident education starting in July 2003. The major points involved limiting duty hours to 80 h/week, limiting work shifts to 24 h and granting at least 1 day off per week, averaged over 4 weeks [3, 4].

Ever since the inception of these regulations though, there have been continuous debates over their intended educational consequences. The regulations while well intentioned may have deleterious educational effects. In the neurosurgical field specifically, there have been concerns about whether or not a trainee will have sufficient exposure and experience in an 80-h week. This is especially important in light of the need for a resident to master a wide range of skills in order to be able to practice in the real world beyond the safety net of residency. Added to such temporal restrictions, neurosurgical training continues to

R. J. Rahme
Department of Neurosurgery, Northwestern Feinberg School and Medicine and McGaw Medical Center, Chicago, IL, USA

C. Krishna · M. G. Sattur · R. J. N. Aoun · M. E. Welz A. Gupta
Department of Neurosurgery, Mayo Clinic, Phoenix, AZ, USA

Precision Neurotherapeutics Lab, Mayo Clinic, Phoenix, AZ, USA

Neurosurgery Simulation and Innovation Lab, Mayo Clinic, Phoenix, AZ, USA
e-mail: Krishna.Chandan@mayo.edu; Mithun.Sattur@mayo.edu; aoun.rami@mayo.edu; Welz.matt@mayo.edu; Gupta.aman@mayo.edu

B. R. Bendok (✉)
Department of Neurological Surgery, Otolaryngology, and Radiology, Mayo Clinic, Phoenix, AZ, USA

Precision Neurotherapeutics Lab, Mayo Clinic, Phoenix, AZ, USA

Neurosurgery Simulation and Innovation Lab, Mayo Clinic, Phoenix, AZ, USA
e-mail: Bendok.bernard@mayo.edu

© Springer International Publishing AG, part of Springer Nature 2018
A. Alaraj (ed.), *Comprehensive Healthcare Simulation: Neurosurgery*,
Comprehensive Healthcare Simulation, https://doi.org/10.1007/978-3-319-75583-0_5

broaden with advances and innovations in open, minimally invasive, and endovascular techniques that a resident must learn. This challenge is compounded with the dilution of cases among an increasing number of academic and private medical centers. With an 80-h work week limit, there are concerns on whether new trainees will ever be able to reach the "10,000-h" proficiency milestone [5]. In addition, during the past two decades, there has been greater attention given to preventing medical errors. The challenges raised by these two forces have put the spotlight on the potential of simulation training to reduce errors and enhance procedural and scenario training. Neurosurgery in particular is a high stakes specialty where the slightest of deviations can lead to detrimental consequences. It is likely to be one of the medical fields to suffer most from the restrictive resident hours. Neurosurgical leadership has therefore invested time and effort into developing potential simulation modules and curricula to circumvent the imposed shortcomings of the new training environment [6–13].

Simulation training and its effectiveness are guided by three major concepts. The first is *deliberate practice*. This is defined as repetitive performance of an intended cognitive and/or psychomotor skill with feedback on specific areas used for improvement. An important parameter of deliberate practice is constantly practicing at more challenging levels with an intention to master a specific skill [14, 15]. Frequent objective feedback from a mentor is critical to deliberate practice. The second is the concept of *proficiency*, defined as the capacity to perform a specific task with reduction of technical error in the least amount of time [16]. Proficiency does not necessarily translate into better surgical outcomes though. There are added factors that are not accounted for in a simulation setting such as, but not limited to, stress and levels of concentration [17]. This leads to the third concept of *automaticity*. Automaticity is defined as the ability to multitask in an operating room. Mastering this skill allows the surgeon to navigate emergent and unpredictable situations that would be difficult to simulate in a lab [16, 18].

History and Evolution of Simulation in Medicine

Training through simulation is not a novel concept. In fact, simulation has been employed as early as the nineteenth century in warfare military training. Military simulations encompass activities such as full-scale field exercises and fully automated abstract computerized models, such as the Rand Strategy Assessment Center (RSAC) [19, 20]. Simulation takes a central role in the aviation sector as well [19]. Flight simulators became a mandatory part of pilot training in the 1930s including military, commercial, and amateur sectors. Similar to the surgical world, mistakes in aviation can be detrimental and lead to loss of human lives. Creating a safe and controlled environment where trainees have repeated exposure to difficult situations is fundamental. It becomes even more crucial when those simulated situations are rare in real life.

As for the medical field, the first simulation training modules utilized actors to portray various clinical encounters. However, it was initially rejected due to lack of validation and high costs. It was not until 1993 that simulation gained wide acceptance after the Medical Council of Canada adopted the use of standardized patient simulation for medical licensure [19]. The National Board of Medical Examiners (NBME) in the United States later endorsed the type of standardized patient examination after two large review articles had validated such an approach. This led to the confirmation of the Step 2 clinical skills examination as an integral part of the US licensing process [21, 22].

The often-emergent nature of interventions and diseases in neurosurgery can make it difficult for new trainees to get a full hands-on experience without risking a poor outcome. This highlights the importance of simulation training specifically for this field. To that objective, there has been a significant push to create simulator models that provide a realistic surgical environment over the last decade. Four types of simulator models have been conceived. The first includes *physical models*. These incorporate synthetic models, as well as mannequins and cadavers. These modules allow the trainee to directly manipulate the tissue and maneuver a device. Physical models have their limitations though, including availability, lack of reproducibility, difficulty in creating specific pathologies, high cost, and difference in tissue consistency when compared to real patients. The second type of simulators consists of *virtual reality modules*. These are computer-generated models that allow a high degree of customizability. Unlike physical models, they can be used multiple times by multiple users since there is no disruption of the actual model. Newer models have haptic feedback, thus, making them even more realistic. The third type of simulation modules are web-based models. Finally, *hybrid simulators* are a combination of the previous three models. Different types of neurosurgical simulators that were conceived include aneurysm clipping [23], microvascular decompression [24], tumor resection [25], various endovascular procedures [26, 27], and spinal instrumentation [28].

Importance of Simulation in Cerebrovascular Neurosurgery

Until recently, neurosurgical resident training has been confined mostly to the operating room with very few opportunities for simulation training due to an absence of validated modules and curricula. In addition, even basic surgical approaches can be complex, and many variants exist that are only introduced late in resident training, decreasing the opportunity for novice surgeons to master these demanding techniques even prior to the 80-h rule. In particular, microvascular anastomosis is one of the most complex and technically challenging surgical skills as it demands high levels of manual dexterity, fine motor skill, and hand-eye coordination, in addition to respect and safe manipulation of the tissue to avoid damage to fragile endothelium and the entire vessel wall. Further, improved proficiency in microanastomosis has been shown to translate to other microsurgical skills [6, 29]. Microanastomosis remains an integral part of the neurosurgical armamentarium, and with the decrease and dilution of the surgical volumes among increasing numbers of

tertiary medical centers, it becomes clear that developing a microanastomosis training model is of paramount importance.

In addition, intracranial access techniques are essential in any neurosurgical procedure. Errors can result in limited exposure, poor operative control, increased infection rates, and thus higher morbidity and mortality rates and sub-optimal esthetic outcomes. In particular to the cerebrovascular and skull base subspecialties, surgical approach to the interpeduncular and ambient cisterns is still a complicated and challenging procedure even in the most experienced of hands. The depth of the structures within the brain, the proximity to vital structures, vascular and neurological, as well as the complexity of the temporal bone anatomy make access to this region extremely delicate and demanding with a very low threshold for error. Repetitive and intensive training is key to achieving mastery with as many as 10,000 h required for proficiency [5], but resident training time is now reduced to an 80-h week. In addition, with the development of endovascular techniques, many pathologies previously treated with an open surgery are now being rerouted to the neuro-interventional suite, further limiting the exposure of residents to complex skull base approaches. Nevertheless, these approaches are still very much needed, and cerebrovascular neurosurgeons need to have these approaches in their armamentarium.

Microsurgical microanastomosis is a very technically demanding procedure with a potentially devastating effect if sub-optimally performed. It is considered to be an integral part of not only neurosurgical training but also of vascular surgery, plastic surgery, and otolaryngology trainings. Residents are typically not exposed to this technique until later in their training program due to the high stakes associated with it. Therefore, simulation training for such a procedure would ensure that residents are not only familiar with the surgical instruments but also with handling and navigating them under an operative microscope and handling the delicate vessel wall. It also ensures that they acquire competency at a basic but essential surgical level.

An added dimension to microvascular anastomosis simulation would be patient specific simulation which could potentially be used in preparation for complex cases for presurgical training.

Microanastomosis Training Models

Regular practice is quintessential to develop, maintain, and improve microsurgical dexterity needed for microvascular anastomosis. Studies have shown that approximately 50 vessel anastomoses are needed for novice surgeons to perform at a level of expert surgeons and achieve similar anastomosis patency [30–33]. Multiple models have been developed throughout the years for training purposes. These models vary from cadavers, both human and animal, to live animals such as rats, to chicken wings, to synthetic physical and virtual models [34–45].

A simulation model has to be reliable, valid, educational, and cost-effective. A reliable model offers a simulated technique that is reproducible and not altered after repeated use as well as when a different reviewer is assessing the results (inter-rater reliability). In terms of validation, there are multiple parameters to be addressed before a simulation exercise is included in a medical curriculum [6, 7, 46].

- *Face Validity* The extent to which the simulation model replicates the real-world scenario. This is typically judged by a panel of experts [6, 7, 46].
- *Content Validity* The extent to which a simulator assesses a specific skill [6, 7, 46].
- *Construct Validity* The extent to which a model is able to assess the level of performance (i.e., differentiate between novice and experts) [7, 46].
- *Concurrent Validity* The extent to which the outcome correlates with previously validated measures [6, 46].
- *Predictive Validity* The extent of transposition of the acquired skill into an operating room and correlation with future performances [5].

Different models have been developed to address these various validity measures, although no model is currently optimal for all measures. For example, human cadavers, though anatomically realistic, lack the hemodynamic and pulsatile characteristics of the live cerebral tissue in the OR. Garrett et al. and Aboud et al. developed dynamic pulsatile cerebral models to circumvent this issue [47, 48]. Based on this concept, Olabe et al. developed an infused human cadaver brain model used for training in various microsurgical techniques including microvascular anastomosis [39]. While this model does in theory address the concept of validity in many of its aspects and does somewhat replicate an OR setting, it does present multiple challenges. Human cadavers can be difficult to obtain, are expensive, and require special biohazard safe labs. In addition, these models require preparation and setup and are therefore time-consuming. Further, similar to all other physical models, it can only be used a limited number of times. Hence increased validation may come at the expense of cost-effectiveness and reproducibility.

Microsurgical training using gauze, 10–0 sutures, and a microscope was proposed by Inoue et al. This model is cheap, requires no preparation, and is widely available. While this model might help with dexterity and comfort of micromovement under the microscope, it clearly lacks the characteristics of an actual vascular bypass procedure. The consistency of gauze clearly does not replicate the different layers of blood vessels [49].

Brachial artery extracted from chicken wings has been proposed as a cheap readily available model for microanastomosis practice [36, 43]. Chicken wings are cheap, easy to purchase, and do not require any special facilities to preserve. Multiple papers have detailed the technique of extracting the artery from the chicken wing [36, 43, 50, 51]. The typical size of the chicken wing brachial artery is about 1.0 mm, similar to the M4 branches of the middle cerebral artery [36, 43]. One of the main issues with this model though is the wide variability of the diameter of the artery as well as its relatively short length [37]. Turkey wing brachial arteries have been tried as an alternative instead. These arteries have a larger diameter – on average about 1.47 mm – and are therefore more easily manipulated and thus perhaps more suited for training for the novice trainee [37]. Similarly to chicken wings, these arteries are readily available, cheap, and do not require any special equipment or facilities. Turkey brachial arteries were found to have less variability in diameter and were longer then chicken brachial arteries and therefore could potentially be used for multiple anastomoses [37]. In addition, Kawashima et al., in a study of 25 cadaver specimens, found that the M4 branches of the middle cerebral artery were larger than 1.5 mm in two thirds of cases and larger then 1 mm in 90% of cases [52]. With chicken brachial arteries sometimes as small as 0.6 mm in diameter, turkey arteries could potentially be better suited for anastomosis training [37]. This model provides a relatively realistic experience even though it does come with limitations. The periadventitial dissection required to extract the vessels is more extensive than for intracranial vessels, which could be time-consuming. Also, even though it is not a biohazard material, the wings are still biodegradable tissue, can be messy, and need to be properly disposed of. Preserving them might also alter the physical characteristics (i.e., frozen) and may make them unusable or at the very least unrealistic. In addition, while stenosis can be assessed post anastomosis, this model does not allow to appropriately evaluate for thrombosis unlike live models [37].

Rats have been used in medical research for decades due to the close similarity of their genetic, biological, and behavioral characteristic to humans, in addition to the fact that many human symptoms and conditions can be replicated in rats. It is therefore not surprising that they have been also used for microsurgical training [51, 53]. Rats are widely available at low cost and have a high resistance to infection [7]. It has even been suggested that these rat models are the "gold standard" for microsurgical training [7]. While this claim might be questionable, live rat models do provide a training experience that closely resembles that of human vessels [37, 51, 54]. When comparing different models through surveys filled by neurosurgery residents and attendings, live rats consistently scored the highest and were found to be the most realistic [37, 51]. Unfortunately, using live animals for training models raises some issues. Live animals require strict adherence to institutional protocols in terms of animal welfare. In addition, it requires maintaining licensures and proper personnel training as well as providing appropriate housing for the animals. Further, rat models cannot be used outside of specialized labs and are therefore not readily available for residents who have limited time to practice. Added to this, there are ethical concerns about using a live animal for training purpoeses [37]. All these issues make using rat models unpractical. In a comparative study, Hwang et al. found that while rat models were the most realistic, they were less practical than chicken wings [51].

Synthetic vessel models are more cost-effective, more readily available, and easier to handle, store, and maintain compared to animal models [6]. Silicone vessels have been used to this end. Even though they might not be as realistic as rat vessels, their practicality makes them an attractive alternative to biological and virtual models. Various designs have been proposed, including portable "microvascular training cards." Therefore these models do not necessitate a formal setting and are cheap, yet they lack the hemodynamic properties and can be tedious to set up [35, 55]. They can be used for end-to-end, side-to-side, and end-to-side anastomosis. In order to replicate the setting of deep anastomosis, trainees can work through a plastic box [34, 35]. In our opinion simulation needs to be cost-effective and amenable to frequent practice. These goals are much easier to achieve with synthetic vessels than rat models.

Validated Assessment Instruments

In a review of the literature pertaining to microsurgical training models and assessment tools performed in 2012, Dumestre et al. reviewed 238 articles, of which only 9 articles were eventually included due to the absence of validation [56].

Similarly, the same authors performed a follow-up review of the literature in 2014 and out of 261 articles, included 10 and 1 abstract in their final review [46]. This was due to either the fact that these articles did not assess microsurgery or lacked an assessment tool. The authors concluded that while there is a large number of simulation models and designs, their utility in resident education is limited due to the lack of validation.

Most current assessment tools are either directly derived from studies in general surgeries or at least based on them. The Imperial College Surgical Assessment Device (ICSAD) is a motion-tracking device initially used in laparoscopic and open general surgery [57–59]. It tracks dual-hand motion of the surgeon in three planes as well as individual hand movement and length of movement. The ICSAD was later validated for microsurgery by comparing its scores to the previously validated Reznick's global rating scales (GRS) showing a decrease in scores with an increase in hand movement and distance traveled [60]. There was also a significant difference in scores between experienced and novice surgeons in terms of hand movement, time to complete task, and path length therefore proving construct validity [61, 62].

Multiple variations of the objective structured assessment of technical skills (OSATS) have also been validated for various specialties, including general surgery, ophthalmology, and microvascular anastomosis [63, 64]. However, the various models were not able to address the different aspects of validity. Nugent et al. [64] evaluated 16 trainees completing microvascular anastomosis and revealed a significant improvement at the end of a 5-day course. However, there was observational bias as the reviewers were not blinded to the trainees. In addition, microsurgical skill performance was correlated with psychomotor aptitude assessments score only in male trainees but not in female trainees [64]. A video-based variation of the OSATS was validated for basic microsurgical suture but failed to prove construct validity as no comparison between different skill levels was performed [61, 62]. Moulton et al. evaluated 38 junior residents and the effect of different practice methods on the acquisition of microvascular anastomosis skill [63]. While they were able to prove content validity for microsurgical anastomosis, construct validity could not be demonstrated due to the lack of comparison between surgeons/trainees of different skill levels.

The University of Western Ontario Microsurgical Skills Acquisition/Assessment (UWOMSA) instrument contains two 5-point Likert scales, the first assessing knot tying and the second evaluating the anastomosis [65]. This tool includes assessment for "quality of knot," "efficiency," "handling," "preparation," "suturing," and "final product." Temple et al. were able to demonstrate criterion, construct, and content validity by evaluating 20 videos of surgical residents and fellows performing knot tying and 17 videos of end-to-end and end-to-side anastomosis [65].

Another assessment tool is the structured assessment of microsurgery skills (SAMS) developed by Chan et al. [66]. This method has three components including a GRS, an error list, and a summative rating (overall performance) as well as free commentary box. The authors were able to demonstrate construct validity with the consultant surgeon scoring consistently higher than the trainees. They also showed predictive validity as well as content validity.

Northwestern Objective Microanastomosis Assessment Tool (NOMAT)

The previously described models and assessment tools, while relevant to acquisition and evaluation of microsurgical skills, were developed and tested in different specialties such as ophthalmology and plastic surgery. The Northwestern Objective Microanastomosis Assessment Tool (NOMAT) was developed and validated specifically for microvascular anastomosis for neurosurgical residents [6, 15, 67]. The NOMAT is a 14-item Likert-type objective assessment scale based on the OSATS. A vascular microanastomosis bench module was developed in the department of neurological surgery at Northwestern University's Feinberg School of Medicine [6]. The initial version of the module consisted of performing 1-mm and 3-mm micro-anastomosis 10-0 nylon sutures (Fig. 5.1). A basic microsurgical tool set in addition to a microscope is part of the setup (Fig. 5.2). The module with the NOMAT was initially tested and validated at Northwestern based on a study on 21 participants of different levels of expertise. The trainees were divided into experienced, exposed, and novice. Trainees had to perform both the 1-mm and the 3-mm anastomosis and were recorded. At the end of the procedure, an infusion pump with red dye was attached to the vessels to determine the patency of the anasto-mosis as well as any leaks or any vascular injury. The vessels were additionally opened axially to

assess the quality of the anastomosis. The de-identified videos were blindly reviewed by expe-rienced vascular neurosurgeons and scored on the NOMAT scale and a subjective rating based on the viability of the anastomosis. Construct validity was demonstrated after the experienced trainees performed significantly better than the exposed and novice trainees on the 1-mm mod-ule [15]. The difference was not significant with the 3-mm vessels though. This was thought to be due to the fact that the microanastomosis on the 1-mm vessels is more delicate and complex and therefore more sensitive at detecting differences in experience. In addition, trainees performed the anastomosis on the 3-mm vessels first. Experienced trainees might have had a faster learning curve and therefore performed better on

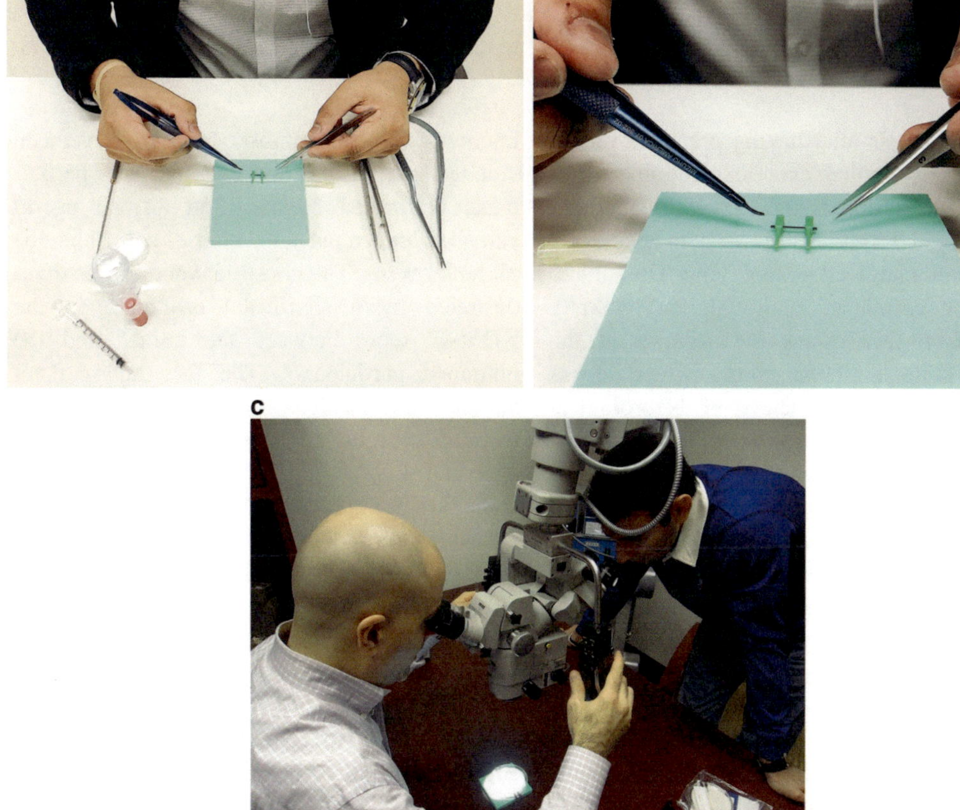

Fig. 5.1 (**a, b**) 1- and 3-mm vessels with infusion pump attachment at each end. (**c**) The initial microanastomosis setup under the microscope. (Used with permission of Mayo Foundation for Medical Education and Research. All rights reserved)

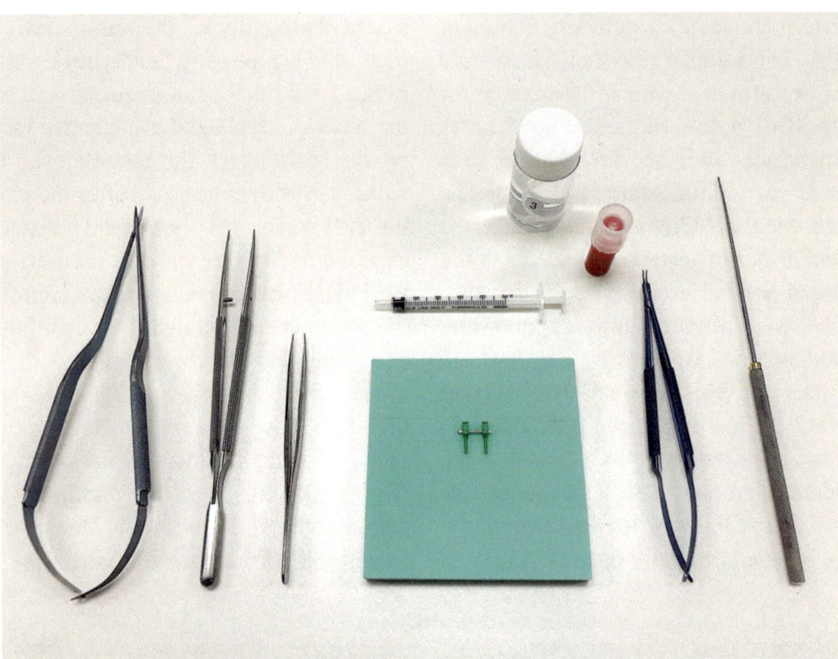

Fig. 5.2 Basic microsurgical tool set used in the NOMAT module. (Used with permission of Mayo Foundation for Medical Education and Research. All rights reserved)

the 1-mm vessels after having practiced on the 3-mm vessels. Further, experienced trainees performed the anastomosis faster with smoother movements and a higher efficiency in needle and tissue handling as well as knot tying. The subjective rating correlated well with the NOMAT score. To further assess the validity of the NOMAT scale, a microanastomosis module was set up at the 2014 Society of Neurological Surgeons (SNS) boot camp [15]. Fifty-four first year residents performed the microanastomosis on the 3-mm model and were scored using the NOMAT tool by 2 postdoctoral fellows and 1 experienced microsurgeon (Fig. 5.3). Combining the results from this study with the initial Northwestern University study, a total of 75 residents were evaluated. The intra-class correlation coefficient revealed high global inter-rater reliability for the NOMAT, which showed that the level of expertise of the rater did not affect the precision nor the validity of this tool.

The NOMAT was used in different studies, further proving its validity [40, 68]. Belykh et al. [40] used the NOMAT to evaluate human and bovine placental vessels as potential models for microvascular anastomosis training. Seventeen "trained" participants and 13 "untrained" participants performed bypasses on a total of 40 extracted human placental arteries and 10 bovine placental veins. The construct validity was demonstrated by a significant difference in the NOMAT score between the trained and the untrained participants. The face and content validity were also demonstrated as the model was thought to highly replicate the real-life experience and was thought to improve microsurgical technique based on subjective surveys filled by the participants. Further analyzing their results, the authors concluded that a score of >50 on the NOMAT correlated with a successful performance of the microanastomosis.

Organized Neurosurgery and Simulation

Due to the changing nature of practicing medicine, the Congress of Neurological Surgeons (CNS) formed a committee in 2010 with a goal of "maximizing neurosurgical education to improve

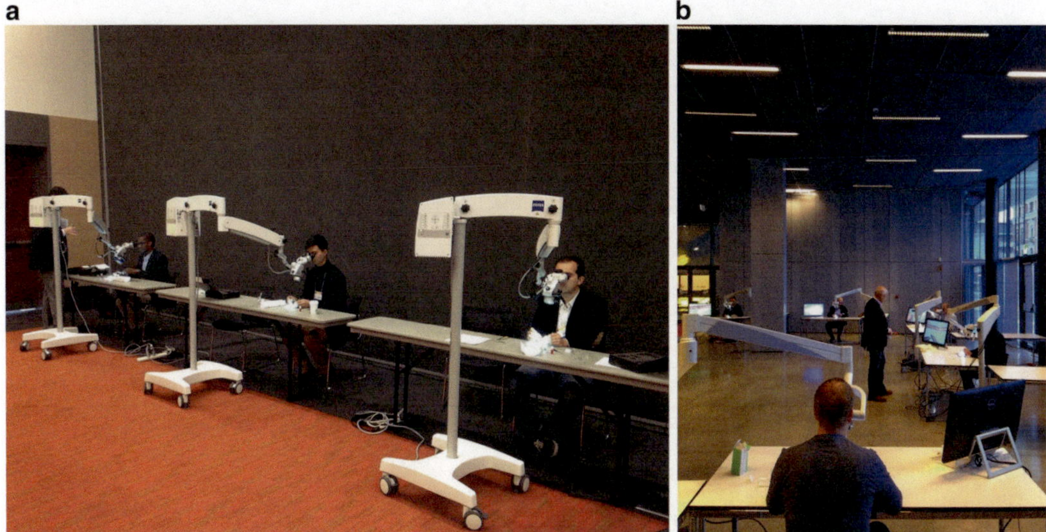

Fig. 5.3 (**a, b**) Participants performing the microvascular anastomosis under the microscope during a microanastomosis course. (Used with permission of Mayo Foundation for Medical Education and Research. All rights reserved)

patient outcomes with the greatest efficiency and safety." This committee came to be known as the CNS Simulation Committee. Its mission is to create a comprehensive neurosurgical simulation initiative geared toward developing and reforming resident education [8]. The committee designed a simulation-based curriculum around the six residency core competencies defined by the ACGME: patient care, medical knowledge, practice-based learning and improvement, interpersonal and communication skills, professionalism, and system-based practice.

The first simulation curriculum was organized during the 2011 CNS annual meeting in Washington, DC. The curriculum covered three main areas: vascular, cranial, and spinal procedures. The vascular curriculum was mainly focused on angiography models and later added a bypass model (Fig. 5.4). Based on resident and participant feedback, the committee then modified and standardized the educational curriculum. The details of the curriculum are beyond the scope of this chapter, but briefly, the simulation modules had predefined goals and objective as requested by the residents. There was a premodule test which was retaken at the end of the course. Didactic sessions were also included in addition to the technical aspects of the simula-

tion. Using this educational model, vascular anastomosis simulation was tested at the 2012 CNS annual meeting [67]. This module included a cognitive and microanastomosis pre-lecture test, a didactic lecture, followed by a cognitive and microanastomosis post-lecture test. The participants were evaluated using the NOMAT. There was a statistically significant improvement between the pre- and post-lecture testing both in the cognitive and technical performance. Although the number of participants was small, the results of this study reinforced the validity of the format of the simulation curriculum as set forth by the CNS committee.

The same module was applied to European residents at the European Association of Neurological Societies resident vascular course which was held in Prague, Czech Republic [69]. Again using the NOMAT as an assessment tool, the study revealed a significant improvement in the hands-on technical portion as well as the didactic portion of the module. These results give more credence to the concept of standardized simulation courses and training for residents. In fact, a survey of program directors of US neurosurgical programs revealed that 72% of program directors believe that simulation would improve patient outcome with almost half stating that

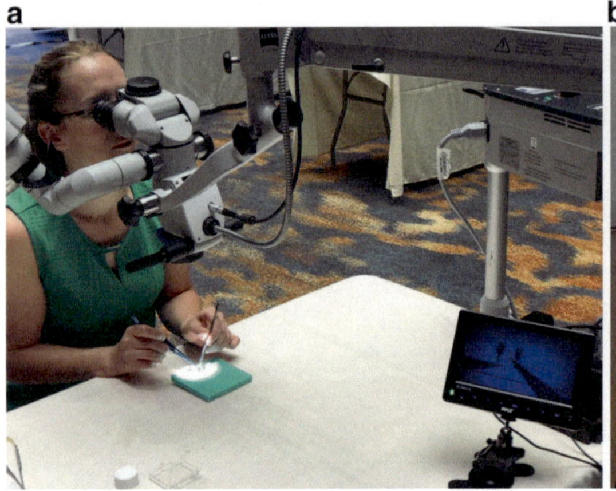

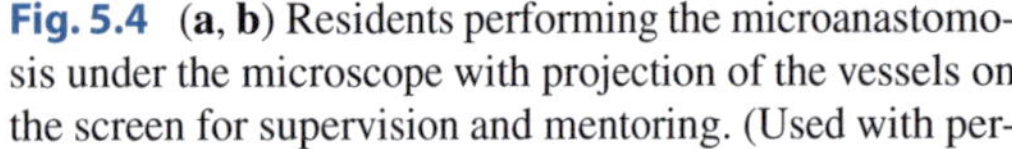

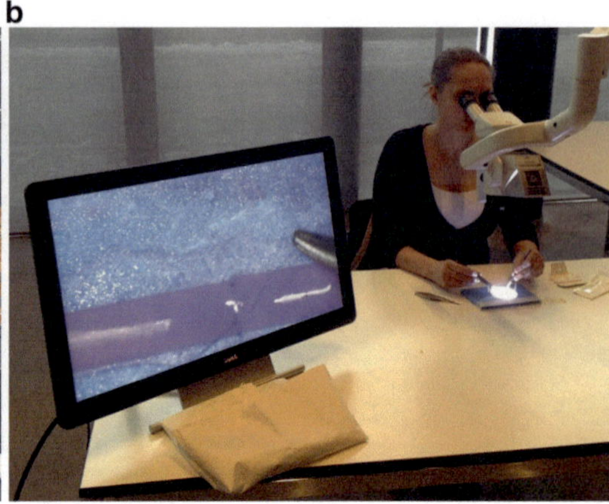

Fig. 5.4 (**a**, **b**) Residents performing the microanastomosis under the microscope with projection of the vessels on the screen for supervision and mentoring. (Used with permission of Mayo Foundation for Medical Education and Research. All rights reserved)

residents should achieve a predefined level of proficiency on simulators before working on patients [70]. In addition, 74% of responders stated that they would make simulation training a mandatory part of residency. To further reinforce the importance and validity of simulation as part of residency training, a survey conducted as part of the SNS boot camp for the postgraduate year 1 residents found a high level of satisfaction and knowledge retention of skills acquired during the boot camp [71].

Conclusion and Future Direction

Simulation in neurosurgery is still in its infancy. Microvascular anastomosis remains perhaps the last frontier of vascular neurosurgery with low volumes and high technical complexity. Multiple simulation models have been developed using a variety of synthetic and biologic material. Each model has its benefits and its drawbacks. The perfect microvascular anastomosis simulation model remains elusive though, and more importantly while promising assessment scales such as the NOMAT have been tested and validated on small numbers of trainees, we still need to correlate the scores and the improvement with the performance in the OR. While huge strides have been made over the last decade, there is still a lot of work ahead to enhance resident education through validated simulation models and modules. The inclusion of simulation-based learning and curricula in the CNS annual meeting is a promising start. Large-scale studies are the next step in determining the exact role and effect of simulation on resident education, as well as on clinical outcomes.

References

1. Carter BN. The fruition of Halsted's concept of surgical training. Surgery. 1952;32(3):518–27.
2. Fabricant PD, Dy CJ, Dare DM, Bostrom MP. A narrative review of surgical resident duty hour limits: where do we go from here? J Grad Med Educ. 2013;5(1):19–24.
3. Accreditation Council for Graduate Medical Education. Report of the ACGME work group on resident duty hours: Accreditation Council for Graduate Medical Education. Chicago: Accreditation Council for Graduate Medical Education;2002.
4. Accreditation Council for Graduate Medical Education: Accreditation Council for Graduate Medical Education. Statement of justification/impact for the final approval of common standards related to resident duty hours. Chicago: Accreditation Council for Graduate Medical Education;2002.
5. Ericsson KA, Krampe RT, Tesch-Römer C. The role of deliberate practice in the Acquisition of Expert Performance. Psychol Rev. 1993;100(3):363–406.
6. Aoun SG, El Ahmadieh TY, El Tecle NE, et al. A pilot study to assess the construct and face validity

of the Northwestern Objective Microanastomosis Assessment Tool. J Neurosurg. 2015;123(1):103–9.

7. Balasundaram I, Aggarwal R, Darzi LA. Development of a training curriculum for microsurgery. Br J Oral Maxillofac Surg. 2010;48(8):598–606.

8. Harrop J, Lobel DA, Bendok B, Sharan A, Rezai AR. Developing a neurosurgical simulation-based educational curriculum: an overview. Neurosurgery. 2013;73(Suppl 1):25–9.

9. Zammar SG, Hamade YJ, Aoun RJ, et al. The cognitive and technical skills impact of the Congress of Neurological Surgeons simulation curriculum on neurosurgical trainees at the 2013 Neurological Society of India meeting. World Neurosurg. 2015;83(4):419–23.

10. Fargen KM, Arthur AS, Bendok BR, et al. Experience with a simulator-based angiography course for neurosurgical residents: beyond a pilot program. Neurosurgery. 2013;73(Suppl 1):46–50.

11. Harrop J, Rezai AR, Hoh DJ, Ghobrial GM, Sharan A. Neurosurgical training with a novel cervical spine simulator: posterior foraminotomy and laminectomy. Neurosurgery. 2013;73(Suppl 1):94–9.

12. Ghobrial GM, Balsara K, Maulucci CM, et al. Simulation training curricula for neurosurgical residents: cervical foraminotomy and durotomy repair modules. World Neurosurg. 2015;84(3):751–755 e751–7.

13. Lobel DA, Elder JB, Schirmer CM, Bowyer MW, Rezai AR. A novel craniotomy simulator provides a validated method to enhance education in the management of traumatic brain injury. Neurosurgery. 2013;73(Suppl 1):57–65.

14. Duvivier RJ, van Dalen J, Muijtjens AM, Moulaert VR, van der Vleuten CP, Scherpbier AJ. The role of deliberate practice in the acquisition of clinical skills. BMC Med Educ. 2011;11:101.

15. Pines AR, Alghoul MS, Hamade YJ, et al. Assessment of the interrater reliability of the congress of neurological surgeons microanastomosis assessment scale. Oper Neurosurg. 2016;Publish Ahead of Print.

16. McCaslin AF, Aoun SG, Batjer HH, Bendok BR. Enhancing the utility of surgical simulation: from proficiency to automaticity. World Neurosurg. 2011;76(6):482–4.

17. Prabhu A, Smith W, Yurko Y, Acker C, Stefanidis D. Increased stress levels may explain the incomplete transfer of simulator-acquired skill to the operating room. Surgery. 2010;147(5):640–5.

18. Stefanidis D, Scerbo MW, Montero PN, Acker CE, Smith WD. Simulator training to automaticity leads to improved skill transfer compared with traditional proficiency-based training: a randomized controlled trial. Ann Surg. 2012;255(1):30–7.

19. Singh H, Kalani M, Acosta-Torres S, El Ahmadieh TY, Loya J, Ganju A. History of simulation in medicine: from Resusci Annie to the Ann Myers Medical Center. Neurosurgery. 2013;73(Suppl 1):9–14.

20. Davis PK, Winnefeld JA, Bankes SC, Kahan JP. Analytic War Gaming with the RAND Strategy Assessment System (RSAS). 1987. http://www.rand.org/pubs/research_briefs/RB7801.html.

21. Barrows HS. An overview of the uses of standardized patients for teaching and evaluating clinical skills. AAMC Acad Med. 1993;68(6):443–51; discussion 451-443.

22. Swanson DB, van der Vleuten CP. Assessment of clinical skills with standardized patients: state of the art revisited. Teach Learn Med. 2013;25(Suppl 1):S17–25.

23. Mashiko T, Otani K, Kawano R, et al. Development of three-dimensional hollow elastic model for cerebral aneurysm clipping simulation enabling rapid and low cost prototyping. World Neurosurg. 2015;83(3):351–61.

24. Oishi M, Fukuda M, Hiraishi T, Yajima N, Sato Y, Fujii Y. Interactive virtual simulation using a 3D computer graphics model for microvascular decompression surgery. J Neurosurg. 2012;117(3):555–65.

25. Delorme S, Laroche D, DiRaddo R, Del Maestro RF. NeuroTouch: a physics-based virtual simulator for cranial microneurosurgery training. Neurosurgery. 2012;71(1 Suppl Operative):32–42.

26. Nguyen N, Eagleson R, Boulton M, Realism d RS. Criterion validity, and training capability of simulated diagnostic cerebral angiography. Stud Health Technol Inform. 2014;196:297–303.

27. Spiotta AM, Rasmussen PA, Masaryk TJ, Benzel EC, Schlenk R. Simulated diagnostic cerebral angiography in neurosurgical training: a pilot program. J Neurointerv Surg. 2013;5(4):376–81.

28. Luciano CJ, Banerjee PP, Sorenson JM, et al. Percutaneous spinal fixation simulation with virtual reality and haptics. Neurosurgery. 2013;72(Suppl 1):89–96.

29. Crosby NL, Clapson JB, Buncke HJ, Newlin L. Advanced non-animal microsurgical exercises. Microsurgery. 1995;16(9):655–8.

30. Lascar I, Totir D, Cinca A, et al. Training program and learning curve in experimental microsurgery during the residency in plastic surgery. Microsurgery. 2007;27(4):263–7.

31. Blackwell KE, Brown MT, Gonzalez D. Overcoming the learning curve in microvascular head and neck reconstruction. Arch Otolaryngol Head Neck Surg. 1997;123(12):1332–5.

32. Hui KC, Zhang F, Shaw WW, et al. Learning curve of microvascular venous anastomosis: a never ending struggle? Microsurgery. 2000;20(1):22–4.

33. Szalay D, MacRae H, Regehr G, Reznick R. Using operative outcome to assess technical skill. Am J Surg. 2000;180(3):234–7.

34. Buis DR, Buis CR, Feller RE, Mandl ES, Peerdeman SM. A basic model for practice of intracranial microsurgery. Surg Neurol. 2009;71(2):254–6.

35. Matsumura N, Hayashi N, Hamada H, Shibata T, Horie Y, Endo S. A newly designed training tool for microvascular anastomosis techniques: microvascular practice card. Surg Neurol. 2009;71(5):616–20.

36. Kim BJ, Kim ST, Jeong YG, Lee WH, Lee KS, Paeng SH. An efficient microvascular anastomosis training model based on chicken wings and simple instruments. J Cerebrovasc Endovasc Neurosurg. 2013;15(1):20–5.

37. Abla AA, Uschold T, Preul MC, Zabramski JM. Comparative use of turkey and chicken wing brachial artery models for microvascular anastomosis training. J Neurosurg. 2011;115(6):1231–5.

38. Olabe J, Olabe J, Roda JM, Sancho V. Human cadaver brain infusion skull model for neurosurgical training. Surg Neurol Int. 2011;2:54.

39. Olabe J, Olabe J, Sancho V. Human cadaver brain infusion model for neurosurgical training. Surg Neurol. 2009;72(6):700–2.

40. Belykh E, Lei T, Safavi-Abbasi S, et al. Low-flow and high-flow neurosurgical bypass and anastomosis training models using human and bovine placental vessels: a histological analysis and validation study. J Neurosurg. 2016;125(4):915–28.

41. Hicdonmez T, Hamamcioglu MK, Tiryaki M, Cukur Z, Cobanoglu S. Microneurosurgical training model in fresh cadaveric cow brain: a laboratory study simulating the approach to the circle of Willis. Surg Neurol. 2006;66(1):100–4. discussion 104

42. Colpan ME, Slavin KV, Amin-Hanjani S, Calderon-Arnuphi M, Charbel FT. Microvascular anastomosis training model based on a Turkey neck with perfused arteries. Neurosurgery. 2008;62(5 Suppl 2):ONS407–410; discussion ONS410–401.

43. Hino A. Training in microvascular surgery using a chicken wing artery. Neurosurgery. 2003;52(6):1495–7; discussion 1497–8.

44. Schoffl H, Hager D, Hinterdorfer C, et al. Pulsatile perfused porcine coronary arteries for microvascular training. Ann Plast Surg. 2006;57(2):213–6.

45. Inoue T, Tsutsumi K, Saito K, Adachi S, Tanaka S, Kunii N. Training of A3-A3 side-to-side anastomosis in a deep corridor using a box with 6.5-cm depth: technical note. Surg Neurol. 2006;66(6):638–41.

46. Dumestre D, Yeung JK, Temple-Oberle C. Evidence-based microsurgical skills acquisition series part 2: validated assessment instruments – a systematic review. J Surg Educ. 2015;72(1):80–9.

47. Garrett HE Jr. A human cadaveric circulation model. J Vasc Surg. 2001;33(5):1128–30.

48. Aboud E, Aboud G, Al-Mefty O, et al. "Live cadavers" for training in the management of intraoperative aneurysmal rupture. J Neurosurg. 2015;123(5):1339–46.

49. Inoue T, Tsutsumi K, Adachi S, Tanaka S, Saito K, Kunii N. Effectiveness of suturing training with 10-0 nylon under fixed and maximum magnification (x 20) using desk type microscope. Surg Neurol. 2006;66(2):183–7.

50. Olabe J, Olabe J. Microsurgical training on an in vitro chicken wing infusion model. Surg Neurol. 2009;72(6):695–9.

51. Hwang G, Oh CW, Park SQ, Sheen SH, Bang JS, Kang HS. Comparison of different microanastomosis training models : model accuracy and practicality. J Korean Neurosurg Soc. 2010;47(4):287–90.

52. Kawashima M, Rhoton AL Jr, Tanriover N, Ulm AJ, Yasuda A, Fujii K. Microsurgical anatomy of cerebral revascularization. Part I: anterior circulation. J Neurosurg. 2005;102(1):116–31.

53. Ilie V, Ilie V, Ghetu N, Popescu S, Grosu O, Pieptu D. Assessment of the microsurgical skills: 30 minutes versus 2 weeks patency. Microsurgery. 2007;27(5):451–4.

54. Onoda S, Kimata Y, Matsumoto K. Iliolumbar vein as a training model for microsurgical end-to-side anastomosis. J Craniofac Surg. 2016;27(3):767–8.

55. Rayan B, Rayan GM. Microsurgery training card: a practical, economic tool for basic techniques. J Reconstr Microsurg. 2006;22(4):273–5; discussion 276.

56. Dumestre D, Yeung JK, Temple-Oberle C. Evidence-based microsurgical skill-acquisition series part 1: validated microsurgical models – a systematic review. J Surg Educ. 2014;71(3):329–38.

57. Taffinder N, Smith SG, Huber J, Russell RC, Darzi A. The effect of a second-generation 3D endoscope on the laparoscopic precision of novices and experienced surgeons. Surg Endosc. 1999;13(11):1087–92.

58. Datta V, Chang A, Mackay S, Darzi A. The relationship between motion analysis and surgical technical assessments. Am J Surg. 2002;184(1):70–3.

59. Datta V, Mackay S, Mandalia M, Darzi A. The use of electromagnetic motion tracking analysis to objectively measure open surgical skill in the laboratory-based model. J Am Coll Surg. 2001;193(5):479–85.

60. Grober ED, Hamstra SJ, Wanzel KR, et al. Validation of novel and objective measures of microsurgical skill: hand-motion analysis and stereoscopic visual acuity. Microsurgery. 2003;23(4):317–22.

61. Ezra DG, Aggarwal R, Michaelides M, et al. Skills acquisition and assessment after a microsurgical skills course for ophthalmology residents. Ophthalmology. 2009;116(2):257–62.

62. Saleh GM, Voyatzis G, Hance J, Ratnasothy J, Darzi A. Evaluating surgical dexterity during corneal suturing. Arch Ophthalmol. 2006;124(9):1263–6.

63. Moulton CA, Dubrowski A, Macrae H, Graham B, Grober E, Reznick R. Teaching surgical skills: what kind of practice makes perfect? A randomized, controlled trial. Ann Surg. 2006;244(3):400–9.

64. Nugent E, Joyce C, Perez-Abadia G, et al. Factors influencing microsurgical skill acquisition during a dedicated training course. Microsurgery. 2012;32(8):649–56.

65. Temple CL, Ross DC. A new, validated instrument to evaluate competency in microsurgery: the University of Western Ontario Microsurgical Skills Acquisition/Assessment instrument [outcomes article]. Plast Reconstr Surg. 2011;127(1):215–22.

66. Chan W, Niranjan N, Ramakrishnan V. Structured assessment of microsurgery skills in the clinical setting. J Plast Reconstr Aesthet Surg. 2010;63(8):1329–34.

67. El Ahmadieh TY, Aoun SG, El Tecle NE, et al. A didactic and hands-on module enhances resident microsurgical knowledge and technical skill. Neurosurgery. 2013;73(Suppl 1):51–6.
68. Belykh E, Byvaltsev V. Off-the-job microsurgical training on dry models: Siberian experience. World Neurosurg. 2014;82(1–2):20–4.
69. Zammar SG, El Tecle NE, El Ahmadieh TY, et al. Impact of a vascular neurosurgery simulation-based course on cognitive knowledge and technical skills in European neurosurgical trainees. World Neurosurg. 2015;84(2):197–201.
70. Ganju A, Aoun SG, Daou MR, et al. The role of simulation in neurosurgical education: a survey of 99 United States neurosurgery program directors. World Neurosurg. 2013;80(5):e1–8.
71. Selden NR, Anderson VC, McCartney S, Origitano TC, Burchiel KJ, Barbaro NM. Society of Neurological Surgeons boot camp courses: knowledge retention and relevance of hands-on learning after 6 months of postgraduate year 1 training. J Neurosurg. 2013;119(3):796–802.

Endovascular Surgical Neuroradiology Simulation

6

Teddy E. Kim, Mark B. Frenkel, Kyle M. Fargen, Stacey Q. Wolfe, and J. Mocco

Introduction

Surgical training is currently undergoing a paradigm shift from traditional apprenticeship-based training to increased use of simulation-based training [1]. This has been driven, in part, by concerns for patient safety issues, work hour restrictions, and limited training opportunities under current apprenticeship models [1]. Regardless of method, the acquisition of efficient, reliable, and safely performed complex psychomotor skills, in addition to surgical judgment to contend with variable anatomy, pathology, and potential complications, is paramount. Given the increasing public interest in physician qualifications, programs such as Maintenance of Certification have been implemented to ensure high standards of medical practice with the goal of improving care, increasing patient safety, and providing better cost-benefit ratios. The assessment of key competencies and procedural skills is challenging, and a written examination may be insufficient in a surgical field as a marker for overall competence [2].

Development of virtual reality simulation-based surgical skills has demonstrated improved performance and transfer of newfound skills in the operating room across multiple specialties [3–7]. In the field of laparoscopic surgery, standardized basic simulated programs such as the Fundamentals of Laparoscopic Surgery has been incorporated into training curricula and is now a prerequisite for certification with the American Board of Surgery [7, 8]. Many surgical specialties have developed unique simulators to suit specialty-specific techniques that are required in each respective surgical training including, but not limited to, laparoscopy, arthroscopy, bronchoscopy, gastrointestinal, genitourinary, gynecologic, temporal bone surgery, robotic surgery, and endovascular surgery [1, 4, 6, 9, 10].

This chapter will focus on the use of simulation in neuroendovascular surgery. We will first review simulator-based training in endovascular surgery, then discuss modern neuroendovascular simulation devices and the available literature on neuroendovascular simulation and procedural performance.

Electronic supplementary material: The online version of this chapter https://doi.org/10.1007/978-3-319-75583-0_6 contains supplementary material, which is available to authorized users.

T. E. Kim (✉) · K. M. Fargen · S. Q. Wolfe
Department of Neurological Surgery, Wake Forest University, Winston-Salem, NC, USA
e-mail: tekim@wakehealth.edu

M. B. Frenkel
Department of Neurosurgery, Wake Forest Baptist Medical Center, Winston Salem, NC, USA

J. Mocco
Department of Neurological Surgery, Mount Sinai Hospital, New York, NY, USA

Simulation-Based Training in Endovascular Surgery

Modern medicine has increasingly evolved toward minimally invasive procedures, and the mastery of endovascular techniques has become crucial in multiple specialties [11]. Catheter-based procedures are widely utilized in endovascular surgery and interventional radiology and are employed for diagnosis as well as therapy. These procedures demand a specialized skill set for successful navigation through three-dimensional vascular trees using two-dimensional on-screen feedback. It can be challenging for trainees to acquire this surgical skill set in the current apprenticeship model, as interventional procedures often allow for just one surgeon at a time [11]. Currently, training is carried out primarily in the patient care setting, occasionally with increased risk to patient safety [12]. For this purpose, virtual reality simulators have been developed to assist with endovascular training.

The unique properties of endovascular procedures provide both a blessing and curse for simulation. On one hand, replicating endovascular procedures on a simulator is relatively simple. Proceduralists never actually "see" the coils as they leave the catheter or the actual movement of the catheter or wire, just image representations on biplanar fluoroscopy. As such, simulators must merely capture catheters and wire movements and then produce a visual representation on a screen that mimics fluoroscopy. These factors therefore make simulation of angiographic cases much more simplistic than open surgical procedures, because all that is needed is wire and catheter input. On the other hand, because endovascular skills in real clinical practice demand mastery of subtle hand motions and understanding load on devices and fluid physiology, the haptics of capturing subtle hand movements and the effect of blood hemodynamic factors on simulated device responsiveness must be so much more realistic to make simulation effective and realistic. This means that developing a generic endovascular simulator is relatively straightforward, but designing a realistic one may actually be incredibly complex.

Fortunately, as technology advances, simulators are becoming more and more realistic.

Training modules such as the vascular interventional system trainer [13] developed in Sweden have been demonstrated to significantly improve operator outcomes in the context of lower extremity occlusive disease, cardiac disease, and carotid disease [11, 14–16]. In a prospective observational cohort study, Lee et al. enrolled 41 medical students in an 8-week elective vascular surgery course where they were trained in renal artery stenting using a high-fidelity endovascular simulator [17]. There was a statistically significant improvement in procedure time, accuracy, and overall performance when comparing pre- and post-training sessions [17]. Similarly, Van Herzeele et al. demonstrated a statistically significant improvement in the performance of 11 experienced endovascular interventionalists after attending a 2-day course for carotid artery stenting using endovascular simulators [18]. Improvement in performance can be seen in total procedural times, contrast use, cannulation time, and target accuracy [11]. These and other studies indicate that training with endovascular simulation can improve the performance of novice as well as experienced interventionalists [19, 20].

See et al. performed a meta-analysis of the endovascular simulation literature and found 23 trials showing statistically significant improvements in procedure time, fluoroscopy time, and contrast volume [21]. Five trials were patient-specific procedure rehearsals, demonstrating that simulation significantly affected the fluoroscopy angle and improved performance metrics, and three were randomized controlled trials revealing both overall and procedure-specific improvements after endovascular simulator training, supporting the idea that there is a beneficial role of simulation in endovascular training [21].

Neuroendovascular Simulators

There are two currently available approaches in neuroendovascular simulation: computerized virtual reality simulators and silicone vascular models, with or without a circulation pump. VR simulators are capable of recording the surgeons actions, translating this into a digital performance assessment with quantitative evaluation [2]. On the silicone vascular flow model, the trainee is able to use the material in its dedicated "wet" environment allowing practice with every step of a procedure.

Flow Models

The Replicator (Vascular Simulations, Stoneybrook, NY; Fig. 6.1) is a replica of the human arterial system including a functional left side of the heart. This advanced flow model replicates individual patients' anatomy and pathology, which can be used to perform and practice neuroendovascular procedures prior to clinical treatment. It duplicates the cardiac cycle with a functional left atrium and ventricle, and "blood flow" passes through a silicone aorta with compliance that recreates the waveforms of a human aorta. The cervical vessels arising from the aortic arch and cerebral vasculature are made from imaging studies of the actual patient, and their pathology, such as an intracranial

aneurysm, can be recreated. Additional modules are underdevelopment, including stroke, carotid stenosis, cerebral arteriovenous malformations, abdominal aortic aneurysms, and aortic and mitral stenosis.

Less sophisticated flow models also exist (Video 6.1), with silicone circuits filled with saline with various pathologies (most commonly, cerebral aneurysms), which allow for use under direct vision, or fluoroscopy, to practice using different technologies such as coils, stents, flow diverters, and embolic agents (Fig. 6.2). These have the benefit of being easily portable and are fairly reasonable and are often used to introduce new interventional products to interventionalists, who can practice the deployment of new stents or compare different coils head-to-head. They do have the drawback of absent pulsatile flow, and the absence of catheter stability from the usual femoral arterial access spanning the vascular tree, with redundant catheter eliminating the typical one-to-one tactile feedback that is necessary for precise movement deployment. Arthur et al. observed a shortened learning curve with use of advanced techniques in a high-fidelity simulation environment such as the Replicator, without compromising patient safety [22, 23].

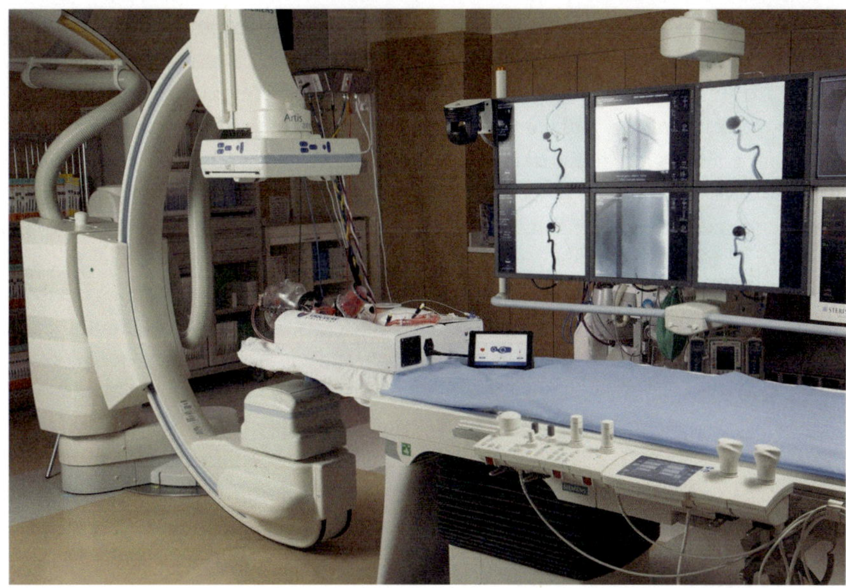

Fig. 6.1 The Replicator simulator (with permission from Vascular Simulations, LLC)

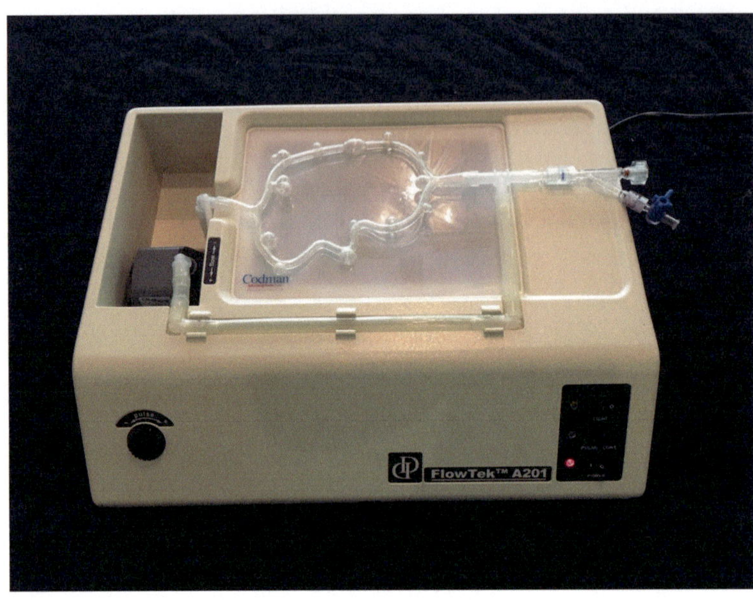

Fig. 6.2 A silicone flow model device with saline pump and simulated aneurysms

VIST- C: Vascular Intervention Systems Training (Mentice, Goteborg, Sweden)

The VIST-C system (Mentice, Goteborg, Sweden) is an endovascular interventional simulator that has a wide variety of applications, from femoral, iliac, aortic, renal, carotid, coronary, to intracerebral vessel simulation (Fig. 6.3). It is a portable, high-fidelity endovascular simulator (Video 6.1). This system makes use of actual endovascular catheters and wires engaged along internal tracking wheels that are introduced through a port, capturing fine movements of the catheter in all planes [24]. Virtual contrast is simulated by the injection of air by a syringe, and advanced haptics provide sensory feedback using force feedback technology [25]. There are a wide variety of training scenarios with actual devices and equipment used in clinical practice to challenge the learner's technical skills, clinical decision-making abilities, and procedural proficiency.

ANGIO Mentor: Simbionix (3D Systems, Littleton, CO)

The Simbionix ANGIO Mentor system (3D Systems, Littleton, CO) provides an interactive biplanar fluoroscopic display for both diagnostic and interventional case scenarios. The system is able to incorporate a wide variety of sheaths, diagnostic catheters, and guide wires and measure their unique mechanical properties in constructing the simulation [26]. The system uses the mechanistic properties of the catheters and wire such as shear and Young's modulus, to measure the wire manipulations by tracking horizontal translation and rolls at a fixed position, and translates this visually onto the screen [26]. Vessels exert varying forces to keep the catheter intraluminally, and software calculates the collision forces of the catheter into the vessel wall [26]. This combined information allows the system to simulate the position of the catheter in the vessel by calculating values such as angulation, friction, and forward loading, for high-end haptic feedback, which realistically mimics actual endovascular interventions.

The system features over 23 different endovascular procedures and 158 patient scenarios and spans multiple disciplines, including interventional cardiology, interventional radiology, vascular surgery, cardiothoracic surgery, electrophysiology, interventional neuroradiology, trauma, and neurosurgery. The PROcedure Rehearsal Studio (3D Systems, Littleton, CO) can

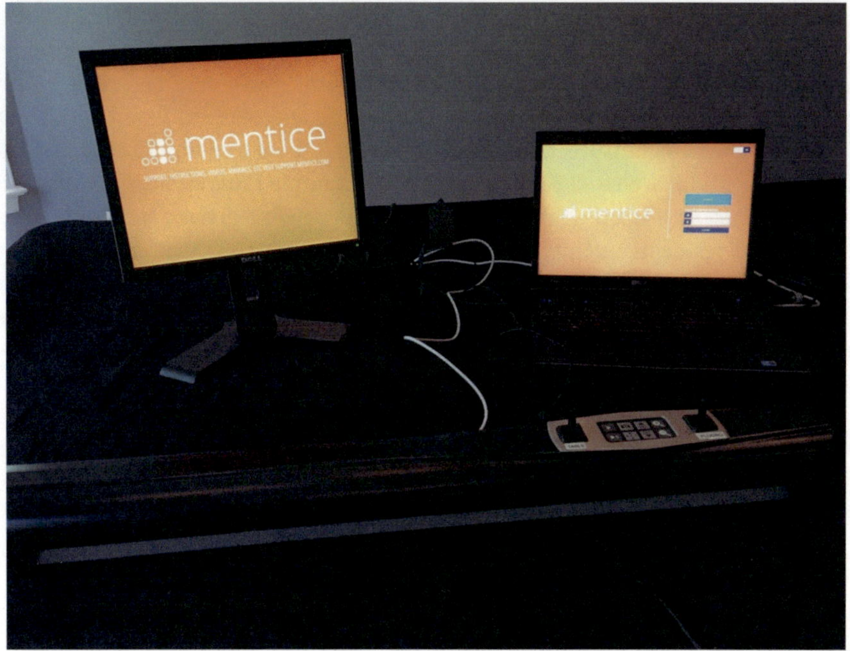

Fig. 6.3 The Mentice simulator with simulated table and foot pedal controls (not shown)

be used to prepare for upcoming interventions creation of a patient-specific 3D model based on scanned images. This 3D model can be exported to a virtual simulation environment or physically printed by 3D printers, for the purpose of simulating, analyzing, and evaluating surgical treatment options.

Compass: Medical Simulation Corporation (Medical Simulation Corporation, Denver, CO)

The Compass (Medical Simulation Corporation, Denver, CO) is a more portable endovascular simulator. It fits into a single case similar to a rolling suitcase and can be checked as luggage on an airplane. It can be set up within minutes and used on a conventional table for single use on a high-fidelity screen or projected to a large screen display for large group training. Tactile feedback is provided with anatomical variations and upon device deployment. A tablet is used to control elements such as contrast injection or C-arm movement.

Endovascular Simulation in Neurosurgical Training

Endovascular techniques are a skill set entirely separate from that of "open" neurosurgical technique. While traditional neurosurgical residency focuses on the use of two-hand instrument and suction techniques under direct visualization (and often with the aid of magnification), endovascular procedures involve the subtle manipulation of wire and catheter with the results visualized on a monitor. While both techniques require considerable repetition to master, importantly mastery of endovascular techniques is not predicated on proficiency in open neurosurgical techniques and vice versa. While this fact seems obvious as interventional neuroradiologists and neurologists perform endovascular surgeries, it represents an important distinction in neurosurgical training. Importantly, the lack of prerequisite skills means that trainees may learn and practice these skills at any point in their training. This is unlike many other specializations within neurosurgery. For example, consider neurosurgery residents that would like to complete an open cerebrovascular microsurgery fellowship to acquire mastery in vascular microneurosurgery. Before being a suitable fellow where surgical nuance can be learned, applicants must first master general neurosurgery to provide a foundation on which new skills can be acquired. Therefore, in-folded fellowships where inexperienced residents attempt to learn complex microneurosurgery are not feasible. However, endovascular skills do not require a foundation of neurosurgical skill and can therefore be learned at any point during neurosurgery residency training. The fact that medical students, residents, and even fully trained attending neurosurgeons may potentially be equally equipped to acquire endovascular skills means that there is a potential role for endovascular simulator learning across the entire training spectrum. This may widen the applicability of an endovascular simulation and may maximize yield for departments looking to employ simulation in their residency training program.

While there is increasing utility of simulation in residency training in interventional radiology and general surgery, simulation in neurosurgical training is lagging slightly behind that of other specialties [24]. However, pilot projects of endovascular simulation show excellent utility for this training modality [24]. With the primary objective of providing education in the fundamental principles of angiography, anatomy identification, catheter selection, fundamentals of catheter and wire interaction, reducing radiation exposure, and basic angiography, Fargen et al. demonstrated that a hands-on simulator course (VIST-C, Mentice, Goteborg, Sweden) for neurosurgery residents with no prior experience increases performance and trainee knowledge, creating a viable means to train residents early on [24]. Pre- and post-training tests, including general principles of angiographic anatomy, procedures, and indications, as well as objective data including fluoroscopy time, time to target vessel cannulation, and volume of contrast used, all showed a statistically significant improvement [24].

Another neurosurgical pilot study by Spiotta et al. used the Simbionix system (Simbionix USA Crop, Cleveland, OH) to assess the utility of endovascular simulation in neurosurgical residents and fellows with varied experience [26]. Each participant was asked the number of angiograms performed and their knowledge of the aortic and cervical vascular anatomy, along with their level of comfort on catheter selection and technique [26]. Residents with limited prior experience were given a short didactic presentation regarding basic anatomy of the aorta and its branches, properties, and geometry of diagnostic catheter and guide wires, basic technique of crossing the arch, and selective catheterization [26]. The residents reported a paucity of exposure to cerebral angiograms (50% having never observed one, 2 with <5 observed, and 1 with >10 observed) [26]. All fellows had performed more than 100 cases [26]. Regardless of prior exposure to angiography, all participants, both residents and fellows, showed an improvement in the trials as demonstrated by fluoroscopy times [26]. There were no serious simulated complications during the training session, although residents with little prior exposure were noted to perform occasional "dangerous" maneuvers, which were corrected with real-time instruction [26].

A similar study format was used to assess training residents in more complex aortic arch anatomy using a secondary curve catheter [27]. The training protocol started with a 5-min didactic session covering basic and complex aortic arch anatomy using a primary and secondary curve catheter and consisted of five trials with all participants showing a statistically significant improvement in overall time required for selective catheterization using a Simmons II catheter [27].

Building off of these pilot studies, a 120-min simulator-based training course was performed at two subsequent Congress of Neurological Surgeons (CNS) annual meetings [24]. Pre-course written and simulator skills assessments were performed in 37 neurosurgical trainees, followed by instructor-guided training on an endovascular simulator. Post-course written and simulator practical assessments were then performed. Posttest written scores were significantly higher than pretest scores ($p < 0.001$), and instructor assessments of practical posttest scores of participants were significantly higher than pretest practical scores for both the CNS 2011 and CNS 2012 groups ($P < 0.001$), again indicating that simulation may be an effective method of teaching certain neuroendovascular skills [22].

Ernst et al. assessed key competencies and analyzed associations between the clinical experience, knowledge, and technical skill [2, 28]. All participants were European interventionalists ($N = 26$) who performed a middle cerebral artery (MCA) M1 segment thrombectomy for acute stroke and embolized a posterior communicating artery aneurysm on the ANGIO Mentor (3D Solutions,) after a brief didactic session. The Replicator (Vascular Simulations, Stony Brook NY) was used for embolization of a MCA bifurcation aneurysm with an intra-saccular flow disrupter (WEBTM Aneurysm Embolization System, Sequent, California) [28].

This study provides an example of a curriculum that reasonably and cost-effectively assesses certain competencies of a neuroendovascular surgeon in terms of theoretical knowledge and practical skills. Time of work experience does not guarantee clinical judgment or expertise; however, there are significant associations between theoretical knowledge and practical skills [2]. Moreover, technical knowledge (i.e., material and techniques) does seem to be associated with technical skill in aneurysm coiling and thrombectomy [2]. The assessment of procedural skills by the use of endovascular simulators has proven to be a feasible approach to yield objective data for evaluating technical competency [2].

Benefits and Limitations

Neuroendovascular surgery is now a clear component of neurosurgical residency training. Recently, there has been increasing emphasis placed upon inclusion of neurointerventional surgical skills within the core neurosurgical competencies, manifested by an increase in the Residency Review Committee case minimums and focus on angiographic skills and knowledge in Intern Boot camps and the written and oral board examinations. Therefore it is important that resident training programs incorporate new methods of educating trainees in neuroendovascular surgery while being compliant to work hour restrictions and not sacrificing training in other areas of neurosurgery [24].

Use of simulation in endovascular training has risen sharply, and technological advances in simulation now more closely resemble real clinical scenarios [24, 29, 30]. New devices with augmented reality simulation, combine simulation with real-world surgical devices, provide haptic feedback and with close resemblance to actual endovascular surgery [24]. Additionally, systems can now recreate actual patient anatomy and pathology, with can be used to size devices and practice treatment configurations prior to actual patient treatment. The literature demonstrates a correlation between technical skill on a simulator and clinical endovascular experience [19, 31–33], suggesting that currently available simulators mimic clinical conditions closely enough to translate into improved clinical skill [33]. Furthermore, there is data that shows even skilled interventionalists have continued benefit from simulation courses [24].

One of the greatest benefits of simulation is repetitive practice in a risk free environment. Learning of sequential steps, with the ability to repeat after correction of any mistake, is a key component to successful technical skill. Simulation allows for education without risk to patient safety, cost of medical equipment, or lab costs and time constraints. This type of learning environment is both beneficial and efficient. Simulators have several other advantages, in that they do not require radiation dose and are customizable on a case-by-case basis. Similar to other disciplines, there is a strong suggestion that skills acquired on the simulator might be transferable to the real patients in the angiography suite [2, 26, 34, 35].

However, there remain significant limitations to simulation-based training. Skills such as material preparation outside the patient cannot be trained and assessed by simulators [2]. Availability and cost remain large limitations, and to date, the haptic feedback, while significantly improved from previous generations of simulators, is still not exactly that of real-world experience. Importantly, electronic simulators do not yet have a means of adequately simulating a fluid medium that incorporates blood stasis, contrast injection, or flushing. A key skill set in endovascular technique, particularly for learners, is the prevention of air or clot embolism. Inadvertent injection of air or stagnation of blood in a catheter with resultant embolism may have dire consequences to patients. Focus on perfect technique in the presence of a hazardous fluid medium is an integral component of learning neurointerventional techniques. Unfortunately, every electronic simulator does not yet have the capability to teach learners this critical skill set. Additionally, because the simulation setting is a risk free environment and often goes unsupervised by faculty, poor technique may fail to generate real clinical consequence and may foster poor habits if no proper feedback is provided to the trainee [24].

The Future

Future studies are needed to confirm the efficacy of simulation in endovascular surgical training and to probe whether simulation is a useful adjunct to traditional training in the endovascular lab. Furthermore, research is needed to validate whether skills acquired on the simulator are transferrable to the clinical setting, and if simulator training actually improves safety and quality of patient care. The accuracy of the simulator is of utmost importance for quality training to take place with the use of neurosimulation platforms. A further step from just using the simulator as a training module is to use the simulator to "practice" difficult cases before the actual procedure. The high-fidelity simulation platform would be ideal for a "trial" treatment of many vascular conditions to assess the quality of the planned procedure; however, one must keep in mind that this is under the assumption that the simulator is an accurate depiction of in vivo conditions. It is an exciting time for neurosimulation with many more developments to come that would further advance endovascular treatment of neurovascular conditions.

References

1. Andersen SA, Konge L, Caye-Thomasen P, Sorensen MS. Retention of mastoidectomy skills after virtual reality simulation training. JAMA Otolaryngol Head Neck Surg. 2016;142:635–40.
2. Dayal AK, Fisher N, Magrane D, Goffman D, Bernstein PS, Katz NT. Simulation training improves medical students' learning experiences when performing real vaginal deliveries. Simul Healthc. 2009;4:155–9.
3. Dawe SR, Pena GN, Windsor JA, et al. Systematic review of skills transfer after surgical simulation-based training. Br J Surg. 2014;101:1063–76.
4. Dawe SR, Windsor JA, Broeders JA, Cregan PC, Hewett PJ, Maddern GJ. A systematic review of surgical skills transfer after simulation-based training: laparoscopic cholecystectomy and endoscopy. Ann Surg. 2014;259:236–48.
5. Sturm LP, Windsor JA, Cosman PH, Cregan P, Hewett PJ, Maddern GJ. A systematic review of skills transfer after surgical simulation training. Ann Surg. 2008;248:166–79.
6. Dorozhkin D, Nemani A, Roberts K, et al. Face and content validation of a Virtual Translumenal Endoscopic Surgery Trainer (VTEST). Surg Endosc. 2016;30:5529–36.
7. Boza C, Leon F, Buckel E, et al. Simulation-trained junior residents perform better than general surgeons on advanced laparoscopic cases. Surg Endosc. 2016;31:135–41.
8. Scott DJ, Ritter EM, Tesfay ST, Pimentel EA, Nagji A, Fried GM. Certification pass rate of 100% for fundamentals of laparoscopic surgery skills after proficiency-based training. Surg Endosc. 2008;22:1887–93.
9. Waterman BR, Martin KD, Cameron KL, Owens BD, Belmont PJ Jr. Simulation training improves surgical proficiency and safety during diagnostic shoulder arthroscopy performed by residents. Orthopedics. 2016;39:1–7.
10. Shore EM, Grantcharov TP, Husslein H, et al. Validating a standardized laparoscopy curriculum for gynecology residents: a randomized controlled trial. Am J Obstet Gynecol. 2016;215:204.e1–204.e11.
11. Narra P, Kuban J, Grandpre LE, Singh J, Barrero J, Norbash A. Videoscopic phantom-based angiographic simulation: effect of brief angiographic simulator practice on vessel cannulation times. J Vasc Interv Radiol. 2009;20:1215–23.
12. Ahmed K, Keeling AN, Fakhry M, et al. Role of virtual reality simulation in teaching and assessing technical skills in endovascular intervention. J Vasc Interv Radiol. 2010;21:55–66.
13. Rodriguez D, Berenguera A, Pujol-Ribera E, Capella J, Peray JL, Roma J. Current and future competencies for public health professionals. Gac Sanit. 2013;27:388–97.

14. Chaer RA, Derubertis BG, Lin SC, et al. Simulation improves resident performance in catheter-based intervention: results of a randomized, controlled study. Ann Surg. 2006;244:343–52.
15. Patel AD, Gallagher AG, Nicholson WJ, Cates CU. Learning curves and reliability measures for virtual reality simulation in the performance assessment of carotid angiography. J Am Coll Cardiol. 2006;47:1796–802.
16. Gallagher AG, Renkin J, Buyl H, Lambert H, Marco J. Development and construct validation of performance metrics for multivessel coronary interventions on the VIST virtual reality simulator at PCR2005. EuroIntervention. 2006;2:101–6.
17. Lee JT, Qiu M, Teshome M, Raghavan SS, Tedesco MM, Dalman RL. The utility of endovascular simulation to improve technical performance and stimulate continued interest of preclinical medical students in vascular surgery. J Surg Educ. 2009;66:367–73.
18. Van Herzeele I, Aggarwal R, Neequaye S, et al. Experienced endovascular interventionalists objectively improve their skills by attending carotid artery stent training courses. Eur J Vasc Endovasc Surg. 2008;35:541–50.
19. Van Herzeele I, Aggarwal R, Choong A, Brightwell R, Vermassen FE, Cheshire NJ. Virtual reality simulation objectively differentiates level of carotid stent experience in experienced interventionalists. J Vasc Surg. 2007;46:855–63.
20. Dawson DL, Meyer J, Lee ES, Pevec WC. Training with simulation improves residents' endovascular procedure skills. J Vasc Surg. 2007;45:149–54.
21. See KW, Chui KH, Chan WH, Wong KC, Chan YC. Evidence for endovascular simulation training: a systematic review. Eur J Vasc Endovasc Surg. 2016;51:441–51.
22. Fargen KM, Arthur AS, Bendok BR, et al. Experience with a simulator-based angiography course for neurosurgical residents: beyond a pilot program. Neurosurgery. 2013;73(Suppl 1):46–50.
23. Arthur A, Hoit D, Coon A, Delgado Almandoz JE, Elijovich L, Cekirge S, Fiorella D. Physician training within the WEB Intrasaccular Therapy (WEB-IT) study. J Neurointerv Surg. 2018;10(5):500–4.
24. Fargen KM, Siddiqui AH, Veznedaroglu E, Turner RD, Ringer AJ, Mocco J. Simulator based angiography education in neurosurgery: results of a pilot educational program. J Neurointerv Surg. 2012;4:438–41.
25. Jensen UJ, Jensen J, Olivecrona GK, Ahlberg G, Tornvall P. Technical skills assessment in a coronary angiography simulator for construct validation. Simul Healthc. 2013;8:324–8.
26. Spiotta AM, Rasmussen PA, Masaryk TJ, Benzel EC, Schlenk R. Simulated diagnostic cerebral angiography in neurosurgical training: a pilot program. J Neurointerv Surg. 2013;5:376–81.
27. Spiotta AM, Kellogg RT, Vargas J, Chaudry MI, Turk AS, Turner RD. Diagnostic angiography skill acquisition with a secondary curve catheter: phase 2 of a curriculum-based endovascular simulation program. J Neurointerv Surg. 2015;7:777–80.
28. Ernst M, Kriston L, Romero JM, et al. Quantitative evaluation of performance in interventional neuroradiology: an integrated curriculum featuring theoretical and practical challenges. PLoS One. 2016;11:e0148694.
29. Lemole GM Jr, Banerjee PP, Luciano C, Neckrysh S, Charbel FT. Virtual reality in neurosurgical education: part-task ventriculostomy simulation with dynamic visual and haptic feedback. Neurosurgery 2007;61:142–8; discussion 8–9.
30. Botden SM, Torab F, Buzink SN, Jakimowicz JJ. The importance of haptic feedback in laparoscopic suturing training and the additive value of virtual reality simulation. Surg Endosc. 2008;22:1214–22.
31. Bech B, Lonn L, Falkenberg M, et al. Construct validity and reliability of structured assessment of endoVascular expertise in a simulated setting. Eur J Vasc Endovasc Surg. 2011;42:539–48.
32. Van Herzeele I, Aggarwal R, Malik I, et al. Validation of video-based skill assessment in carotid artery stenting. Eur J Vasc Endovasc Surg. 2009;38:1–9.
33. Tedesco MM, Pak JJ, Harris EJ Jr, Krummel TM, Dalman RL, Lee JT. Simulation-based endovascular skills assessment: the future of credentialing? J Vasc Surg. 2008;47:1008–1; discussion 14.
34. Stolarek I. Procedural and examination skills of first-year house surgeons: a comparison of a simulation workshop versus 6 months of clinical ward experience alone. N Z Med J. 2007;120:U2516.
35. Smith CC, Huang GC, Newman LR, et al. Simulation training and its effect on long-term resident performance in central venous catheterization. Simul Healthc. 2010;5:146–51.

Part III

Biological Models Simulation

Biological Models for Neurosurgical Training in Microanastomosis

7

Evgenii Belykh, Michael A. Bohl, Kaith K. Almefty, Mark C. Preul, and Peter Nakaji

Abbreviation

STA   Superficial Temporal Artery
IACUC   Institutional Animal Care and Use Committee

Introduction

Cerebral arteries differ from arteries in the extracranial vasculature by having a thinner wall and by lacking an external elastic membrane. These differences make intracranial vessels more susceptible to certain vascular pathologies [1], such as moyamoya disease, atherosclerotic occlusions, intracranial aneurysms, and arteriovenous malformations. Each of these pathologies poses unique surgical challenges, and cerebro-

vascular neurosurgeons must be proficient in the microsurgical treatment of all of them. As a result, neurosurgeons must become proficient in a large number of complex microvascular surgical skills. Furthermore, these skills are often needed in emergent situations, in which the difference between a good and a poor outcome can be measured in seconds and minutes; thus, developing speed is also essential. Microvascular techniques must therefore be developed in advance so that the neurosurgeon is prepared when presented with a cerebrovascular problem or emergency. However, given the increasingly regulated work-hour rules for residents, the demand on training centers to deliver faster care, and the increasing number of patients being treated by endovascular techniques, it can be difficult for residents to obtain the practical experience necessary to become proficient in these techniques. Therefore, simple and accessible models for microvascular training are increasingly providing a key means to develop, refine, and preserve this surgical skill set.

Developing adequate simulation models for cerebrovascular procedures requires replication of the peculiarities of the surgical environment. Such situational conditions include a craniotomy that limits surgical freedom and provides a surface for hand support, narrow surgical corridors with or without [2] brain retractors, eloquence of the surrounding brain, fragility and softness of the surrounding brain tissue, and the presence of

E. Belykh
Department of Neurosurgery, Barrow Neurological Institute, St. Joseph's Hospital and Medical Center, Phoenix, AZ, USA

Department of Neurosurgery, Irkutsk State Medical University, Irkutsk, Russia

M. A. Bohl · K. K. Almefty · M. C. Preul · P. Nakaji (✉)
Department of Neurosurgery, Barrow Neurological Institute, St. Joseph's Hospital and Medical Center, Phoenix, AZ, USA
e-mail: Neuropub@barrowneuro.org

© Springer International Publishing AG, part of Springer Nature 2018   91
A. Alaraj (ed.), *Comprehensive Healthcare Simulation: Neurosurgery*,
Comprehensive Healthcare Simulation, https://doi.org/10.1007/978-3-319-75583-0_7

cerebrospinal fluid. Another important dimension in the surgical environment is timing, as most cerebrovascular procedures are a race against time because temporary clips or vessel compromise can result in irreversible brain ischemia or stroke. Small perforating arteries contribute an additional layer of complexity to the surgical environment.

In addition to these anatomical variables, the microsurgical environment presents specific dynamic conditions, such as surface tension, magnetism, tensile strength of adventitia, adhesions, and contractility of vessels. Finally, the tools of the neurosurgeon must be considered; these include the operating microscope, long bayoneted instruments, microdissectors, and other instruments unique to microsurgery. Together, these variables create an environment with which all neurosurgeons must become familiar before being able to safely perform intracranial microsurgical procedures.

It is a well-accepted rule that microanastomosis skills should be perfected in the laboratory before being applied during surgery on a real patient. Participating in a microsurgical training course and learning basic microsurgical skills and principles should serve as the starting point for further training in the laboratory. Microanastomosis practice should consist of three integral parts. First, trainees should attend an annual microsurgical course, where they can learn new techniques on high-fidelity models, with expert faculty assistance readily available. During future courses, trainees can reassess their techniques and experience gained during the past year and get coaching and feedback from experts. Second, they should perform daily self-driven exercises on readily available models [3]. Simple biological or artificial models can be used for this useful approach to maintaining and improving basic microsurgical techniques (Fig. 7.1). Third, they should practice microsurgery in the operating room where learned techniques should be safely applied to dissect the arachnoid membrane, handle cerebral arteries and veins, and suture microvascular anastomoses. This combination of teaching modalities represents an ideal algorithm for

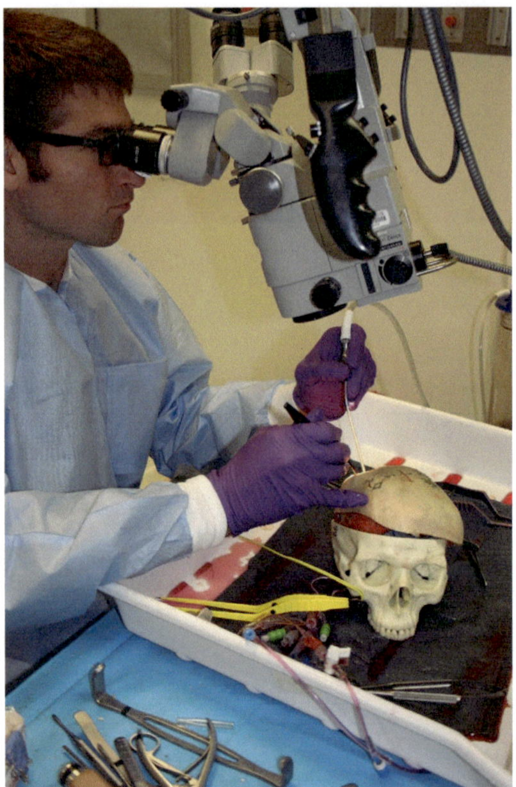

Fig. 7.1 Microvascular surgery practice on a placenta model during the bypass course at Barrow Neurological Institute. (Used with permission from Barrow Neurological Institute, Phoenix, Arizona)

training and maintenance of manual skills (Fig. 7.2). A number of training models exist for daily self-driven practice, including both dry and wet materials representing low-fidelity and high-fidelity simulations, respectively. Training with these models should be developed in a graduated fashion, beginning first with dry material before progressing to wet training on biological simulation models. This chapter focuses on biological simulation models for microvascular surgical training.

Laboratory for Biological Models

The addition of biological models to resident laboratory education requires adequate facilities with the necessary equipment, supplies, and material for safely handling and disposing of

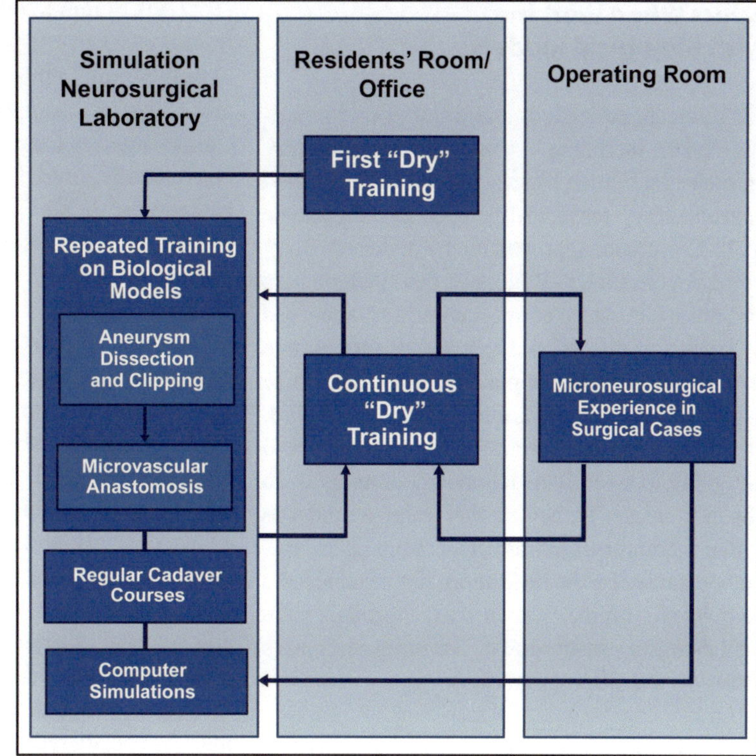

Fig. 7.2 Algorithm of microneurosurgical manual skill training. The training begins with dry suturing training, followed by annually repeating courses that include a bypass course, and a microsurgical anatomy and surgical approaches to the brain course. Ideally, rapidly available practice modules are placed in the residents' room for individual practice. Finally, microneurosurgical manual skills are refined and combined with the knowledge of microsurgical anatomy in the operating room. (Used with permission from Barrow Neurological Institute, Phoenix, Arizona)

human and animal tissue. In a survey of 100 US neurosurgical residency programs (65% response rate), 95.4% of residency program directors believed that a dissection laboratory should be an obligatory component of a neurosurgical training program [4]. In addition to using the laboratory to learn microsurgical anatomy, trainees can use it to safely gain proficiency and comfort working under the operating microscope with microsurgical instruments. The laboratory should comply with institutional regulations, and when possible, it should be located near other research departments for collaboration and to decrease costs via shared equipment. Surgical rooms with additional appropriate equipment and resources are necessary for animal survival experiments and for work with larger laboratory animals.

Although the list of necessary laboratory equipment varies by the type of training being conducted, basic neurosurgical instruments and operating microscopes should be standard. Additional standard equipment includes a working table; a sink with a water faucet; good venti-lation; shelves for books, instruments, supplies, and educational materials; and cabinets for chemicals.

Ideally, a neuroscience research laboratory should include a sterile operating room for survival experiments on small and large animals, an angiography suite for endovascular research and training, a skull base laboratory for anatomical studies, and a laboratory for interdisciplinary basic science projects and cell work. Additional facilities may include a room with computer workstations for trainees to use, walk-in freezers to store cadavers, an autoclave and instrument cleaning room, a conference room, a large dissection hall for instructional courses, and staff offices. There also may be a practice laboratory that contains the necessary equipment for basic microsurgical training on both silicone and biological models (such as turkey wings or chicken wings) [5]. This practice laboratory provides a convenient and rapidly available setup for training that could be performed almost every day [3].

Ethics When Working with Biological Models

All research, education, and training on biological models, including live and nonlive laboratory animals and human tissues, should be conducted appropriately, respectfully, and in accordance with the protocol approved by the dedicated institutional committee. Protocols that include rats and other laboratory animals should be approved by an institutional animal care and use committee (IACUC). Protocols for placenta usage should be approved by an institutional review board. Obtaining appropriate training for personnel who are going to work with laboratory animals is an absolute necessity before the trainees undergo actual laboratory training. Such training is usually organized by the institution, but it can also be completed online, such as through the Collaborative Institutional Training Initiative (https://www.citiprogram.org/).

Microsurgical Practice on Poultry Arteries

Fresh or frozen poultry are an excellent source of small vessels for microvascular practice. Chicken wing arteries were initially used for anastomosis practice after a report by Hino [6]. Later, arteries from turkey wings were used, and they are now preferred because the arteries are longer and of larger diameter than those from chickens (1.47 ± 0.14 mm in the turkey vs 1.07 ± 0.25 mm in the chicken) [5]. These vessel dimensions closely resemble those of human middle cerebral and superficial temporal arteries (Fig. 7.3) [5]. Carotid arteries from the turkey neck can also be conveniently used [7]. Poultry arteries can be catheterized in situ [8] or dissected out and then connected to a pressurized line or syringe to simulate blood flow.

A vessel that is 4–6 cm in length and 1.5 mm in diameter is useful for a wide spectrum of microvascular exercises, including all types of anastomoses (end to side, end to end, and side to side), microsurgical creation of aneurysms, and aneurysm clip application. The chicken wing can also be used to practice dissection skills under endoscopic visualization [9]. We have also successfully used small-diameter (1.5 mm) arteries from turkey wings to practice the manipulation and suturing of arteries under three-dimensional endoscopic visualization.

Several properties of dead nonhuman tissues must be considered when these tissues are used in microsurgical training. Differences in the vessel wall structure of the human cerebral arteries and the animal peripheral arteries provide different tactile feedback. Nonetheless, such biological models provide much greater fidelity than artificial models. Another important consideration is that small poultry arteries can become dry and stiff much faster and more readily than arteries in live models, thus requiring frequent moistening. Isotonic solutions are better than plain water for

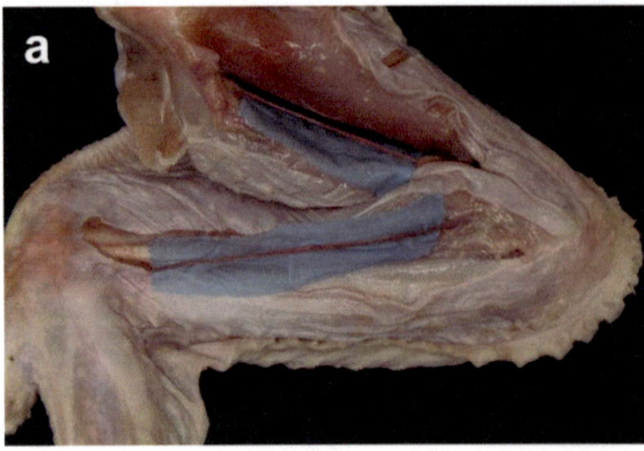
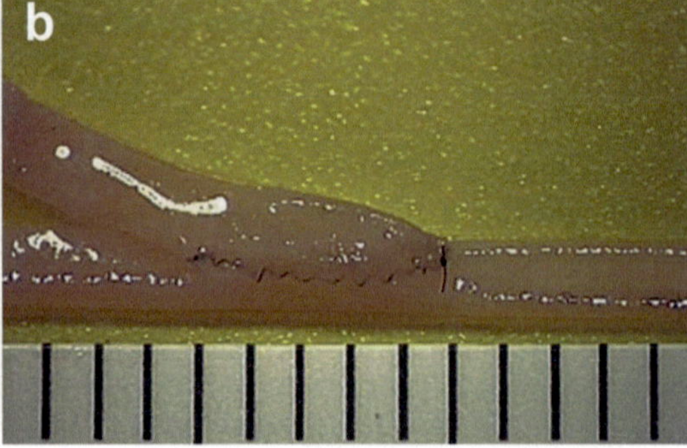

Fig. 7.3 Turkey wing model for microvascular practice. (**a**) Overview of dissected artery. (**b**) Completed end-to-side anastomosis. ((**a**) is used with permission from Barrow Neurological Institute, Phoenix, Arizona; (**b**) is used with permission from Abla et al. [5])

moistening chicken and turkey tissue specimens because the water leads to tissue swelling. A moistened cottonoid placed close to the working area can help to keep the area wet, and it will prevent excessive pooling of liquid. Poultry tissue can be frozen and thawed several times; however, it will increasingly become soft and flabby, which decreases its simulative quality. This model is convenient for biological training because it is easily accessible from commercial vendors to consumers (e.g., grocery stores), only a short time is needed to dissect the vessel and begin practice, and no regulatory supervision is necessary from an IACUC or an institutional review board.

Microsurgical Practice on Placental Vessels

Human placenta is one of the most realistic biological models on which to practice microsurgical tasks on small vessels (Fig. 7.4). The average human placenta weighs 500 g and has two surfaces, a fetal surface and a maternal surface. The fetal surface is covered by a thin amniotic layer that resembles the arachnoid membrane. Arteries and veins diverge radially from the place of the umbilical cord attachment on the fetal surface beneath the amniotic membrane.

A study comparing the quantitative histologic properties of human and bovine placentas showed that they are adequate substitutes for tissue models of brain vasculature [10]. This study found that the diameter of distal human placental arteries closely approximates the size of the M2–M4 segments of the middle cerebral arteries and the superficial temporal artery (STA) (Fig. 7.5). The thickness of the arterial media layer of 1-mm diameter distal placental arteries approximates the dimensions of the media layer of the M4, and the thickness of the media layer of 1.8-mm diameter placental arteries approximates the dimensions of the media layer of the STA. In addition, reticular fiber layers of placental arteries approximate those of arteries in the cerebrovasculature. The thickness of the reticular fiber layers of distal placental arteries approximates the thickness of the reticular fiber layer of the M4, and the thickness of the reticular fiber layers of 1.8-mm diameter placental arteries approximates the dimensions of the reticular fiber layers of the STA. The same study examined the differences between trained neurosurgeons and untrained course participants when using this model, and data confirmed the validity of the placenta model as a microvascular anastomosis training tool [10].

Most hospitals have maternity departments from which screened placentas can be obtained. Preparation of a placenta for microsurgical training takes approximately 5 min and includes removing the excess amniotic membranes, washing to remove excess blood, and catheterizing and flushing the two arteries and the vein of the umbilical cord. Additional preparation may include the creation of aneurysms on the placental vessels by inserting and inflating endovascular

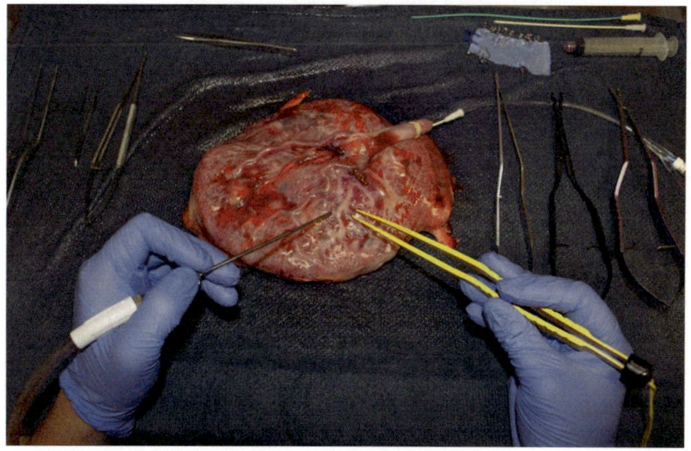

Fig. 7.4 Human placenta model for microvascular practice. The placenta is cleaned and connected to pressurized flow. Microdissection is practiced with a suction device and a bipolar device. (Used with permission from Barrow Neurological Institute, Phoenix, Arizona)

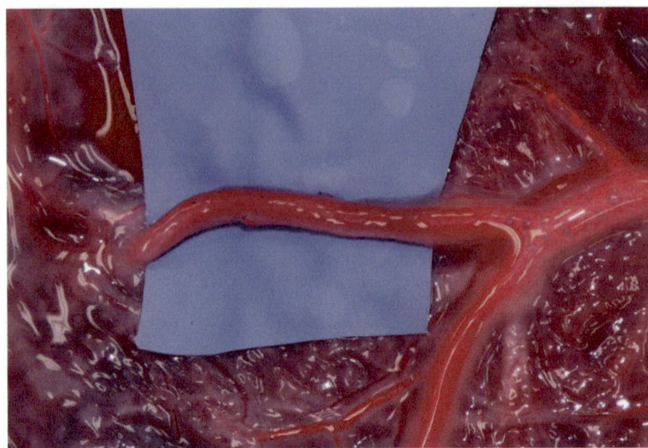

Fig. 7.5 A dissected segment of a human placental artery. (Used with permission from Barrow Neurological Institute, Phoenix, Arizona)

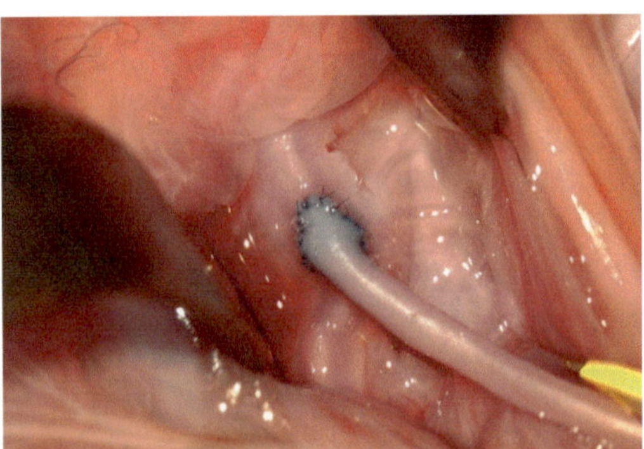

Fig. 7.6 Completed end-to-side anastomosis of the placental arteries. Self-retaining retractors are used to create a working corridor through the overlying second placenta. (Used with permission from Barrow Neurological Institute, Phoenix, Arizona)

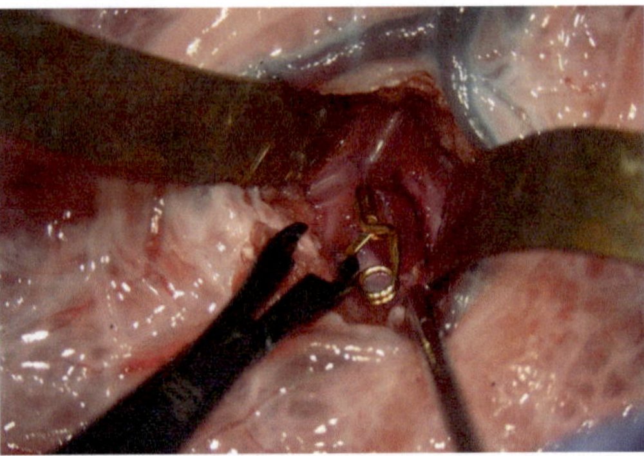

Fig. 7.7 Simulation of an aneurysm clipping using a placental artery, with a corridor through a second placenta used to simulate a craniotomy and the transsylvian approach. (Used with permission from Barrow Neurological Institute, Phoenix, Arizona)

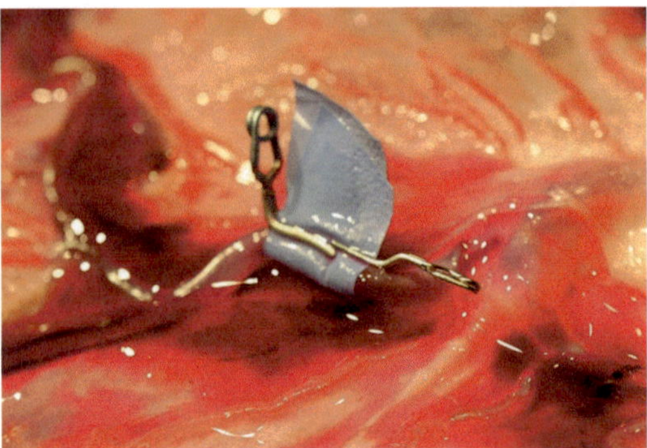

Fig. 7.8 Clip-wrapping technique practice using a placental artery. (Used with permission from Barrow Neurological Institute, Phoenix, Arizona)

balloons. Placentas can also be connected to pressurized containers of colored dye to make the arteries look and feel perfused. Additionally, two or more placentas can be stacked to simulate working through a narrow corridor, mimicking cerebral surgery.

The placenta model as a material for microsurgical practice has recently gained attention. Multiple reports describe exercises using it, such as various microvascular anastomoses (Fig. 7.6) [10, 11], aneurysm creation and subsequent clipping (Fig. 7.7) or wrapping (Fig. 7.8) [12, 13], and simulation of brain tumor microdissection [14].

The major advantage of this model is that the fresh human placenta has all the tensile properties of human tissue. Moreover, arteries on the fetal surface of the placenta are quite similar to human cerebral arteries, and they are covered with the amniotic membrane, which allows a similar experience to working with cerebral vessels that are covered with arachnoid membrane (Fig. 7.9). The walls of placental and cerebral arteries have similar histologic structures. The

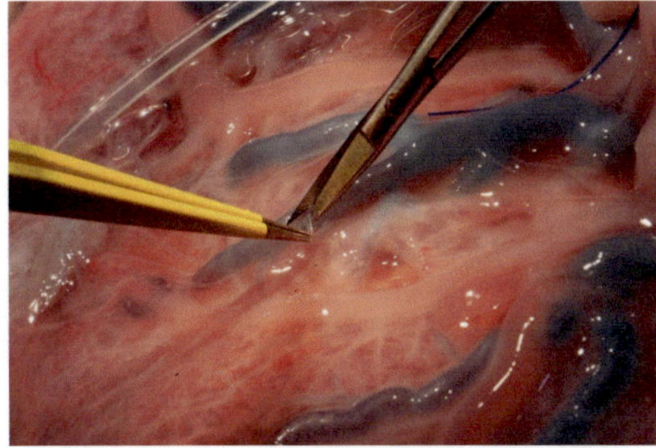

Fig. 7.9 Sharp dissection of the thin amniotic membrane, which resembles dissection of the arachnoid membrane. (Used with permission from Barrow Neurological Institute, Phoenix, Arizona)

limitations of the placental model include restricted usage time (usually about 1–2 weeks). A placenta can and should be used numerous times or by numerous trainees before it begins to decay and has to be discarded. In addition, human placentas carry a risk of infection; donors should be adequately screened before obtaining their consent for use of the placenta, and exposure of the trainees should be minimized by the use of blood-proof gloves, gowns, and splash protection. A final limitation of the placental model is that it does not simulate human brain anatomy or cerebrospinal fluid.

Bovine placentas can also be used as a biological model, and they afford a plethora of vessels for training. The average bovine placenta weighs about 5 kg and consists of about 100 cotyledons distributed on the amnionic membrane that are connected with the umbilical cord by long arterial and venous vessels of various diameters (Fig. 7.10). The large placental branches are similar in size to human

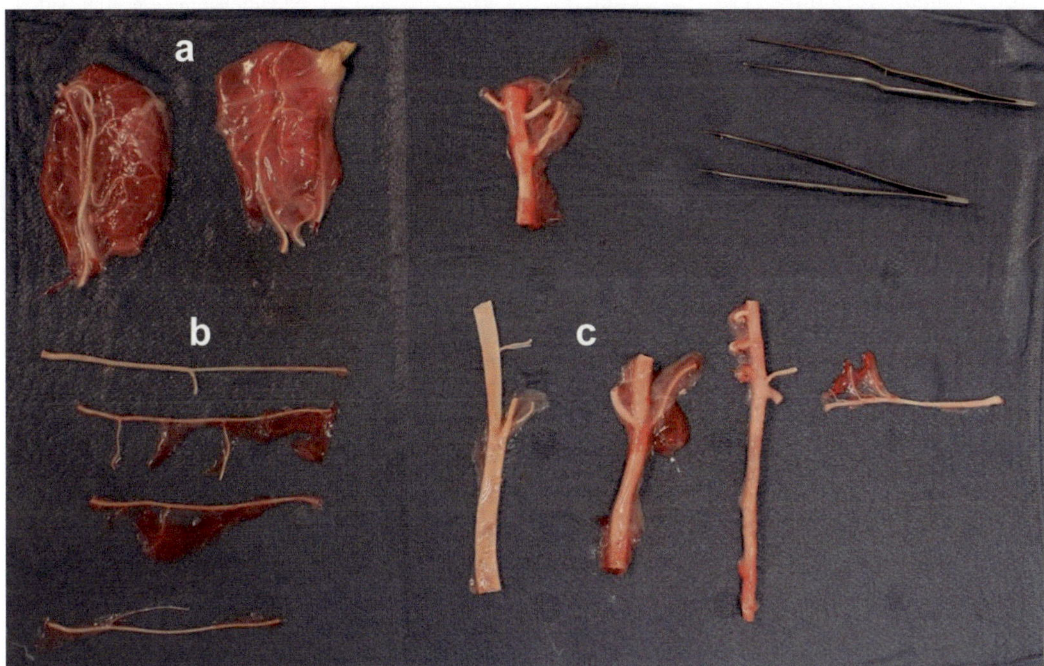

Fig. 7.10 Examples of several vascular segments dissected from a single bovine placenta, including separate cotyledons (**a**) and long small-diameter branches (**b**) that approximate a radial artery graft. Larger vascular segments (**c**) approximate human carotid arteries. (Used with permission from Barrow Neurological Institute, Phoenix, Arizona)

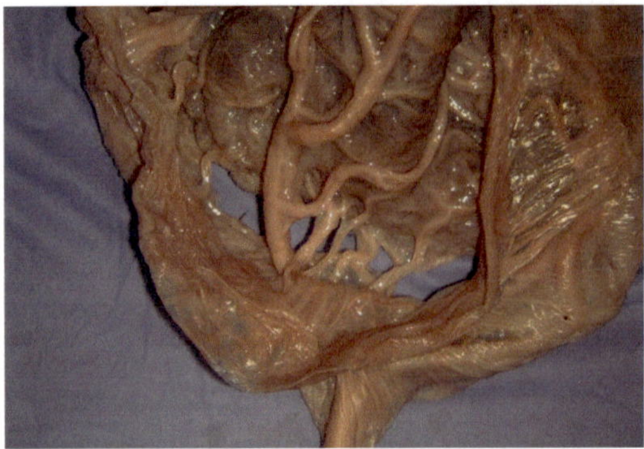

Fig. 7.11 Simulation of the arteriovenous malformation dissection on the cotyledon of fixed bovine placenta. The nodule of vessels is partly dissected from the surrounding tissue with preserved feeding vessels. (Used with permission from Barrow Neurological Institute, Phoenix, Arizona)

carotid arteries, and the small placental arteries approximate the size of the human radial artery, which is frequently used as a vascular graft in neurosurgical bypasses.

Bovine placental arteries can successfully be used as a biological model to simulate carotid endarterectomies [15] or complex bypass procedures that include anastomosing arteries of different sizes. Cotyledons of bovine placenta can be dissected from the surrounding tissue to simulate dissection of arteriovenous malformations from brain parenchyma (Fig. 7.11). Each cotyledon is a rich tree of vasculature with several "feeders" and outflow vessels that should be recognized during removal. Resection is performed in a circumferential fashion, similar to actual arteriovenous malformation surgery.

Microsurgical Practice on Laboratory Rats

The common laboratory rat is an excellent model for practicing microsurgical skills and has been used for this purpose for decades. Microsurgical practice using laboratory rats is possible after IACUC approval and special training on how to work with and care for laboratory animals.

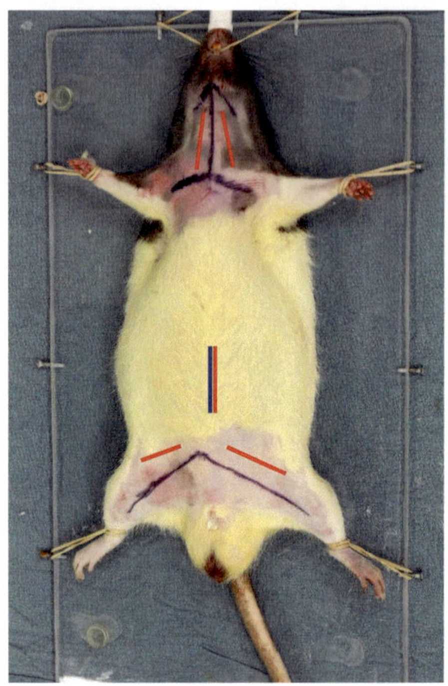

Fig. 7.12 Anesthetized rat placed on a specialized board. The skin near the incision areas is shaved. Projections of the vessels that are commonly used for microsurgical practice are shown. (Used with permission from Barrow Neurological Institute, Phoenix, Arizona)

Appropriate laboratory and animal-keeping facilities are required, as well as anesthetic drugs and a restriction table, in addition to the standard microneurosurgical instrument set. Anastomosis practice is usually performed as a termination procedure; however, a survival protocol may also be implemented.

Carotid arteries, jugular veins, aortas, vena cava, and iliac arteries of adult rats are typically used for microanastomosis practice (Fig. 7.12). Arterial aneurysms can also be surgically created by suturing blunt vessel segments in an end-to-side fashion [16]. Neurosurgical bypasses are usually created on vessels 1–2 mm in diameter, which corresponds to the size of the carotid arteries of a rat (Fig. 7.13). Anastomosing vessels that are less than 1 mm in diameter, such as the femoral vessels of the rat, are less relevant for neurosurgical procedures, but the additional

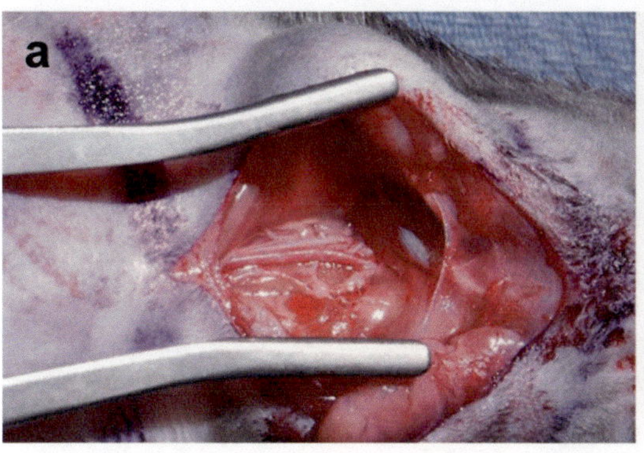

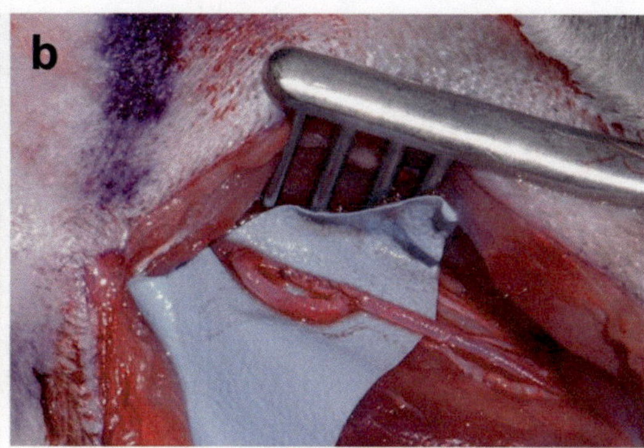

Fig. 7.13 Microvascular practice on the right carotid artery of the rat. (**a**) The common carotid artery and bifurcation are dissected. (**b**) Two end-to-side anastomoses are created, forming a loop by using arterial graft harvested from the contralateral carotid artery. (Used with permission from Barrow Neurological Institute, Phoenix, Arizona)

challenge will improve surgical skill in working with small vessels.

The main advantage of the rat model is its unique opportunity to assess the functional outcome of the anastomosis under physiological conditions, including bleeding, thrombosis, appropriate use of anticoagulants, and arterial spasm. Working with a live biological model may also provide a more stressful situation than a nonlive model, making it closer to the actual operating room experience. However, the histologic properties of the rat's arteries and veins differ from human cerebral vessels because they are peripheral vessels and have a thick adventitial layer.

The disadvantages of this model include the necessity for strict adherence to the approved protocol, adequate facilities to work with animals, and the need for drugs and specialized surgical equipment with their associated costs. Therefore, we recommended that young neurosurgeons and residents participate in research projects that require microsurgical procedures on small laboratory animals. Additionally, they can practice microanastomosis on laboratory animals that have been euthanized according to experimental protocols; this is in accordance with the "reduction" principle of ethics.

Human Cadaveric Heads as a Model for Bypass Procedures

Practicing neurosurgical dissections on fixed and color-injected cadaveric heads (Fig. 7.14) is probably the best way to learn surgical neuroanatomy. In addition, practice on cadaveric heads may be skill oriented. Several modifications have been proposed to increase the similarity of cadaveric heads to live surgery. These modifications include the use of light fixation to allow brain retraction, simulation of the pulsatile flow in blood vessels by cannulating vessels and attaching the tubing to a peristaltic pump, and simulation of cerebrospinal fluid flow by inserting a catheter in the subarachnoid space [17].

Whole cadaveric heads are not always available, so donated cadaveric brains with preserved carotid and vertebral arteries can be used for microvascular practice [18]. Cerebral veins and sinuses are usually damaged during brain extraction and are difficult to preserve. It is important to cannulate all four major arteries and flush out all blood and thrombi with a large volume of tap water as soon as possible after death. Washing can be done with large syringes. However, excess pressure should be avoided to prevent arteries from bursting. After light fixation, brains with preserved vascula-

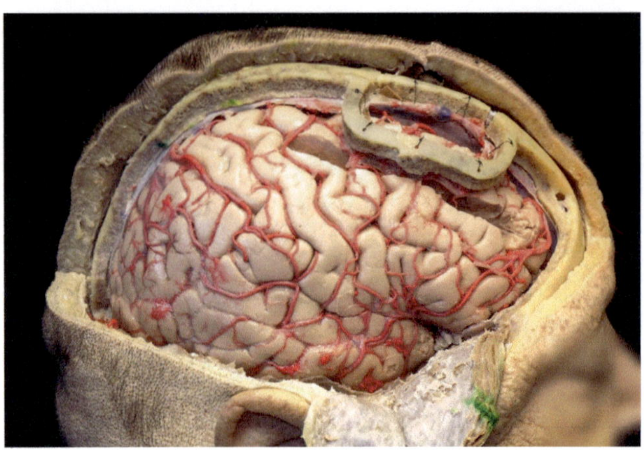

Fig. 7.14 Fixed and silicone-injected cadaver head used for microsurgical dissection. (Used with permission from Barrow Neurological Institute, Phoenix, Arizona)

ture may be used not only for learning anatomy but also for simulating arterial anastomoses on different arterial segments and for aneurysmal clip application in an anatomically relevant environment. Placed in an artificial or real cranium, this model suitably simulates the technical challenges of actual human intracranial bypass procedures [19].

The main advantage of human cadaveric models for surgical training is their anatomical and tactile similarity to human brain tissue, with the possibility for simulating an entire procedure and not just the anastomosis itself. Such "live cadavers" have been used to simulate and practice high-flow extracranial-intracranial bypass procedures [20]. Limitations of such comprehensive cadaveric models are the significant cost, effort, and time required for preparation, management, and documentation.

Benefits of Available Biological Models

Biological models are most similar to human tissue in task-related conditions and tactile feedback for neurosurgical practice. Arteries from all biological models have similar connective tissue and adventitial adhesions and can be used in wet conditions similar to those encountered in the operating room. Practicing on chicken wing arteries under wet conditions, with arteries immersed in water, may provide additional training challenges and significantly improve time to complete the anastomosis [21]. As with most things the neurosurgeon does, preparation is a key step for the successful performance of a bypass. Biological models present unique opportunities for practicing all the preparatory steps and actual microsuturing. The importance of preparation cannot be overemphasized, as it determines whether the anastomosis will be an effortless, smooth procedure or an anguished struggle of dealing with wayward vessels and sutures. Biological models provide a necessary environment for practicing the cleaning of the surgical field, preparation of a bloodless operative field, adequate drainage of the cerebrospinal fluid, tailoring of vessel ends, and appropriate clipping. During the suturing itself, only a biological model can provide the feeling of resistance and puncture of real tissue and the fragile thin intima that should be protected as much as possible.

Adequate biological models also allow trainees to practice the management of inadvertent events with a high degree of realism. Practicing for complications, such as the rupture of an aneurysm or the thrombosis of an anastomosis, can develop crucial skills before actual surgery is ever performed.

Biological models can also be used in combination with other simulation technologies for procedure simulation and team practice. In such cases, biological models make simulation realistic for all training participants, including residents and scrub nurses [17].

Limitations of Biological Models and Ways to Overcome Them

Nearly every biological model for cerebrovascular anastomosis training lacks surrounding tissues that would simulate fragile nearby brain tissue. These models also lack restrictions related to the craniotomy window or complex anatomical locations. This aspect is important because it influences the hand position of the neurosurgeon during surgery and ultimately influences microsurgical performance. Most of these conditions can be simulated by artificial three-dimensional printed models. For example, a mannequin of a patient's head with an open craniotomy allows practice of the placement of any biological or artificial vessel [22].

Some complex biological models, such as cadaveric heads or live animals, require significant management and documentation work. Successful implementation of such models often requires additional funding, as well as collaboration with hospital and research administrators.

Conclusion

Although not used often, bypass skills are essential and critical when needed. Such skills should be developed before they will ever be required in surgery. Results of these training and validation experiments, supplemented by insights from modern neurophysiological data, provide background and recommendations for evidence-based approaches toward the development of neurosurgeon-oriented microsurgical training. A number of well-developed and validated biological models exist for training in microvascular anastomosis. Cerebrovascular training curricula that include microsurgical anastomosis practice may be implemented in virtually any neurosurgical department for the training of residents and fellows.

Acknowledgments The authors thank the Neuroscience Publications staff at Barrow Neurological Institute in Phoenix, Arizona, for their kind assistance in the preparation of this manuscript.

References

1. Krings T, Mandell DM, Kiehl TR, et al. Intracranial aneurysms: from vessel wall pathology to therapeutic approach. Nat Rev Neurol. 2011;7(10):547–59.
2. Sun H, Safavi-Abbasi S, Spetzler RF. Retractorless surgery for intracranial aneurysms. J Neurosurg Sci. 2016;60(1):54–69.
3. Belykh E, Byvaltsev V. Off-the-job microsurgical training on dry models: Siberian experience. World Neurosurg. 2014;82(1–2):20–4.
4. Kshettry VR, Mullin JP, Schlenk R, Recinos PF, Benzel EC. The role of laboratory dissection training in neurosurgical residency: results of a national survey. World Neurosurg. 2014;82(5):554–9.
5. Abla AA, Uschold T, Preul MC, Zabramski JM. Comparative use of turkey and chicken wing brachial artery models for microvascular anastomosis training. J Neurosurg. 2011;115(6):1231–5.
6. Hino A. Training in microvascular surgery using a chicken wing artery. Neurosurgery. 2003;52(6):1495–7; discussion 7–8.
7. Colpan ME, Slavin KV, Amin-Hanjani S, Calderon-Arnuphi M, Charbel FT. Microvascular anastomosis training model based on a turkey neck with perfused arteries. Neurosurgery. 2008;62(5 Suppl 2):ONS407-10; discussion ONS10-1.
8. Olabe J, Olabe J. Microsurgical training on an in vitro chicken wing infusion model. Surg Neurol. 2009;72(6):695–9.
9. Jusue-Torres I, Sivakanthan S, Pinheiro-Neto CD, Gardner PA, Snyderman CH, Fernandez-Miranda JC. Chicken wing training model for endoscopic microsurgery. J Neurol Surg B Skull Base. 2013;74(5):286–91.
10. Belykh E, Lei T, Safavi-Abbasi S, et al. Low-flow and high-flow neurosurgical bypass and anastomosis training models using human and bovine placental vessels: a histological analysis and validation study. J Neurosurg. 2016;125(4):915–28.
11. Romero FR, Fernandes ST, Chaddad-Neto F, Ramos JG, Campos JM, Oliveira E. Microsurgical techniques using human placenta. Arq Neuropsiquiatr. 2008;66(4):876–8.
12. Oliveira Magaldi M, Nicolato A, Godinho JV, et al. Human placenta aneurysm model for training neurosurgeons in vascular microsurgery. Neurosurgery. 2014;10(Suppl 4):592–600; discussion 600–1.
13. Belykh EG, Byval'tsev VA, Nakadzhi P, Lei T, Oliviero MM, Nikiforov SB. A model of the arterial aneurysm of the brain for microneurosurgical training. Zh Vopr Neirokhir Im N N Burdenko. 2014;78(2):40–5; discussion 5.
14. Oliveira MM, Araujo AB, Nicolato A, et al. Face, content, and construct validity of brain tumor microsurgery simulation using a human placenta model. Neurosurgery. 2015;12:61–7.

15. Belykh EG, Lei T, Oliveira MM, et al. Carotid endarterectomy surgical simulation model using a bovine placenta vessel. Neurosurgery. 2015;77(5):825–9; discussion 9–30.

16. Marbacher S, Marjamaa J, Abdelhameed E, Hernesniemi J, Niemela M, Frosen J. The Helsinki rat microsurgical sidewall aneurysm model. J Vis Exp. 2014;92:e51071.

17. Aboud E, Aboud G, Al-Mefty O, et al. "Live cadavers" for training in the management of intraoperative aneurysmal rupture. J Neurosurg. 2015;123(5):1339–46.

18. Olabe J, Olabe J, Sancho V. Human cadaver brain infusion model for neurosurgical training. Surg Neurol. 2009;72(6):700–2.

19. Olabe J, Olabe J, Roda JM, Sancho V. Human cadaver brain infusion skull model for neurosurgical training. Surg Neurol Int. 2011;2:54.

20. Russin JJ, Mack WJ, Carey JN, Minneti M, Giannotta SL. Simulation of a high-flow extracranial-intracranial bypass using a radial artery graft in a novel fresh tissue model. Neurosurgery. 2012;71(2 Suppl Operative):ons315–19; discussion ons 319–20.

21. Shimizu S, Sekiguchi T, Mochizuki T, et al. Moist-condition training for cerebrovascular anastomosis: a practical step after mastering basic manipulations. Neurol Med Chir (Tokyo). 2015;55(8):689–92.

22. Takeuchi M, Hayashi N, Hamada H, Matsumura N, Nishijo H, Endo S. A new training method to improve deep microsurgical skills using a mannequin head. Microsurgery. 2008;28(3):168–70.

Pseudoaneurysm Surgery Simulation Using the "Live Cadaver" Model for Neurosurgical Education

Emad Aboud, Talal Aboud, Jaafar Basma, Hassan Saad, Wei Hsun Yang, Ghaith Aboud, and Ali Krisht

Introduction

With the increasing popularity of endovascular strategies and minimal invasive treatment, fewer aneurysms are treated with open surgery in the modern era [1], although it remains a critically important procedure and a challenging surgery. Surgical treatment of aneurysms requires a certain level of skill and experience to achieve excellent results after surgery and to avoid complications, one of which is intraoperative aneurysmal rupture, a devastating crisis that can jeopardize a patient's life and neurologic functions [2].

The reduced number of working hours for residents and the trend toward minimal or even noninvasive treatment of cerebral aneurysms have resulted in residents' decreased exposure to live surgery and hands-on experience in the operating room. This decrease becomes increasingly relevant when surgeons encounter complications, especially vascular injuries and the intraoperative rupture of cerebral aneurysms. After completion of their training, neurosurgery residents will face complicated cases and intraoperative aneurysmal rupture in their practice while they are on their own. To develop competency in managing cerebral aneurysms, compensatory mechanisms should be adopted to cover the decreased hands-on experience in the OR; thus, significant training will now have to occur in a laboratory setting [3, 4].

Simulation and laboratory training are the best compensation mechanisms to address this loss of expertise and skill. This fact was realized by Yasargil and other pioneers early on with the introduction of microneurosurgery. In his landmark book, *Microneurosurgery*, Yasargil stated: "In delicate organs such as the central nervous system, the surgeon's individual skills play a crucial role in determining patient outcome. Hence, the emphasis has been placed on laboratory training, preparing surgical trainees for the operating room experience" [5]. To simulate a real surgical procedure, one must imitate and include all elements of live surgery. John Hunter, the noted Scottish surgeon of the eighteenth century, is believed to have said that surgery is anatomy plus hemostasis. Training models that do include these elements are ideal for higher-level training and bridging the gap between laboratory environment and the operating room.

Electronic supplementary material: The online version of this chapter https://doi.org/10.1007/978-3-319-75583-0_8 contains supplementary material, which is available to authorized users.

E. Aboud (✉) · T. Aboud · H. Saad · W. H. Yang
G. Aboud · A. Krisht
Department of Neurosurgery, Arkansas
Neuroscience Institute, Little Rock, AR, USA
e-mail: EAboud@stvincenthealth.com

J. Basma
Department of Neurosurgery University of Tennessee
Health Science Center, Memphis, TN, USA

© Springer International Publishing AG, part of Springer Nature 2018
A. Alaraj (ed.), *Comprehensive Healthcare Simulation: Neurosurgery*,
Comprehensive Healthcare Simulation, https://doi.org/10.1007/978-3-319-75583-0_8

Although training models and simulators currently available provide a wide range of opportunities to practice skills and play a role in surgical training, they do not successfully replicate all the characteristics of the living human cerebral vasculature, particularly the combination of real human anatomy with lifelike circumstances [6–8]. In this chapter we will describe a more realistic aneurysm model, called the "live cadaver" model, which allows repetitive training under lifelike conditions for residents and other trainees to practice surgical clipping of cerebral aneurysms using human cadaveric head specimens, especially prepared for this purpose (Fig. 8.1). This model is in practical use in training courses and on a daily basis in several training facilities in the United States.

Preparation of the "Live Cadaver" Model

Preparing the Head Specimen

Cadaveric specimens were preserved with alcohol-based disinfectant and ethylene glycol. Suitable tubes were used to cannulate the major vessels in the neck and the subarachnoid spaces through the spinal canal, and the vascular tree was irrigated with normal saline to drain clots and blood remnant (Fig. 8.2a, b). The vessels were then connected to artificial blood reservoir "serum bags that were wrapped with pressure bags," and the pressure applied to the arterial reservoir was maintained at 120–130 mmHg and to the venous reservoir at 10–15 mmHg. The arterial reservoir was further connected through the pressure bag to a pump that provided pulsating pressure; pumps used for this purpose were the intra-aortic balloon pump (System 90/97, Datascope Corp., Fairfield, NJ, and the HART

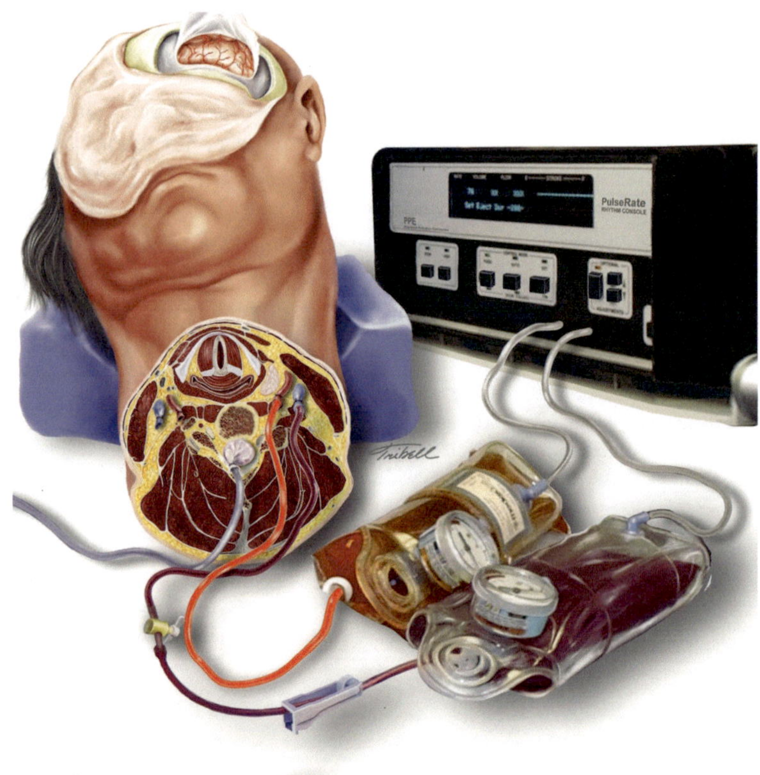

Fig. 8.1 Artistic illustration showing the connections and the settings of the "live cadaver" model. (Published with permission of the University of Arkansas for Medical Sciences)

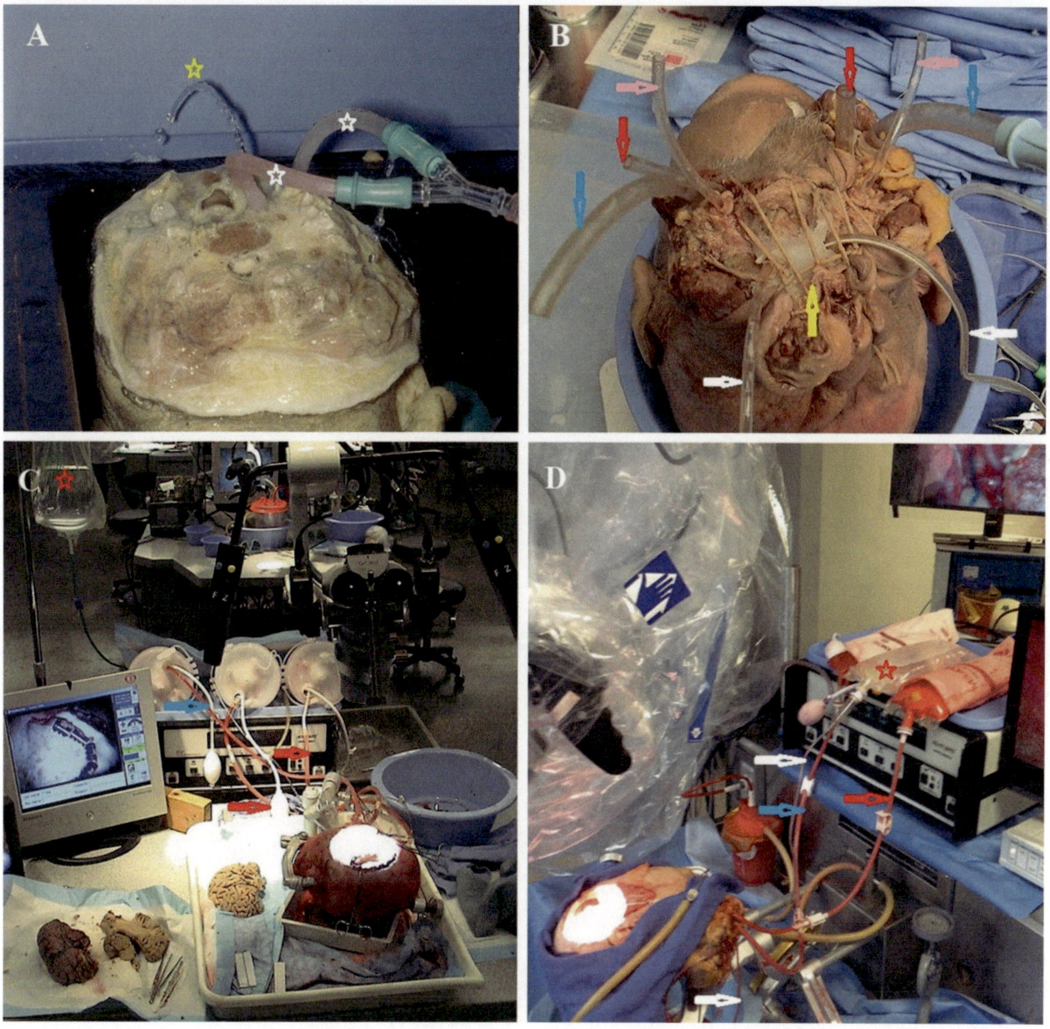

Fig. 8.2 (**a**) Irrigation of the vascular tree, injecting N saline via connecting tubes in the jugular vein and carotid artery (white stars); notice the fluid jet coming out of the contralateral vessels (yellow star). (**b**) Final cannulation; we can see tubes to the jugular veins (blue arrows), carotid arteries (red arrows), vertebral arteries (pink arrows), and (white arrows) indicate the tubes to the arachnoid spaces through the spinal canal (yellow arrow). (**c**, **d**) Settings of the working stations; notice the CSF simulant reservoir (red star) and the connection to the reservoirs

MATE, TCI, Thermo Cardiosystems Inc., Woburn, MA). The pulsation rate of the pump was kept on 80 pulses per minute. One of the tubes in the spinal canal was connected to a reservoir of clear liquid and hung on a serum pole to simulate cerebrospinal fluid (CSF) and sat at a rate of 15–20 cm per hour (Fig. 8.2c, d). The tip of the other tube in the spinal canal was kept 10–12 cm above the level of the foramien of Monrow and left open to drain excess fluid. More details about preparing and operating the model have been published elsewhere [9]. Blood simu-

lant can be prepared using water-based paints, or it can be purchased as a prepared formula for training purposes. When the pump is turned on, the blood simulant fills into the vessels, fluctuates in the arteries with the pulses of the pump, and is kept static under fixed pressure in the veins.

In these settings, the human anatomy is presented in more lifelike circumstances that allow a true simulation of surgical procedures in terms of bleeding, the pulsation of arteries, and the softness of tissue.

Creating Pseudoaneurysms

Pseudoaneurysms can be created either by an instructor or by the trainee himself; in both cases a wide pterional craniotomy was made to allow all possible approaches through this route, the sylvian fissure and basal cisterns were opened exploring all visible vessels in the field, and the artery of interest was dissected and prepared to create the aneurysm. During this the pump is on, blood is filling the vessels under pressure, and CSF is filling the subarachnoid spaces. The trainee will need to coagulate the vessels while cutting the skin and deal with bone bleed, coagulate dural vessels, and cut the arachnoid and drain CSF as the same as with live patients in the OR. This by itself is an exciting experience, especially for residents in their early residency.

Venous grafts are harvested from the neck, either in the same or different specimen. During harvest, a thin layer of the loose fatty tissue was left attached to the wall (to seal the hole in the dome while simulating aneurysmal rupture). The graft was cut into the desired length, usually 10–15 mm, and was then turned inside out, so that the inner surface becomes the outside. One end of the graft was sutured with 8.0 or 9.0 sutures, and the graft was then inverted again to its original position so that the sutures were hidden inside the aneurysmal sac and the loose tissue attached to the wall covered the suture line on the outside, so the dome had a rounded shape. At this point, the aneurysm was ready to be sutured in place. An arteriotomy that fits the diameter of the aneurysm's base was made on the parent artery, and the aneurysm was sutured to the edges of the arteriotomy with 8.0 sutures (Fig. 8.3).

At bifurcations, the base of the aneurysm was shaped to be part of the bifurcating branches on one or both sides to allow for reconstruction. Care was taken to keep the contour and configuration of the parent artery as it was and to spare the adjacent branches. In cases of ophthalmic and posterior communicating aneurysms, we sutured the aneurysm in intimate proximity to these vessels to make clipping and reconstruction more challenging and to simulate the surgical anatomy encountered during aneurysm surgery (Fig. 8.4).

Once sutured into place, the aneurysm was tested to check the filling of the sac and blood flow in distal and adjacent vessels and to detect any leak from the base. If such a leak occurred, additional sutures were placed.

Training Exercises

Trainees of all levels have practiced neurovascular procedures under lifelike conditions nearly identical to that of live surgery. They were able to use suction, bipolar coagulation, micro-Doppler, and all other instruments and devices normally used in the operating room. We will describe here two exercises: aneurysm clipping and management of intraoperative aneurysmal rupture (Fig. 8.5).

The head specimen harboring the aneurysm was placed and fixed with head holders. Then, the blood reservoirs were placed to be slightly higher than the specimen to prevent air embolism and enable control of the simulated blood pressure. The clear liquid reservoir (CSF simulant) was hung on a serum pole with a controlled flow around 18–20 cc per hour, and the pump was placed to the side of the working station.

Aneurysm Clipping Exercises (See Video 8.1)

In general, an instructor first demonstrates clipping of the aneurysm and the management of an intraoperative rupture. Then, trainees practice clipping and reconstruction techniques and the management of intraoperative rupture. Before each training exercise, the spaces around the aneurysm and neighboring cisterns were filled with clotted blood simulant (Luna Products & Engineering, Blacksburg, VA, USA) to simulate a real subarachnoid hemorrhage. Trainees navigate their way to the aneurysm following the anatomical landmarks to achieve proximal control and then reach out to the aneurysm, dissect the dome from the surroundings, and prepare the neck of the aneurysm for clipping as the same as in a live surgery (Fig. 8.6).

Fig. 8.3 (**a**) The venous graft, (**b**) turning the graft inside out, (**c**) suturing one end of the graft, (**d**) inverting back the graft to its original position to form the aneurysm sac (blue star), (**e**) the edges of the arteriotomy (white arrows) on the right carotid artery (yellow star), (**f**) suturing the aneurysm (blue star) to the edges of the arteriotomy, (**g**) the suture line (yellow arrows) delineating the aneurysm base, (**h**) the final formation of the aneurysm

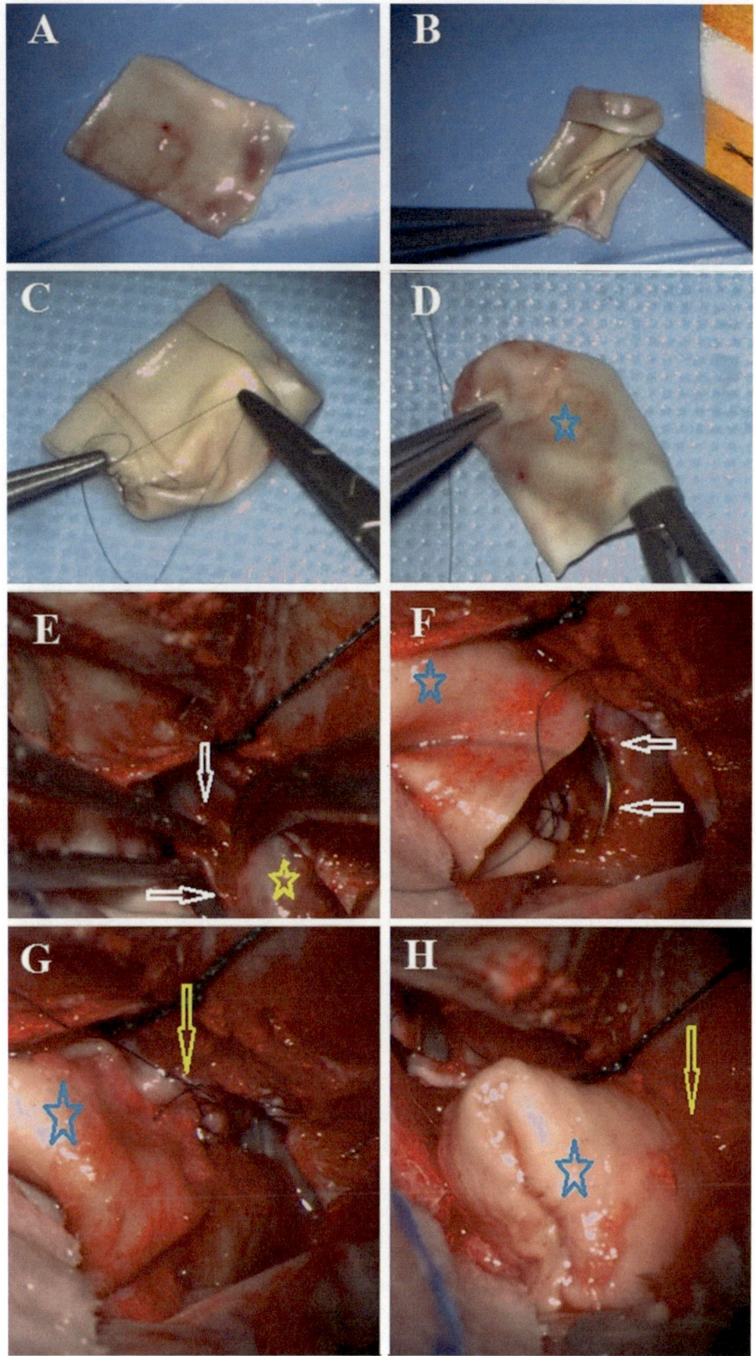

For advanced training, more sticky materials were injected around the aneurysm to make the dissection more challenging, materials such as Tisseel Baxter Healthcare Corporation, Westlake Village, CA, USA. Also, more complicated aneurysms usually created that need reconstruction and multiple clips. In some occasions, when an angiogram was previously made, trainees will study the images and discuss clipping strategy with the instructor. Of course, trainees will have the opportunity to repeat the exercise again either on the same specimen or on different aneurysms prepared in other specimens.

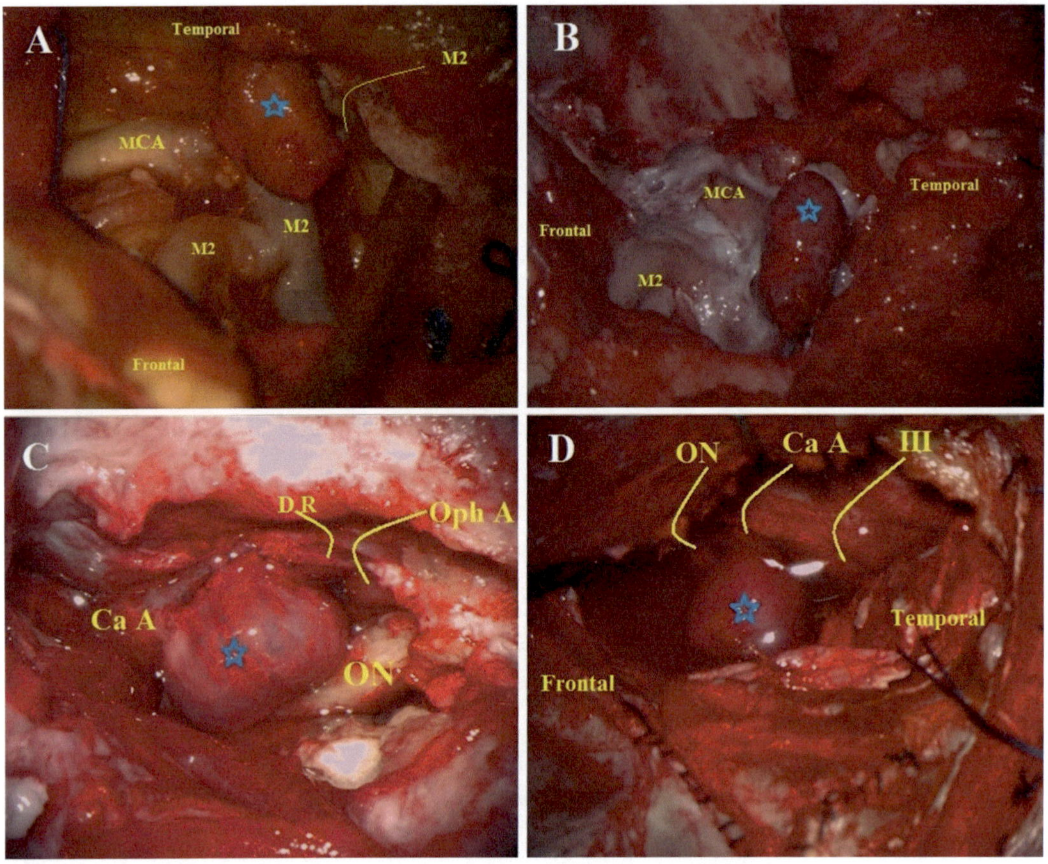

Fig. 8.4 Aneurysms made in different locations: (**a**, **b**) right MC; (**c**, **d**) left and right paraclinoid aneurysms, respectively MCA middle cerebral artery, M2 branches of the MCA beyond the bifurcation over the insula, Ca A carotid artery, DR dural ring, Oph A ophthalmic artery, ON optic nerve, III, third nerve

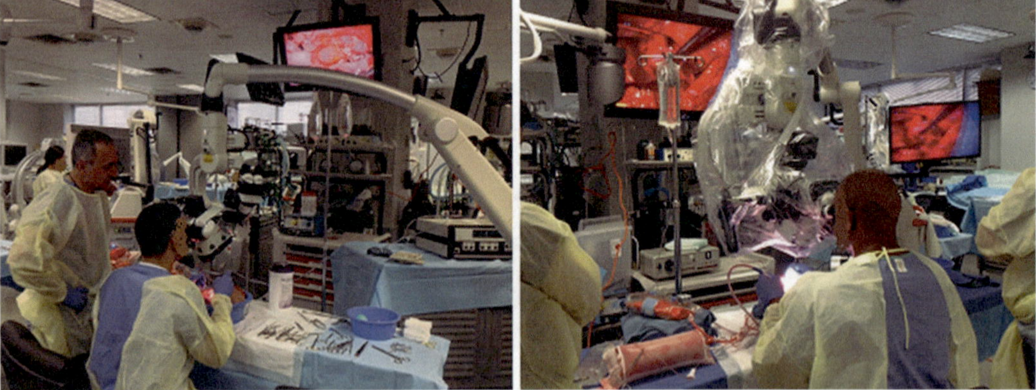

Fig. 8.5 Trainees practicing aneurysmal clipping and management of rupture under supervision; the surgical field can be seen on the overhead monitors

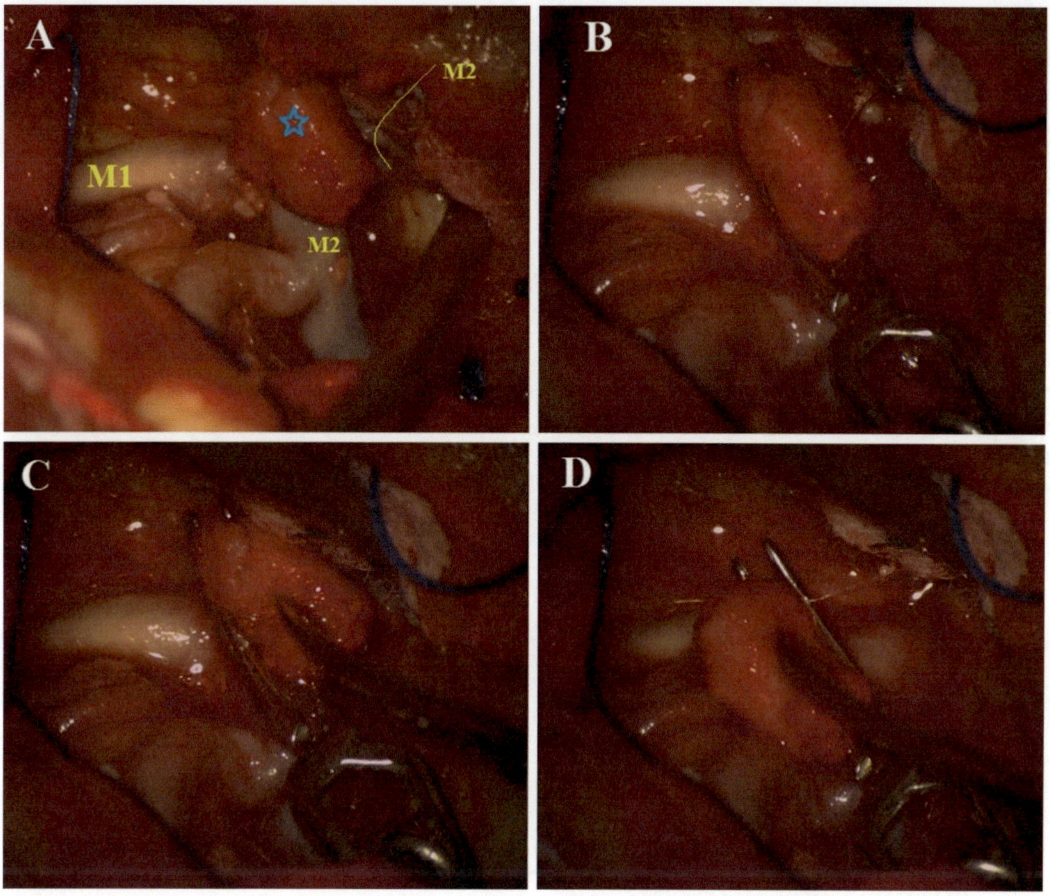

Fig. 8.6 Aneurysm clipping: (**a**) right MCA aneurysm, (**b**) the clip on position, (**c, d**) making sure that no aneurysm left under the clip

Trainees were able to practice clipping procedures under supervision in a risk-free environment where they can repeat the same step several times until they get it done the right way. For residents who have never clipped an aneurysm before, this was a golden opportunity to test their abilities and explore this experience. For other trainees who have clipped aneurysms, this was another chance to refine their skills in certain stages of the procedure and challenge themselves facing difficulties that we tend to add during the training sessions, especially the management of intraoperative rupture.

Management of Intraoperative Rupture (See Video 8.2)

After practicing clipping and all its maneuvers, a small hole was made on the side of the dome of each aneurysm. No bleeding can happen under low pressure due to the presence of the tissue kept attached to the venous graft when the aneurysm was made, and the loose tissue covers the hole so the aneurysm will be filled by blood simulant with some oozing which makes the exercise even more challenging. But if the pressure is raised, profuse bleeding will occur.

Trainees followed the same training scenario to clip the aneurysm while the field is filled with clotted blood simulant. As they were dissecting around the aneurysm or trying to apply the clip, we suddenly raised the pressure and made the aneurysm bleed profusely. To achieve that, we connected an additional blood simulant reservoir through a three-way cannula to the arterial side in addition to the original arterial reservoir and kept it closed but under high pressure up to 220 mmHg, while the original reservoir is under normal or even low pressure just enough to keep the filling of the aneurysm and the vessels. Under this pressure the hole that previously existed in the aneurysm will not bleed, but when we open the additional reservoir and pump the blood simulant under high pressure, the aneurysm will bleed as it has ruptured, and the blood simulant will fill the surgical field (Fig. 8.7).

When the bleeding occurs, trainees were instructed to follow sequence of actions that will control the bleeding in a short time without any additional injury. They practiced pressure control and temporary tamponade, using additional section to allow visualization, clipping the bleeding point or the visible part of the aneurysm dome, proximal control of the bleeding by clipping the parent vessel, bipolar coagulation control in some cases, and working under simulated cardiac arrest.

This was an exciting experience for residents of all levels of training as such an opportunity is rarely available in the OR.

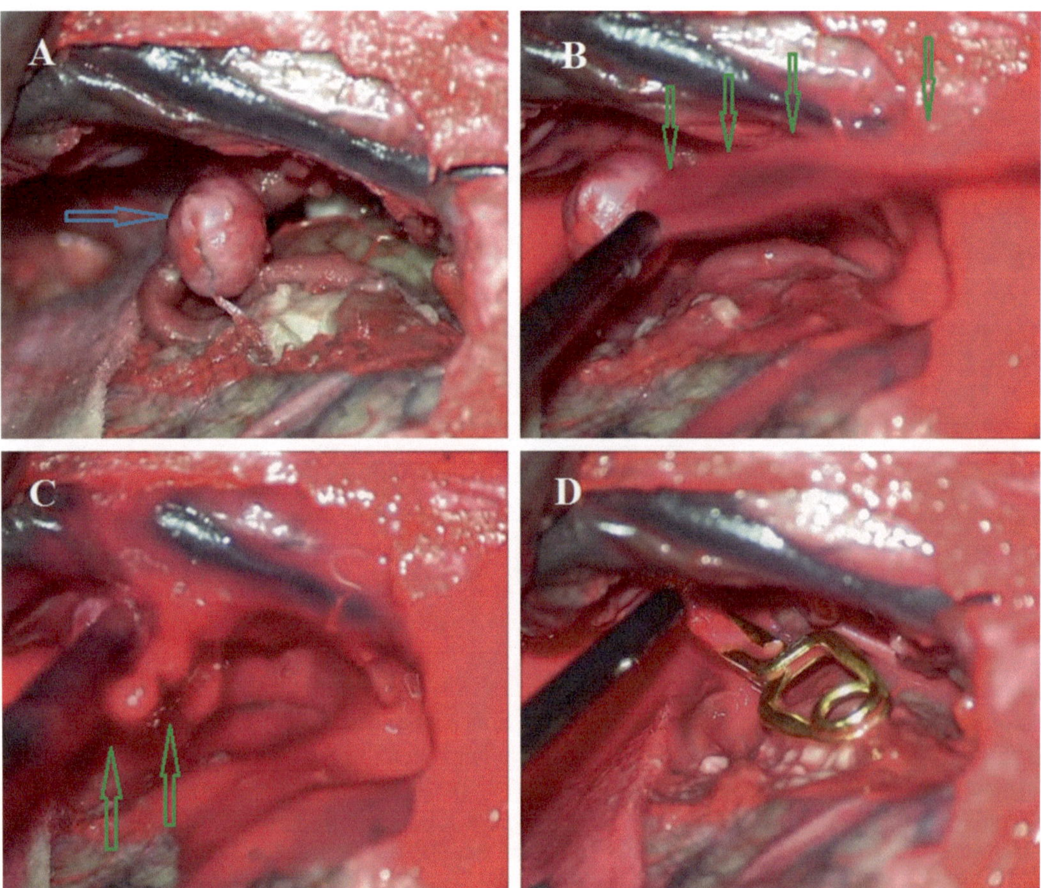

Fig. 8.7 Management of rupture: (**a**) right MCA aneurysm (blue arrow), (**b, c**) bleeding jet from the aneurysm dome (green arrows) and suction control of the bleeding, (**d**) temporary clip on the bleeding point

Model Evaluation

Trainees were enthusiastic to work on a cadaver that could bleed. They welcomed the opportunity to clip cerebral aneurysms and to manage intraoperative aneurysmal rupture, a procedure that they may not have encountered yet. Most of the participants in our courses stated that the live cadaver session was the part of the course they liked the most. The live cadaver model enabled trainees to practice aneurysmal clip placement and all maneuvers and techniques to control intraoperative aneurysmal rupture, including tamponade, suction, proximal and distal vascular control, temporary clip placement, coagulation, and hypotension or simulation of cardiac arrest (the pressure in the specimen can be controlled through adjustment of the pressure in the arterial reservoir). In a previously published study, 91 (27 faculty members and 64 participants) completed a questionnaire to rate their personal opinions of the live cadaver model (Table 8.1) [10]. Most either agreed or strongly agreed that the model was a true simulation of the conditions of live surgery on cerebral aneurysms and represented a realistic simulation for aneurysmal clip placement and intraoperative rupture.

Training Procedures and Applications of the "Live Cadaver" (See Video 8.3)

Training exercises using the "live cadaver" model is not limited to pseudoaneurysm applications; the model can be used for practicing all neurosurgical procedures. Here we will describe some examples on the capabilities of this model and other procedures that we made.

To achieve the maximum benefit from the specimen and perform all possible procedures before the vessels were damaged, we advise to start with minimal invasive procedures such as endovascular interventions and endoscopic techniques and other procedures that could be performed on the surface before working deep into the brain and the skull base.

Endoscopic Procedures

After a frontal burr hole had been made, the sheath of the endoscope was introduced toward the lateral ventricle. The optic apparatus was introduced after the introducer had been pulled out, and the choroid plexus and the septal and thalamic veins

Table 8.1 The questionnaire administered after completion of the training course

Question	Strongly disagree (%)	Disagree (%)	Neutral (%)	Agree (%)	Strongly agree (%)
This model was a true simulation of the conditions of live surgery on aneurysms.		1.09	2.19	28.57	68.13
This model promotes the acquisition of microsurgical skills.			6.59	21.97	71.42
This model offers benefits not available in existing training models.			6.59	21.97	71.42
The tissue characteristics in this model are very similar to those of living tissues	3.29	1.09	3.29	32.96	59.34
The scenario of aneurysm clipping and intraoperative rupture is realistic			7.69	30.76	61.53
This model could significantly improve current training in the management of intraoperative cerebrovascular complications				24.17	75.82
This model could add significantly to training in microneurosurgical techniques				26.37	73.62
This model will be a valuable addition to the medical device development and testing process	1.09	2.19	7.69	23.07	65.93
This model is superior to existing models for cerebral revascularization		1.09	4.39	27.47	67.03

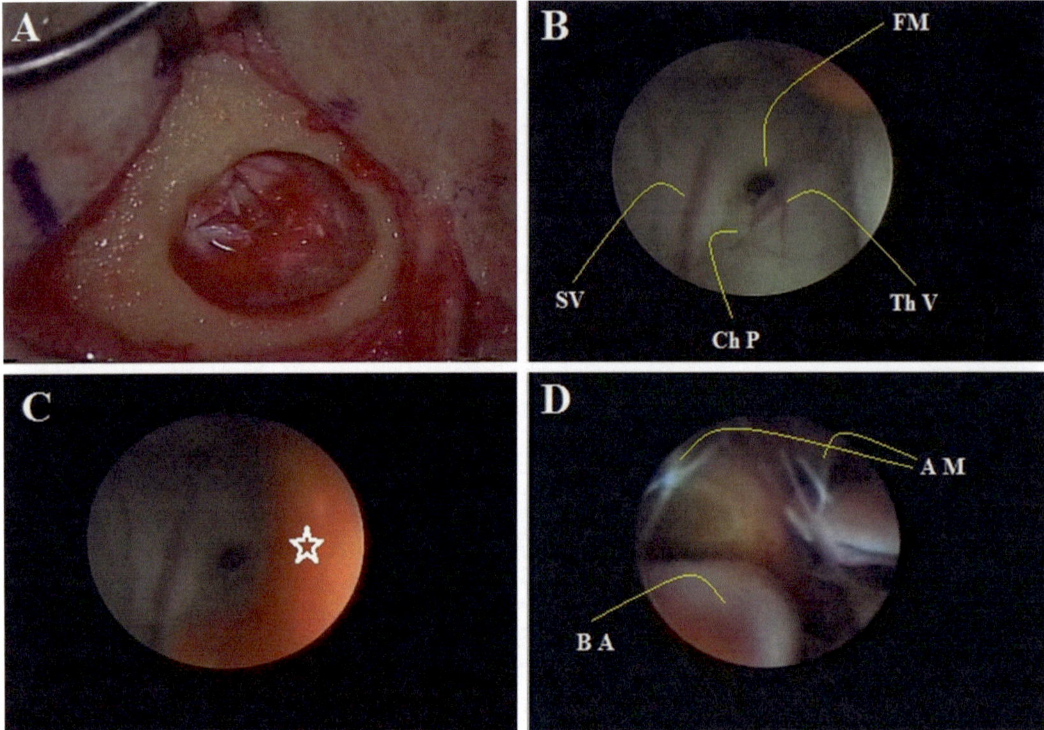

Fig. 8.8 During third ventriculostomy. (**a**) In the burr hole, notice the CSF and oozing from the edges of the incisions. (**b**, **c**) Inside the third ventricle, notice some bleeding coming from the pathway of the endoscope through the brain paranchima. (**d**) In the interpeduncular cistern, the basilar and arachnoid membranes can be seen. FM foramen of Monro, SV septal vein, Th V thalamic vein, Ch P choroid plexus, B A basilar artery, A M arachnoid membranes

led the way to the foramen of Monro (Fig. 8.8). The endoscope passed the foramen into the third ventricle, and the mammillary bodies and the infundibular recess were identified. The floor of the third ventricle was perforated in front of the BA bifurcation in the area of the tuber cinereum. The BA trunk and branches, which were filled and pulsating, were identified in the interpeduncular cistern. Practicing irrigation and clearing of liquid inside the ventricles were achieved, as were observing the pulsation of the BA and identifying the liquid flow through the fenestra.

Craniotomy

A large scalp flap was made to allow a variety of approaches. The STA was preserved for practicing an STA–MCA bypass. Bleeding vessels were ligated, coagulated, or clamped using Raney clips. According to the intended procedure, a variety of craniotomies were performed with care taken to preserve the underlying dura mater. The edges of the bone were waxed to control oozing points. The dura mater was opened, and leaking vessels were coagulated (Fig. 8.9).

Cisternal and Vascular Dissection

The exposed brain was extremely lifelike (Fig. 8.10); the arteries were light red and pulsating, the veins were dark red and filled, and a clear fluid simulated the release of cerebrospinal fluid when the arachnoid was opened. We split the sylvian fissure and followed the branches of the MCA down to the carotid and basal cisterns, dissecting the branches of the circle of Willis and exposing all neurovascular structures in the skull base.

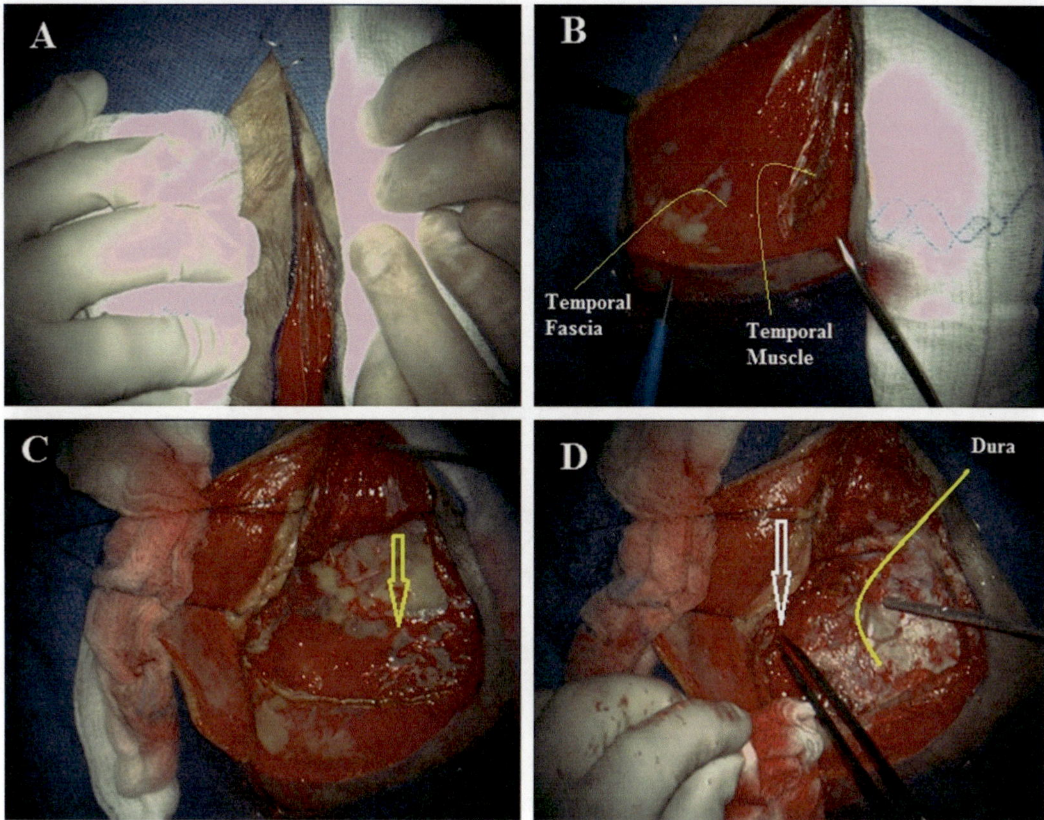

Fig. 8.9 (**a**) Skin incision; (**b**) after raising the skin flab; (**c**) after raising the temporal muscle, notice bleeding from a bony crack in the field (yellow arrow); (**d**) coagulating the dural vessels

Vascular Suturing and Anastomosis

A variety of exercises were performed, starting with the establishment of an STA–MCA bypass (end-to-side anastomosis) and including repair of a longitudinal incision or a partial arterial defect and a transected artery (end-to-end anastomosis), as well as segmental arterial replacement. These procedures were performed on the cortical branches of the MCA and the M2 and M3 branches deep within the fissure. We used various segments of these branches. Each segment was dissected for approximately 1 cm of its length from the overlying arachnoid membrane. Small branches were coagulated and disconnected to free the segment. Two vascular clips were applied on both sides of the segment, and arteriotomies were performed according to the kind of repair or anastomosis desired. After

suture completion, the temporary clips were released, establishing flow under pressure and allowing detection of the integrity and patency of the anastomoses (Fig. 8.11).

Thrombectomy

Some specimens had a remnant of thrombus inside the branches of the MCA; this provided the opportunity to perform a thrombectomy and resuture the vessel (Fig. 8.12).

Resection of Artificial Tumors

Gelatinous material was injected into different locations of the basal cisterns and within the parenchyma to represent a tumor mass so that

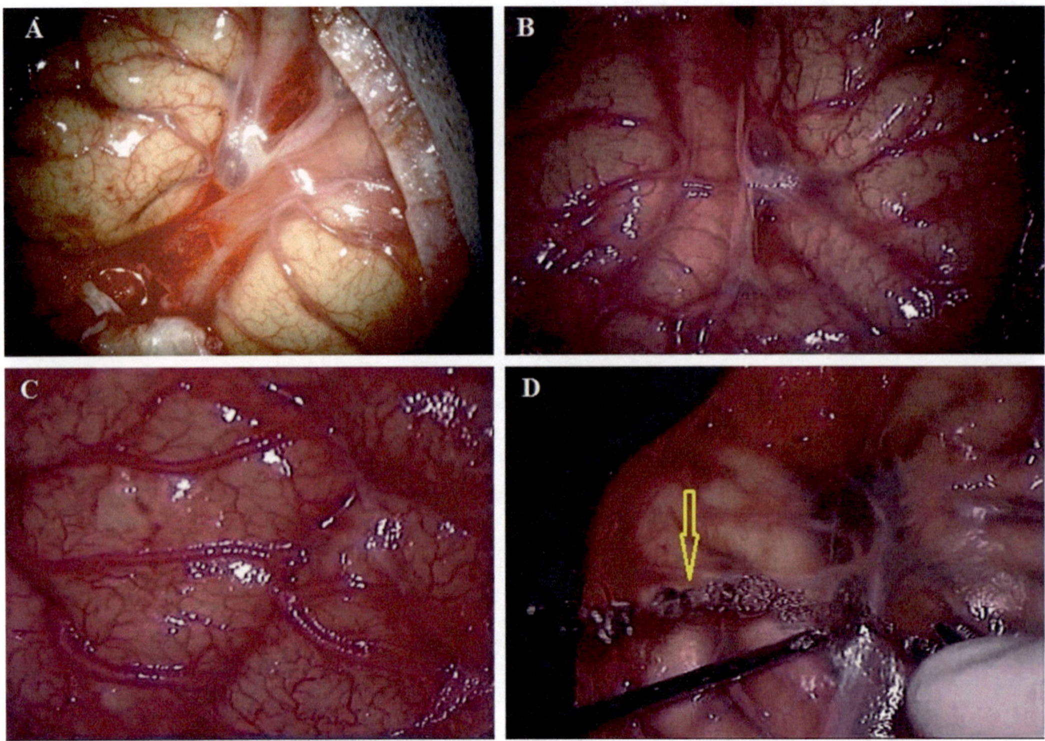

Fig. 8.10 (**a–c**) Different views of the brain surface; notice the filling of the cortical vessels. (**d**) Notice the CSF escaping the subarachnoid space while opening the sylvian fissure (yellow arrow)

the trainee could practice resection of these masses while preserving neurovascular structures (Fig. 8.13). Skull base approaches, intraparenchymal resections, and other procedures that we usually practice in cadavers prepared using traditional methods were practiced as well.

We also applied this method in a whole-brain specimen obtained at autopsy. In this case both CAs were cannulated, allowing a variety of vascular exercises on the major branches (Fig. 8.14).

Clearly, the "live cadaver" model can be used for all kinds of surgical procedures; some has been already practiced and under evaluation such as carotid endarterectomy, endoscopic skull base surgery, transsphenoidal approaches with internal carotid artery injury, endovascular procedure, and spinal surgery with repair of durotomy.

Future of the "Live Cadaver" Model

Cadavers provide trainees with an excellent opportunity and a safe environment to learn basic open vascular surgery principles and improve their operative confidence and consequently patient safety [11–14]. Some authors described cadaver models as "the gold standard for technical skills training" [15].

Adding the lifelike conditions of the living body to cadaver models makes it even more valuable; this combination is a unique feature of the "live cadaver" model not available in any existing training model. It allows trainees to practice surgical procedures as if they were performing a real surgery in the operating room, using the same instruments and techniques, such as suction, bipolar coagulation, echo Doppler ultrasonography, flow measurement, and other devices common to the operating room.

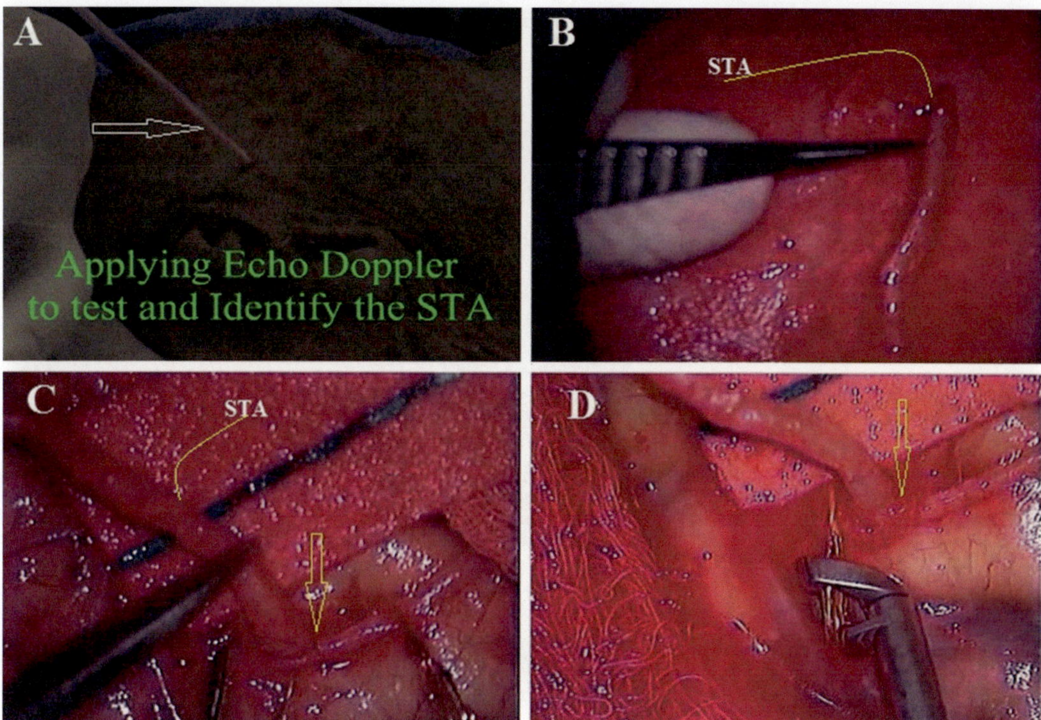

Fig. 8.11 STA–MCA anastomosis. (**a**) Detecting the STA using micro-Doppler (white arrow). (**b**) The STA is dissected and prepared. (**c**, **d**) suturing the STA to a cortical branch in the temporal region; the suture line is shown (yellow arrow) and covered with surgicel at the end

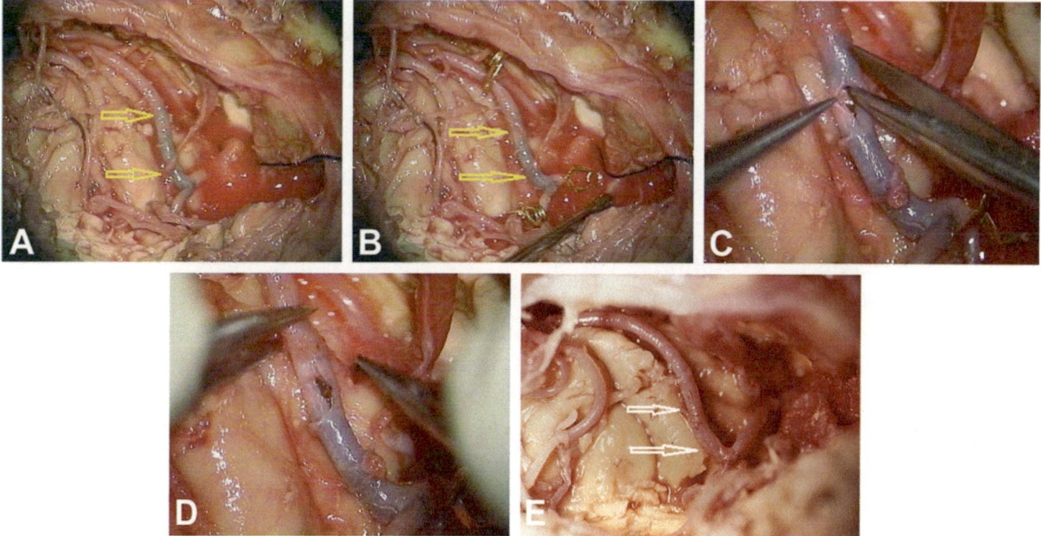

Fig. 8.12 Thrombectomy: (**a**, **b**) thrombosis filling a segment of M2 branch of the middle cerebral artery (yellow arrows), (**c**, **d**) evacuating the clots, (**e**) reestablishing the flow at this segment of the artery (white arrows). (Reprinted with permission from Ref. [9] (AANS))

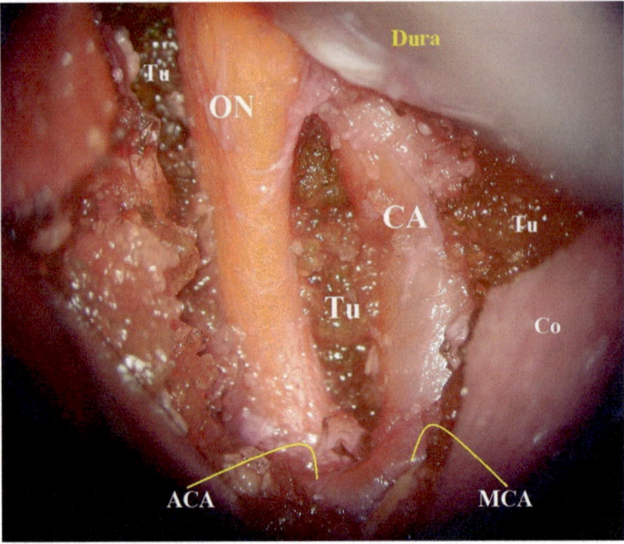

Fig. 8.13 Artificial tumor wrapping the neurovascular structures in the cellar and paracellar region. ON optic nerve, CA carotid artery, Tu tumor, ACA anterior cerebral artery, MCA middle cerebral artery, Co cotton

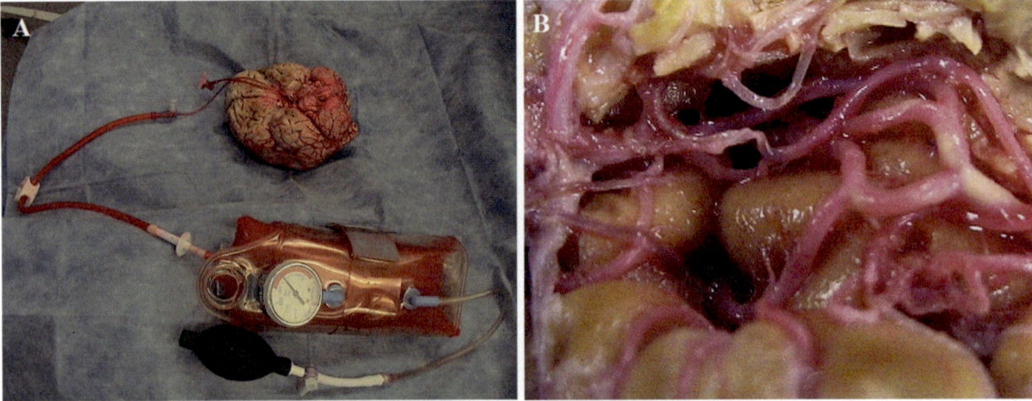

Fig. 8.14 (**a**) Isolated brain is cannulated through the carotid arteries and connected to the reservoir, (**b**) MCA branches over the insula, suitable for all types of micro suturing and bypass exercises

Health hazard associated with the use of cadavers is prominent with fresh tissue. Any hazard can be minimized by following universal precautions and performing serologic testing before cadaver use. For neurovascular exercises we usually use lightly preserved cadavers; the model was successfully tested by Benet et al. for a novel embalming technique that provides an optimal retraction profile and lifelike physical properties while preventing microorganism growth and brain decay [16]. Lightly embalmed cadavers allow for the preservation of lifelike tissues and offer more durability for long-term repeated use [17].

These embalming techniques work better for the brain than fresh or cryopreserved specimens.

Settings and preparations of the model may seem to be lengthy and demanding but in fact, they are not. Preliminary preparation is the same traditional preparation for cadaveric dissection; the only difference is the final cannulation of the vessels and irrigation, which can be achieved within 90 min in most cases. We started giving instructions to our providers to do the cannulation the way we need instead of the traditional cannulation they used to do as this will reduce the preparation time and efforts. Preparing the aneurysm model is time-consuming but by itself is part of the training. The preparation basically includes performing a surgical approach, followed by fine and microdissection of the vessels and neural structure, and then performing a micro-anastomosis to create the aneurysm.

For future use of the "live cadaver," we are working on the development of a new review course for the final years of neurosurgery residents where they spend a full week performing all possible neurosurgical procedures that they have already learned and the ones that they didn't have the chance to practice and finally be able to create their own aneurysms in different locations and practice clipping and managing complications. Such advanced training would be a transitional step forward, and the "live cadaver" would be the first surgical case for every surgery resident before he moves to his own practice. To facilitate use of our model, we designed a special pump contained in a compact box along with blood reservoirs *(US 6790043)* [18].

In the meantime, with few modifications, cardiac pumps that are no longer for clinical use work very well, tubes, cannulas and other accessories are readily available in any medical facility, and blood simulant can be either purchased as prepared formula or locally made with tap water and water-based coloring materials.

Needless to say, the live cadaver model can be used to practice all types of procedures in other surgical disciplines. We described the use of the whole cadaver for training with traumatic injuries and penetrating wounds and for practicing airway management [19, 20].

Conclusion

Pseudoaneurysms created in real human vasculature allows for true simulation of the conditions of live surgery on cerebral aneurysms and intraoperative aneurysmal rupture and provides a great opportunity for residents and trainees to practice these procedures in a realistic surgical environment. The "live cadaver" model combines the actual human anatomy with lifelike conditions. This model could significantly improve the current training in aneurysm surgery and in neurosurgery at large, particularly procedures and conditions that residents have no adequate exposure to during their residency.

Acknowledgments We thank Ronalda Williams for her editorial assistance and Ron Tribell for his artistic work.

References

1. Liu A, Huang J. Treatment of intracranial aneurysms: clipping versus coiling. Curr Cardiol Rep. 2015;17(9):628.
2. Batjer H, Samson D. Intraoperative aneurysmal rupture: incidence, outcome, and suggestions for surgical management. Neurosurgery. 1986;18:701–7.
3. Batjer H: Comment on Lawton MT, Du R: Effect of the neurosurgeon's surgical experience on outcomes from intraoperative aneurysmal rupture. Neurosurgery. 2005;57:9–15.
4. Chowdhry SA, Spetzler RF. Genealogy of training in vascular neurosurgery. Neurosurgery. 2014;74(Suppl 1):S1989–203.
5. Yasargil MG. Microneurosurgery, vol. I. New York: Thieme Stratton; 1984. p. 6.
6. Alaraj A, Luciano CJ, Bailey DP, Elsenousi A, Roitberg BZ, Bernardo A, Banerjee PP, Charbel FT. Virtual reality cerebral aneurysm clipping simulation with real-time haptic feedback. Neurosurgery. 2015;11(Suppl 2):52–8.
7. Singh H, Kalani M, Acosta-Torres S, El Ahmadieh TY, Loya J, Ganju A. History of simulation in medicine: from Resusci Annie to the Ann Myers Medical Center. Neurosurgery. 2013;73(Suppl 1):9–14.
8. Mori K, Yamamoto T, Nakao Y, Esaki T. Development of artificial cranial base model with soft tissues for practical education: technical note. Neurosurgery. 2010;66(6 Suppl Operative):339–41.
9. Aboud E, Al-Mefty O, Yasargil MG. New laboratory model for neurosurgical training that simulates live surgery. J Neurosurg. 2002;97:1367–72.
10. Aboud E, Aboud G, Al-Mefty O, Aboud T, Rammos S, Abolfotoh M, Hsu SP, Koga S, Arthur A, Krisht A. "Live cadavers" for training in the management of intraoperative aneurysmal rupture. J Neurosurg. 2015;123(5):1339–46.
11. Reed AB, Crafton C, Giglia JS, Hutto JD. Back to basics: use of fresh cadavers in vascular surgery training. Surgery. 2009;146:757–62.
12. Jansen S, Cowie M, Linehan J, Hamdorf JM. Fresh frozen cadaver workshops for advanced vascular surgical training. ANZ J Surg. 2014;84(11):877–80.
13. Mitchell EL, Sevdalis N, Arora S, Azarbal AF, Liem TK, Landry GJ, Moneta GL. A fresh cadaver laboratory to conceptualize troublesome anatomic relationships in vascular surgery. J Vasc Surg. 2012;55(4):1187–94.

14. Benet A, Plata-Bello J, Abla AA, Acevedo-Bolton G, Saloner D, Lawton MT. Implantation of 3D-printed patient-specific aneurysm models into cadaveric specimens: a new training paradigm to allow for improvements in cerebrovascular surgery and research. Biomed Res Int. 2015;2015:939387.

15. Anastakis DJ, Regehr G, Reznick RK, et al. Assessment of technical skills transfer from the bench training model to the human model. Am J Surg. 1999;177:167–70.

16. Benet A, Rincon-Torroella J, Lawton MT, S'anchez JJG. Novel embalming solution for neurosurgical simulation in cadavers: laboratory investigation. J Neurosurg. 2014;120(5):1229–37.

17. Anderson SD. Practical light embalming technique for use in the surgical fresh tissue dissection laboratory. Clin Anat. 2006;19:8–11.

18. Aboud ET. Method and apparatus for surgical training. U S Patent No US 6,790,043. Sep 2004.

19. Aboud ET, Krisht AF, O'Keeffe T, Nader R, Hassan M, Stevens CM, et al. Novel simulation for training trauma surgeons. J Trauma. 2011;71:1484–90.

20. Aboud ET, Aboud G, Aboud T. "Live cadavers" for practicing airway management. Mil Med. 2015;180(3 Suppl):165–70.

Use of Cadaveric Models in Simulation Training in Spinal Procedures

Theodosios Stamatopoulos, Vijay Yanamadala, and John H. Shin

Introduction

The practice of spinal surgery is thought to have originated in ancient Egypt, around 3000 BC [1]. Neurosurgery is a specialty that requires a high level of skill, not only because of the complex anatomy of the structures of the central and peripheral nervous system but also due to the irreversible damage that can be easily caused to the patient. Spine surgeons often experience the situation of an obvious MRI or CT image of spine pathologic condition with a rather demanding and complex operation. Our clinical experience has shown that patients in neurosurgery can be at a very critical condition, so there is need for experienced and qualified surgeons, who can operate accurately and precisely. In an interesting study by Moby et al. at the University of Texas Medical Branch, 415 out of 3505 members of the American Academy of Neurological Surgeons were questioned whether they had operated on a wrong level of the spine [2]. Interestingly, it had shown that over half of them had made a mistake during their career. But also, in the same study, researchers also found that the annual risk of wrong spine-level operation dramatically reduced over the years of practice. Additionally, the introduction of novel techniques and equipment for spine surgery has opened avenues for physicians to search for new ways to upgrade their skills. Several types of surgical laboratories have been organized, where the intraoperative conditions are being simulated. In the past decades, there has been an increasing interest in this type of training, and after trying different variations of models, human and animal cadaveric models have steered the spine surgery training at a new direction internationally. Thus, with the unmeasurable help of body donors, senior and junior trained doctors could have a highly educative experience. Cadavers offer an exact specimen of the human body and offer young surgeons a great medium to practice their dissection skills. In cadaveric *spine surgery simulation*, surgeons are trained to perform cervical, thoracic, and lumbar spine procedures maintaining the mechanics and stability of the *spine* and more importantly the *spinal cord* along with its *nerve roots*.

T. Stamatopoulos (✉)
Department of Neurosurgery, Massachusetts General Hospital, Harvard Medical School, Boston, MA, USA

CORE-Center for Orthopedic Research at CIRI-AUTh, Aristotle University Medical School, Thessaloniki, Hellas, USA

V. Yanamadala · J. H. Shin
Department of Neurosurgery, Massachusetts General Hospital, Harvard Medical School, Boston, MA, USA

Why Do We Need the Cadaveric Models in Training for Spine Surgery?

Spine is the tree of life. Respect it. (Martha Graham)

© Springer International Publishing AG, part of Springer Nature 2018
A. Alaraj (ed.), *Comprehensive Healthcare Simulation: Neurosurgery*,
Comprehensive Healthcare Simulation, https://doi.org/10.1007/978-3-319-75583-0_9

Although Martha was not a neurosurgeon but a dancer, what she said is absolutely true.

Role of Spine

The spine holds the load of the upper body and hosts the spinal cord – the pathway through which messages from the brain are transferred to the rest of the body and backward. The vertebral column is very complicated and difficult to understand as a structure. It is formatted by *vertebrae* which stand in line one above each other shaping a type "S" column, *the vertebral column*, which consists of 24 vertebrae and the sacrum (7 cervical, 12 thoracic, 5 lumbar, and the sacrum) forming four curvatures (cervical, thoracic, lumbar, and sacral). Between the vertebrae, there are the *intervertebral discs* which connect them and absorb and spread the loads from each other. Impressively, each vertebra is unique and differs from the rest, and yet, with the tone of the muscles and its' strong ligaments, spine is stable and allows three-dimensional movements of the trunk [3]. Spine is also divided into three columns: posterior, middle, and anterior [4]. More importantly, the spine holds the body in the right position and hosts the *spinal cord* with the exiting *nerve roots*, which give motion and feeling to the body.

Learning on Cadavers

Knowing that nerve tissue is very sensitive, it is clear that accuracy when operating on the spine is a prerequisite, because every neural injury can lead to devastating and irreversible consequence. Sclafani JA. et al. showed that this precious technical proficiency in minimally invasive spinal procedures such as trans-foraminal interbody fusions is very difficult to gain. Specifically, the complication rate decreases dramatically after 30 operations and the operation time after the 15th operation on average [5]. In another study, Gonzalvo A. et al. proved that it takes approximately 25 cases, meaning 80 screws for a resident, to correctly place the pedicle screws, indicating that this type of procedure is difficult

to learn [6]. It is obvious that the lack of experience leads to longer operation time and, in this way, raises the cost of each surgery. Unfortunately, residents may not be able to reach this number of cases throughout their training, and indicatively the curriculum in medicine, e.g., in the United Kingdom and United States, offers little exposure to the fields of neurosurgery during the final years of medicine [7]. Additionally, it has been proven that students understand better the anatomy through cadaveric dissection [8]. Kshettry VR et al. found that the 93.8% of neurosurgery programs in the United States include cadaveric dissection during the training – 77% of them practice spinal instrumentation – and more importantly it was clear that "educators believe that cadaveric dissection is an integral part of the training" [7]. The Congress of Neurological Surgeons (CNS) has established a committee in 2010 to organize the education of the residents, for them to be better prepared for operations (Fig. 9.1.). The residents are now educated and perform the same operation several times in simulation models; therefore, they are more experienced when they get involved in the operating room (OR) later in their training [9] (Table 9.1). Thus, every budding spine surgeon should be encouraged to train on cadaveric models as early as possible, to understand the peculiar anatomy of the spine and augment their surgical skills.

About Cadavers

From ancient times, around the early third century BC, cadaveric dissection was carried out by Greek Physicians Herophilus of Chalcedon and Erasistratus of Chios. Da Vinci later on, at 1506 AD, studied the human body in detail [10]. In recent years, the cadaveric dissection is part of the anatomy lesson in most medical schools around the globe, and students sometimes take part voluntarily [8]. Apart from it, the cadavers have been used by physicians from all the specialties to sharpen their skills. Nowadays, the body donation rate is still low because very few people are eager to donate their or their family member's body to science. Through certain procedures,

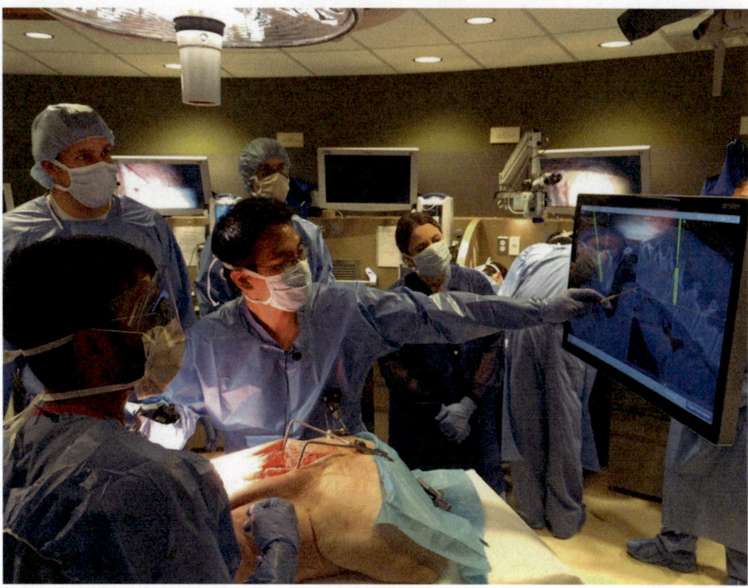

Fig. 9.1 Residents learn the anatomy and correct pedicle screw positioning

experts can conserve the bodies for a long period of time at a very good and acceptable condition, which is problem solving because this gives a great quality of tissue to learn on and provides the time to schedule the next training course [11, 12]. There are four techniques mainly used (fresh frozen, formalin, Theil's, and saturated salt solution method); each of them has its value [12]. There are differences on the quality of tissue they offer for training. On the one hand, there is no significant difference in the range of motion (ROM) and softness of the tissue and joints between Theil's and saturated salt solution embalming method. On the other hand, the fresh frozen method seems to be the most popular of them, as it offers the closest-to-fresh specimen to operate on. It always depends on the facility restrictions of the laboratory which preservation method is being used, though [12]. Tomlinson JE et al. showed that trainees were more satisfied by the Theil's technique for preservation of the body when they were asked to place pedicle screws in the cadaver and evaluate the cadaver's quality [13].

Additionally, we did not find any studies or laboratories globally which conduct *pediatric* cadaveric training except synostosis models, which is made of rubber [14]. Specifically in the United Kingdom, the minimum age at which someone is allowed to donate his body to science is 17 years old. The cadaveric dissection is being done with respect to the underlying person and only for educational reasons. Summarizing, with the help of the technology on preserving the quality of the tissue, training on cadavers will help us minimize the morbidity and mortality of the surgery in general.

Setting Up the Training Lab

There are many cadaveric training laboratories that offer the opportunity to neurosurgeons or orthopedic surgeons to expertise on the classic techniques or get to know the new instruments and new approaches, which are emerging in spine surgery [7]. If no human cadavers are available, sheep or pigs can be used [11, 15]. The sheep's spine provides an acceptable specimen for practicing due to similarities in the anatomy, so the techniques can be repeated likewise in humans especially for lumbar procedures [16–18]. Sheep are preferred for transthoracic routes, while pigs are suggested for anterior transabdominal approaches [10]. Fresh tissues in spine surgery are mandatory because they closely mimic the actual consistency of soft tissues while performing dissections. Animal cadavers are easily available in rural areas and provide a useful and cheap educational tool [10].

Table 9.1 Advantages and disadvantages of cadaveric spine surgery [18, 19]

Advantages	Disadvantages
Reveal the stress of the patient that the surgeon is learning on him	Ethical restrictions on humans and animals
Enhance skills and experience, learn how to use mechanical strength	Difficulty in reoperation
Learn the anatomy and anatomical landmarks	Not equal to living human
Have guidance from experienced surgeons – valuable time for discussion	Can operate on animal tissue
Lack of intraoperative stress – have the chance of mistake	Operate in a "safe environment" – no mistakes have clinical complications
Operate with up-to-date equipment and become familiar with the new techniques	Courses can be expensive and are held at specific places
Become increasingly familiar with the theater setup	All the spine pathology may be not available
The trainee is being evaluated continuously	Some procedures are being done with assumptions
Training on cases that they may not have the chance to during the residency	The stability of the spine is not being tested postoperatively as it would be in real life
The cost/time of each surgery is being reduced	Minimal neural intraoperative damage cannot be detected
Better quality of service in medicine	

Theater-like conditions are mandatory, as well as up-to-date technical infrastructure. C-arm mobile X-ray or computer-assisted image-guided technology helps the trainees visualize each case before and after the operation. Preoperative imaging and discussion of each case individually with experienced surgeons stimulates potential decision-making situations and encourages trainees to think about choosing the right surgical approach and the appropriate instruments depending on the local anatomy.

In summary, the combination of the infrastructure with the special surgical equipment, along with the guidance of the right trainers, leads to very qualified physicians.

Theoretical Part

As the courses are organized to fully train spine surgeons from both surgical and theoretical aspect, all cadaveric workshops include lessons during which trainees can enhance their knowledge. Surgeons are educated through lectures highlighting series of aspects and controversial cases questioning whether the patient should have an operation or not and how (which procedure and approach). Orthopedic and neurological surgeons exchange their experience on spine surgery as in some cases they operate together. A fundamental skill of a surgeon is to know when *not* to lead a patient to surgery; therefore, these discussions provide trainees with valuable principals. Through these courses, spine surgeons have the opportunity to discuss rare and difficult cases, types of patients who need specific management and follow-up, as well as the latest techniques in spine surgery. It is known that on the ground that spine surgery is very elective and that the new guidelines are being introduced by surgeons who operate at international medical centers, cadaveric courses offer unique opportunity for meaningful discussion. Berjano P. et al. in his study stated that learners were very satisfied by discussing cases with experts, as they had the chance to have a useful case-based conversation, but more importantly, nearly 70% of them changed their opinion on the appropriate treatment [19]. Thus trainees can assess their level of knowledge and get valuable guidance on cases that they haven't experienced before throughout their career. Unfortunately, there are discussed cases that may not be seen on cadavers such as revisions, malignancies or spine metastases, fractures (osteoporotic or pathologic), infections, scoliosis and deformities, and many special cases. In this way, next to high qualified and experienced surgeons, through a one-to-one teaching procedure and hands-on training, there is the time needed for the trainees to better understand the procedures and gain the necessary experience required.

Beyond that, the cadaveric laboratories are equipped with new high-quality neurosurgical equipment. New tools are being presented and tested by the trainees, demonstrating their use, the developments they have, and how they will make the surgery safer. In this way, surgeons are getting used to handling these instruments in a safe environment and under right guidance. More importantly, as technology develops rapidly and new innovative equipment is being promoted to surgical practice all the time, this exposure to new technology is more than necessary. In this way, any chance of intraoperative mistakes in the real operation is being minimized.

Additionally, trainees experience real-time operative simulation in OR setup. Strict attention to patient positioning is being paid as any mistake can change the outcome of a surgery [20]. Major postoperative complications such as visual loss, perioperative peripheral nerve injury, or even death can occur because of bad patient positioning [20–22, 33] (Table 9.2). It is being made clear that the surgical courses on cadavers sharpen the attitude, boosts the confidence and the surgical skills of trainees, and builds up the surgical personality of orthopedic and neurological surgeons [22, 23].

Table 9.2 Complications associated with inappropriate prone patient positioning in spine surgery

Complication category	Complication
Hemodynamic	Pressure on the inferior vena cava, pressure of the chest (cardiac dysfunction), acute renal failure
Ophthalmologic	Ischemic optic neuropathy (posterior and anterior), central retinal artery occlusions, cortical blindness
Neurologic	Pneumocephalus, acute cervical myelopathy, spinal cord compression (infraction), CN VI palsy, brachial plexopathy, ulnar nerve palsy, lateral femoral cutaneous nerve neuropathy, meralgia paresthetica
Myocutaneous	Acute rhabdomyolysis, ischemic limb due to arterial compression, compartment syndrome, pressure ulcers, femoral head avascular necrosis, shoulder dislocation
Abdominal	Abdominal compartment syndrome, acute bowel ischemia

Practical Part: Hands On

Thus far, technology has not yet offered us the means to functionally conserve neither the *spinal cord* nor the *nerves* in a condition at which we could practice on this very sensitive part of the spine with *intraoperative neurophysiological monitoring* (Fig. 9.1.). However, there have been cadaveric studies on spinal cord anatomical variations, so this can be educational for the trainees; surgeons can only learn from it as an anatomical structure and the anatomical landmarks of the spinal cord [24, 25].

In fact, the cadaveric muscles, joints, and vertebrae are in an acceptable condition. When the fresh frozen, the Theil's, and the saturated salt solution method are used, the muscles and the joints are softer and have wider ROM than when formalin is used [12]. This makes the Theil's method ideal for screw insertion training [13]. Apart from international courses, which use cadaveric models, cadaveric dissection is a part of the program of many scientific congresses. Trainees learn to identify the anatomical structures and the anatomical landmarks at each part of the spine. In conclusion, nowadays we have the means to take advantage of chemistry, conserve the bodies in an acceptable condition, and learn on human and animal cadavers, conducting dissections and a wide variety of procedures on the cadaveric spine.

Learning on the Cadaveric Cervical Spine

Applied Cervical Spine Surgery on Cadavers

The most commonly conducted cervical spine (CS) operations aim to cure spinal cord compression and spinal instability. Operating on CS can be very demanding, as out of the seven cervical vertebrae (C1–C7), two of them, C1/atlas and C2/axis, have unique shape and the neck hosts vital anatomical structures and nerves. And yet, after operating in the cervical spine, the neck must be functional, with a satisfactory ROM. Cadaveric

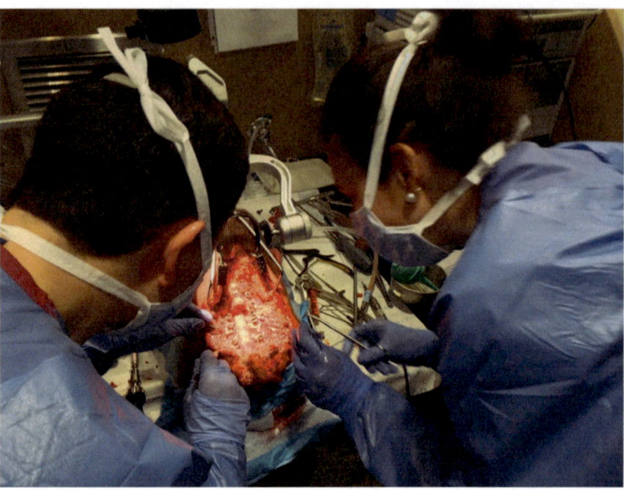

Fig. 9.2 Trainees learn the anatomical landmarks and the surgery of the cervical spine

Table 9.3 Operation being learned on cadaveric cervical spine

Types of operations on cadaveric cervical spine
Trans-oral odontectomy
C1–C2 fusion and plates
Occiput C1–C2 stabilization
Cervical lateral mass screw and plate fixation
Posterior cervical micro discectomy
Cervical corpectomy
Anterior cervical micro foraminotomy – laminoforaminotomy
Anterior cervical discectomy approach
Decompressive procedures – durotomy

Table 9.4 Complications of cervical spine surgery

Complications when operating on cervical spine [26]
Carotid or vertebral artery injury, which may result to stroke
Excessive bleeding
Neural root injury (recurrent laryngeal, superior laryngeal, and hypoglossal nerve injuries)
Damage to the spinal cord (about 1 in 10,000), resulting in paralysis
Quadriplegia
Leakage of cerebral spinal fluid
Pneumocephalus
Damage to the esophagus, trachea, or vocal cords
Nonunion
Screw malposition
Spinal instability
Chronic neck or arm pain
Persistent swallowing or speech disturbance

spine surgery training includes all these principals as it offers close-to-reality conditions [25] (Fig. 9.2). Trainees are being taught anatomy along with the anatomic landmarks and the fundamental skills that every spine surgeon should acquire. Special attention is being given to the C1 and C2 surgery, as their unique shape and role requires high level of accuracy and experience, by specialized surgeons. Most CS procedures can be stimulated on cadavers, so they should be included in spine surgery education (Table 9.3), The bodies can be decapitated or not, depending on the laboratory [11]. At the present, most CS procedures are being educated on cadavers.

The neck hosts vital organs; surgical approaches in spine surgery can be very demanding. Complications after cervical spine surgery (CSS) can be fatal, so the surgeons' excellence is manda-

tory (Table 9.4). Postoperative pitfalls are avoided through careful analysis of the spinal anatomy and pathology, right selection of the patients who are led to the OR and right technique conduction.

Learning on the Thoracic and Lumbar Cadaveric Spine

The thoracic spine (TS) and the lumbar spine (LS) are formed by 12 and 5 vertebrae, respectively. These two parts of the spine are often referred together as many of the surgical procedures include both.

Applied Thoracic Spine Surgery on Cadavers

TS has unique characteristics. On the one hand, TS surgery includes fewer chances of postoperative complications due to the stability of the thorax and thus less mechanical forces on the operated area. On the other hand, though, the narrow anatomical distances and relations of the nerve roots with the pedicles make TS surgery tough [27]. At TS surgery, the most common pathologies that can be stimulated on cadavers are spinal cord compression of any cause (tumor, disc herniation, etc.) and TS stabilization arthrodesis. Scoliosis and deformities of the TS are not usually seen on cadaveric workshops; however, the correcting operation can be simulated on them following the basic spine surgery principles (Table 9.5). The altered anatomy and the difficultly, sometimes to recognize the anatomical landmarks in such cases, show the value of this type of training [28]. At specific laboratories there is special course on scoliosis and deformities and potentially tumor extraction, with specific assumptions. Impressively, it was found that 10% of the adult deformity surgery presented postoperative complications. Although this rate depends on many factors, surgeons need to improve their skills and minimize the risk of the surgery.

TS arthrodesis and spinal cord decompressions are often followed by spine fusion with screws and rods stabilization, if stability is compromised. However, learning to correctly insert the screws in the pedicle needs experience and assistance using intraoperative imaging such as fluoroscopy or CT guidance. This so commonly applied surgical procedure seems to be difficult to learn, and especially at TS, there is experience required. Burgeson RK. et al. studied the time and the experience that a resident needed, regardless of his year of training, to learn how to insert 297 screws in the thoracic pedicle. He used 15 cadavers for his study, and the results demonstrated that after a certain amount of screws on the fourth cadaver for each surgeon, their skills improved significantly, indicating the necessity of this type of training simulation [29]. The same result was proven by Yong Jung's study, as the chances of misplacing pedicle screws using free-hand technique decrease over the years of experience [30]. Experience and right guidance seem to be major factors in improving the skills in spine surgery and minimizing the chances of perioperative complications [31, 32] (Table 9.6). Cadaveric TS training has its' unique value, as apart from learning of the approaches posteriorly, trainees have the chance to perform laparoscopic TS (Figs. 9.3 and 9.4.).

In summary, TS surgery can also be successfully stimulated on cadavers, aiding the trainees to boost their surgery skills and confidence.

Applied Lumbar Spine Surgery on Cadavers

LS is the part of the spine that most commonly presents with pathological conditions.

Table 9.5 Operations being learned at cadaveric thoracic spine

Types of operations being learned on cadaveric thoracic spine
Thoracic pedicle screws
Surgical approach to thoracic inlet
Surgical approach to thoracic vertebrae – anterior/anterolateral/posterior
Thoracic wedge osteotomy
Thoracoscopic discectomy

Table 9.6 Complications of thoracic spine surgery

Complications when operating on thoracic spine
Pedicle fractures
Screw misplacement
Screw loosening or pull-out
Dural lesions
Nerve root irritation
Sense and motor deficits
Partial bilateral drop foot
Lower extremity paraplegia
Pleural effusion
Pneumothorax – hemothorax
Thoracic aorta impingement
Injury of the right coronary artery
Cerebrospinal fluid leakage

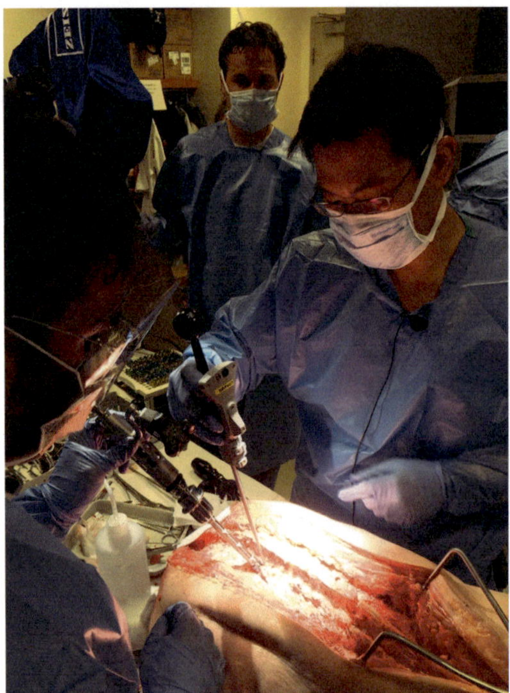

Fig. 9.3 Thoracic and lumbar spinal fusion. Trainee's hands-on practice. Under supervision, the thoracic and lumbar screws are being placed with fluoroscopic guidance

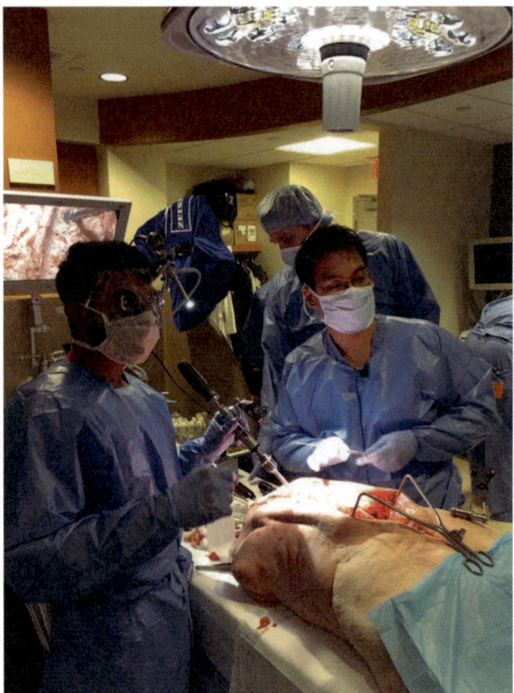

Fig. 9.4 Thoracic and lumbar spinal fusion. Trainee's hands-on practice. Under supervision, the thoracic and lumbar screws are being placed with fluoroscopic guidance

Lumbar disc herniation is one of the most common diagnosis in the United States reaching almost 2% of the population. When surgical discectomy is needed, lateral, posterolateral, or posterior approach can be used. In these procedures, as they are routine for the spine surgeons, there is less tolerance for mistakes (Table 9.7), so the training on cadavers can give the experience needed to the residents. They can perform difficult approaches at the lumbar spine and get used with the anatomy in general.

In addition, decompression and stabilization procedures are being done, covering most the cases, such as laminotomies, laminectomies, laminoplasty, foraminotomy, as well as fusion and lumbar interbody cages. Although the mechanical stability of the spine cannot be tested as it would be in real life, surgeons can effectively improve their performance. Furthermore, the complications of lumbar spine surgery are being pointed out to the trainees (Table 9.8.).

Table 9.7 Operations on cadaveric lumbar spine

Types of operations being learned on cadaveric lumbar spine
Pedicle screws
Interbody fusion – translateral posterior surgical approaches
En bloc discectomy
Endoscopic discectomy
Percutaneous spinal fixation procedures
Lumbar interbody cages
Lumbar puncture

Minimally Invasive Surgery on Cadavers

As long as endoscopic and robotic surgery are increasing in use in clinical practice, there will be need for training in these new surgical techniques.

Thus, minimally invasive surgery (MIS) has drawn the attention of surgeons the last decades.

Table 9.8 Complications of lumbar spine surgery

Complications after operating on lumbar spine [33]
Dural tear
Motor loss of the lower limb – nerve palsy
Increased leg or low back pain
Screw malposition
Screw/rod breakage or looseness
Pedicle fracture
Cerebrospinal fluid leakage
Adjacent disc herniation

Undoubtedly, patients prefer smaller surgical incisions as they offer less postoperative pain and a small scar. A systematic review comparing MIS versus open posterior lumbar interbody fusion stated that there is less blood loss, quicker decrease in postoperative pain, and better functional recovery in patients with MIS [34]. On account of this, the MIS is steering surgery in new techniques making it mandatory for all surgeons to change their surgical approach. Additionally, MIS is associated with less postoperative pain and less complications during and after surgery [37]. However, surgical skills are acquired basically by experience and not theoretically. Sclafani et al. found that the complication rate of the MIS lumbar micro discectomy is reduced after the 30th operation [35]. Cadaveric courses offer this opportunity to spine surgeons as they can practice these techniques in the safety of the laboratory environment and learn from the specialists on a one-to-one basis.

Abuzayed B et al. practiced thoracoscopic spinal procedures as sympathectomy, discectomy, and corpectomy through lateral approach and so indicated this technique for complicated cases, which are not suitable for the usually used approach [36]. Accordingly, Isaacs RE et al. used successfully a posterolateral approach to perform micro endoscopic discectomy without entering in the chest cavity, on cadavers, pointing out that this approach is safe for the patients as it caused minimal damage to the surrounding soft tissue [37].

Research on Cadaveric Spine

Except for surgical training, cadavers offer us the opportunity for academic research on them. Anatomic dissections add extra knowledge through a better understanding of the anatomy and the dynamics of the spine [38]. Liu J and his team reviewed the published literature on the variation of the cervical vertebrae anatomical dimensions, concluding that there are differences between men and women and more impressively between Asian and European/American population. This is a fact that a spine surgeon should certainly take into consideration before leading a patient to the OR [38].

Several laboratories are also testing new techniques and surgical approaches on cadavers. When a new technique is applied, it must be tested on anatomical and technical aspects. Human body cadavers are an excellent medium for surgeons to practice their dissection skills. The importance of such cadaveric spinal surgery training was being demonstrated in Srikantha U et al.'s study, where MIS for atlantoaxial fusion was tested in four fresh frozen cadavers before it was applied to living patients, successfully [39]. Additionally, Ludwig CS et al. compared three techniques on pedicle screw placement on cadavers – (1) using anatomical landmarks, (2) using visual and tactile cues after laminoforaminotomy, and (3) using computer-assisted guidance – and proved that taking into consideration the cervical spine anatomy, the anatomical variations, and the anatomical structures of the neck, pedicle screw placement is demanding and should be under image-assisted guidance [40]. In Dixon's D et al. study which was conducted on fresh frozen cadavers, it was found that dynamic surgical guidance during screw insertion in cervical spine aids the surgeon at real-time circumstances, showing the route of the screw and thus avoiding any complications as shown above [41]. At another study, first Kessler and his team studied the use of ultrasound guidance on cadavers to find the correct space for lumbar puncture preoperatively, a skill which can easily be used as an alternative of intraoperative X-ray when less radiation is required [28].

Cadavers are additionally used as a mean to test and study the biomechanics of implants which are used for spinal reconstructions. In Jerry Y. Du et al.'s meta-analysis on the biomechanics of different types of screw constructs which are used to stabilize the C1–C2 levels of the CS and which were applied on cadavers, it was shown that the currently used techniques have significant differences in stability, so their use and effectiveness should be clinically evaluated [42]. Majid K. et al. used CS of 14 cadavers to test the biomechanics and stability of extender plates when loads can be applied mechanically highlighting the need for further research on the materials which are used on the spine [43]. Accordingly, Reis MT et al. showed that the 4-screw cage or the standard plate with cage is more stable than the 2-screw cage especially at extension and axial rotation of the CS [44].

First, Junhui et al. studied the correlation of mechanical properties of the lumbar discs with endplates and suggested that the quality of the endplate is affected by the disc degeneration over the years and decompression surgeries. This finding indicates that the extraction of the lumbar intervertebral disc changes the stresses of the adjacent vertebra, contributing to potentially more degenerative changes [45].

Studies like these help surgeons to acquire a better understanding of the spine, test ex vivo the instrument and the implants which are being used, and help them have better postoperative results. However, in the aforementioned studies, it was clearly stated that the number of the cadavers in each of them was not enough for safe conclusions, so further studies are needed.

Conclusion: Discussion

In conclusion, cadaveric spine surgery training and research are nowadays a necessary part of the neurosurgery training regardless of the level of skills or experience. Despite the assumptions and disadvantages of this type of training, evidence shows significant impact on the surgeon's performance. It is better from an ethical perspective to be more qualified over the years and provide better quality of medical practice. Surgery is making steps forward in terms of surgical techniques and new equipment, so spine surgeons need to follow these changes. To respond to this call for new knowledge and better training, many surgical skill courses on cadavers have been organized. Studies show that cadaveric spine surgery training contributes to the development of surgical personalities, in terms of knowledge and skills. Thus, the American Association of Neurosurgical Surgeons, the European Association of Neurosurgeons, and many hospital-based and university-based laboratories around the globe have organized this type of courses regularly. It is essential for the surgeon to be qualified, build his attitude, and make right choices.

References

1. Perez-Cruet MJ, Balabhadra RSV, Samartzis D, Kim DH. Historical background of minimally invasive spine surgery. In: Kim DH, Fessler RG, Regan JJ, editors. Endoscopic spine surgery and instrumentation. New York: Thime; 2004. p. 3–18. Attaching top medical students to a career in Neurosurgery.
2. Mody MG, Nourbakhsh A, Stahl DL, Gibbs M, Alfawareh M, Garges KJ. The prevalence of wrong level surgery among spine surgeons. Spine. 2008;33:194–8.
3. Spinal disorders: fundamentals of diagnosis and treatment. Am J Neuroradiol. 2009.; https://doi.org/10.3174/ajnr.a1299.
4. Denis F. The three column spine and its significance in the classification of acute thoracolumbar spinal injuries. Spine. 1983;8:817–31.
5. Sclafani JA, Kim CW. Complications associated with the initial learning curve of minimally invasive spine surgery: a systematic review. Clin Orthop Relat Res. 2014;472:1711–7.
6. Gonzalvo A, Fitt G, Liew S, de la Harpe D, Turner P, Ton L, Rogers MA, Wilde PH. The learning curve of pedicle screw placement: how many screws are enough? Spine. 2009;34:E761–5.
7. Kshettry VR, Mullin JP, Schlenk R, Recinos PF, Benzel EC. The role of laboratory dissection training in neurosurgical residency: results of a national survey. World Neurosurg. 2014;82:554–9.

8. Nwachukwu C, Lachman N, Pawlina W. Evaluating dissection in the gross anatomy course: correlation between quality of laboratory dissection and students' outcomes. Anat Sci Educ. 2015;8:45–52.

9. Harrop J, Lobel DA, Bendok B, Sharan A, Rezai AR. Developing a neurosurgical simulation-based educational curriculum: an overview. Neurosurgery. 2013;73(Suppl 1):25–9.

10. Jones R. Leonardo da Vinci: anatomist. Br J Gen Pract. 2012;62:319.

11. Smith A, Gagliardi F, Pelzer NR, Hampton J, Chau AM, Stewart F, Mortini P, Gragnaniello C. Rural neurosurgical and spinal laboratory setup. J Spine Surg. 2015;1:57–64.

12. Hayashi S, Naito M, Kawata S, Qu N. History and future of human cadaver preservation for surgical training: from formalin to saturated salt solution method. Anat Sci Int. 2016. https://doi.org/10.1007/s12565-015-0299-5.

13. Tomlinson JE, Yiasemidou M, Watts AL, Roberts DJ, Timothy J. Cadaveric spinal surgery simulation: a comparison of cadaver types. Global Spine J. 2016;6:357–61.

14. Coelho G, Warf B, Lyra M, Zanon N. Anatomical pediatric model for craniosynostosis surgical training. Childs Nerv Syst. 2014;30:2009–14.

15. Benneker LM, Gisep A, Krebs J, Boger A, Heini PF, Boner V. Development of an in vivo experimental model for percutaneous vertebroplasty in sheep. Vet Comp Orthop Traumatol. 2012;25:173–7.

16. Gragnaniello C, Abou-Hamden A, Mortini P, Colombo EV, Bailo M, Seex KA, Litvack Z, Caputy AJ, Gagliardi F. Complex spine pathology simulator: an innovative tool for advanced spine surgery training. J Neurol Surg A Cent Eur Neurosurg. 2016;77:515–22.

17. Suslu H. A practical laboratory study simulating the percutaneous lumbar transforaminal epidural injection: training model in fresh cadaveric sheep spine. Turk Neurosurg. 2012;22:701–5.

18. Turan Suslu H, Tatarli N, Hicdonmez T, Borekci A. A laboratory training model using fresh sheep spines for pedicular screw fixation. Br J Neurosurg. 2012;26:252–4.

19. Berjano P, Villafañe JH, Vanacker G, Cecchinato R, Ismael M, Gunzburg R, Marruzzo D, Lamartina C. The effect of case-based discussion of topics with experts on learners' opinions: implications for spinal education and training. Eur Spine J. 2016. https://doi.org/10.1007/s00586-016-4860-2.

20. Kamel I, Barnette R. Positioning patients for spine surgery: avoiding uncommon position-related complications. World J Orthop. 2014;5:425–43.

21. Stambough JL, Dolan D, Werner R, Godfrey E. Ophthalmologic complications associated with prone positioning in spine surgery. J Am Acad Orthop Surg. 2007;15:156–65.

22. DePasse JM, Palumbo MA, Haque M, Eberson CP, Daniels AH. Complications associated with prone positioning in elective spinal surgery. World J Orthop. 2015;6:351–9.

23. Chambers SB, Deehan DJ. Cadaveric surgical training improves surgeon confidence. The Bulletin of the RCS. 2015.

24. Turnbull IM, Brieg A, Hassler O. Blood supply of cervical spinal cord in man: a microangiographic cadaver study. J Neurosurg. 1966;24:951–65.

25. Breig A, Turnbull I, Hassler O. Effects of mechanical stresses on the spinal cord in cervical spondylosis: a study on fresh cadaver material. J Neurosurg. 1966;25:45–56.

26. Harrop JS, Aarabi B, Shaffrey C, Dvorak M, Fisher C. Early versus delayed decompression for traumatic cervical spinal cord injury: results of the Surgical Timing in Acute Spinal Cord Injury Study (STASCIS). PLoS One. 2012;7:e32037.

27. Ebraheim NA, Jabaly G, Xu R, Yeasting RA. Anatomic relations of the thoracic pedicle to the adjacent neural structures. Spine. 1997;22:1553.

28. Kessler J, Moriggl B, Grau T. The use of ultrasound improves the accuracy of epidural needle placement in cadavers. Surg Radiol Anat. 2014. https://doi.org/10.1007/s00276-013-1243-9.

29. Bergeson RK, Schwend RM, DeLucia T, Silva SR. How accurately do novice surgeons place thoracic pedicle screws with the free hand technique? Spine. 2008. https://doi.org/10.1097/BRS.0b013e31817b61a.

30. Oh CH, Yoon SH, Kim YJ, Hyun D, Park H-CC. Technical report of free hand pedicle screw placement using the entry points with junction of proximal edge of transverse process and lamina in lumbar spine: analysis of 2601 consecutive screws. Korean J Spine. 2013;10:7–13.

31. Gautschi OP, Schatlo B, Schaller K, Tessitore E. Clinically relevant complications related to pedicle screw placement in thoracolumbar surgery and their management: a literature review of 35,630 pedicle screws. Neurosurg Focus. 2011;31:E8.

32. Lonner BS, Auerbach JD, Estreicher MB, Kean KE. Thoracic pedicle screw instrumentation: the learning curve and evolution in technique in the treatment of adolescent idiopathic scoliosis. Spine. 2009. https://doi.org/10.1097/BRS.0b013e3181b4f7e8.

33. Shriver MF, Zeer V, Alentado VJ, Mroz TE, Benzel EC, Steinmetz MP. Lumbar spine surgery positioning complications: a systematic review. Neurosurg Focus. 2015;39:E16.

34. Goldstein CL, Phillips FM, Rampersaud YR. Comparative effectiveness and economic evaluations of open versus minimally invasive posterior or transforaminal lumbar interbody fusion: a systematic review. Spine. 2016;41(Suppl 8):S74–89.

35. Shriver MF, Xie JJ, Tye EY, Rosenbaum BP, Kshettry VR, Benzel EC, Mroz TE. Lumbar microdiscectomy complication rates: a systematic review and meta-analysis. Neurosurg Focus. 2015;39:E6.

36. Abuzayed B, Tuna Y, Gazioglu N. Thoracoscopic anatomy and approaches of the anterior thoracic spine: cadaver study. Surg Radiol Anat. 2012. https://doi.org/10.1007/s00276-012-0949-4.

37. Isaacs RE, Podichetty VK, Sandhu FA, Santiago P, Spears JD, Aaronson O, Kelly K, Hrubes M, Fessler RG. Thoracic microendoscopic discectomy: a human cadaver study. Spine. 2005;30:1226–31.

38. Liu J, Napolitano JT, Ebraheim NA. Systematic review of cervical pedicle dimensions and projections. Spine. 2010;35:E1373–80.

39. Srikantha U, Khanapure KS, Jagannatha AT, Joshi KC, Varma RG, Hegde AS. Minimally invasive atlantoaxial fusion: cadaveric study and report of 5 clinical cases. J Neurosurg Spine. 2016:1–6.

40. Ludwig SC, Kramer DL, Balderston RA, Vaccaro AR, Foley KF, Albert TJ. Placement of pedicle screws in the human cadaveric cervical spine: comparative accuracy of three techniques. Spine. 2000;25:1655–67.

41. Dixon D, Darden B, Casamitjana J, Weissmann KA, Cristobal S, Powell D, Baluch D. Accuracy of a dynamic surgical guidance probe for screw insertion in the cervical spine: a cadaveric study. Eur Spine J. 2016. https://doi.org/10.1007/s00586-016-4840-6.

42. Du Jerry Y, Aichmair A, Kueper J, Label TWDR. Biomechanical analysis of screw constructs for atlantoaxial fixation in cadavers: a systematic review and meta-analysis. J Neurosurg Spine. 2015;22(2):151–61.

43. Majid K, Moldavsky M, Khalil S, Gudipally M. An in-vitro biomechanical study evaluating cervical extension plates for stabilizing degenerated adjacent levels. Clin Spine Surg. 2016. https://doi.org/10.1097/BSD.0b013e3182a26734.

44. Reis MT, Reyes PM, Crawford NR. Biomechanical assessment of anchored cervical interbody cages: comparison of 2-screw and 4-screw designs. Neurosurgery. 2014;10(Suppl 3):412–7; discussion 417.

45. Liu J, Hao L, Suyou L, Shan Z, Maiwulanjiang M. Biomechanical properties of lumbar endplates and their correlation with MRI findings of lumbar degeneration. J Biomech. 2016;49:586–93.

Konstantin V. Slavin and Dali Yin

Introduction

Low back pain with or without radiculopathy is estimated to affect 70% of adults during a lifetime in developed countries [1] and is a major health problem globally [2, 3]. Low back pain can result in functional limitations and consequent disability [4] that produce significant medical and economic burden on individuals and society. In the USA, more than $100 billion are used to treat patients with chronic neuropathic pain each year [5, 6]. Medications and corrective surgery have demonstrated some efficacy for management of chronic pain. However, therapeutic effectiveness is not always achieved with these treatments, which, on other hand, may result in some serious adverse effects. Therefore, there is an obvious need for a neurosurgeon to learn alternative surgical techniques for the treatment of chronic pain, therefore reducing related disability.

Spinal cord stimulation (SCS) has been developed as an established treatment for chronic neuropathic pain [7, 8]. The advantages of SCS include effectiveness, reversibility, minimal invasiveness, and low complication rate, which make it more popular than before for pain management. With the improvements in leads and battery of SCS system, it has become the most commonly used surgical intervention for chronic pain. Approximately 14,000 patients around the world undergo SCS implantation each year [9]. More than 60,000 SCS systems have been implanted in the USA over the past 15 years, many with very successful results [9]. Recently, two technological innovations, percutaneous paddles and wireless SCS devices, have been developed, and these would raise the level of neurosurgical interest in percutaneous lead insertion. Despite the advanced technology and large number of surgeries involved, 30% of implanted patients fail to achieve long-term pain relief in the follow-up period [10]. Many factors influence the success rates in SCS, including physician experience, surgical technique, patient selection, and postoperative follow-up care [9]. It has been shown that surgeons' experience and surgical skills positively impact on morbidity and mortality [11, 12]. However, SCS is not part of standard neurosurgical educational curriculum, and training for placement of SCS system is nonmandatory. Since implantation and management of SCS systems are a multidisciplinary teamwork, any physicians in this regard should be familiar with patient selection, implantation, and follow-up. To increase its applicability, guidelines and training requirements for SCS device have been issued by the North American Neuromodulation Society (NANS) for neurosurgeons, orthopedic surgeons, anesthesiologists, physiatrists, neurologists, and others [9].

K. V. Slavin (✉) · D. Yin
University of Illinois at Chicago, Department of
Neurosurgery, Chicago, IL, USA
e-mail: kslavin@uic.edu; daliyin@uic.edu

© Springer International Publishing AG, part of Springer Nature 2018
A. Alaraj (ed.), *Comprehensive Healthcare Simulation: Neurosurgery*,
Comprehensive Healthcare Simulation, https://doi.org/10.1007/978-3-319-75583-0_10

Neurological surgery requires years of training to obtain the knowledge and technical skills in order to provide high-quality patient care that is safe and effective. Learning through observation and operation in the operating room (OR) has been the majority of surgical training, which has faced too many issues, including patient safety, work hour limitations, and cost of OR time [13]. On the other hand, surgeons must practice to improve their skills and to maintain proficiency. SCS is a relatively simple neurosurgical procedure; however, it requires training to maximize therapeutic benefit while minimizing surgical risks to patients. Moreover, high level of functioning in patients with chronic neuropathic pain and a small number of surgeons who perform SCS has prevented such hands-on training in the OR. Therefore, improvement in SCS training and education is very important for both surgeon and patient safety. Fortunately, simulation technology offers opportunities to teach surgeons and allow them to practice surgical procedures outside the OR [14]. It can provide surgeons with appropriate training to obtain surgical skills, techniques, and knowledge before practicing procedures on the real patients.

Simulation Training

Simulation allows surgeons to use models to practice surgical procedures in a controlled setting. It has played an important role in providing appropriate education and training for neurosurgeons who can obtain surgical skills and knowledge without compromising care quality or patient safety. It is clear that the ideal place for the initial acquisition and refinement of surgical skills, including SCS, is not in the operating room. Moreover, it is necessary for neurosurgeons to learn surgical technical skills to provide safe patient care. Simulation-based training enables surgeons to reproduce the SCS techniques in a protected environment for not only residency and fellows but also practitioners.

Simulation is currently used in different ways in the education, including virtual reality (such as computer simulators), physical models (such as cadaveric models and synthetic models), and mixed-reality simulator with focus on technical and nontechnical skills and knowledges. The benefits of simulation have been demonstrated in neurosurgical training, which provides surgeons with opportunities to refine techniques and enhances the safety and efficacy of surgical procedures before the actual clinical practice. Surgical techniques used in SCS simulation include [1] identification of anatomical landmarks, [2] the use of fluoroscopy for placement of SCS electrodes, and [3] generator implantation. Simulation would be an efficient learning strategy for SCS procedure. Importantly, surgeons can go back to simulation training repeatedly until they feel comfortable to perform SCS procedure. The SCS simulation can help surgeons to place electrodes effectively, thus reducing postoperative complications.

In our practice, we have used percutaneous permanent leads and "tunnel trial" technique for implantation of SCS system. It is usually done in a standard operating room. This technique allows us to avoid having the patient go through electrode insertion twice. The main advantage of this approach is that the same lead used during the trial will be also used as permanent electrode for SCS. Moreover, the lead insertion becomes easier with exposure of the deep fascia, therefore making access to the epidural space less complicated and more predictable. Here, in this book chapter, we described the simulation of SCS step by step for treatment of chronic pain, which may be able to provide surgeons and pain specialists with a no-risk learning environment for improved performance of this procedure. Surgeons can be trained using physical models for SCS technique. The details are described as following.

Chronic Pain: Indications and Patient Selection

SCS is mainly used to treat neuropathic pain, such as failed back surgery syndrome (FBSS), complex regional pain syndrome (type I, reflex sympathetic dystrophy, and type II, causalgia), peripheral neuropathy, spinal arachnoiditis, lumbar radiculitis, and severe ischemic pain from perivascular disease. FBSS is the most common indication for SCS. For patients with neuropathic pain, MRI and/or CT are necessary to rule out pathologies that can be treated surgically.

In the use of SCS, appropriate patient selection is a major determinant of successful outcome. Patients are selected based on correct diagnosis, failure with conservative therapy, psychological evaluation, medical evaluation, patient expectations, and SCS trial demonstrating pain relief. Understanding of what factors predict a good outcome from SCS is critical in counseling patients.

Surgical Techniques of SCS Procedure

NANS offers cadaver training course of SCS procedures at an annual meetings.

There are medical labs in Medtronic, St. Jude, and Boston Scientific, which provide a realistic environment that enables a surgeon to simulate SCS procedures under the guidance of their experts. We have used "tunnel trial" technique for SCS procedure, which includes insert of permanent percutaneous electrode(s) from the beginning. This SCS surgical technique includes two stages of the procedures, with stage one of electrode implantation, and stage two of electrode internalization and implantation of SCS generator.

Stage I: Electrode Implantation

Implantation of electrodes is performed under monitored anesthetic care. The patient is placed in prone position (Fig. 10.1). The AP view of the lumbar spine is obtained with C-arm to determine incision site (Fig. 10.2). After injection of local anesthetic, a 2-cm straight incision is made, and a pocket is created under the skin and above the fascia by dissection of soft tissue (Fig. 10.3).

First, A 18-gauge Tuohy needle is inserted into the epidural space (Fig. 10.4), usually at the level of L2–L3 under fluoroscopic guidance (Fig. 10.5) with the loss of resistance technique. Then guide wire is inserted through the needle

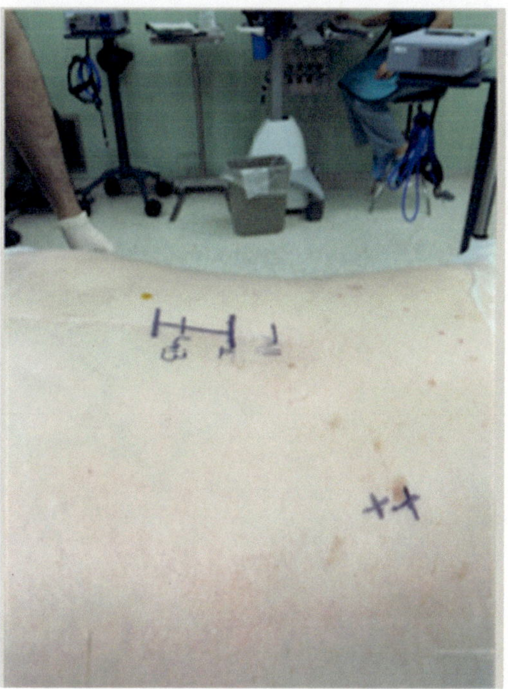

Fig. 10.1 Patient positioned prone on the operating table

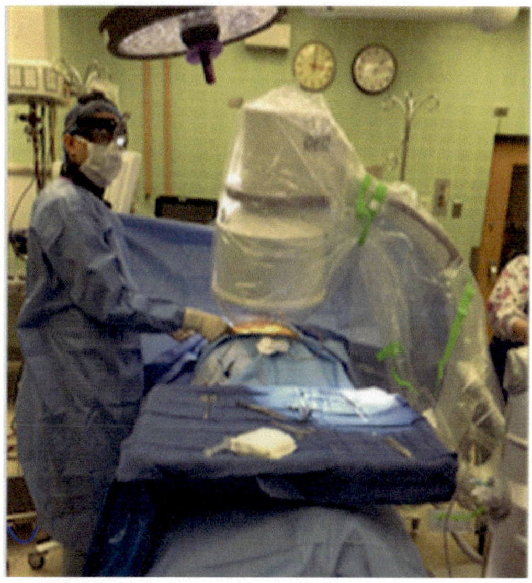

Fig. 10.2 Levels of surgery are confirmed with C-arm fluoroscopy

and removed after confirmation. The first percutaneous electrode is inserted through the needle into the epidural space (Fig. 10.6) and advanced up to the target level, such as T8–T9 under live

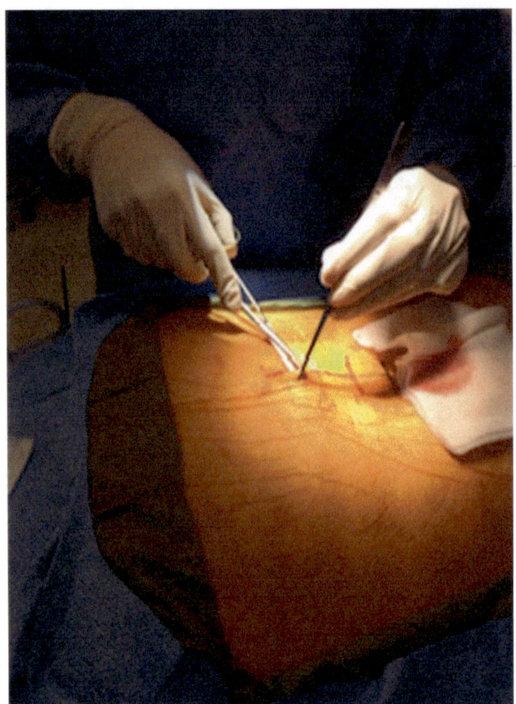

Fig. 10.3 A pocket is created under the skin and above the fascia

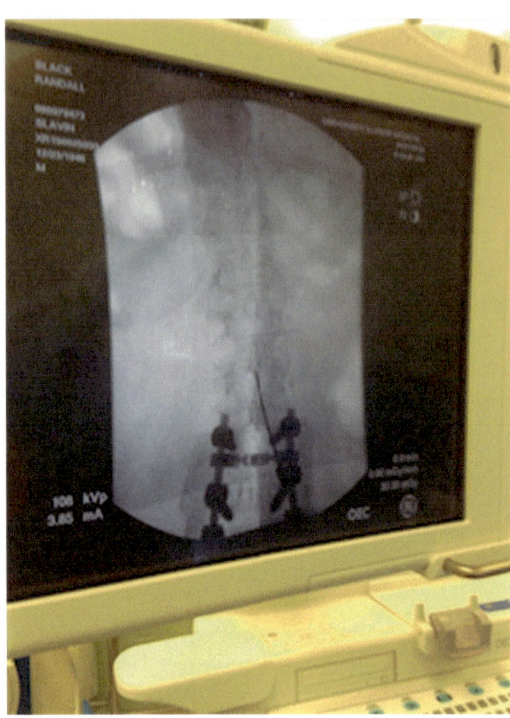

Fig. 10.5 Fluoroscopic image of paramedian needle insertion

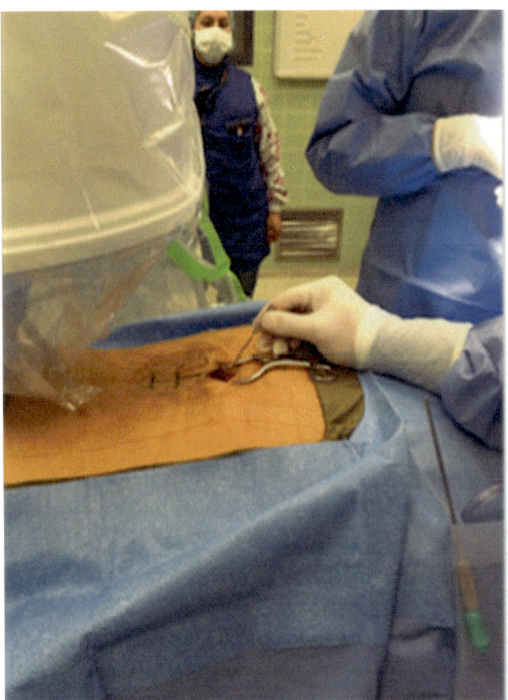

Fig. 10.4 Paramedian needle insertion

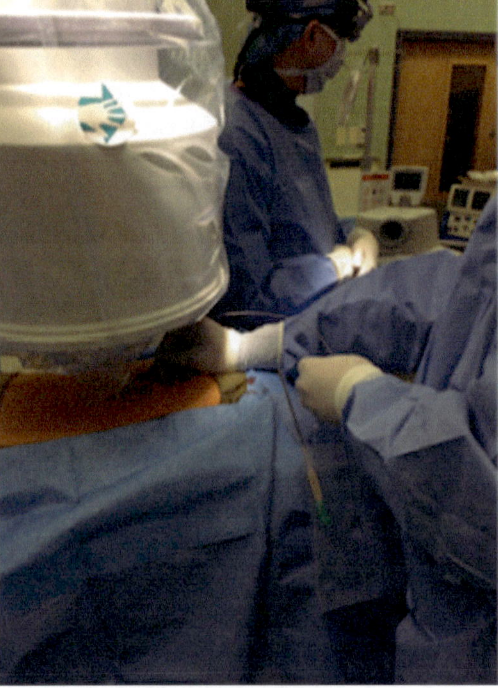

Fig. 10.6 Percutaneous electrode is inserted through a needle

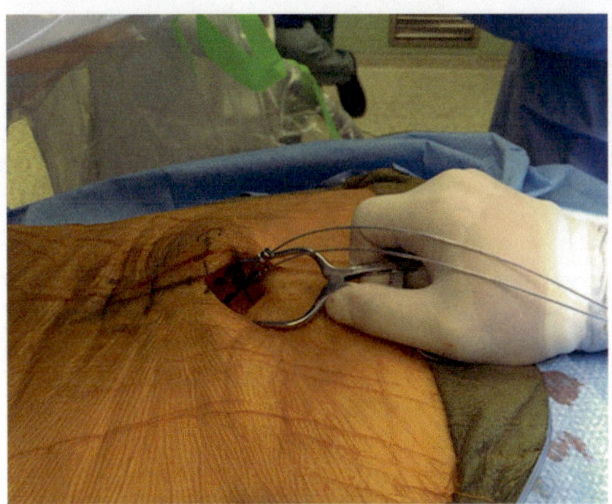

Fig. 10.7 The second percutaneous electrode is inserted through the needle and advanced parallel to the first one all the way to the target level

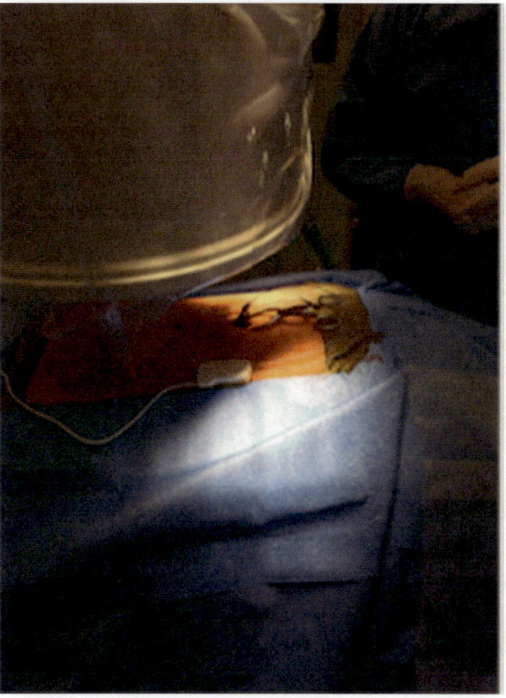

Fig. 10.8 Electrodes are connected to the screening cable for intraoperative stimulation trial

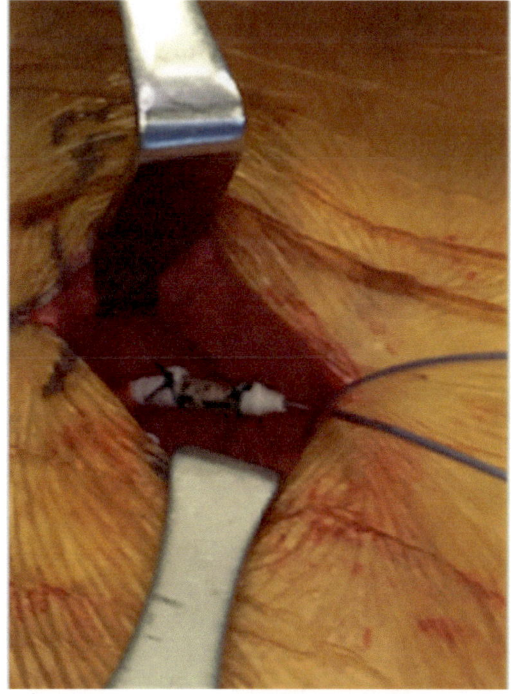

Fig. 10.9 Electrodes are anchored to the fascia. Two nonabsorbable sutures are placed over each anchor, which is fixed onto the fascia

fluoroscopy. Similarly, the second percutaneous electrode is placed through the needle and advanced parallel to the first one, all the way to the desired level (Fig. 10.7).

After the electrodes are positioned side by side in the posterior epidural space, the intraoperative stimulation trial is started. The patient sedation is stopped prior to initiation of intraoperative testing. The electrodes are connected to temporary extension wires and screening device (Fig. 10.8). By asking the patient about his/her sensations, different configurations and stimulation parameters are tested until the patient described good coverage of his/her painful areas. Repositioning of electrodes may need to be performed to adjust the distribution of paresthesias. Once the intraoperative trial is completed, the position of the electrodes is recorded with C-arm fluoroscopy. The needles are removed, and the electrodes are anchored to the fascia (Fig. 10.9).

Two temporary extension cables are tunneled subcutaneously on the opposite side of the proposed generator location and brought to the skin surface 10 cm away from the original midline incision (Fig. 10.10). Extension cables are connected to SCS electrodes. The excess of the electrodes is coiled above the fascia but below the connection with the temporary cables (Fig. 10.11) to protect the electrodes during internalization. The incision is closed in layers with 2-0 Vicryl for the subcutaneous tissues and 3-0 nylon for the skin (Fig. 10.12). A nylon suture is used to affix

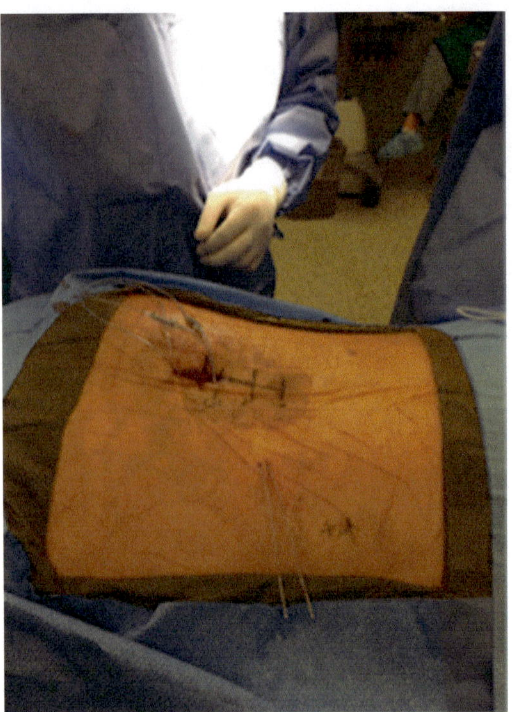

Fig. 10.10 Tunneling for extension cables and connection between electrodes and extension cables

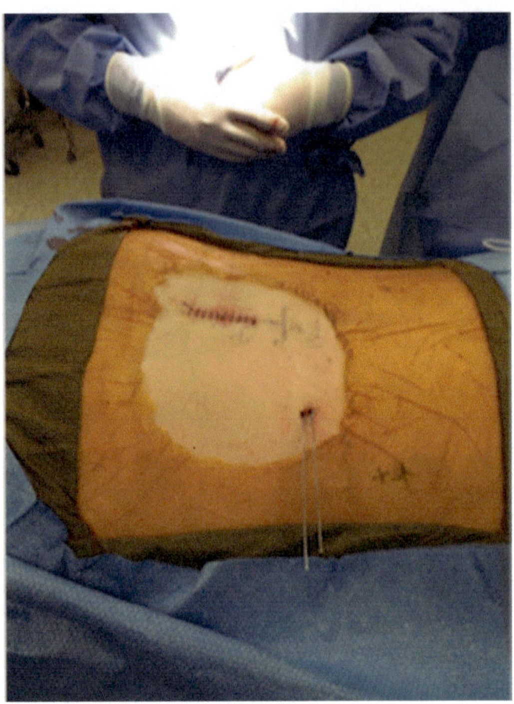

Fig. 10.12 Skin incision closure

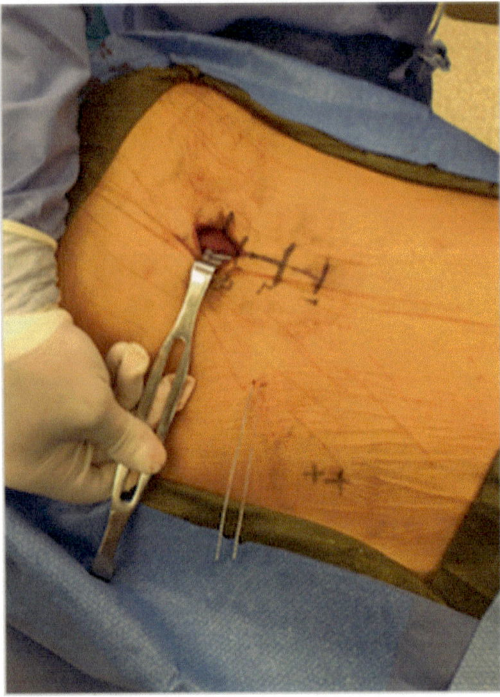

Fig. 10.11 The excess of the electrodes is coiled above the fascia but below the connector with the temporary cables

the temporary extension cables onto the skin to prevent dislodgement and to minimize the risk of infection (Fig. 10.12). Extension cables are connected to the screening cable, and the impedance of all contacts of electrodes is checked and confirmed to be within normal range.

The patient can test the device for about 7 days to confirm that the paresthesia is perceived in a good place and the pain relief is adequate. If the trial is successful, patient will have electrode internalization and implantation of implantable pulse generator (IPG). On the other hand, if the trial fails, lead/anchor/extension cable needs to be removed in the OR.

Stage II: Electrode Internalization and Implantation of SCS Generator

This procedure is performed under general anesthesia. If the patient is not a driver, the generator is usually implanted in the right side of abdominal area to avoid the seatbelt line. In cases like this, patient is intubated and placed in lateral decubitus position with his/her right side up. This allows access to both lumbar and anterior abdominal regions. After prep, draping, and application of local anesthetic, first the suture line in the lumbar region is reopened carefully, and the electrodes and extension cables are identified. The extension cables are cut and removed. The electrodes are inspected for integrity and checked for length to determine abdominal incision site for accommodation of generator. In some cases, extension cables may be needed.

A second incision is then made on the right side of the abdomen between the 12th rib and iliac crest. The pocket for the generator is made under the subcutaneous plane above the fascia, with the thickness of layer of tissue above the generator less than 2.0 cm. The electrodes are passed through a special passer between lumbar and abdominal incisions, connected to a generator, and secured with setscrews. The generator is then placed into the pocket, attached to the underlying fascia with nonabsorbable sutures. Finally, SCS device is interrogated to confirm that the impedance of all contacts is within normal limits. Incisions are then closed. Our preference is to put the generator into the abdominal wall because of easier recharging and programming, as well as less discomfort during sitting and lying down. Moreover, the abdominal IPG placement may cause less stress to electrodes and extension cables, therefore reducing the risk of migration or fracture.

In summary, this book chapter provides information about simulation of SCS procedure for treatment of chronic neuropathic pain. Through this simulation-based training, we hope it would enhance a surgeon's knowledge, skills, and performance in SCS procedure.

References

1. Andersson GBJ. Epidemiological features of chronic lowback pain. Lancet. 1999;354(9178):581–5.

2. Hoy D, Brooks P, Blyth F, Buchbinder R. The epidemiology of low back pain, best practice and research. Clin Rheumatol. 2010;24(6):769–81.

3. Adams MA. Biomechanics of back pain. Acupunct Med. 2004;22(4):178–88.

4. Vos T, Flaxman AD, Naghavi M, Lozano R, Michaud C, Ezzati M, et al. Years lived with disability (YLDs) for 1160 sequelae of 289 diseases and injuries 1990–2010: a systematic analysis for the Global Burden of Disease Study 2010. Lancet. 2012;380(9859):2163–96.

5. Katz JN. Lumbar disc disorders and low-back pain: socioeconomic factors and consequences. J Bone Joint Surg Am. 2006;88(2):21–4.

6. Luo X, Pietrobon R, Sun SX, Liu GG, Hey L. Estimates and patterns of direct health care expenditures among individuals with back pain in the United States. Spine. 2004;29(1):79–86.

7. Slavin K. Epidural spinal cord stimulation: indications and technique. In: Schulder M, editor. Handbook of functional and stereotactic surgery. New York: Marcel Dekker; 2002. p. 417–30.

8. Burchiel KJ, Slavin KV. Peripheral neuropathic pain syndromes. In: Batjer HH, Loftus CM, editors. Textbook of neurological surgery. Philadelphia: LWW; 2003. p. 3013–22.

9. Henderson JM, Levy RM, Bedder MD, Staats PS, Slavin KV, Poree LR, North RB. NANS training requirements for spinal cord stimulation devices: selection, implantation, and follow-up. Neuromodulation. 2009;12(3):171–4.

10. De La Cruz P, Fama C, Roth S, Haller J, Willocj M, Lange S, Pilitsis J. Predictors of spinal cord stimulation success. Neuromodulation. 2015;18(7):599–602.

11. Bilimoria KY, Phillips JD, Rock CE, et al. Effect of surgeon training, specialization, and experience on outcomes for cancer surgery: a systematic review of the literature. Ann Surg Oncol. 2009;16:1799–808.

12. Holm T, Johansson H, Cedermark B, Ekelund G, Rutqvist LE. Influence of hospital- and surgeon-related factors on outcome after treatment of rectal cancer with or without preoperative radiotherapy. Br J Surg. 1997;84:657–63.

13. Alaraj A, Lemole MG, Finkle JH, Yudkowsky R, Wallace A, Luciano C, Banerjee PP, Rizzi SH, Charbel FT. Virtual reality training in neurosurgery: review of current status and future applications. Surg Neurol Int. 2011;2:52.

14. Alaraj A, Charbel FT, Birk D, Tobin M, Luciano C, Banerjee PP, Rizzi S, Sorenson J, Foley K, Slavin K, Roitberg B. Role of cranial and spinal virtual and augmented reality simulation using immersive touch modules in neurosurgical training. Neurosurgery. 2013;72(Suppl 1):115–23.

Introduction to Haptics

Edwing Isaac Mejia Orozco
and Cristian Javier Luciano

Introduction to Haptics

Haptics refers to the studies of the sense of touch. It enables to "touch" virtual objects simulated in a virtual environment. Haptics is to touching, as visual is to seeing and auditory is to hearing. Therefore, haptic devices allow humans to "feel" computer-generated objects.

Haptics is an interdisciplinary field that merges concepts from computer science, mechanical design, physics, and human perception. The term haptics was introduced in the early twentieth century from the area of psychophysics. Later, on the decade of 1970–1980, haptics was focused on telerobotics. During the early 1990s the first commercially available haptic device was born, named SensAble PHANToM. In the last 20 years, haptics became an active field of research and development worldwide [1].

Unlike computer graphics, which enables a unidirectional interaction, haptics is symmetrical and bidirectional. Examples of devices that pro-

vide this type of dual interaction are robotic tele-manipulators, exoskeletons, physical rehabilitation and exercise machines, intelligent assistance devices, advanced prosthetics, and "near-field" telerobotics, to name a few [2].

The unidirectional interaction on usual computer interaction is shown on Fig. 11.1, where the user provides input commands to the computer, and this device processes the data and prepares a new graphics rendered on the display device. This is a close loop, but there is no other feedback provided to the user besides the images displayed [2].

Haptics is a dual cycle interaction, meaning that there are two control closed loops. In other words, the difference with the previous type of unidirectional interaction is that there is not only a one cycle as with computer graphics. Haptics takes into consideration that there is a machine closed loop taking place on the haptic device and another closed loop on the sensory system of the human. Figure 11.2 describes better this type of dual cycle interaction that is used in haptics [2].

Haptics rendering is a term utilized to describe how the computer generates the forces to be applied by the haptic device. Haptics rendering cycle is a closed loop based on the user's hand movement (input) and the detection of such movements to recreate the forces (output) Fig. 11.3 [1].

E. I. Mejia Orozco (✉)
Department of Research and Development,
Holo Surgical S.A., Warsaw, Poland
e-mail: edwing.mejia-orozco@fulbrightmail.org

C. J. Luciano
Bioengineering, Biomedical and Health
Information Sciences, University of Illinois
at Chicago, Chicago, IL, USA

© Springer International Publishing AG, part of Springer Nature 2018
A. Alaraj (ed.), *Comprehensive Healthcare Simulation: Neurosurgery*,
Comprehensive Healthcare Simulation, https://doi.org/10.1007/978-3-319-75583-0_11

Fig. 11.1 Unidirectional interaction. (Adapted from Mansor et al. [2])

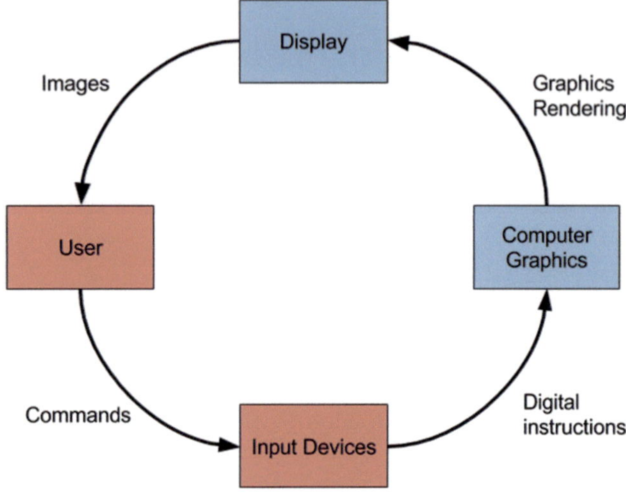

Fig. 11.2 Dual cycle interaction. (Adapted from Mansor et al. [2])

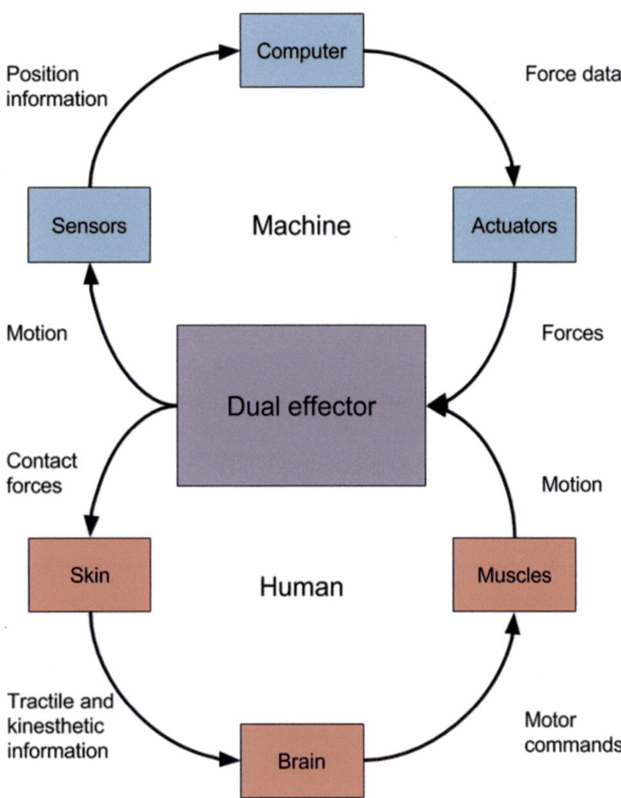

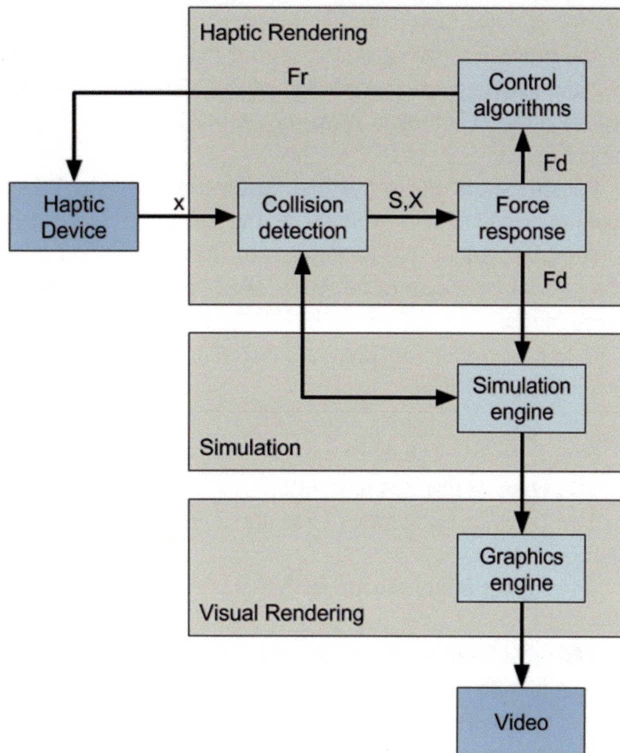

Fig. 11.3 Haptics rendering cycle. (Adapted from Salisbury et al. [1])

Haptics Disciplines

Haptics is divided in three disciplines (Fig. 11.4):

- Human haptics
- Machine haptics
- Computer haptics

Human Haptics

Human haptics merges human perception, cognition, and neurophysiology. Human perception is achieved by both tactile (skin) and kinesthetic (muscle and bone) stimuli. The tactile sensation includes perception of temperature, texture, slip,

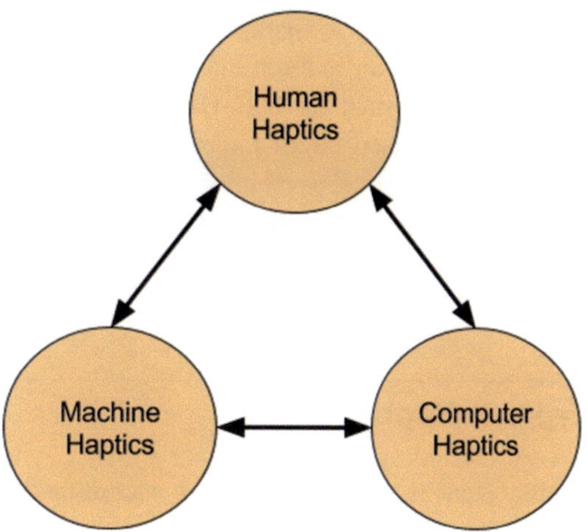

Fig. 11.4 Haptics disciplines. (Adapted from Salisbury et al. [3], CS277 Lecture January 2011)

vibrations, force, and pain. Kinesthetics consists on the process involved in controlling the muscles and knowing where each part of the body is based on the information from the nervous system [3].

Kinesthesia is the sense that detects bodily position, weight, or movement of the muscles, tendons, and joints. The perception of the shape of an object by means of touch is called "tactual stereognosis."

In human perception, there are different types of receptors [3, 4]:

- Four types of mechanoreceptors
- Two types of thermos receptors
- Two types of nociceptors (free nerve endings for pain)
- Three types of kinesthetic receptors

The sense of touch relies on a vast number of sensors in both the skin and the musculoskeletal system that work in conjunction with the motor control system to enable sensing of mechanical stimuli. Haptics does not utilize an extensive bandwidth. The stimuli can be sensed temporally at 1 Khz and with a spatial discrimination of 1 mm. There is an extraordinary sensitivity to certain stimuli such as 300 Hz for vibration (0.1 um and raised edges under 1 um). While haptics does not excel as a high-bandwidth channel for structured information such as characters, words, or text, it does excel at 3D object recognition [3, 4].

Types of Haptic Devices

Haptic devices can be classified according to Salisbury et al. [3, 4] by:

- Kind of stimulus: This represents the type of pressure, force, or sensation that the device provides. It can be an array of pins that move vertically or laterally. There are also shear displays that provide a sensation of different friction on the fingers.
- Degrees of freedom: They represent the number of possible movements that the device can

perform. It can be one such as the one found on pedals or steering wheels and two for mice, stylus, and joysticks. It can reach up to six degrees of freedom like the ones for teleoperators and training phantoms.

- Transmission type: For tactile response, they can be (1) by impedance, as increasing the force on which the user needs to apply to move a device, or (2) by admittance, which uses an active sensor to provide a larger range of forces.
- Grounding location: It refers to where the device is placed for a point of interaction; the categories are divided in grounded or exoskeletal. A grounded device is not a wearable device; an example would be a joystick. The exoskeleton can be several types of wearable devices such as the ones developed by CyberForce, UTAH/Sarcos Research Arm, Rutgers Master, and PERCRO Human Interface. There are also hybrid wearable and exoskeleton devices, such as the inertial reaction device used on video game controllers, which provide vibration depending on the effect.
- Others: sensing quality, actuator quality, and bandwidth communication.

Components of a Haptic Device

Typical haptic devices are mainly composed of actuators and sensors.

(A) *Sensors* allow haptic device to "feel" the interaction with the user. Either force or capacitive field sensors are used by the controller of the device to know when the user is in contact with the haptic device. Force sensor generally consists of a "spring" that changes its electromechanical properties based on the deformation obtained after the force has being applied. Encoders are also sensors in the haptic device. They are generally placed on the shaft of an electrical motor to determine its position, speed, and acceleration. They used to determine the location of each movable part of the arm of the haptic

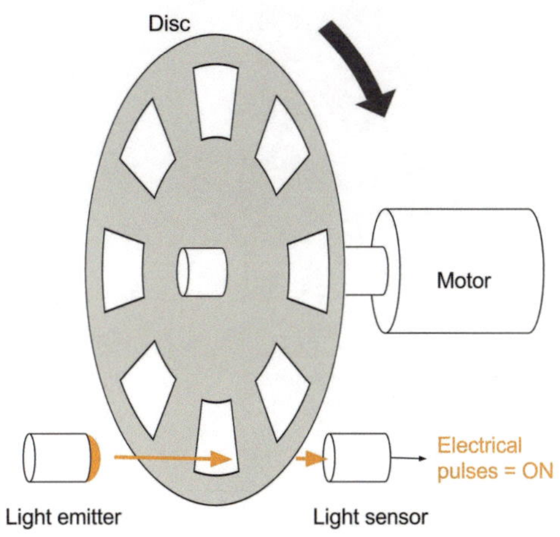
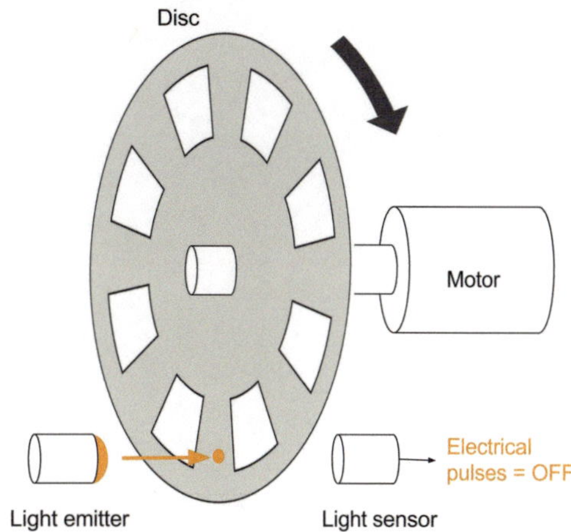

Fig. 11.5 How the encoders work on a referential frame

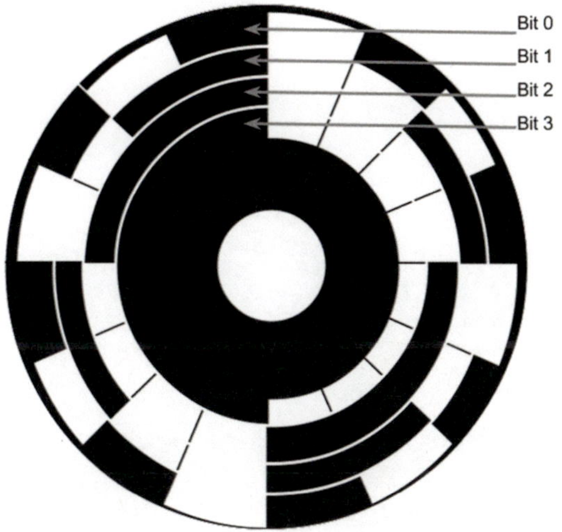

Fig. 11.6 Absolute encoder: can tell the position of the shaft in an absolute frame of reference

device. There are two main types of encoders: (1) optical and (2) magnetoresistive [5].

(1) In optical encoders, a focused beam of light is aimed at a photodetector that gets pulses of light and interrupted light after a certain number of degrees. The encoders can detect a finite number of degrees on an absolute or a referential frame [5] (Figs. 11.5 and 11.6).

(2) Magnetoresistive sensors are built using materials that change their electrical resistance when an external magnetic field is applied. Capacitive field sensors usually have a charge that is placed on specific points that change their properties the reception based on the presence of the external physical elements that divide them. When a user touches something or there is a collision, the electrical field gets disturbed, and a "contact" event is perceived. There are components where a resistance depends on the angle between the magnetization vector of the ferromagnetic material and the direction of the current flow (Fig. 11.7).

(B) *Actuators* allow the user to feel the force applied by the haptic device. Examples of typical actuators are (1) DC brushed motors, (2) brushless motors, (3) servomotors, and (4) pneumatic and hydraulic motors.

(1) DC brushed motors have an armature that rotates inside a field magnet or coil. The armature has a commutator that changes the polarity of the armature windings on each rotation one or two times. The change in polarity forces the rotation to take place on the shaft. After each change in polarity, the shaft rotates more degrees. The brushes keep the same polarity, and those are the ones that transmit the polarity to the windings placed on the commutator [6] (Fig. 11.8).

(2) In brushless motors, the windings do not rotate. There are permanent magnets

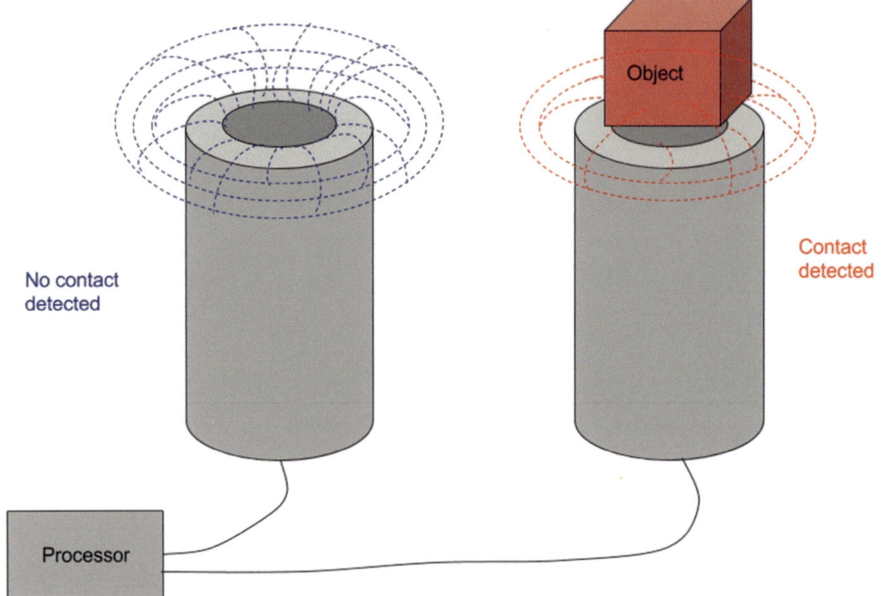

Fig. 11.7 Capacitive sensor

Fig. 11.8 DC brushed motor showing the commutator and brushes

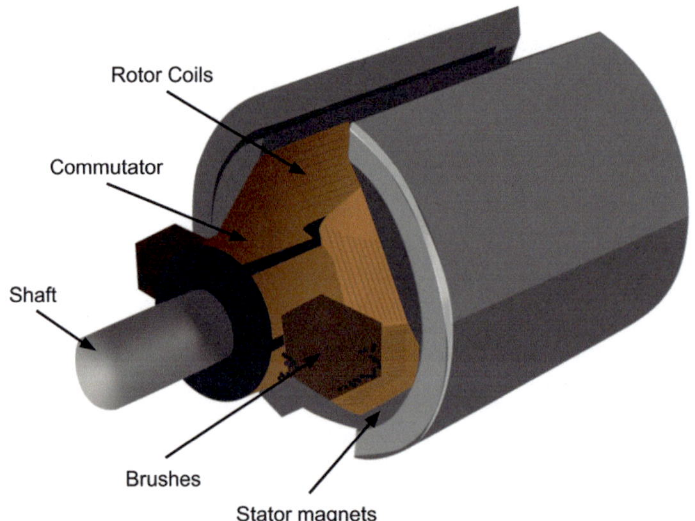

attached to the shaft. The windings change the polarity and attract the permanent magnets of the shaft to a different position. These changes of polarity on the electromagnets that are the windings enable the rotation of the shaft. The brushless motors do not wear that easily over time, so these motors are usually used to provide vibration feedback on the elements of haptic devices that require long period of work and reliability. These vibration feedback elements are also used on video game controllers [6] (Fig. 11.9).

(3) There are also servomotors that work by a combination of a controller, an encoder, and an internal motor. The servomotors use an electrical pulse of variable width

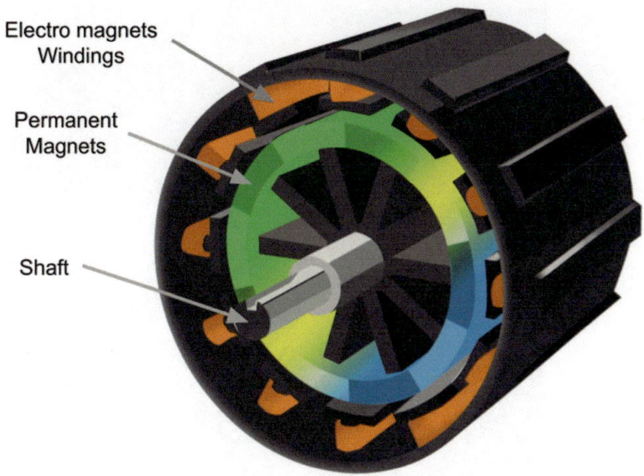

Fig. 11.9 Brushless motor

or pulse width modulation (PWM) as a control signal that activates the internal motor to provide and keep the desired position. Generally, the servomotors reach between 0° and 180°. These are the motors used in the joints of the haptic devices and robotic arms [7].

(4) In pneumatic and hydraulic motors, the flow of different fluids inside a chamber can change the pressure, texture, and strength of a surface. These pumps consist of a motor that controls the flow of fluid or air through the pump based on the pressure feedback that it receives. These types of actuators are used on small devices that have a touchable surface that changes based on the element it simulates.

Examples of Haptic Devices

HaptX created a haptic glove named HaptX GloveTM that allows the user to feel the texture and temperature of different objects using several small actuators. The company is also currently working on an exoskeleton that will enable fully immersive environment for the user into a virtual world. This project will be beneficial for teaching applications and the game industry [8] (Fig. 11.10).

Dexmo, developed by Dexta Robotics, is a haptic device that works similarly to a hand glove, with multiple actuators attached to each finger that allow the user to feel the virtual objects. When coupled with a second device, via Dexmo+Handuino interface, it can measure the resistance provided by real objects and reproduce a virtual replica of the object [9] (Fig. 11.11).

Gloveone is a wearable glove that has a haptic actuator for each finger as well. This glove provides sensations based on the relative position of the virtual represented hand and the virtual environment [10] (Fig. 11.12).

Geomagic Touch X and *Geomagic Touch* (Figs. 11.13 and 11.14), formerly known as SensAble Desktop and Omni, respectively, are two 6-DOF haptic devices manufactured by Geomatic. Being the most popular commercially available haptic devices used for research and development, they provide a relatively strong force feedback in a compact size [11, 12].

Examples of Haptic Medical Simulators

PalpSim was developed by Bangor University and Istituto Italiano di Technologia (Italian Institute of Technology) and their medical partner Royal Liverpool University Hospital. PalpSim is a device that shows a virtual environment on the screen and allows interaction with the user using a palpable surface and a haptic device that works as a syringe or another surgical instrument. The palpable surface detects the force and

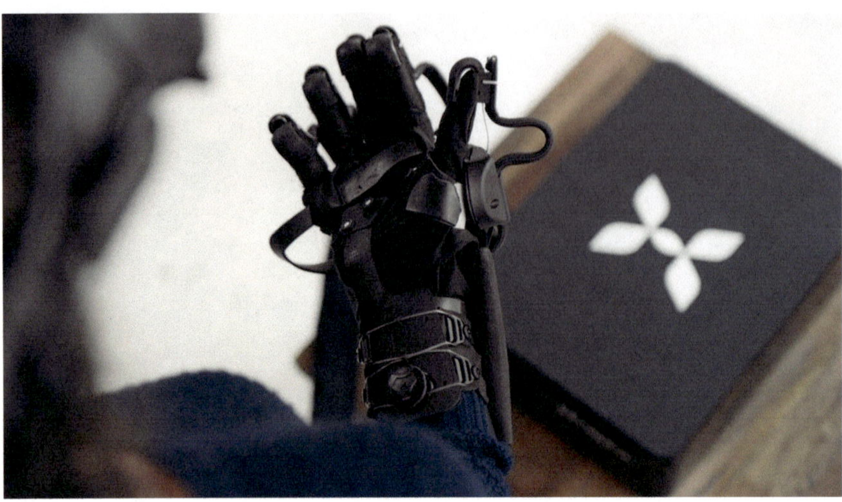

Fig. 11.10 AxonVR. (Courtesy of HaptX Inc., ©2018 [8], used with permission)

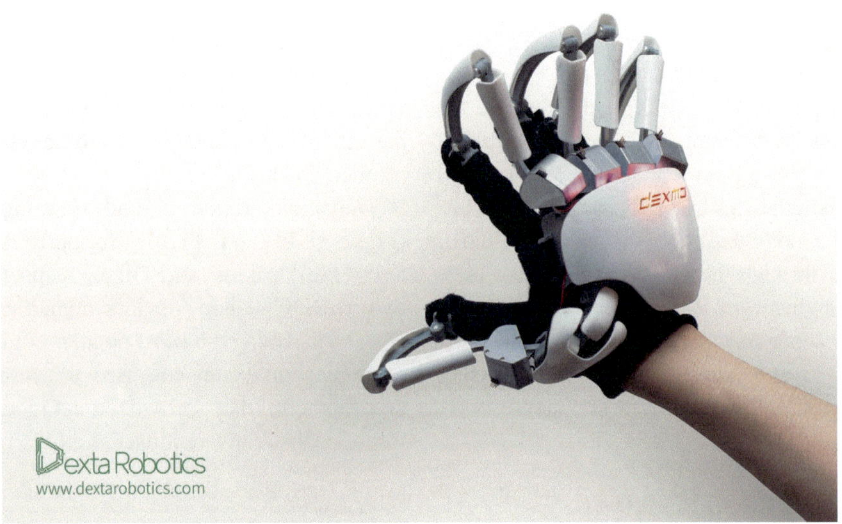

Fig. 11.11 Dexmo. (Courtesy of Dexta Robotics Inc., 2018 [9], used with permission)

updates the force that needs to be applied back to the user. Therefore, there is a real-time interaction that is being shown on a haptic or touchable display, a haptic device, and a visual display [13] (Fig. 11.15).

The *Bimanual Haptic Simulator for Medical Training*, developed by Virtual Reality Group, RWTH Aachen University, uses two haptic devices to simulate bimanual surgical procedures. One haptic device is used to palpate the anatomical 3D model and the other one to handle a virtual needle. A projection screen positioned behind the haptic devices shows the virtual patient, the virtual representations of the surgeon's hands, and the virtual instruments [14] (Fig. 11.16).

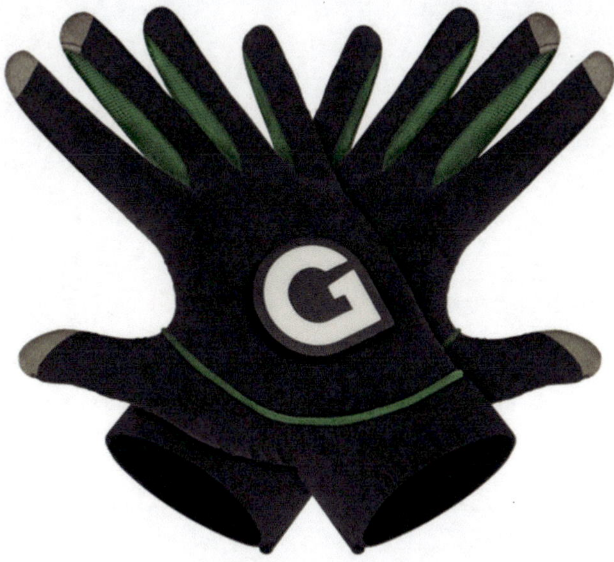

Fig. 11.12 Gloveone. (Courtesy of NeuroDigital Technologies, 2018 [10], used with permission)

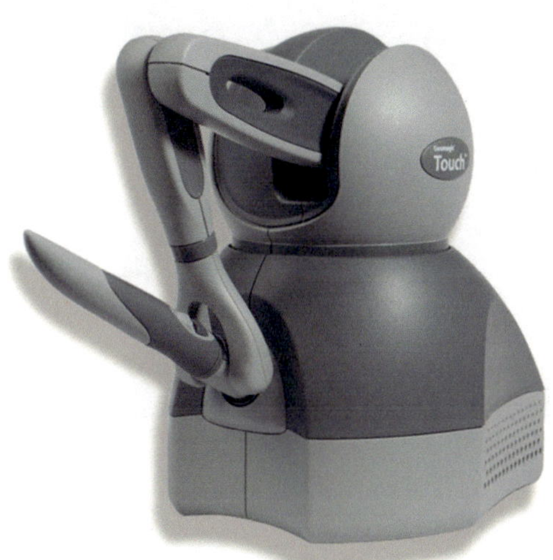

Fig. 11.13 Geomagic Touch. (Courtesy of 3D Systems, 2018 [11], used with permission)

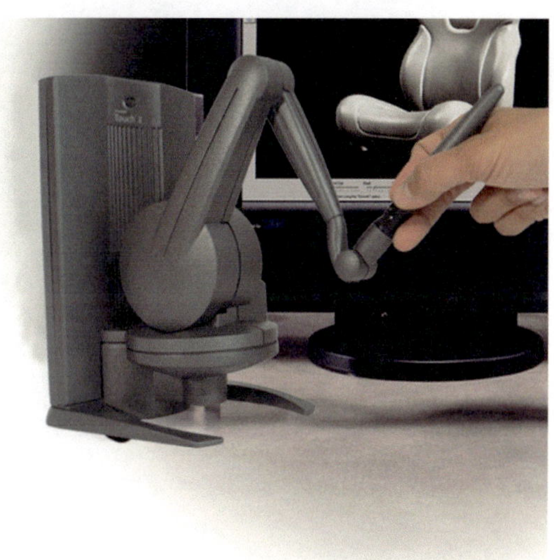

Fig. 11.14 Geomagic Touch X. (Courtesy of 3D Systems, 2018 [12], used with permission)

ImmersiveTouch developed by the University of Illinois at Chicago is a 3D augmented reality and haptic simulator for medical procedures. ImmersiveTouch combines one or two haptic devices, a 3D monitor, an electromagnetic tracker, and a half-silvered mirror to create an augmented reality environment. The haptic devices allow the user to manipulate virtual representations of the virtual instruments and interact with the virtual patient anatomy. The tracking device determines the position and orientation of the user's head to display the proper 3D perspective and perfectly match virtual and real objects in the augmented reality environment [15] (Fig. 11.17).

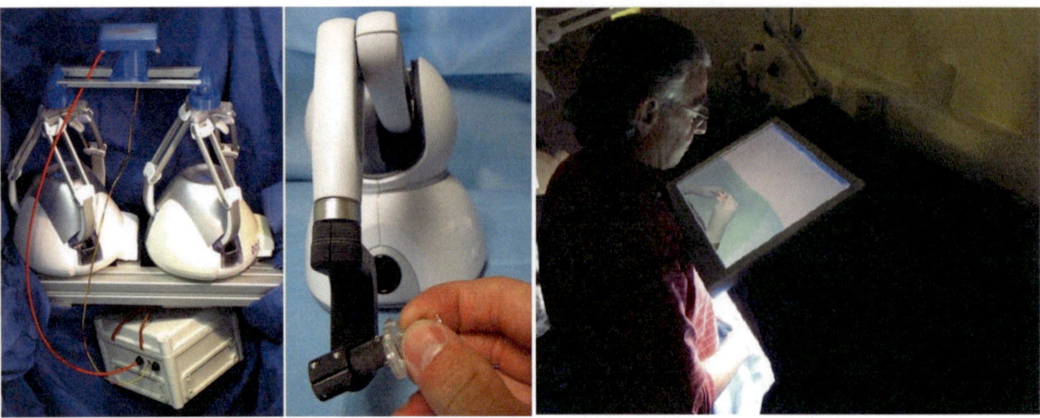

Fig. 11.15 PalpSim. (Courtesy of Tim Coles, 2011 [13], used with permission)

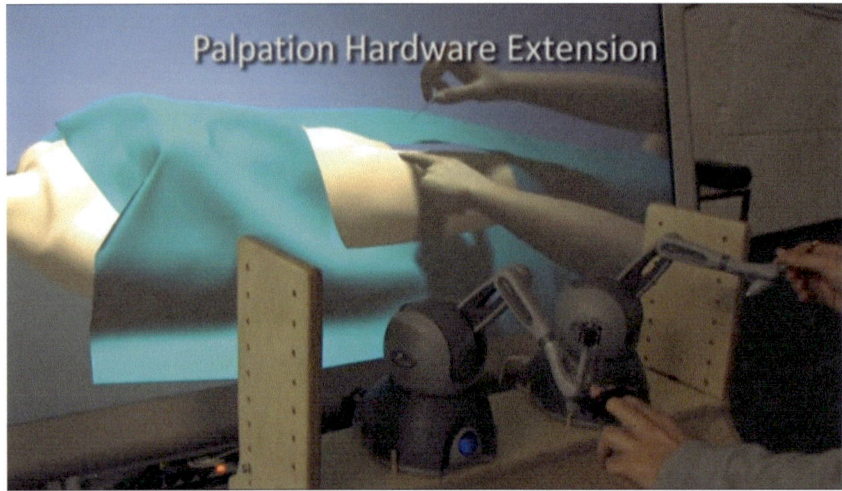

Fig. 11.16 Bimanual haptic simulator for medical training. (Courtesy of Ullrich et al. [14], used with permission)

Fig. 11.17
Immersivetouch
simulator. (Luciano
et al. [15], used with
permission)

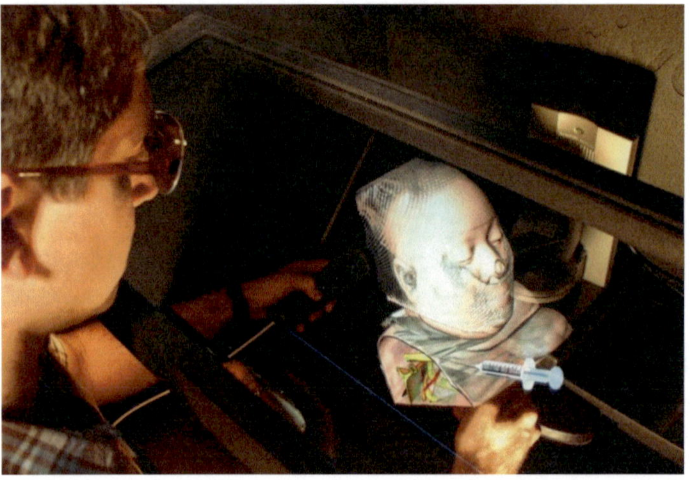

Conclusions

Haptics-based medical simulation is currently an active field of research in the scientific community and will continue to be for the next decades. Realistically simulating those tactile and kinesthetic sensations perceived during surgery, while interacting with intricate patient anatomy and with an extensive range of soft and hard body tissues, is technologically challenging, but it has without a doubt the potential to improve surgical training.

Even though the basic principles presented in this chapter about human-computer interaction, actuators, and sensors that enable humans to perceive force and torque will most likely remain fundamentally unchained, both haptic exoskeletons and grounded stand-alone devices, as well as the multidisciplinary areas of human perception, and machine and computer haptics, will continue to evolve.

Advanced medical simulation and training that coherently provide multiple stimuli, from visual to auditory to touch, have already shown promising results. We envision they will continue to increase their levels of realism and sophisticated human-computer interaction to enhance medical education, with the ultimate goal of improving surgical outcomes and increasing patient safety.

References

1. Salisbury K, Conti F, Barbagli F. Haptic tendering: introductory concepts. IEEE Comput Graph Appl. 2004;24(2):24–32.
2. Mansor NN, Jamaluddin MH, Shukor AZ. Concept and application of virtual reality haptic technology: a review. J Theor Appl Inf Technol. 2017;95(14):3320–36.
3. Salisbury, K, Barbagli, F, Conti, F. CS277 Lecture 01. Stanford University. 2011 Jan 4. Retrieved August 2017, from https://web.stanford.edu/class/cs277/resources/lectures/CS277-L01-Introduction.pdf
4. Salisbury, K, Barbagli, F, Conti, F. CS 277 – Experimental Haptics Lecture 2 Haptic rendering, force fields. Stanford University. 2011 Jan 6. Retrieved August 2017, from https://web.stanford.edu/class/cs277/resources/lectures/CS277-L02-ForceFields.pdf
5. Craig, K. Actuators and sensors in mechatronics (N. Y. University, Producer). 2017. Retrieved December 24, 2017, from Optical Encoders: http://engineering.nyu.edu/mechatronics/Control_Lab/Criag/Craig_RPI/SenActinMecha/S&A_Optical_Encoders.pdf
6. Lawlor. CS 480: Robotics & 3D printing. 2017. Retrieved December 24, 2017, from motor types & control schemes: https://www.cs.uaf.edu/2015/fall/cs480/lecture/09_11_motor_control.html
7. New York University, Polytechnic Institute of NYU. Lecture 8 Servomotors. 2017. Retrieved December 24, 2017, from http://engineering.nyu.edu/mechatronics/smart/pdf/SMART2010/PDFLectrues/Lectures(Day4).pdf
8. HaptX Inc. HaptX Inc. Haptics Enterprise. 2018. Retrieved January 3, 2018, from https://axonvr.com/#haptics-enterprise
9. Dexta Robotics Inc. Dexmo. 2018. Retrieved October 22, 2017, from http://www.dextarobotics.com/
10. Neuro Digital Technologies. Glove One. 2018. Retrieved October 22, 2017, from https://www.neurodigital.es/gloveone/
11. 3D Systems. Touch. 2018. Retrieved October 23, 2017, from https://www.3dsystems.com/haptics-devices/touch
12. 3D Systems. Touch X. 2018. Retrieved October 23, 2017, from https://www.3dsystems.com/haptics-devices/geomagic-touch-x
13. Coles TR. Investigating augmented reality Visio-haptic techniques for medical training (Doctoral dissertation); 2011.
14. Ullrich S, Rausch D, Kuhlen, T. Bimanual haptic simulator for medical training: system architecture and performance measurements. In: Joint Virtual Reality Conference of EGVE -Euro VR; 2011.
15. Luciano, C, Banerjee, P, Fiorea, L, Dawe G. Design of the immersivetouch: a high-performance haptic augmented virtual reality system. In: 11th International Conference on Human-Computer interaction. Las Vegas, NV; 2005 July.

Competency Assessment in Virtual Reality-Based Simulation in Neurosurgical Training

12

Laura Stone McGuire and Ali Alaraj

Competency Assessment Post-simulation in Neurosurgical Training

Interest in implementing VR simulation in graduate medical education has grown over the past decade, especially within surgical specialties. For instance, the use of VR simulators in general surgery training has been well-studied, and research examining its use for laparoscopic cholecystectomy practice demonstrated that those groups who practiced with the simulator were less likely to have errors or make critical mistakes and completed the procedure quicker [1].

Similarly, the inclusion of VR simulators in neurosurgical training has expanded recently, and its goals are multifold. VR simulation provides a safe environment to practice technical skills with no risk to the patient, which becomes an increasingly important objective as advocacy for transparency in patient surgical outcomes and the involvement of residents in cases has progressed [2, 3]. The development of surgical skills among trainees on a lifelike model for a variety of procedures within a safe environment to improve patient outcomes encaptures the overall purpose of incorporating VR simulation into

residency [4]. Multiple VR simulators have been produced in an effort to address these needs, including but not limited to Surgical Theater ®, NeuroTouch ®, Simbionix ® ANGIO Mentor ™, and ImmersiveTouch ®. These technologies will be discussed in more detail in other chapters. Additionally, the Congress of Neurological Surgeons (CNS) established a Simulation Committee in 2010 and recently published an overview of a simulator-based educational curriculum, including vascular, cranial, and spine components [5]. This committee aimed to create both virtual reality and physical simulations to maximize resident education, improving outcomes both safely and efficiently, and using an algorithm to standardize assessments among participants.

Procedures

VR simulators overall provide training on a variety of neurosurgical procedures along a spectrum of complexity, and the performance of these procedures as well as structured curriculums has been studied among neurosurgical residents. Among spine-based techniques, a 90-min curriculum on the anterior cervical discectomy and fusion with written and practical pretests, didactics and hands-on training, and subsequent posttests has been published, indicating improvement from baseline scores among participants [6]. Another study examined a 2-h educational

L. S. McGuire · A. Alaraj (✉)
Department of Neurosurgery, University of Illinois
at Chicago, Chicago, IL, USA
e-mail: lmcguir1@uic.edu; Alaraj@uic.edu

© Springer International Publishing AG, part of Springer Nature 2018
A. Alaraj (ed.), *Comprehensive Healthcare Simulation: Neurosurgery*,
Comprehensive Healthcare Simulation, https://doi.org/10.1007/978-3-319-75583-0_12

curriculum for posterior cervical decompression, including laminectomy and foraminotomy exercises, and demonstrated improved posttest didactic and technical scores [7]. Additionally, the CNS Simulation Committee developed a simulation model for durotomy and cerebrospinal fluid leak repair both within the lumbar spine [8] and cervical spine [9].

Simulated endovascular procedures have similarly been studied. A 2-h resident simulator-based course on diagnostic cerebral angiography available at two CNS annual meetings showed significant improvement in posttest-written assessment and practical skill scores [10]. Additionally, another small, pilot study assessed technical skills in performing a diagnostic cerebral angiogram on the Simbionix ® ANGIO Mentor ™ system, and participants improved procedure and fluoroscopy time over five attempts [11]. A study of VR-based simulation for endovascular aneurysm repair, also using Simbionix ® ANGIO Mentor ™, demonstrated faster procedural times, better device sizing, and fewer complications after training with the simulator [12]. Furthermore, simulated carotid artery stenting improved procedural and overall fluoroscopy times, as well as successful cannulation of the common carotid artery and sizing and deployment of embolic protection device [13]. A longitudinal analysis of participants over 30 days with five participants showed overall performance improvement in diagnostic cerebral angiogram, embolectomy, and coil embolization, as measured by total procedure time, fluoroscopy time, contrast dose, packing densities, number of coils used, and number of stent-retriever passes [14].

Many simulated cranial procedures have also been designed, from ventriculostomy placement to cerebral aneurysm clipping and brain tumor resection. The CNS Simulation Committee implemented a trauma module at two annual meetings, including ventriculostomy and craniotomy procedures; participants performing ventriculostomies demonstrated improved burr hole placement, catheter location, and procedure completion time [15], and those participating in craniotomies for traumatic brain injury bettered their incision planning, burr hole placement, and

craniotomy size [16]. Similarly, utilizing the ImmersiveTouch ®, neurosurgical residents improved their ability to perform ventriculostomy, with an increase in successful first-pass attempts [17]; in using a novel mixed-reality simulator, residents placed ventriculostomy catheters more accurately and in less time after practicing with the device [18]. VR simulators have also implemented in vascular procedural training; for instance, using the ImmersiveTouch ® virtual reality platform with real-time sensory haptic feedback to rehearse cerebral aneurysm clipping, neurosurgical residents reported usefulness of the simulation in preparing for surgery [19]. An application of the NeuroTouch ® VR simulator for practicing the endoscopic endonasal transsphenoidal approach has also been developed [20], and a study on simulated practice of endoscopic endonasal procedures using this platform showed improved operative performance among residents [21]. Several additional studies have also examined the NeuroTouch ® platform in simulated brain tumor resection [22–24]. The National Research Council of Canada published their conceptual framework for a simulation-based curriculum utilizing the NeuroTouch ®, which developed five standardized training modules for technical skill acquisition in neurosurgical oncology, including ventriculostomy, endoscopic nasal navigation, tumor debulking, hemostasis, and microdissection [25].

Skills Development and Performance Metrics

Advocates of the incorporation of virtual reality simulation into neurosurgical education argue that VR simulators strengthen cognitive task processing, technical skills, and understanding of operative and neuroanatomy [4]. Advancing technology has become increasingly realistic as the VR platforms have become both more immersive and interactive, adding haptic feedback to visual and audio cues. Simulators such as Simbionix ® ANGIO Mentor ™, NeuroTouch ®, and ImmersiveTouch ® include tactile feedback to represent the force required of the user to perform a particular task with a specific instrument and to replicate the texture of the tissue. Better visualization of operative anatomy improves understanding of relationship between key structures; current technology, including the Surgical Theater ®, allows cut-throughs and specific tissue selection to view the neuroanatomy, including patient-specific imaging data and reconstructions, which may prove useful not only in the study of the pertinent structures but also in the design of surgical approaches.

VR simulators offer longitudinal tracking of learning and improvement among objective performance assessments, which represents another advantage of simulator-based training within neurosurgical residency. Further, simulator-based curriculums can be incrementally designed, providing increasing number of tasks with growing complexity and layering of possible complications. The NeuroTouch ® platform provides reports on specific computer-generated metrics, which derived 13 performance metrics and categorized into tier 1, tier 2, or tier 3 [23]. Tier 1 metrics aim to evaluate safety and quality and include volume of tumor and brain resected as well as blood loss. Tier 2 metrics assess motor skills, such as instrument tip path length, time taken to resect the brain tumor, pedal activation frequency, and sum of applied forces. Advanced tier 2 and tier 3 metrics measure complex motor and cognitive bimanual skills interactions, including sum of forces applied to different tumor regions, instrument tips average separation distance, efficiency index, simulated aspirator path length index, coordination index, and simulated ultrasonic aspirator bimanual forces ratios [23, 24, 26]. These metrics have further been studied to assess proficiency among varying level of experience, from novice to expert, which enabled the authors to establish goal benchmarks for neurosurgical residents [27].

In several published studies, a variety of VR simulator platforms appropriately discriminate among level of expertise, which further enhances their utility in neurosurgical education and competency assessment. Seventy-one residents participated in a study of the simulation-based training in percutaneous trigeminal rhizotomy using the ImmersiveTouch ®; as PGY level increased, the distance from ideal entry point decreased, as well as the distance from the target, and more senior residents had better final scores [28]. Another study assessing performance in brain tumor resection on the NeuroTouch ® device with eight different lesions varying in color, stiffness, and border complexity successfully differentiated from novice and expert participants [23]. Using the Simbionix ® ANGIO Mentor ™ to assess performance in carotid artery stenting, a study of 33 participants in 82 simulated procedures appropriately discriminated between operator experience with metrics of fluoroscopy time, incomplete coverage of the lesion by the stent, and coverage of the lesion with devices other than a 0.014-in. wire prior to filter deployment [29].

Limitations of Simulation in Training

Although VR simulation provides many advantages in neurosurgical training and certainly enhances graduate medical education, it does not replace hands-on experience of live, real-time operating. The simulated procedures are not perfectly realistic, but haptic and visual feedback have improved drastically over recent years. The cases are also not truly three-dimensional; however, with the advancement of holographic technologies, such as the Microsoft HoloLens, this limitation may be short-lived. Furthermore, current simulators are generally not patient-specific, which limits their utility in operative planning and practice; however, recent technological advancements, including newer iterations of Surgical Theater ®, may incorporate patient-specific details, allowing for improved preoperative anatomical visualization. Furthermore, although the benefits of VR-based simulators in neurosurgical education may be easily recognized, the literature on these technologies and on educational curriculums based on them is limited to small studies and affected by publication bias. Larger studies to validate VR simulators in neurosurgical education are required.

To date, only one publication illustrates the cost and financial feasibility of including simulation in neurosurgical training. To quantify the total costs and benefits of incorporating simulation-based curricula remains a challenging task. Gasco et al. discuss the development of a simulation program for neurosurgical residents at the University of Texas Galveston [30]. Within this study, 180 procedures among six residents were analyzed, and both junior and senior residents self-reported improvement in performing procedures following simulations. This simulation program included cadaver simulations, physical simulators, and computer-based platforms and cost $341,978.00 initially with $27,876.36 annually afterward, although industry collaboration defrayed expenses through academic grants and equipment rentals. In this study, costs comprehensively included materials, equipment, space, and operating room time, which do not necessarily translate from one program to another, depending on the resources available and the specific program contents of the simulation curriculum (i.e., strictly computer-based versus cadaver and physical simulators).

Conclusion and Future Directions

Although simulations are not formally included in neurosurgical training across residency programs, one might easily imagine the incorporation of VR-simulated case scenarios into board examinations. Many studies are ongoing to confirm the validity of VR simulators in a variety of neurosurgical procedures and among trainees, and as these simulators continue to improve, an expansion of their use in graduate medical education becomes more likely. As imaging quality improves, computing power expands, and simulation software advances, the application of VR simulators in neurosurgery will similarly grow, especially as patient-specific data may be incorporated into future procedure simulations. Currently, VR simulators provide an avenue for basic procedural skill acquisition among residents. In the future, as support from national professional societies and industry spreads and new technologies emerge, simulators will become more affordable, readily available, and effective adjuncts to neurosurgical education.

References

1. Carter FJ, Schijven MP, Aggarwal R, Grantcharov T, Francis NK, Hanna GB, Jakimowicz JJ. Consensus guidelines for validation of virtual reality surgical simulators. Simul Healthc. 2006;1(3):171–9.
2. Lim S, Parsa AT, Kim BD, Rosenow JM, Kim JY. Impact of resident involvement in neurosurgery: an analysis of 8748 patients from the 2011 American College of Surgeons National Surgical Quality Improvement Program database. J Neurosurg. 2015;122(4):962–70.
3. Kim DH, Dacey RG, Zipfel GJ, Berger MS, McDermott M, Barbaro NM, Shapiro SA, Solomon RA, Harbaugh R, Day AL. Neurosurgical education in a changing healthcare and regulatory environment: a consensus statement from 6 programs. Neurosurgery. 2017;80(4S):S75–82.
4. Konakondla S, Fong R, Schirmer CM. Simulation training in neurosurgery: advances in education and practice. Adv Med Educ Pract. 2017;8:465–73.
5. Harrop J, Lobel DA, Bendok B, Sharan A, Rezai AR. Developing a neurosurgical simulation-based educational curriculum: an overview. Neurosurgery. 2013;73(Suppl 1):25–9.
6. Ray WZ, Ganju A, Harrop JS, Hoh DJ. Developing an anterior cervical diskectomy and fusion simulator for neurosurgical resident training. Neurosurgery. 2013;73(Suppl 1):100–6.
7. Harrop J, Rezai AR, Hoh DJ, Ghobrial GM, Sharan A. Neurosurgical training with a novel cervical spine simulator: posterior foraminotomy and laminectomy. Neurosurgery. 2013;73(Suppl 1):94–9.
8. Ghobrial GM, Anderson PA, Chitale R, Campbell PG, Lobel DA, Harrop J. Simulated spinal cerebrospinal fluid leak repair: an educational model with didactic and technical components. Neurosurgery. 2013;73(Suppl 1):111–5.
9. Ghobrial GM, Balsara K, Maulucci CM, Resnick DK, Selden NR, Sharan AD, Harrop JS. Simulation training curricula for neurosurgical residents: cervical foraminotomy and durotomy repair modules. World Neurosurg. 2015;84(3):751-5.e1–7.
10. Fargen KM, Arthur AS, Bendok BR, Levy EI, Ringer A, Siddiqui AH, Veznedaroglu E, Mocco J. Experience with a simulator-based angiography course for neurosurgical residents: beyond a pilot program. Neurosurgery. 2013;73(Suppl 1):46–50.
11. Spiotta AM, Rasmussen PA, Masaryk TJ, Benzel EC, Schlenk R. Simulated diagnostic cerebral angiography in neurosurgical training: a pilot program. J Neurointerv Surg. 2013;5(4):376–81.

12. Saratzis A, Calderbank T, Sidloff D, Bown MJ, Davies RS. Role of simulation in endovascular aneurysm repair (EVAR) training: a preliminary study. Eur J Vasc Endovasc Surg. 2017;53(2):193–8.

13. Gosling AF, Kendrick DE, Kim AH, Nagavalli A, Kimball ES, Liu NT, Kashyap VS, Wang JC. Simulation of carotid artery stenting reduces training procedure and fluoroscopy times. J Vasc Surg. 2017;66(1):298–306.

14. Pannell JS, Santiago-Dieppa DR, Wali AR, Hirshman BR, Steinberg JA, Cheung VJ, Oveisi D, Hallstrom J, Khalessi AA. Simulator-based angiography and endovascular neurosurgery curriculum: a longitudinal evaluation of performance following simulator-based angiography training. Cureus. 2016;8(8):e756.

15. Schirmer CM, Elder JB, Roitberg B, Lobel DA. Virtual reality-based simulation training for ventriculostomy: an evidence-based approach. Neurosurgery. 2013;73(Suppl 1):66–73.

16. Lobel DA, Elder JB, Schirmer CM, Bowyer MW, Rezai AR. A novel craniotomy simulator provides a validated method to enhance education in the management of traumatic brain injury. Neurosurgery. 2013;73(Suppl 1):57–65.

17. Yudkowsky R, Luciano C, Banerjee P, Schwartz A, Alaraj A, Lemole GM Jr, Charbel F, Smith K, Rizzi S, Byrne R, Bendok B, Frim D. Practice on an augmented reality/haptic simulator and library of virtual brains improves residents' ability to perform a ventriculostomy. Simul Healthc. 2013;8(1):25–31.

18. Hooten KG, Lister JR, Lombard G, Lizdas DE, Lampotang S, Rajon DA, Bova F, Murad GJ. Mixed reality ventriculostomy simulation: experience in neurosurgical residency. Neurosurgery. 2014;10(Suppl 4):576–81; discussion 581.

19. Alaraj A, Luciano CJ, Bailey DP, Elsenousi A, Roitberg BZ, Bernardo A, Banerjee PP, Charbel FT. Virtual reality cerebral aneurysm clipping simulation with real-time haptic feedback. Neurosurgery. 2015;11(Suppl 2):52–8.

20. Rosseau G, Bailes J, del Maestro R, Cabral A, Choudhury N, Comas O, Debergue P, De Luca G, Hovdebo J, Jiang D, Laroche D, Neubauer A, Pazos V, Thibault F, Diraddo R. The development of a virtual simulator for training neurosurgeons to perform and perfect endoscopic endonasal transsphenoidal surgery. Neurosurgery. 2013;73(Suppl 1):85–93.

21. Thawani JP, Ramayya AG, Abdullah KG, Hudgins E, Vaughan K, Piazza M, Madsen PJ, Buch V, Sean Grady M. Resident simulation training in endoscopic endonasal surgery utilizing haptic feedback technology. J Clin Neurosci. 2016;34:112–6.

22. Gélinas-Phaneuf N, Choudhury N, Al-Habib AR, Cabral A, Nadeau E, Mora V, Pazos V, Debergue P, DiRaddo R, Del Maestro RF. Assessing performance in brain tumor resection using a novel virtual reality simulator. Int J Comput Assist Radiol Surg. 2014;9(1):1–9.

23. Alotaibi FE, AlZhrani GA, Mullah MA, Sabbagh AJ, Azarnoush H, Winkler-Schwartz A, Del Maestro RF. Assessing bimanual performance in brain tumor resection with NeuroTouch, a virtual reality simulator. Neurosurgery. 2015;11(Suppl 2):89–98; discussion 98.

24. Azarnoush H, Alzhrani G, Winkler-Schwartz A, Alotaibi F, Gelinas-Phaneuf N, Pazos V, Choudhury N, Fares J, DiRaddo R, Del Maestro RF. Neurosurgical virtual reality simulation metrics to assess psychomotor skills during brain tumor resection. Int J Comput Assist Radiol Surg. 2015;10(5):603–18.

25. Choudhury N, Gélinas-Phaneuf N, Delorme S, Del Maestro R. Fundamentals of neurosurgery: virtual reality tasks for training and evaluation of technical skills. World Neurosurg. 2013;80(5):e9–19.

26. Alotaibi FE, AlZhrani GA, Sabbagh AJ, Azarnoush H, Winkler-Schwartz A, Del Maestro RF. Neurosurgical assessment of metrics including judgment and dexterity using the virtual reality simulator NeuroTouch (NAJD Metrics). Surg Innov. 2015;22(6):636–42.

27. AlZhrani G, Alotaibi F, Azarnoush H, Winkler-Schwartz A, Sabbagh A, Bajunaid K, Lajoie SP, Del Maestro RF. Proficiency performance benchmarks for removal of simulated brain tumors using a virtual reality simulator NeuroTouch. J Surg Educ. 2015;72(4):685–96.

28. Shakur SF, Luciano CJ, Kania P, Roitberg BZ, Banerjee PP, Slavin KV, Sorenson J, Charbel FT, Alaraj A. Usefulness of a virtual reality percutaneous trigeminal rhizotomy simulator in neurosurgical training. Neurosurgery. 2015;11(Suppl 3):420–5; discussion 425.

29. Weisz G, Smilowitz NR, Parise H, Devaud J, Moussa I, Ramee S, Reisman M, White CJ, Gray WA. Objective simulator-based evaluation of carotid artery stenting proficiency (from assessment of operator performance by the carotid stenting simulator study [ASSESS]). Am J Cardiol. 2013;112(2):299–306.

30. Gasco J, Holbrook TJ, Patel A, Smith A, Paulson D, Muns A, Desai S, Moisi M, Kuo YF, Macdonald B, Ortega-Barnett J, Patterson JT. Neurosurgery simulation in residency training: feasibility, cost, and educational benefit. Neurosurgery. 2013;73(Suppl 1):39–45.

Ralf A. Kockro and Luis Serra

Introduction to Neurosurgery

Neurosurgery is the surgical treatment of disorders, which affect any portion of the nervous system including the brain, the skull base, and the spinal cord. Most neurosurgical interventions are reaching into a highly complex anatomical space, especially when targeting the skull base for tumors, when dealing with vascular structures and cranial nerves or when reaching into the ventricular system, the deep brain, or the brain stem. Often the surgeon is confronted with an enormous spacious complexity and additionally faces the challenge to identify and dissect on the optimal surgical corridor and to apply the right strategy and technique to accomplish the surgical aim.

Electronic supplementary material: The online version of this chapter https://doi.org/10.1007/978-3-319-75583-0_13 contains supplementary material, which is available to authorized users.

R. A. Kockro (✉)
Department of Neurosurgery, Hirslanden Hospital, Zurich, Switzerland
e-mail: ralf@kockro.com

L. Serra
Galgo Medical SL, Barcelona, Spain
e-mail: luis.serra@galgomedical.com

Planning of Neurosurgery: The Key to Minimal Invasiveness

During surgery, the neurosurgeon must navigate a safe route through a highly complex three-dimensional space – a procedure that requires careful preplanning and a comprehensive understanding of the patient's intracranial structures and anatomy. It is thus crucial that before embarking in such navigation, the surgeon plans the path with whatever information is made available at that time. Preoperative planning is a crucial step toward successful neurosurgery.

The aim of the planning is to let the surgeon critically reflect – and later perform – on the ideal approach according to the individual pathoanatomy of the patient as well as the individual personal experience, attitude, and capability of the surgeon, ideal in the sense of minimizing exploratory dissection, brain retraction, and the exposure of neuronal structures not relevant to the surgical mission.

Tools for Planning a Neurosurgical Intervention

When undertaking surgical planning, the neurosurgeon usually relies on a series of radiological images derived from preoperative investigations such as magnetic resonance imaging (MRI) with all its subdomains as MR angiography (MRA) or

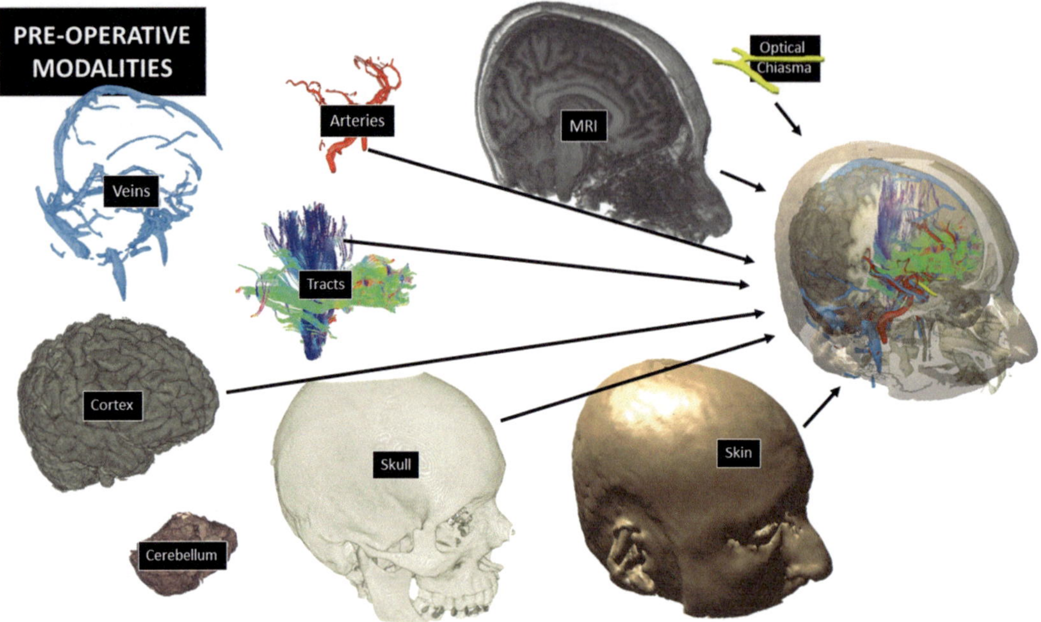

Fig. 13.1 Multiple imaging modalities are needed to obtain the complete picture of a patient

diffusion tensor imaging (DTI), computed tomography (CT), and X-ray angiography (Fig. 13.1). No single imaging modality is sufficient to provide the full view of the patient's condition: MRI is the most complete for soft tissue but lacks the detail of the bone. CT provides good bone imaging and, with contrast injected, good detail of the vessels but lacks soft tissue detail. Comprehensive planning of a surgical approach needs imaging contributions from all the different imaging modalities, and these must be combined into one unique 3D mental model of the site of the operation – since only a 3D model can fully reveal the accurate spatial relationships between intracranial structures. Building this mental 3D model is a significant challenge involving the integration of numerous multimodal images, and it is further complicated by the fact that the images vary in slice thickness, scale, and patient orientation.

Computer-based 3D neurosurgical planning tools emerged in the early 1980s when computer technology began to allow acceptable graphics rendering. Although pioneering attempts faced long processing times and were restricted to CT data, they were found to be useful in enhancing the surgeon's 3D perception. The 3D reconstructions were presented as static screen photographs from different angles. Since then, 3D image reconstructions built from CT, MRA, and CTA image sequences have been successfully used to plan craniofacial surgery and vascular neurosurgery.

There are certain key features that a surgical planning system must have to try to minimize the number of intraoperative surprises and maximize the safety of the procedure.

Easy to Interact 3D Views

The surgical planning system should naturally provide 3D views, from any angle, so that the surgeon can explore the best approach to the lesion: the approach with the least structural obstacles liable to get damaged and result in neurological deficit along the surgical path. Most planning systems do that, but unfortunately, the neurosurgeon must interact with the reconstructed 3D image in an awkward, nonintuitive 2D way – by moving a screen-bound cursor with a mouse, with the help of the keyboard. This is a considerable restriction given the complex manipulations that the surgeon must perform on the 3D image for surgery planning. For example, simulating the removal of bone to access a surgical target or manipulating the image to simulate surgical views, these interactions can be tortuous using a mouse and keyboard.

These 3D manipulations should allow selecting a target point and simulating the surgical viewpoint. It should be easy to add and remove structures from view, to peel them away so that the surgeon can see beyond the surrounding brain or vessels, and know what lies behind.

The planning should allow zooming in and out along a trajectory as though it was the surgical microscope, to anticipate obstacles along the way, and should provide these views stereoscopically, involving both eyes to get a clear understanding of the depth relationships between structures.

Simulation Tools in 3D

In addition to these visualizations resulting from the manipulations, the surgeon would like to perform certain simulations on the data of the patient, that is, try different scenarios to help decide the best approach.

It would be important, first of all, to easily measure distances (from bone to the lesion, within the lesion space, also distances along the skin and bone) and to get a sense of the constraints that will be faced during the intervention. It should also be desirable to annotate key landmark points. The annotations are helpful to measure progress during surgery (say, at a particular vessel bifurcation), as well as maintain overall orientation, especially since the orientation of an intraoperative viewpoint varies depending on head and microscope position.

It is also key to locate the best position for the craniotomy and to decide on its size and exact extent. And use that craniotomy to judge if access will be unimpeded. And if not, widen it, or relocate it, until the best position and size are found. The craniotomy is key in that once done, it fixes the rest of the surgical procedure and determines how much access there is to the lesion.

The Dextroscope in the Virtual Reality Technology Context

There are a number of approaches to achieve the surgical planning goals specified above (for a comprehensive review of the field, see Alaraj et al. [1, 2]). They could be classified either by their emphasis on *education* (medical knowledge as well as skills training) or on *patient-specific clinical decision-making*. All systems ultimately aim at complementing the education of neurosurgeons using computers, so that skills and decisions can be rehearsed ahead of the critical time of the intervention. But given the limitations of the current technology, they have to focus either on:

1) *Surgical Skills*, to deliver a generic and realistic training scenario (say, the sequence of steps in temporal bone surgery, including both the hand movements necessary to carry out drilling, the simulation of different bones, and the sensation of touching soft tissue). The difficulty of automatically converting DICOM data to correct biomechanical models results in having to rely on generic patient models.

2) *Decision-Making*, to provide accurate 3D information on a specific patient for the planning of the surgery. The difficulty of knowing the patient's biomechanical tissue properties results in "rigid" 3D data with which to plan the approach for the specific individual.

Although no doubt the ultimate VR simulation should combine both in a single system, the difficulty at this stage of extracting detailed mechanical computer models from patient-specific DICOM data has forced this division of work. A survey of the literature by Malone et al. [3] revealed that surgical simulators are evolving from platforms used for preoperative planning and anatomic education into programs that aim to simulate essential components of key neurosurgical procedures, bounded by graphics/volume rendering, model behavior/tissue deformation, and haptic feedback.

Surgical skills simulators were pioneered by O'Toole et al. [4] and Hill et al. [5], and they used a similar ergonomic setup to the Dextroscope (with the addition of force feedback). Commercial examples of surgical skills simulators are the NeuroTouch [6] or the ImmersiveTouch [1] systems. They all use haptic devices that transmit force feedback to the user so that the impression of touching tissue can be conveyed. Examples of decision-making systems are any of the planning software available in current commercial navigation systems (Brainlab, Germany or Medtronic Inc., CO, USA) or more recently the surgical theater system. Here is a short overview.

Other examples of surgical skills simulators are:

- *TempoSurg* (Spiggle & Theis Medizintechnik GmbH, Overath, Germany): University of Hamburg group created TempoSurg with otolaryngology applications in mind. Nevertheless, the model simulates temporal and petrous bone surgical approaches that are relevant to cranial base neurosurgery.
- University of Illinois, Chicago, introduced *ImmersiveTouch* (Immersive Touch Inc., Chicago, Illinois), a VR environment with haptic feedback based on a mirrored 3D image or a helmet. Modules exist for the simulation of some neurosurgical procedures like ventriculostomy, craniotomy, pedicle screw placement, and cataract surgery.
- *NeuroTouch*: A virtual reality medical simulation platform developed by the National Research Council Canada and currently under license to CAE Inc. (a manufacturer of patient simulators for the practice of technical skills, diagnosis, and interprofessional team training for emergency care) under the name CAE NeuroVR. The system makes use of two side-by-side monitors to produce a stereoscopic effect uses and engages the user with two haptic feedback devices. It is intended for training and has modules for tumor debulking, soft tissue dissection, bipolar hemostasis, and transnasal–transsphenoidal path simulation.

Examples of decision-making planning systems are:

- *Surgical theater* (Israel) offers planning (SRP) and navigation (SNAP) software. SRP provides interactive, immersive reconstruction that can be seen on a touchscreen and through the use of a VR headset, such as Oculus Rift® or HTC Vive®. SNAP enhances the surgeon's current operating room workflow by enhancing the existing surgical navigation system along with other tools and technologies while using the capabilities of VR. The surgeon interacts with the 3D data using the mouse or a video game console.
- Surgical planning modules incorporated into neurosurgical navigation systems like *CURVE* (Brainlab, Germany) and *StealthStation* (Medtronic Inc, CO). These modules are operated with mouse and keyboard on a regular monitor. Image segmentation and measurement tools allow the planning and simulation of surgical access routes and viewpoints.

The Dextroscope: A Tailored Virtual Reality Approach

The Dextroscope was intended to address the needs of neurosurgical planning. It automatically integrates imaging sequences from multiple modality sources into a single, 3D dataset representing the virtual patient that will be operated. And then it provides an interactive environment to allow the surgeons to manipulate this virtual patient and plan the ideal surgical trajectory – for example, by simulating interoperative viewpoints or the removal of bone and soft tissue.

The Dextroscope was designed to be a practical variation of virtual reality which introduced an alternative to the prevalent trend of full immersion of the 1990s. Instead of immersing the whole user into a virtual reality, it just immersed the hands of the neurosurgeon into the patient data. There is no justifiable need for more. The Dextroscope started as a research project in the mid-1990s with the name The Virtual Workbench

[7–14] and started commercialization in 2000 with the incorporation of the company Volume Interactions Pte Ltd.

Technical Setup of the Dextroscope

In the Dextroscope, a stereoscopic image (involving left and right eye views) is displayed on a monitor and reflected via a mirror into the user's eyes (see Fig. 13.2). The user works from a seated position with forearms positioned on comfortable armrests. Wearing a pair of stereoscopic glasses – synchronized with the display – the user looks into the mirror to see a stereoscopic image that seems to float behind the mirror. When reaching with both hands behind the mirror, the user experiences the sensation of having the hands in the same workspace as the 3D object. The fact that object and hand movements take place in the same apparent position allows for careful, dexterous work (Fig. 13.3).

In one hand the user holds an ergonomically shaped handle with a switch that, when pressed, allows the 3D image to be moved freely as if it were an object held in real space. The other hand holds a pencil-shaped stylus that is used to select a variety of tools from a virtual control panel and perform detailed manipulations and operations on the 3D image (Fig. 13.4). The virtual workspace provides a set of tools for volume exploration, image segmentation, and color and transparency adjustment. With a virtual fork, objects can be uncoupled from their surroundings for closer inspection. Drawing and measurement tools are applicable at any point and angle in 3D space. Virtual drilling and suctioning enable the simulation of surgical corridors. A selection of aneurysm clips of different sizes and shapes can be picked and virtually tested when planning the clipping of an aneurysm.

While working the user does not see the real stylus, handle, or the hands as they are hidden behind the mirror that is totally opaque. Instead, the user sees computer-generated imagery calibrated to appear in exactly the same position as the real handle and real stylus. The virtual images change as the user selects different tools (a drill, a measurement tool) and works on the virtual patient data model.

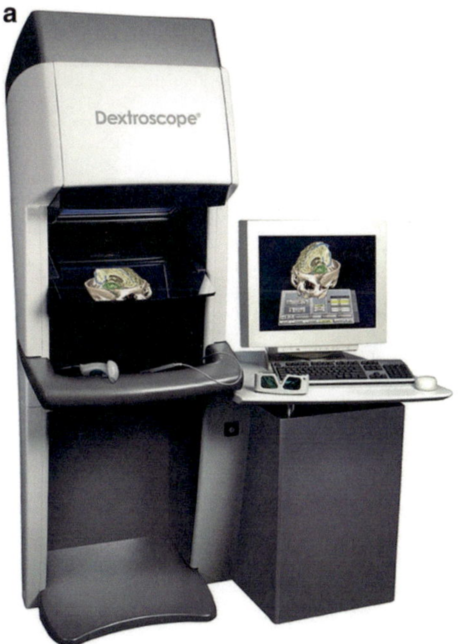

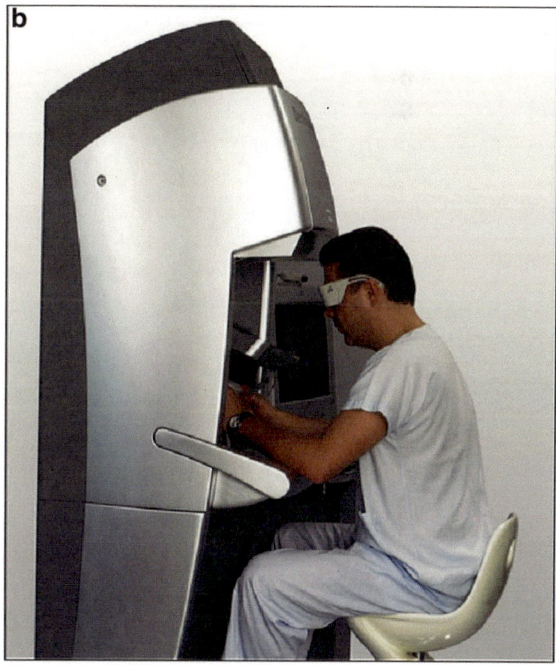

Fig. 13.2 (**a, b**) The Dextroscope virtual reality environment

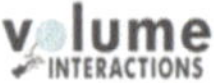

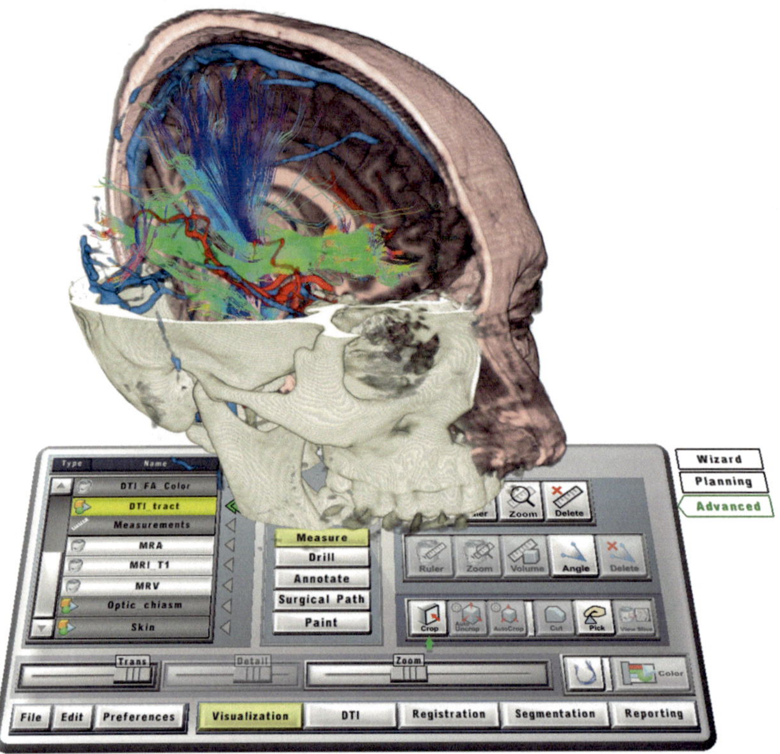

Fig. 13.3 A view of the Dextroscope imagery, showing the brain cortex (extracted from MRI T1), the vessels (extracted from MRI T1 with contrast), white matter tracts (extracted from DTI, labels, TMS points, and the control interface at the *bottom*)

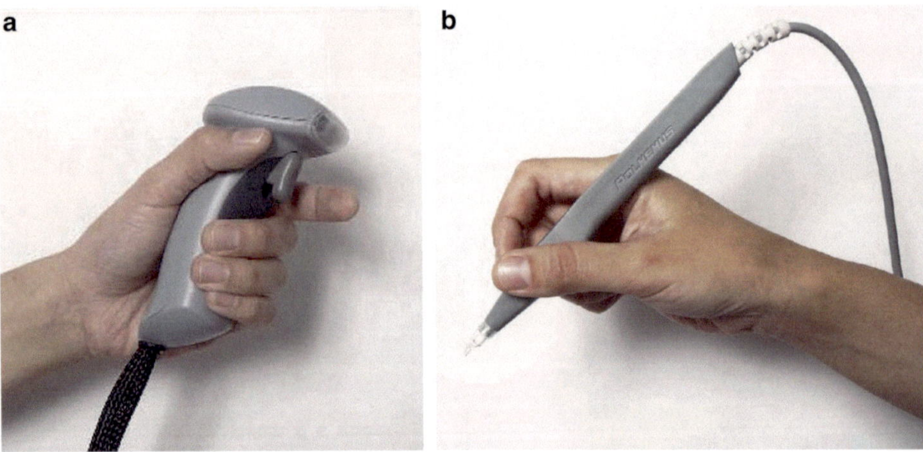

Fig. 13.4 The handle (**a**) and stylus (**b**)

This setup allows to intuitively interact and manipulate the 3D data using the hands in a similar manner to how they would manipulate a real object. Apart from being much faster and natural than using a mouse and keyboard, this setup also provides the surgeon with a greater degree of control over the 3D image – with the hands literally being able to reach inside to manipulate the image interior. The 3D image is now no longer just a passive image but an active 3D virtual representation of the patient's anatomy. This high degree of interactivity and control is particularly useful when working with complex datasets containing numerous imaging modalities (MRI, MRA, CT, DTI, etc., each with its own orthogonal image planes) and their additional segmentations (tumor, vessels, and white matter tracts). In these cases, interpretation of the structures within the 3D image is particularly difficult and requires an interactive investigation of the image rather than passively looking at static views.

Stereo Real-Time Visualization

The Dextroscope interactivity will be of little use if it were not for the real-time volume-rendering implementation in the software. The volume rendering is additionally multimodal in that it can render more than one volume simultaneously to produce final images that correctly match what would be seen if two volumes were to be shown to the naked eye. Furthermore, the display is stereoscopic and needs to render images for the right and left eyes.

Ergonomics of 3D Interaction

Background on 3D Interaction

Schmandt [15] pioneered the manipulation of 2D icons over a surface that was an integral part of the 3D space. The interaction with the surface icons was done using a 2D "graphics tablet" which was made to coincide with the virtual surface where the icons appeared. Schmandt also experimented with 3D interactions using a 3D tracker, although the two modes (2D and 3D)

were not properly integrated together. Subsequent work by Sowizral on the virtual tricorder [16] introduced the idea of using passive haptic feedback on a small handheld board within a head-mounted display environment.

Handheld boards or "pen-and-tablet" interfaces are a response to the frustrations experienced by researchers in trying to interact with menus floating in space [16–18]. This method seems to be gaining popularity in the VR community since it provides an unequivocal and inexpensive way to operate on buttons. Handheld boards provide the necessary passive haptic feedback while holding the buttons. Perhaps their main shortcoming is having to devote one hand to hold the board itself. Floating menus, on the other hand, use some kind of virtual pointer combined with physical button-click to manipulate widgets. Using these types of interfaces is hard to perform precise movements, such as dragging a slider to a specific location or selecting from a pick list. The difficulty comes from the fact that the user is pointing in free space, without the aid of anything to steady the hands.

Take for example Deering [19] who uses a hybrid 2D/3D menu widgets organized in a disk layout. Menus pop up in a fixed position relative to the current position of a 6 DOF wand and are then selected by hand relative movements. His approach tries to compromise the advantages of 2D window interfaces with 3D work, but the lack of support in 3D interactions still detracts from its usability.

The Dextroscope Approach

To be applicable in clinical routine, a virtual reality environment must be easy and comfortable to use and support shared sessions where many medical experts work together to discuss the same patient. The "classic" head-mounted display usually associated with virtual reality does not meet these needs – being cumbersome to wear and poorly suited to group working interaction where users frequently wish to switch between the virtual reality environment and the real world to interact with their colleagues. In contrast, the Dextroscope provides an open and robust environment in which the user works in a normal seated position wearing stereoscopic glasses that do not require exact positioning on the user's head and so can be quickly removed and replaced again. With arms resting in a relaxed position, the user perceives the stereoscopic virtual image within natural reach – delicate work can now be performed for hours without strain. A second monitor lets observers easily view the virtual reality environment and see exactly what the user sees.

The Dextroscope uses a 3D/2D paradigm of interaction that combines precise 3D manipulation of volumetric data with unambiguous interaction with widgets (Fig. 13.5). The interactions take place within the Dextroscope console, a 90 cm wide, 70 cm deep, and 40 cm high physical encasing, which holds the stereoscopic screen display and provides housing for the input device system. The encasing is designed to provide comfortable support for the arms and a smooth bottom surface against which the tip of the stylus can rest.

Precise 3D interaction is ensured by a combination of resting the lower arms on the armrest and pivoting the hands around the wrist. The position and orientation of the user's hands are obtained by a radio-frequency tracking system (manufactured by Polhemus Inc. (Colchester, Vermont)). This tracking system controls two 3D input devices, one for each hand and each

including a single button switch. One input device is shaped like a pen for dexterous work (the stylus) and the other like a joystick (the handle), to control the pose of the patient data. While resting the arm, the wrist can easily access a space of interaction of 20–30 cm^3, accurately and comfortably. By sliding the arms along the armrest, a wider space is available. This approach was found to simplify the command structure while remaining expressive.

Unambiguous 2D interaction is achieved by providing passive haptic feedback by means of a virtual control panel whose position coincides with the physical surfaces encasing the system. The stylus interacts with the widgets as though it was a mouse, in a similar fashion to [16]. The physical surfaces provide a hard medium against which the stylus switch can be pressed firmly and unequivocally to operate virtual buttons, sliders, and curves. The virtual control panel only pops up when the tip of the stylus touches the physical surfaces surrounding the 3D space (e.g., the top of the table) and remains invisible otherwise. This eliminates confusion by keeping the screen clear from cluttering objects while boosting graphics performance (fewer objects to redraw). The physical surface is smooth so that the tip of the stylus slides effortlessly over it enabling sliders and multiple buttons to be operated comfortably.

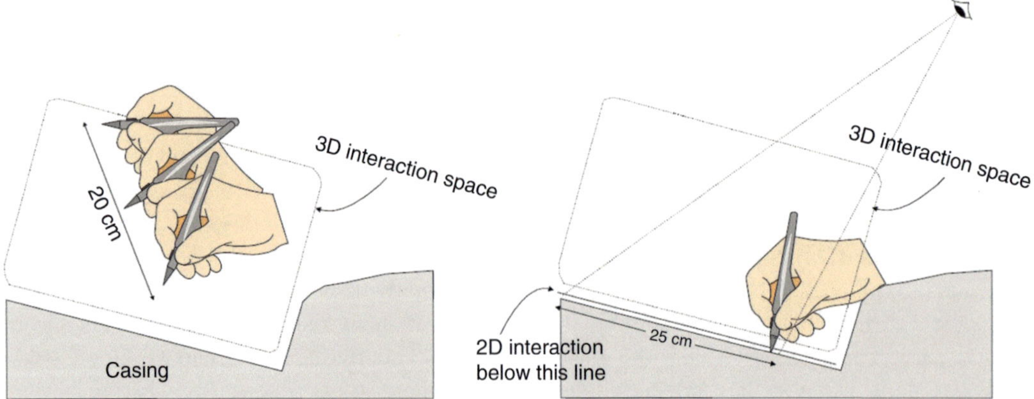

Fig. 13.5 Schematic view of 3D and 2D interactions in the Dextroscope. *Left*, in 3D, the user's forearm rests on the casing, which provides a smooth surface that allows reaching into the 3D space with the hand, doing wrist-based 3D interactions. *Right*, to interact with the virtual control panel, the user touches the base of the casing with the stylus, which shows the 3D panel, and relies of "passive haptic feedback" to firmly select buttons and sliders

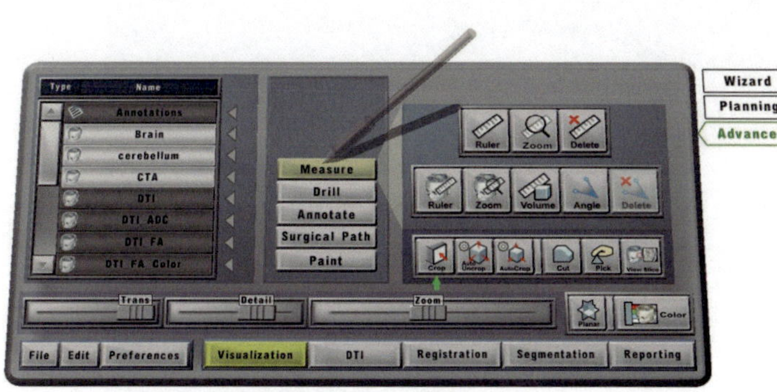
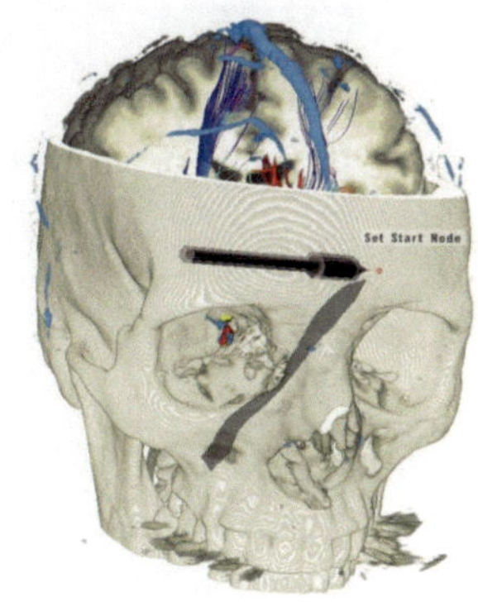

Fig. 13.6 Depth cues. The use of a shadow cast over objects (both volume data and the virtual control panel) helps the user to judge distances to objects and eases 3D interactions. (**a**) Stylus casting shadow over virtual control panel; (**b**) Stylus casting a shadow over the skull to position a measurement point

The use of shadows cast by the stylus provides additional depth cues that help with interactions. When the shadow is cast over the 3D objects, say the skull, it helps judge distances and reinforces the depth perception that stereoscopy provides. This facilitates, for example, placing a point over a surface to do a measurement or make a craniotomy. When used over the virtual control panel, it makes it easier to understand distances to buttons, the angle of the stylus with respect the panel, etc. (see Fig. 13.6).

The Virtual Control Panel

The virtual space is divided by software into two regions: one close to the surface of the encasing system and the other the rest of the space (refer to Fig. 13.5).

The user interacts with virtual 3D objects in the reach-in manner common to most virtual reality systems. The user moves the stylus toward the object of interest, and when reached, the switch on the stylus is pressed to indicate the desired action (grab, delete, resize, etc.). While the control panel is enabled, the 3D objects floating above it can either be fully displayed or be displayed in lower resolution to speed up the interactions with the 2D panel or be made invisible.

The virtual control panel contains 3D widgets such as buttons, sliders, curve-control panels, list boxes, and file dialogs (see Fig. 13.7).

Widgets are grouped by function, such as visualization, registration, segmentation, and reporting.

The virtual control panel area visible at any one time is approximately 50 cm × 25 cm. The angle of inclination of the physical surface is chosen to maximize the visible area of interaction. A 0° surface (parallel to the floor) forces the user to stretch the arm to reach the buttons further away. And a 90° one reduces the amount of available 3D space to interact. Therefore we used a compromise angle of 25° one to bring the control panel closer, for easier reach.

Preparing the Virtual Patient: 3D Image Reconstruction

The Dextroscope reconstructs 3D images from any tomographic data acquisition in DICOM format including most sequences of MRI (MRA, MRV, f-MRI, DTI), CT, CTA, PET, SPECT, and exported series of rotational X-ray angiography in tomographic format. The data is first loaded and previewed in the standard 2D interface where adjustments are made to thresholds, contrast, and brightness. Filters may be applied and cropping performed. Subsequently, the user can launch the virtual reality application to interact with the loaded data in the Dextroscope 3D interface console itself.

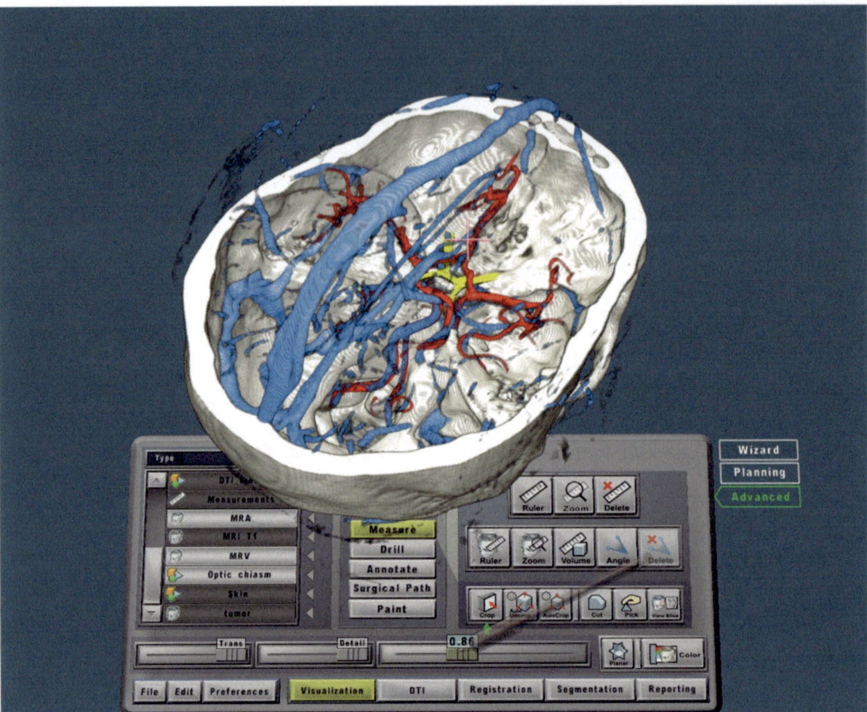

Fig. 13.7 Screen capture from the Dextroscope. This image shows a moment during the planning of a typical neurosurgical procedure involving several imaging modalities: MRI (to visualize the tumor and nerves), MRA (arteries, in *red*), MRV (veins, in *blue*) and CT (for the skull, *white*). The optical chiasm from the MRI is segmented (*yellow*). At the *bottom*, there is the virtual control panel

Virtual Reality Tools for Planning and Simulation

Within the Dextroscope virtual reality environment, there is an extensive set of virtual tools to work with the 3D patient data. Here is a list of some of the most relevant.

Image Fusion

To get the planning started, it is essential to ensure that all the data image modalities (which come from different scanners and for which the patient's head may have been at different orientations) are co-registered into the same coordinate space. A 3D interface for *registration* module is provided in the Dextroscope for this purpose. This module allows to co-register automatically any modality to any other modality: CT to MRI, MRI to MRA, tomographic series of X-ray angiography to CT, etc. The basic algorithm is based on the mutual information algorithm [20].

Segmentation Tools

Segmentation means extracting surgically relevant structures from the original DICOM data. This stage is required since the structures of interest for the surgeon (vessels, tumor) contained in original raw data DICOM do not come separated from each other, and they need to be in order to be suitable for exploration in the VR environment. Typical structures that can be segmented are tumors, blood vessels, aneurysms, the skull base, cranial nerves, or the ventricular system. Segmentation is done either automatically when structures are clearly demarcated by their image intensity or semiautomatically involving some user interaction.

Automatic Segmentation Tools

The Dextroscope provides automatic tools to isolate (segment) the cortex from a T1 MRI; arteries or veins from MRA, MRV, or CTA; or the ventricles from T2 MRI.

Other automatic tools just need the user to point at the desired structure to segment, for example, to point at the surface of the skin (from CT or MRI) to get a mesh of the skin or a tumor that has good contrast from surrounding tissue or a vascular segment from a vessel tree (e.g., containing an aneurysm). Also, color management is automated to perform manual coloring operations on any structure.

Semiautomatic Segmentation Tools

When there is no significant density contrast between a tumor and the surrounding tissue, an outlining tool, the contour editor, is available to let the surgeon decide the extent of the tumor. The outlining tool lets the surgeons draw outlines over the original scan slices (see Fig. 13.8). Although the drawing is done on a slice-by-slice basis, the volume of interest remains in context during the outlining, facilitating the appreciation of the shape of the tumor. This gives context to the contour operation and helps decide what to include or not in the contour based on the 3D visualization [21].

DTI Tractography

Although the processing of the MRI DTI data to extract all the possible tracts is automatic, the actual selection of individual tracts or groups of tracts (the tractography) that pass through a specific region of interest depends on what region needs to be inspected. The Dextroscope provides a 3D interface that allows the surgeon to define a cube-shaped region of interest in 3D space by bringing in anatomical context from the MRI orthogonal planes and other segmentations (like a tumor) (see Fig. 13.9). As the ROI is moved freely in 3D, the tracts intersected by the ROI appear in real time giving immediate feedback to the surgeon to fully understand their paths.

Measurement Tools

The Dextroscope provides manual tools for distance measurements between two points, which can be selected naturally with the stylus, just by pointing directly to the point of the structure of interest. In addition, curved measurements can be made along surfaces such as the bone or the skin, the latter are useful to bring planning measure-

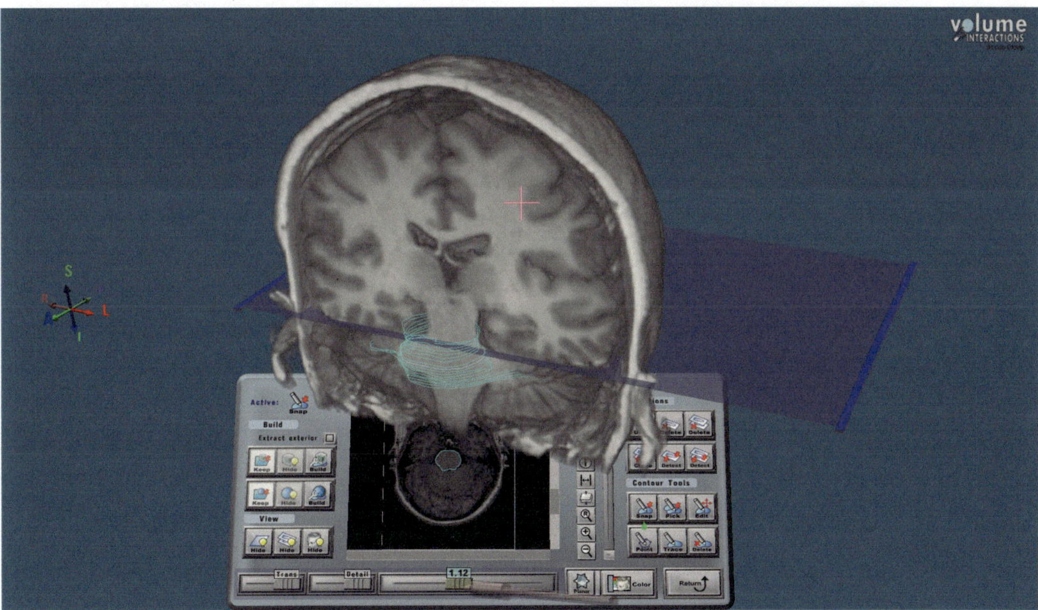

Fig. 13.8 Contour editor 3D interface. Interface showing the MRI floating above the contouring panel, which is part of the control panel, and where the contours are being drawn with the stylus working firmly against the base casing of the Dextroscope. The resulting contours are seen within the context of the MRI in 3D

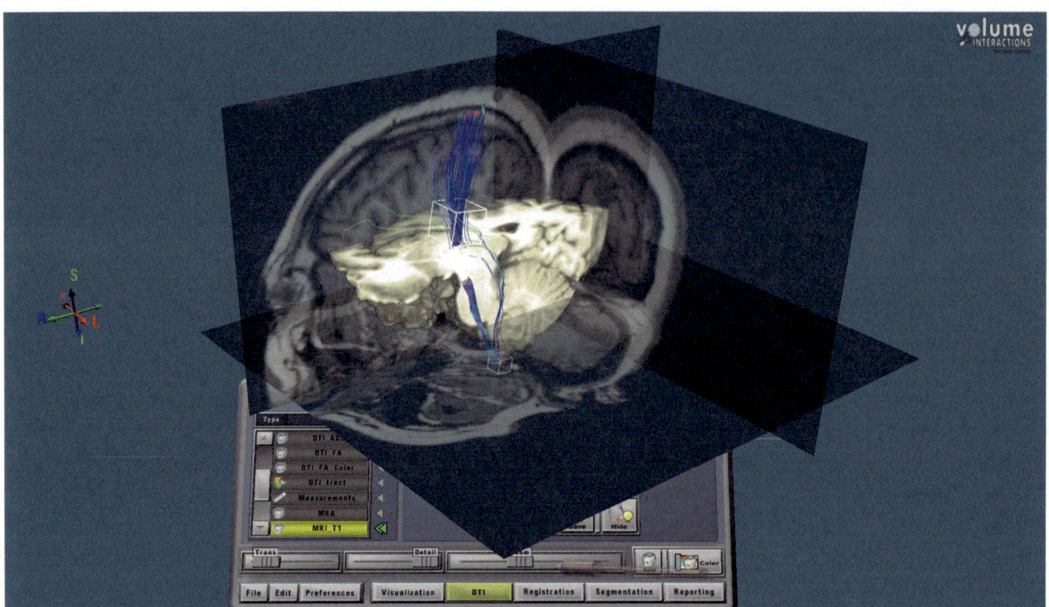

Fig. 13.9 DTI 3D interface. Each cube serves as region of interest (ROI) through which tracts pass. Two ROIs define the space through which a tract must pass. The segmented brain provides additional context to the ROI positioning

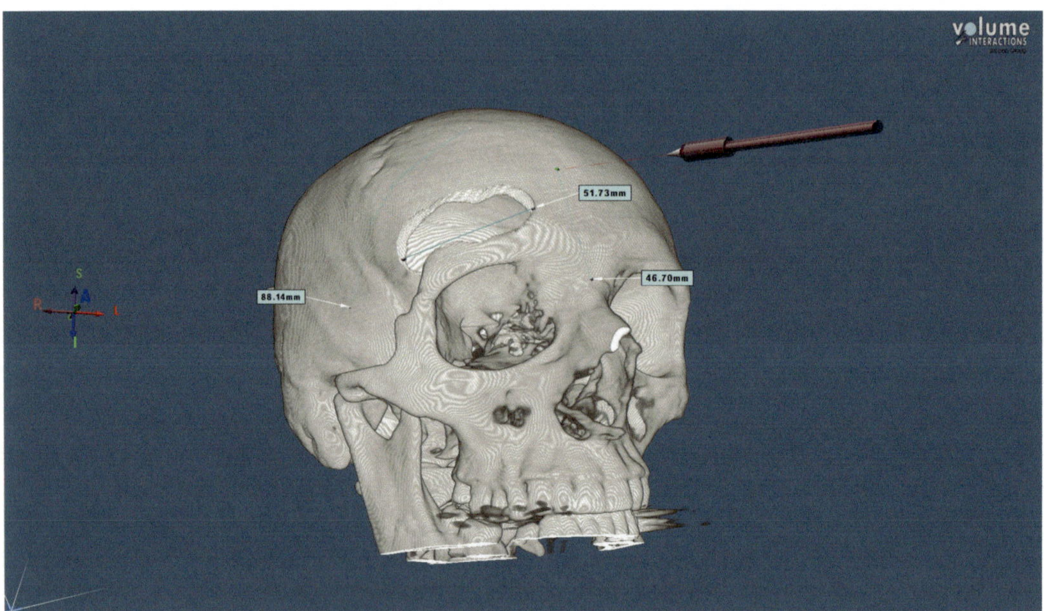

Fig. 13.10 Measurements in 3D. They can be *straight lines* (as seen in the craniotomy) or geodesic over a surface like the skull

ments into the operating room to locate the position of the craniotomy [22]. Volumetric measurements of selected structures like a tumor are also supported, as well as angles (see Fig. 13.10).

Volume Editing ("Drill") Tools

In order to simulate bone or tissue removal, the Dextroscope provides an interactive "virtual drill" tool. The tool works by changing the voxel

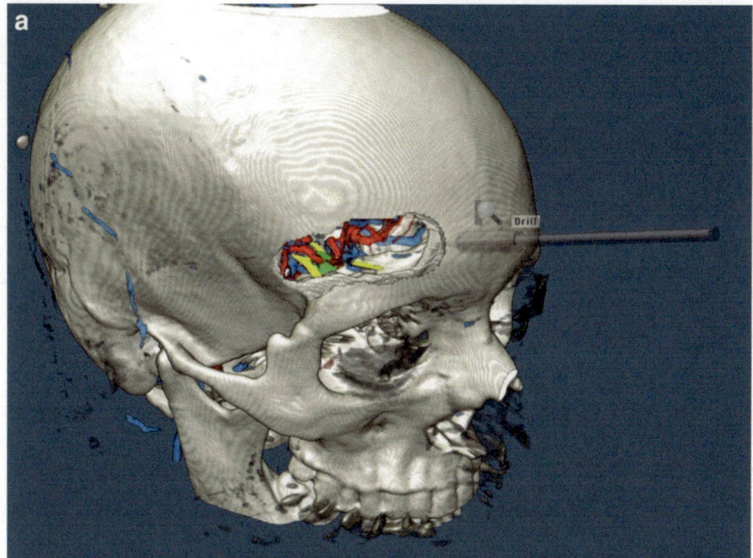

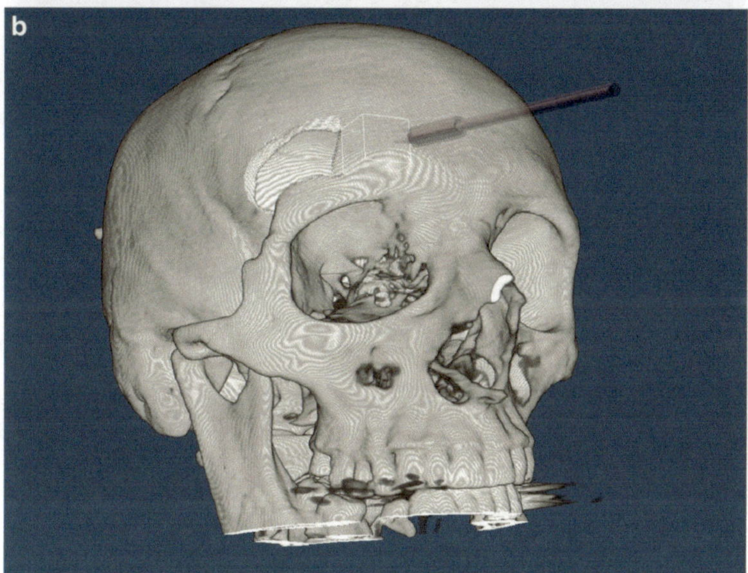

Fig. 13.11 The drill tool making a craniotomy on the bone of the CT (**a**). And the restorer (**b**) closing the previous craniotomy

properties of the volume data so that they change from visible to invisible. If applied to bone tissue, the drill appears to make a craniotomy to simulate views into a surgical corridor toward the lesion (see Fig. 13.11). The drill can be undone by using the "restore" tool which simply changes the voxel properties to the original value.

Approach Tool/Line of Sight Setting

The approach tool allows the user to define a trajectory to the lesion. It involves specifying in 3D the target and entry points (see Fig. 13.12). Once defined, the tool allows the surgeon to align the view to the trajectory, rotate around the line of the path to get the head orientation that will later be used to operate, and slide the point of view along the trajectory to simulate what would be seen by the surgical microscope. The magnification of the view can also be adjusted.

Simulation of Clip Placement

For the planning of aneurysm surgery, a variety of virtual clips is available. Original aneurysms clips (Aesculap, Germany) were scanned with a high-resolution CT and then individually segmented in 3D. The clips can be picked up with

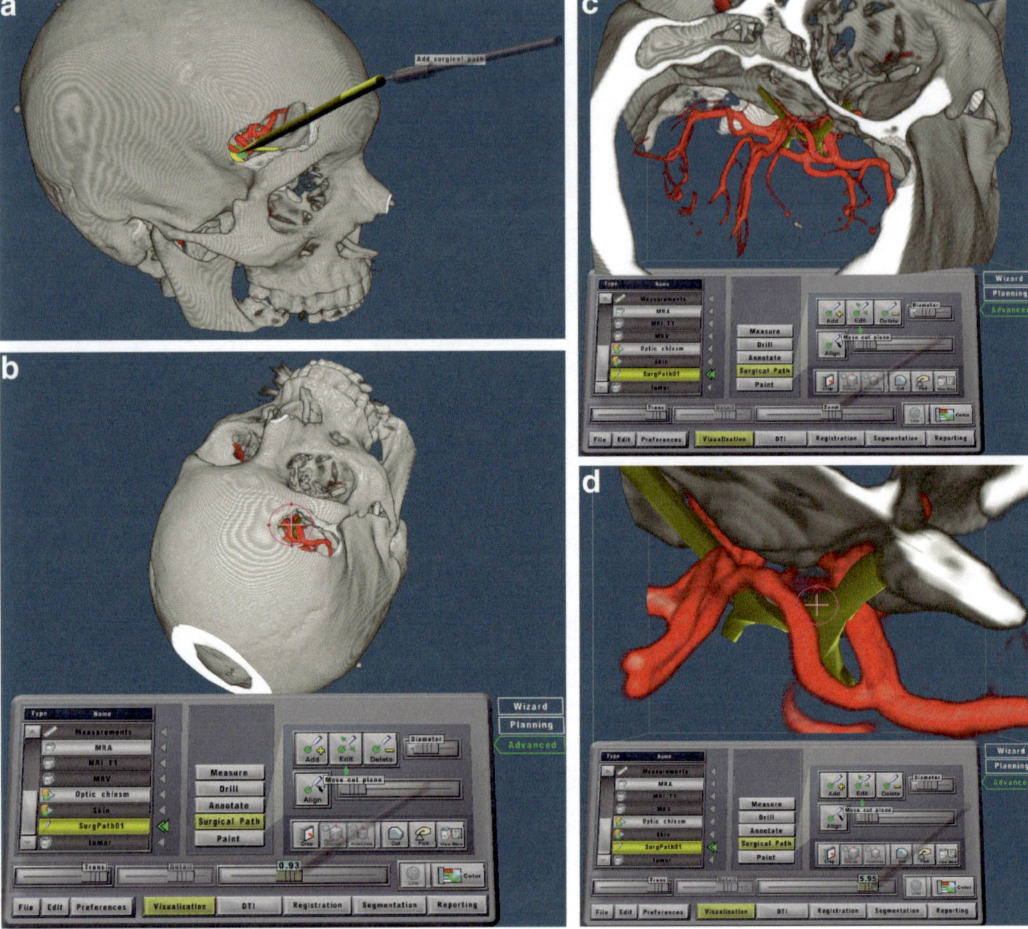

Fig. 13.12 The surgical planning interface. (**a**) Positioning the target and entry points to define a path within the 3D image. (**b**) Aligning the view along the path. (**c**) Zooming along the path simulating a microscope view. (**d**) Reaching the target point of the path

the virtual stylus representing a forking instrument and then virtually be placed over the neck of an aneurysm. This allows approximating the ideal shape, size, and position of one or several clips in order to completely obliterate an aneurysm.

See Video 13.1

The Dextrobeam and DextroVision

The Dextrobeam

The 3D visualization and interactive demonstration capabilities of the Dextroscope make it useful as a tool for medical educators with which to convey 3D information to medical students. But in order to reach a larger group of people such as in a classroom or auditorium, a variation of the Dextroscope was manufactured called Dextrobeam. The Dextrobeam is an interaction console which serves as a platform for 3D interaction and is intended to work in combination with a large stereoscopic projection screen [23–26]; see Fig. 13.13.

The software running on the Dextrobeam is the same as the one running on the Dextroscope, but it is calibrated to work in a different space: by directly looking at a screen instead of through a mirror that reflected the images. The way the interaction with the 3D data is carried out in the same way, and the user can transition from work-

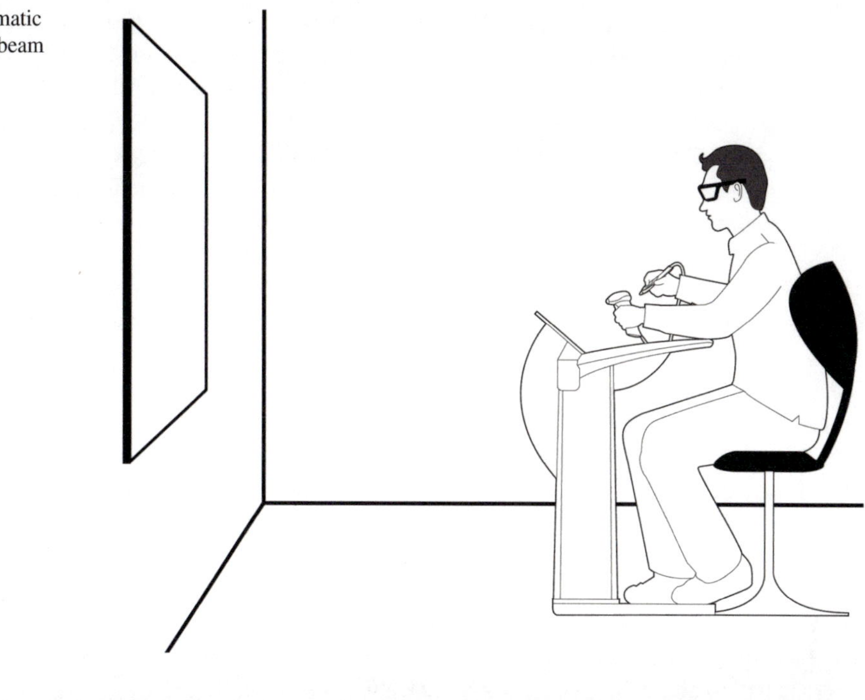

Fig. 13.13 A schematic showing the Dextrobeam setup

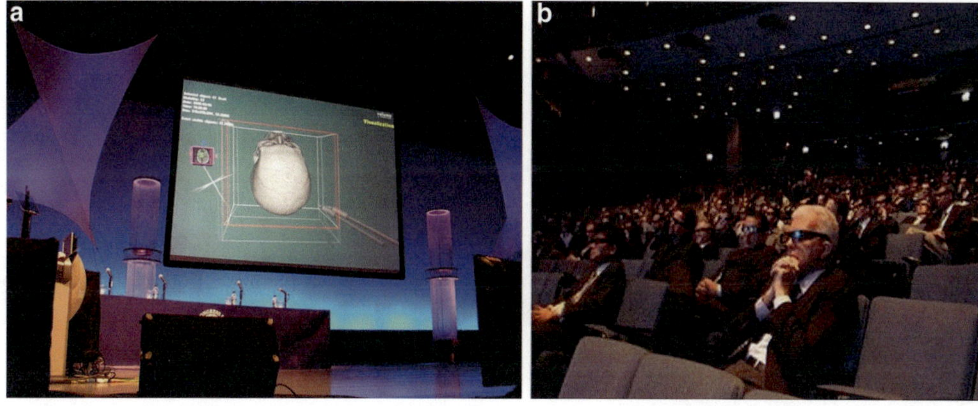

Fig. 13.14 The Dextrobeam at the Congress of Neurological Surgeons, 2006. The projection screen (**a**) and the audience wearing stereoscopic glasses (**b**)

ing on the Dextroscope to the Dextrobeam without having to learn a new interface:

Working without the reflecting mirror can be done in two different ways. One way is using a stereoscopic projection system with which to reach a large audience (see Dextrobeam below). Another is working in front a computer monitor (see DextroVision below).

The Dextrobeam was used successfully as a neurosurgical teaching platform in several CNS (Congress of Neurological Surgeons) presentations (see Fig. 13.14), as well as presentations by several teams around the world. We can highlight the following:

- Dept. Neurosurgery, Johannes Gutenberg University Mainz (Germany). In Mainz, courses are conducted on a regular basis to teach clinical neuroanatomy and demonstrate planning of minimally invasive procedures.
- Dept. Neurosurgery, St Louis Hospital (MO, USA). The neurosurgeons in St Louis have been using the Dextrobeam to support their

Practical Anatomy and Surgical Education's hands-on cadaver workshops.

- Dept. Neurosurgery, National Neuroscience Institute and National University Hospital (Singapore). The neurosurgical team is conducting courses using the Dextrobeam to teach anatomy and surgical approaches.

The DextroVision

The DextroVision represents the transition from the Dextrobeam to a lighter, configuration to be used on the user's desktop. It uses the 3D interface of the Dextrobeam but uses whatever tabletop is available to the user, as long as it is free from metallic interference. This saves space since it only uses a small footprint but sacrifices the ergonomics of the interaction of the Dextroscope. The tracking system is embedded into a specially designed box to house the electronics and the RF emitter. The box also serves as a base on top of which to place a stereoscopic computer monitor (Fig. 13.15). In the figure, a laptop's docking station is used in between the box and the monitor, which enabled to make the system portable.

The virtual control panel still appears inclined toward the user since a flat panel coinciding with the table would be at an angle difficult to view. This mismatch of real surface versus virtual surface has not been a problem (it is effectively like the 2D mouse which moves on a flat table but appears on a plane perpendicular to it) and brings the benefits of a reduced space that compensates for the loss of 3D interaction ergonomics.

The DextroVision was never commercialized.

Fields of Application and Illustrative Cases

The Dextroscope has been used for the patient-specific planning of a broad variety of neurosurgical procedures since 2000 [24, 23, 25]:

- Aneurysms [27–30]
- Cerebral arteriovenous malformations [26, 31, 32]
- Cranial nerve decompression (in cases of trigeminal neuralgia and hemifacial spasm) [33–35]
- Cavernomas [36, 37]
- Meningiomas (skull base, convexity, falcine, or parasagittal) [24, 26, 38–41]
- Ependymomas or subependymomas [29, 42]
- Transnasal approaches [43–45]
- Keyhole approaches [46–48]
- Epilepsy surgery [49]

It has also been reported for deep brain and skull base tumors [50, 51] (pituitary adenomas, craniopharyngiomas, arachnoid cysts, colloid cysts, cavernomas [37, 52] hemangioblastomas, chordomas, epidermoids, gliomas [53], jugular schwannomas, aqueductal stenosis, stenosis of Monro foramen, hippocampal sclerosis) [24, 26, 29, 51].

In addition, spine pathologies such as cervical spine fractures, syringomyelia, and sacral nerve root neurinomas have been evaluated [29].

For other uses of the Dextroscope in neurosurgery, refer to [22, 54–56, 56–64].

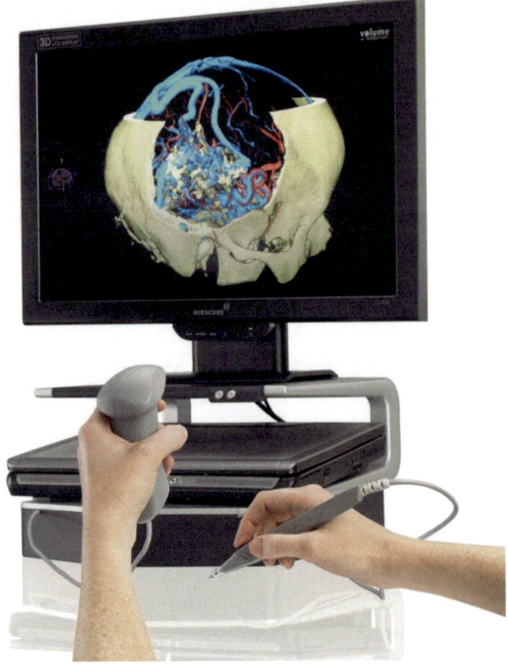

Fig. 13.15 The DextroVision

The Dextroscope was also used for the planning of the separation of the several craniopagus twins. The first separation was done in 1998 in South Africa, and was successful, and was led by a team headed pediatric neurosurgeon Dr Benjamin Carson of the Johns Hopkins Medical Institutions. Subsequently, in 2001, Drs Keith Goh and Chumpon Chan used the Dextroscope for the planning of the successful separation of craniopagus twins from Nepal at the Singapore General Hospital [65–67].

In 2004, at the Johns Hopkins Children's Centre in Baltimore, a 100-member medical team led again by Ben Carson used Dextroscope to plan the surgery to separate conjoined twin sisters [67]. Its contribution was reported to be crucial – illustrating the complex hemodynamic network of the twin's brains and helping plan approaches to the minute divisions that ensured proper circulation. In 2007 a team from King Fahad National Guard Hospital in Riyadh, Saudi Arabia, also used the Dextroscope in the planning of the separation of craniopagus twins.

The usefulness of the system increases with the complexity of the surgical task, especially when aiming at minimizing the invasiveness or optimizing the approach.

Vascular Neurosurgery: A Core Application of the Dextroscope

Aneurysms

The surgical obliteration of an intracranial aneurysm is a delicate maneuver and prone to manifold considerations and limitations. The understanding of the unique architecture of an aneurysm is by far the most important factor determining the success and the clinical outcome of aneurysm surgery. This includes the shape and size of the aneurysm's neck and dome as well as its relationship to feeding and draining vessels and neighboring structures. In addition, the surgeon needs to anticipate the most suitable sizes, shapes, and positions of clips while also taking into account the limitations of the surgical corridor. The software available on PACS workstations or neuro-navigation systems is able to display 3D images of an aneurysm and its surrounding vasculature. However, the surgical corridor, dependent on other intracranial or bony structures, cannot be reliably simulated with these systems, and it is thus sometimes difficult to conceive the spatial relations of the aneurysm as it will appear in the surgical view.

The Dextroscope VR environment integrates the preoperative available tomographic imaging information and allows it to be presented in its inherent, 3D form. In 2007, Wong et al. [30] reported the use of the Dextroscope for the planning of aneurysm clipping in a total of 13 cases and concluded that preoperative simulation "enhances the understanding of the surgical anatomy" and "provides an opportunity for preoperative rehearsal." This group did not, however, report on clinical or radiological outcomes. In 2016, Kockro et al. [28] reported on a retrospective consecutive series of clipping of 115 aneurysms including 85 incidental, unruptured aneurysms in 77 patients and 30 ruptured aneurysms in 28 patients which were all planned with the Dextroscope. For the unruptured aneurysms, the mortality of the surgical procedure was 0%, and morbidity (modified Rankin score mRS >2) was 2.6%. The rate of complete aneurysm obliteration on postoperative imaging was 91.8%. For the ruptured aneurysms, the mortality was 3.6%, the morbidity (mRS>2) 7.1% and the rate of complete aneurysm clipping was 90%. This data shows that virtual reality planning is associated with excellent clinical outcomes while maintaining rates of complete aneurysm closure equivalent to benchmark cohorts. Interestingly a subgroup of surgeons, the ones that were beginners in the field of cerebrovascular surgery, showed comparable of even superior clinical results as compared to their experienced colleagues. See Fig. 13.16 for case illustration.

AVMs Arteriovenous Malformations (Arteriovenous Malformations)

The surgical excision of a cerebral arteriovenous malformation is clearly one of the most techni-

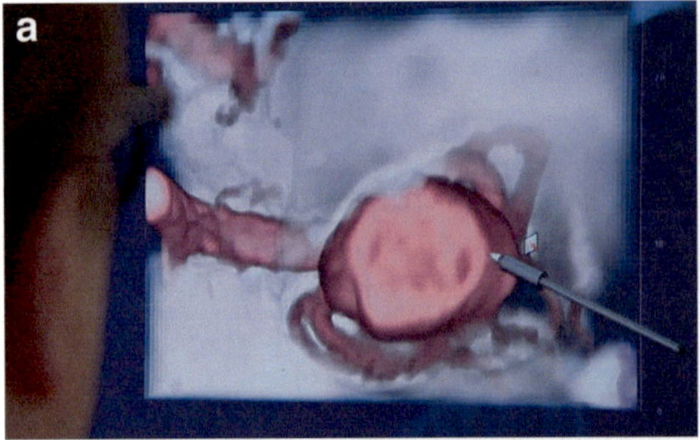
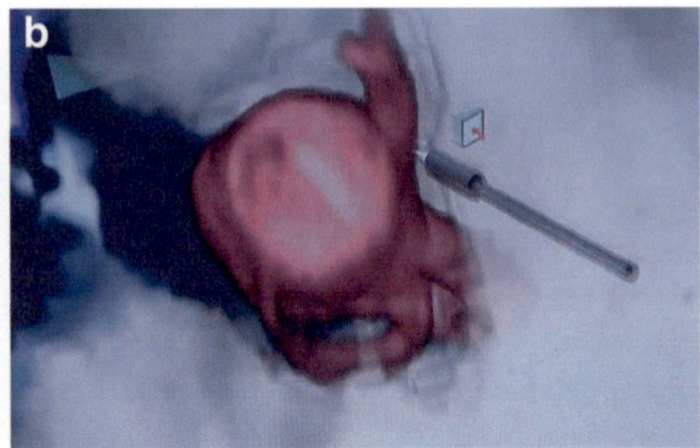
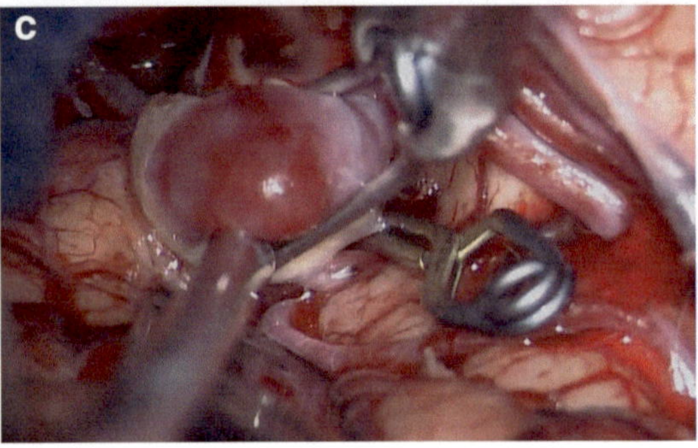

Fig. 13.16 Aneurysm case: Large left-sided aneurysm of the middle cerebral artery (MCA). (**a**) Shows a view over the surgeon's shoulder on a screen. The aneurysm dome is exposed in the Sylvian fissure, and the MCA main trunk leading toward the aneurysm is clearly visible. The aneurysm dome is partially cropped; the virtual pen, serving as volume exploration and pointing tool, is seen on the right. (**b**) Shows a view from more posterior, exposing the branching M2 superior and inferior trunks. The clip positioning of the clip parallel to the axis of the M2 trunks is being planned. (**c**) Intraoperative view. A temporary clip on the MCA main trunk has been placed and the aneurysm clip is being placed as virtually planned

cally challenging neurosurgical procedures. Imperative to surgical success is the precise understanding of the vascular architecture forming the malformation. The individual surgical strategies of reaching the malformation, dissecting the nidus, and obliterating the feeders and draining veins rely directly on the anticipation of vascular spatial relationships, and hence surgical planning by simulating intraoperative perspectives is particularly useful in these cases. Preoperative planning is especially difficult if the mental 3D picture of the lesion needs to be established based on 2D angiography or MRA/CTA. Although MRA and CTA may be displayed in 3D on PACS or navigation workstations, a comprehensive surgical planning is limited by the rather simple segmentation and manipulation tools. A stereoscopic display with an intuitive 3D interface greatly aids the planning procedure by enhancing comprehensive spatial understanding [26, 31, 32]. See Fig. 13.17 for case illustration.

Microvascular Decompression Surgery

A variety of clinical symptoms is caused by the compression and irritation of cranial nerves by one or several arteries or veins. The most common vascular compression syndrome is trigeminal neuralgia, caused by a vessel branch or loop of usually the superior or anterior inferior cerebellar artery conflicting with the trigeminal nerve. The second most common cranial nerve compression syndrome is a hemifacial spasm, caused by vascular compression of the facial nerve. The only therapeutic option of vascular compression syndromes that solves the problems origin rather than inflicting damage on the involved cranial nerve is microsurgical decompression surgery. During this surgical procedure, the vessel, which is compressing a cranial nerve, is carefully dissected off the nerve and its arachnoid surrounding, and subsequently a Teflon pad is positioned between the nerve and the vessel. A precise understanding of the three dimensionality

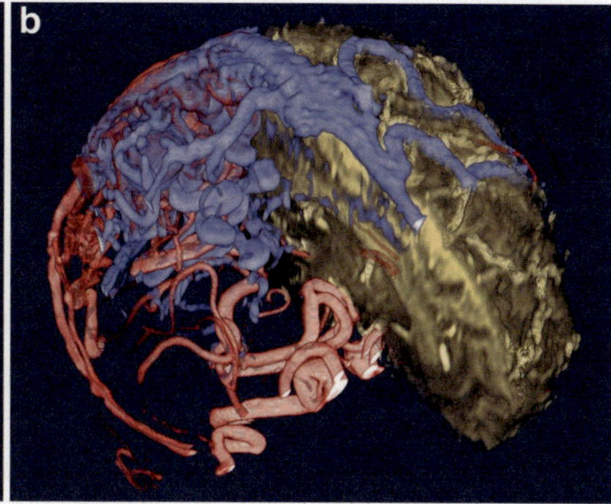

Fig. 13.17 AVM case. Large right parieto-occipital AVM, fused MR angiographic (*red*) and MR venographic (*blue*) images. (**a**) View from *right* superior–posterior–lateral, showing the bilateral middle meningeal arteries and the *right* occipital artery as the superficial feeders. The arterialized, enlarged vessels of the nidus mainly drain into the sagittal sinus. (**b**) View from anterior. The enlarged and curvy *right*-posterior cerebral artery is seen as the deep feeding vessel; the anterior portion of the venous drainage is clearly displayed

of the neurovascular conflict simplifies the surgery by reducing the amount of exploratory dissection and increasing the accuracy of placing the decompression pad (see Fig. 13.18 for case illustration).

Cavernomas

Cavernomas are benign vascular lesions comprising of a magnitude of small venous cavernous structures separated by thin tissue formations. Cavernomas can cause hemorrhages extending into the surrounding brain tissue, and they are often the origin of seizures. Symptomatic cavernomas need to be considered for microsurgical removal, and complete excision often leads to complete relief of symptoms. While the actual microsurgery of excising the cavernoma might be a straightforward procedure, the identification of a suitable path toward a cavernomas can be an enormous challenge, especially when reaching into the deep brain or the brain stem. The planning of deep-seated cavernoma surgery, therefore, requires spatial consideration of all surrounding structures, and the success of surgery is highly dependent on detailed approach planning (see Fig. 13.19 for case illustration).

Installations

The Dextroscope and the Dextrobeam systems were in operation at the medical institutions listed in Table 13.1.

DEX-Ray: Extension into the Operating Room

Image-guidance technology is now pervasive in neurosurgery. It is usually referred as surgical navigation, computer-assisted surgery, navigated surgery, or stereotactic navigation. Similar to a car or mobile Global Positioning Systems (GPS), image-guided surgery systems, like *Curve Image Guided Surgery* and *StealthStation*, use cameras or electromagnetic fields to capture and relay the patient's anatomy and the surgeon's precise movements in relation to the patient to computer monitors in the operating room. These sophisticated computerized systems are used before and during surgery to help orient the surgeon with three-dimensional images of the patient's anatomy.

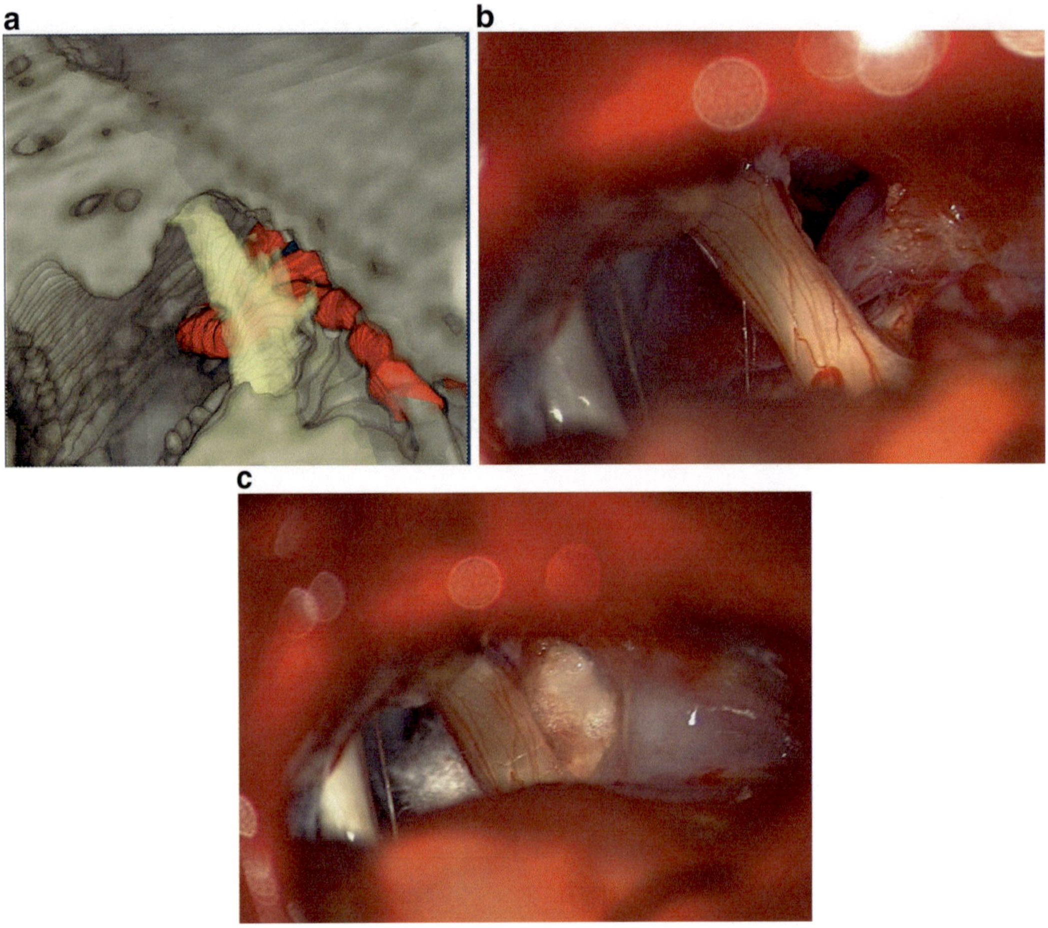

Fig. 13.18 Microvascular decompression case. *Left-*sided trigeminal neuralgia. (**a**) Simulated view toward the *left* trigeminal nerve, which is rendered semitransparent. Behind the nerve a descending and branching superior cerebellar artery is shown to compress the nerve; (**b**) The intraoperative view with the offending vessel exactly as virtually anticipated; (**c**) Shows the Teflon pad being placed between the nerve and the artery

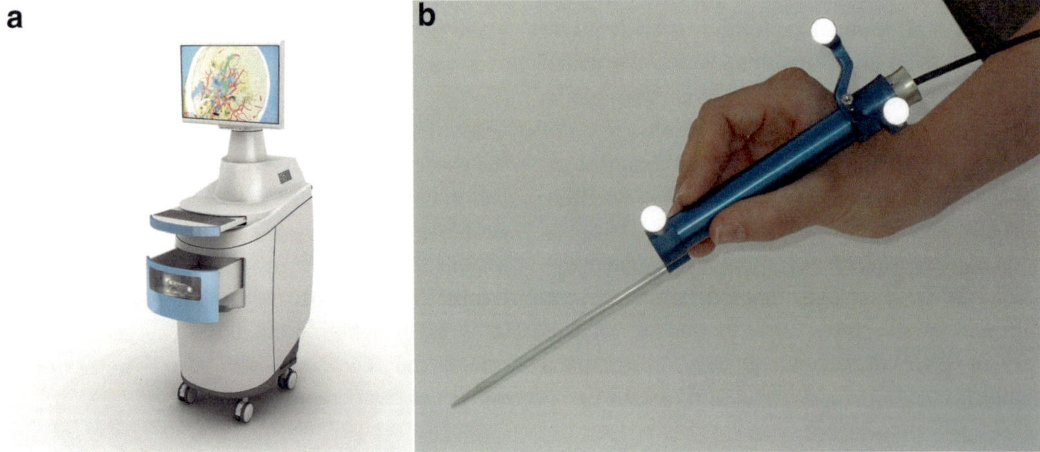

Fig. 13.19 The DEX-Ray system showing the stereoscopic monitor and the drawer housing the camera probe (**a**) and (**b**) the camera probe being held the hand

Table 13.1 Users of the Dextroscope technology

Medical/research institution	Main use
Hirslanden Hospital (Zurich, Switzerland)	Neurosurgery planning, teaching
Johannes Gutenberg University Hospital (Mainz, Germany)	Neurosurgery planning, teaching, and medical education
Hospital del Mar (Barcelona, Spain)	Neurosurgery planning
Stanford University Medical Center (San Francisco, USA)	Neurosurgery and cranio-maxillofacial surgery planning
St Louis University Hospital (St Louis, USA)	Neurosurgery planning, teaching
Johns Hopkins Hospital (Baltimore, USA)	Radiology research
Rutgers New Jersey Medical School (Newark, USA)	Neurosurgery, ENT, planning, and teaching
Hospital of the University of Pennsylvania (Philadelphia, USA)	Neurosurgery and cardiovascular radiology planning
Weill Cornell Brain and Spine Center (New York, USA)	Neurosurgery planning
Université Catholique de Louvain, Cliniques Universitaires St-Luc (Brussels, Belgium)	Neurosurgery planning
Istituto Neurologico C. Besta (Milan, Italy)	Neurosurgery planning
Royal London Hospital (London, UK)	Neurosurgery planning
Faculty of Medicine, University of Barcelona (Barcelona, Spain)	Neurosurgery planning, research, and neuroanatomy
Inselspital (Bern, Switzerland)	ENT planning
School of Medicine, University of Split (Split, Croatia)	Neurophysiology research
National Neuroscience Institute (Singapore)	Neurosurgery planning
SINAPSE Institute (Singapore)	Neurosurgery research
Prince of Wales Hospital (Hong Kong)	Neurosurgery and orthopedics planning
Hua Shan Hospital (Shanghai, China)	Neurosurgery planning
Chong Qing 3rd Military Hospital (Chong Qing, China)	Medical education
Advanced Surgery Training Centre of the National University Hospital (Singapore)	Medical education
Fujian Medical University (Fuzhou, China)	Neurosurgery and maxillofacial surgery planning

DEX-Ray is a navigation system which enables intraoperative image guidance by means of real-time overlay of 3D patient information over a video stream obtained by a camera integrated into a handheld pointer [68]; see Fig. 13.20. It is thus an augmented reality neurosurgical navigation system. The handheld probe functions as a viewing, pointing, and interaction device allowing the switching on or off of 3D patient information. The probe also enables the changing of magnification and altering of transparency to fine tune the see-through effect of the image. It was developed as an intraoperative extension of the Dextroscope.

The camera looks over the probe's tip into the surgical field (see Fig. 13.21). The camera's video stream is augmented with co-registered, multimodality 3D graphics and landmarks obtained during neurosurgical planning with 3D workstations. The handheld probe functions as a navigation device to view and point at and as an interaction device to adjust the 3D graphics.

DEX-Ray has been tested to be accurate in the laboratory. DEX-Ray has been tested clinically in over 140 cases at the NNI in Singapore (comparing it to the StealthStation from Medtronic) and at the Hospital Clinic in Barcelona, Spain (comparing it with Vector Vision from Brainlab). The results indicate that navigation with DEX-Ray improves the image interpretation issues present in conventional navigation [68].

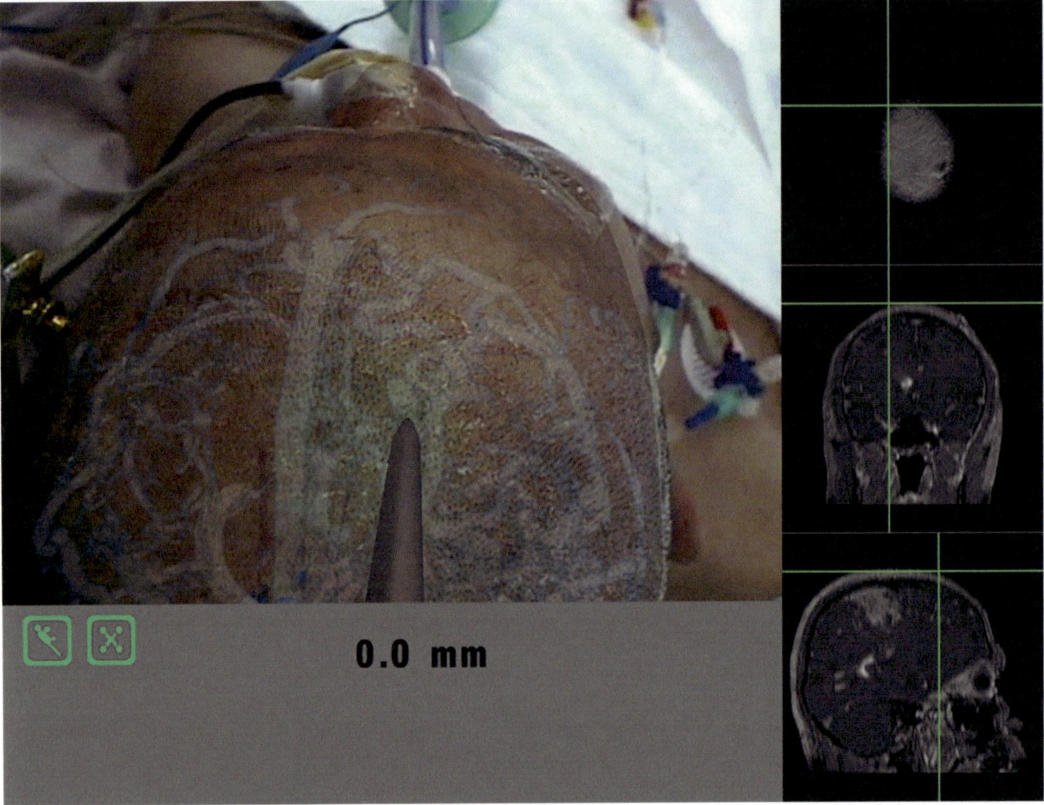

Fig. 13.20 The display of DEX-Ray showing the probe's view and the augmented vasculature overlaid over the video image

DEX-Ray provided accurate and real-time video-based augmented reality display. The system could be seamlessly integrated into the surgical workflow. The see-through effect revealing 3D information below the surgically exposed surface proved to be of significant value, especially during the macroscopic phase of an operation, providing easily understandable structural navigational information. Navigation in deep and narrow surgical corridors was limited by the camera resolution and light sensitivity.

The system was perceived as an improved navigational experience because the augmented see-through effect allowed direct understanding of the surgical anatomy beyond the visible surface and direct guidance toward surgical targets.

Dextroscope and Other Surgical Specialties

The Dextroscope has been applied also outside of neurosurgery to benefit any patient presenting a surgical challenge: an anatomical or structural complexity that requires planning of the surgical (or interventional) approach. See, for example, ENT, orthopedic, trauma, and craniofacial [69–74], cardiology [75], and liver surgery [76, 77].

Furthermore, the Dextroscope virtual reality environment helps bridge the gap between radiology and surgery – by allowing the radiologist to easily demonstrate to surgeons important 3D structures in a way that surgeons are familiar with.

Conclusion

Moving from the second to the third dimension of imaging data analysis for surgery planning has contributed greatly to the outcome of modern surgery. Three-dimensional patient-specific volumetric models fusing together different imaging modalities (CT, CTA, MRI, MRA, DTI) enable surgeons to better understand the patient's anatomy and plan complex operations.

Accurate fusion of multimodal image data is essential for 3D surgery planning systems, as are powerful software tools such as data segmentation. However, an essential ingredient often overlooked by most planning systems is that the 3D patient models should be manipulated by the surgeon in an easy, intuitive, and flexible manner. Most surgical planning systems utilize mouse and keyboard for this purpose – a 2D means of working with a 3D object. This 2D interface approach is nonintuitive, cumbersome, and because of the potential ambiguity arising when directing 3D movements using a 2D device, can often result in unintended position and orientation of the data.

The ideal planning environment would perfectly resemble the conditions faced during surgery, with the difference that virtual structures can be safely viewed from all angles, can be made to be *see-through* to understand what lies beneath, and can be manipulated without causing damage. In short, ideal planning allows perfect anticipation of all parameters and stages that define the surgical procedure. This minimizes guesswork and exploratory dissection and significantly increases patient safety. Ultimately the virtual surgical planning scenario could be superimposed to the surgical field in a way that allows operating while constantly being surrounded by a 3D synthetic environment providing information about all structures beyond the visible walls of the surgical cavity. Combined with the right microsurgical instruments, surgery would then turn into a succession of well anticipated and controlled steps, leaving little room for error and enabling the surgeon to safely implement the most effective surgical strategies.

Acknowledgments The Dextroscope, Dextrobeam, DEX-Ray, and DextroVision were developed by Volume Interactions Pte Ltd, a company member of the Bracco Group (Milan, Italy). Volume Interactions was based in Singapore and was a spin-off from the Kent Ridge Digital Labs (now Institute for Infocom Research) in Singapore.

The Dextroscope and Dextrobeam products received USA FDA 510(K)-Class II (2002) clearance, CE Marking-Class I (2002), China SFDA Registration-Class II (2004) and Taiwan Registration-type P (Radiology) (2007). DEX-Ray and DextroVision were research prototypes.

References

1. Alaraj A, Lemole MG, Finkle JH, Yudkowsky R, Wallace A, Luciano C, et al. Virtual reality training in neurosurgery: review of current status and future applications. Surg Neurol Int [Internet]. 2011 Apr 28.; [cited 2015 Jan 4];2. Available from: http://www.ncbi.nlm.nih.gov/pmc/articles/PMC3114314/.
2. Alaraj A, Tobin MK, Birk DM, Charbel FT. Simulation in neurosurgery and neurosurgical procedures. In: MD AIL, MD SDJ, MD ADS, MD AJS, editors. The comprehensive textbook of healthcare simulation [Internet]. New York: Springer; 2013 [cited 2015 Jan 4]. p. 415–23. Available from: http://link.springer.com/chapter/10.1007/978-1-4614-5993-4_28.
3. Malone HR, Syed ON, Downes MS, D'Ambrosio AL, Quest DO, Kaiser MG. Simulation in neurosurgery: a review of computer-based simulation environments and their surgical applications. Neurosurgery. 2010 Oct;67(4):1105–16.
4. O'Toole R, Playter R, Krummel T, Blank W, Cornelius N, Roberts W, et al. Assessing skill and learning in surgeons and medical students using a force feedback surgical simulator. In: Medical Image Computing and Computer-Assisted Intervention – MICCAI'98 [Internet]. Berlin, Heidelberg: Springer; 1998 [cited 2017 Jun 5]. p. 899–909. Available from: https://link.springer.com/chapter/10.1007/BFb0056278.
5. Hill JW, Holst PA, Jensen JF, Goldman J, Gorfu Y, Ploeger DW. Telepresence interface with applications to microsurgery and surgical simulation. Stud Health Technol Inform. 1998;50:96–102.
6. Delorme S, Laroche D, DiRaddo R, Del Maestro RF. NeuroTouch. Neurosurgery. 2012 Sep;71:ons32–42.
7. Poston T, Serra L. Dextrous virtual work. Commun ACM. 1996 May;39(5):37–45.
8. Poston T, Serra L, Lawton W, Chua BC. Interactive tube finding on a virtual workbench. In: Second International Symposium on Medical Robotics and Computer Assisted Surgery (MRCAS 95), Baltimore, Maryland, November [Internet]. 1995 [cited 2013 Jan 1]. p. 5–7. Available from: http://citeseerx.ist.psu.

edu/viewdoc/download?doi=10.1.1.33.5243&rep=rep1&type=pdf.

9. Poston T, Serra L. The virtual workbench: Dextrous VR. In: Virtual Reality Software and Technology [Internet]. World Scientific; 1994 [cited 2017 May 7]. p. 111–21. Available from: http://www.worldscientific.com/doi/abs/10.1142/9789814350938_0010.

10. Serra L, Nowinski WL, Poston T, Hern N, Meng LC, Guan CG, et al. The Brain Bench: virtual tools for stereotactic frame neurosurgery. Med Image Anal. 1997 Sep;1(4):317–29.

11. Serra L, Poston T, Hern N, Choon CB, Waterworth JA. Interaction techniques for a virtual workspace. Proc ICATVRST'95. 1995;79–80.

12. Serra L, Poston T, Hern N, Pheng Ann H, Beng Choon C. Virtual space editing of tagged MRI heart data. In: Computer Vision, Virtual Reality and Robotics in Medicine [Internet]. 1995 [cited 2013 Jan 1]. p. 70–76. Available from: http://www.springerlink.com/index/m434v81hr1423221.pdf.

13. Serra L, Hern N, Choon CB, Poston T. Interactive vessel tracing in volume data. In: Proceedings of the 1997 Symposium on Interactive 3D Graphics [Internet]. New York: ACM; 1997 [cited 2013 Jan 8]. p. 131-ff. (I3D '97). Available from: http://doi.acm.org/10.1145/253284.253320.

14. Serra L, Kockro R, Guan C, Hern N, Lee E, Lee Y, et al. Multimodal volume-based tumor neurosurgery planning in the virtual workbench. Med Image Comput Comput Assist Interv. 1998:1007–15.

15. Schmandt C. Spatial input/display correspondence in a stereoscopic computer graphic work station. In: Proceedings of the 10th Annual Conference on Computer Graphics and Interactive Techniques [Internet]. New York: ACM; 1983. p. 253–61. (SIGGRAPH '83). Available from: http://doi.acm.org/10.1145/800059.801156.

16. Sowizral HA. Interacting with virtual environments using augmented virtual tools. In: 1994. p. 409–416. Available from: https://doi.org/10.1117/12.173904.

17. Fuhrmann A, Loffelmann H, Schmalstieg D, Gervautz M. Collaborative visualization in augmented reality. IEEE Comput Graph Appl. 1998 Jul;18(4):54–9.

18. Billinghurst M, Baldis S, Matheson L, Philips M. 3D palette: a virtual reality content creation tool. In: Proceedings of the ACM Symposium on Virtual Reality Software and Technology [Internet]. New York: ACM; 1997. p. 155–156. (VRST '97). Available from: http://doi.acm.org/10.1145/261135.261163.

19. Deering MF. The HoloSketch VR sketching system. Commun ACM. 1996 May;39(5):54–61.

20. Wells WM, Viola P, Atsumi H, Nakajima S, Kikinis R. Multi-modal volume registration by maximization of mutual information. Med Image Anal. 1996 Mar;1(1):35–51.

21. Chia WK, Serra L. Contouring in 2D while viewing stereoscopic 3D volumes. Stud Health Technol Inform. 2006;119:93–5.

22. Stadie AT, Kockro RA, Serra L, Fischer G, Schwandt E, Grunert P, et al. Neurosurgical craniotomy localization using a virtual reality planning system versus intraoperative image–guided navigation. Int J Comput Assist Radiol Surg. 2011 Sep 1;6(5):565–72.

23. Ferroli P, Tringali G, Acerbi F, Aquino D, Franzini A, Broggi G. Brain surgery in a stereoscopic virtual reality environment: a single institution's experience with 100 cases. Neurosurgery. 2010 Sep;67(3 Suppl Operative):ons79–84; discussion ons84.

24. Kockro RA, Serra L, Tseng-Tsai Y, Chan C, Yih-Yian S, Gim-Guan C, et al. Planning and simulation of neurosurgery in a virtual reality environment. Neurosurgery. 2000 Jan;46(1):118–35; discussion 135–7.

25. Matis GK, Silva DO d A, Chrysou OI, Karanikas M, Pelidou S-H, Birbilis TA, et al. Virtual reality implementation in neurosurgical practice: the "can't take my eyes off you" effect. Turk Neurosurg. 2013;23(5):690–1.

26. Kockro RA, Stadie A, Schwandt E, Reisch R, Charalampaki C, Ng I, et al. A collaborative virtual reality environment for neurosurgical planning and training. Neurosurgery. 2007 Nov;61(5 Suppl 2):379–91; discussion 391.

27. Guo Y, Ke Y, Zhang S, Wang Q, Duan C, Jia H, et al. Combined application of virtual imaging techniques and three-dimensional computed tomographic angiography in diagnosing intracranial aneurysms. Chin Med J (Engl). 2008;121(24):2521.

28. Kockro RA, Killeen T, Ayyad A, Glaser M, Stadie A, Reisch R, et al. Aneurysm surgery with preoperative three-dimensional planning in a virtual reality environment: technique and outcome analysis. World Neurosurg. 2016 Dec;96:489–99.

29. Stadie AT, Kockro RA, Reisch R, Tropine A, Boor S, Stoeter P, et al. Virtual reality system for planning minimally invasive neurosurgery. Technical note. J Neurosurg. 2008 Feb;108(2):382–94.

30. Wong GKC, Zhu CXL, Ahuja AT, Poon WS. Craniotomy and clipping of intracranial aneurysm in a stereoscopic virtual reality environment. Neurosurgery. 2007 Sep;61(3):564–8; discussion 568–9.

31. Ng I, Hwang PYK, Kumar D, Lee CK, Kockro RA, Sitoh YY. Surgical planning for microsurgical excision of cerebral arterio-venous malformations using virtual reality technology. Acta Neurochir (Wien). 2009 May;151(5):453–63; discussion 463.

32. Wong GKC, Zhu CXL, Ahuja AT, Poon WS. Stereoscopic virtual reality simulation for microsurgical excision of cerebral arteriovenous malformation: case illustrations. Surg Neurol. 2009 Jul;72(1):69–72; discussion 72–3.

33. Du Z-Y, Gao X, Zhang X-L, Wang Z-Q, Tang W-J. Preoperative evaluation of neurovascular relationships for microvascular decompression in the cerebellopontine angle in a virtual reality environment. J Neurosurg [Internet]. 2009 Oct 23 [cited 2010 Jun 3]; Available from: http://www.ncbi.nlm.nih.gov/pubmed/19852542.

34. González Sánchez JJ, Enseñat Nora J, Candela Canto S, Rumià Arboix J, Caral Pons LA, Oliver D, et al. New stereoscopic virtual reality system application

to cranial nerve microvascular decompression. Acta Neurochir. 2010 Feb;152(2):355–60.

35. Liu X-D, Xu Q-W, Che X-M, Yang D-L. Trigeminal neurinomas: clinical features and surgical experience in 84 patients. Neurosurg Rev. 2009 Oct;32(4):435–44.

36. Cerebrovascular Diseases in Children: Anthony J. Raimondi: 9781461276760 [Internet]. [cited 2017 Jun 10]. Available from: https://www.bookdepository.com/Cerebrovascular-Diseases-Children-Anthony-J-Raimondi/9781461276760.

37. Stadie A, Reisch R, Kockro R, Fischer G, Schwandt E, Boor S, et al. Minimally invasive cerebral cavernoma surgery using keyhole approaches – solutions for technique-related limitations. Minim Invasive Neurosurg. 2009 Feb;52(01):9–16.

38. Khu KJ, Ng I, Ng WH. The relationship between parasagittal and falcine meningiomas and the superficial cortical veins: a virtual reality study. Acta Neurochir. 2009;151(11):1459–64.

39. Low D, Lee CK, Tay LL, Ng WH, Ang BT, Ng I. Augmented reality neurosurgical planning and navigation for surgical excision of parasagittal, falcine and convexity meningiomas. Br J Neurosurg. 2010 Feb;24(1):69–74.

40. Tang H, Sun H, Xie L, Tang Q, Gong Y, Mao Y, et al. Intraoperative ultrasound assistance in resection of intracranial meningiomas. Chin J Cancer Res. 2013;25(3):339–45.

41. Tang H-L, Sun H-P, Gong Y, Mao Y, Wu J-S, Zhang X-L, et al. Preoperative surgical planning for intracranial meningioma resection by virtual reality. Chin Med J (Engl). 2012 Jun;125(11):2057–61.

42. Anil SM, Kato Y, Hayakawa M, Yoshida K, Nagahisa S, Kanno T. Virtual 3-dimensional preoperative planning with the dextroscope for excision of a 4th ventricular ependymoma. Minim Invasive Neurosurg. 2007 Apr;50(2):65–70.

43. Wang S-S, Li J-F, Zhang S-M, Jing J-J, Xue L. A virtual reality model of the clivus and surgical simulation via transoral or transnasal route. Int J Clin Exp Med. 2014;7(10):3270–9.

44. Wang S-S, Xue L, Jing J-J, Wang R-M. Virtual reality surgical anatomy of the sphenoid sinus and adjacent structures by the transnasal approach. J Craniomaxillofac Surg. 2012 Sep;40(6):494–9.

45. Di Somma A, de Notaris M, Stagno V, Serra L, Enseñat J, Alobid I, et al. Extended endoscopic endonasal approaches for cerebral aneurysms: anatomical, virtual reality and morphometric study. BioMed Res Int [Internet]. 2014 Jan 19 [cited 2014 Feb 5];2014. Available from: http://www.hindawi.com/journals/bmri/2014/703792/abs/.

46. Reisch R, Stadie A, Kockro R, Gawish I, Schwandt E, Hopf N. The minimally invasive supraorbital subfrontal key-hole approach for surgical treatment of temporomesial lesions of the dominant hemisphere. Minim Invasive Neurosurg. 2009 Aug;52(4):163–9.

47. Fischer G, Stadie A, Schwandt E, Gawehn J, Boor S, Marx J, et al. Minimally invasive superficial tempo-ral artery to middle cerebral artery bypass through a minicraniotomy: benefit of three-dimensional virtual reality planning using magnetic resonance angiography. Neurosurg Focus. 2009 May;26(5):E20.

48. Reisch R, Stadie A, Kockro RA, Hopf N. The keyhole concept in neurosurgery. World Neurosurg. 2013 Feb;79(2 Suppl):S17.e9–13.

49. Serra C, Huppertz H-J, Kockro RA, Grunwald T, Bozinov O, Krayenbühl N, et al. Rapid and accurate anatomical localization of implanted subdural electrodes in a virtual reality environment. J Neurol Surg A Cent Eur Neurosurg. 2013 May;74(3):175–82.

50. Wang S-S, Zhang S-M, Jing J-J. Stereoscopic virtual reality models for planning tumor resection in the sellar region. BMC Neurol. 2012;12:146.

51. Yang DL, Xu QW, Che XM, Wu JS, Sun B. Clinical evaluation and follow-up outcome of presurgical plan by Dextroscope: a prospective controlled study in patients with skull base tumors. Surg Neurol. 2009 Dec;72(6):682–9.

52. Chen L, Zhao Y, Zhou L, Zhu W, Pan Z, Mao Y. Surgical strategies in treating brainstem cavernous malformations. Neurosurgery. 2011 Mar;68(3):609–21.

53. Qiu T, Zhang Y, Wu J-S, Tang W-J, Zhao Y, Pan Z-G, et al. Virtual reality presurgical planning for cerebral gliomas adjacent to motor pathways in an integrated 3-D stereoscopic visualization of structural MRI and DTI tractography. Acta Neurochir. 2010 Nov;152(11):1847–57.

54. de Notaris M, Palma K, Serra L, Enseñat J, Alobid I, Poblete J, et al. A three-dimensional computer-based perspective of the skull base. World Neurosurg. 2014 Dec;82(6S):S41–8.

55. Franzini A, Messina G, Marras C, Molteni F, Cordella R, Soliveri P, et al. Poststroke fixed dystonia of the foot relieved by chronic stimulation of the posterior limb of the internal capsule. J Neurosurg. 2009 Dec;111(6):1216–9.

56. Gu S-X, Yang D-L, Cui D-M, Xu Q-W, Che X-M, Wu J-S, et al. Anatomical studies on the temporal bridging veins with Dextroscope and its application in tumor surgery across the middle and posterior fossa. Clin Neurol Neurosurg. 2011 Dec;113(10):889–94.

57. Kockro RA, Hwang PYK. Virtual temporal bone: an interactive 3-dimensional learning aid for cranial base surgery. Neurosurgery. 2009 May;64(5 Suppl 2):216–29; discussion 229–30.

58. Kockro RA. Neurosurgery simulators – beyond the experiment. World Neurosurg. 2013 Nov;80(5):e101–2.

59. Lee CK, Tay LL, Ng WH, Ng I, Ang BT. Optimization of ventricular catheter placement via posterior approaches: a virtual reality simulation study. Surg Neurol. 2008 Sep;70(3):274–7; discussion 277–8.

60. Robison RA, Liu CY, Apuzzo MLJ. Man, mind, and machine: the past and future of virtual reality simulation in neurologic surgery. World Neurosurg. 2011;76(5):419–30.

61. Shen M, Zhang X-L, Yang D-L, Wu J-S. Stereoscopic virtual reality presurgical planning for cerebrospi-

nal otorrhea. Neurosci Riyadh Saudi Arab. 2010 Jul;15(3):204–8.

62. Shi J, Xia J, Wei Y, Wang S, Wu J, Chen F, et al. Three-dimensional virtual reality simulation of periarticular tumors using Dextroscope reconstruction and simulated surgery: a preliminary 10-case study. Med Sci Monit Int Med J Exp Clin Res. 2014;20:1043–50.

63. Stadie AT, Kockro RA. Mono-Stereo-Autostereo. Neurosurgery. 2013 Jan;72:A63–77.

64. Yang D-L, Che X, Lou M, Xu Q-W, Wu J-S, Li W, et al. Application of dextroscope virtual reality system. In: Anatomical research of inner structures in petrosal bone. [cited 2013 Apr 4]; Available from: http://www.iioab.org/Vol2(4)2011/2(4)16-22.pdf.

65. Goh KYC. Separation surgery for total vertical craniopagus twins. Childs Nerv Syst ChNS Off J Int Soc Pediatr Neurosurg. 2004 Aug;20(8–9):567–75.

66. R.A. Kockro RA, Goh K, Chan C, Hern N, Lee E, Chia GL, Serra L. Pre-Operative Planning Of The Separation Of Craniopagus Twins In A Collaborative Virtual Reality Environment. Proceedings of the XVIII Congress of the European Society for Pediatric Neurosurgery, Kiruna, Sweden, 14-18 June 2002. Child's Nerv Syst. 2002;18:252–3.

67. Johns Hopkins Magazine [Internet]. [cited 2017 May 28]. Available from: http://pages.jh.edu/%7Ejhumag/0205web/separate.html.

68. Kockro RA, Tsai YT, Ng I, Hwang P, Zhu C, Agusanto K, et al. Dex-ray: augmented reality neurosurgical navigation with a handheld video probe. Neurosurgery. 2009 Oct;65(4):795–807; discussion 807–8.

69. Caversaccio M, Eichenberger A, Häusler R. Virtual simulator as a training tool for endonasal surgery. Am J Rhinol. 2003 Oct;17(5):283–90.

70. Corey CL, Popelka GR, Barrera JE, Most SP. An analysis of malar fat volume in two age groups: implications for craniofacial surgery. Craniomaxillofac Trauma Reconstr. 2012 Dec;5(4):231–4.

71. Kwon J, Barrera JE, Jung T-Y, Most SP. Measurements of orbital volume change using computed tomography in isolated orbital blowout fractures. Arch Facial Plast Surg. 2009 Dec;11(6):395–8.

72. Kwon J, Barrera JE, Most SP. Comparative computation of orbital volume from axial and coronal CT using three-dimensional image analysis. Ophthal Plast Reconstr Surg. 2010 Jan;26(1):26–9.

73. Li Y, Tang K, Xu X, Yi B. Application of Dextroscope virtual reality in anatomical research of the mandible part of maxillary artery. Beijing Da Xue Xue Bao. 2012 Feb 18;44(1):75–9.

74. Pau CY, Barrera JE, Kwon J, Most SP. Three-dimensional analysis of zygomatic-maxillary complex fracture patterns. Craniomaxillofac Trauma Reconstr. 2010 Sep;3(3):167–76.

75. Correa CR, Litt HI, Hwang W-T, Ferrari VA, Solin LJ, Harris EE. Coronary Artery findings after left-sided compared with right-sided radiation treatment for early-stage breast cancer. J Clin Oncol. 2007 Jul 20;25(21):3031–7.

76. Chen G, Yang S-Z, Wu G-Q, Wang Y, Fan G-H, Tan L-W, et al. Development and clinical application of 3D operative planning system of live in virtual reality environments. Zhonghua Wai Ke Za Zhi. 2009 Nov;47(21):1620–6.

77. Chen G, Li X, Wu G, Wang Y, Fang B, Xiong X, et al. The use of virtual reality for the functional simulation of hepatic tumors (case control study). Int J Surg. 2010;8(1):72–8.

Role of Immersive Touch Simulation in Neurosurgical Training

Denise Brunozzi, Sophia F. Shakur, Amanda Kwasnicki, Rahim Ismail, Fady T. Charbel, and Ali Alaraj

Introduction

Neurosurgery is one of the most technically demanding surgical specialties, characterized by sophisticated procedures that require refined skills and a high level of competency. 19.1% of neurosurgeons in the United States have malpractice claims brought against them every year, causing it to be one of the most litigious among all medical subspecialties [1]. Learning the precise and delicate surgical techniques necessary to reach expertise requires many years of directed, hands-on training. Currently, creating a comprehensive training program that meets all the educational requirements is a challenge; constantly evolving, minimally invasive techniques and increasing demand for expert-level surgical care prove difficult training environments, particularly when combined with work-hour restrictions and high operative costs.

At the end of the nineteenth century, the Halstedian model marked the first major shift in surgical training: patient contact gained a central role, and the need for a standardized curriculum was recognized [2]. *Operative experience* was the gold standard in twentieth-century training, based on the three-step model of "watch-perform-teach." The trainee learns by watching experienced individuals perform the task, applying what he understood to complete the task independently, and teaching what he learned to someone else, thus providing a direct transfer of information and knowledge from teacher to trainee.

Although this direct apprenticeship model has been the mainstay since the previous century, it has its own limitations. Besides possible harm to patients by the trial-and-error approach, extreme variability exists among patient anatomy, case variety, and mentor availability. Furthermore, educational opportunities may potentially take a higher priority than patient safety and procedure efficacy, which physicians must always put first [2, 3, 4].

Indirect apprenticeship provides the necessary foundation for surgical training and complements to the operative experience in order to achieve a more graded and enhanced education for trainees. Additionally, it is less ethically burdensome as it provides an overall safer surgical experience for the patient. Due to technological advances, a large volume of resources is now available to supplement surgical education. Textbooks, videos, and lectures are easily accessible and attainable, providing extensive anatomical detail and vast technical insights that can be obtained independently of the operative room. However, these modes of learning lack of the basic, hands-on components of the operative experience and

D. Brunozzi · S. F. Shakur · A. Kwasnicki · R. Ismail
F. T. Charbel · A. Alaraj (✉)
Department of Neurosurgery, University of Illinois at
Chicago, Chicago, IL, USA
e-mail: alaraj@uic.edu

graded tactile feedback that is required to master surgical skills. The gap between these two training models has been filled by simulation, a widely used educational tool in the medical field. Simulation is defined as the technique of imitating the behavior of certain situations or processes by means of a suitable analogous situation or apparatus, particularly for the purpose of study or personnel training [1, 5, 6].

Simulation in the medical field has historical roots dating back from early animal and human cadaver dissections in the sixth century BC, primarily performed to learn anatomy [1].

Simulation in medicine has gained a critical role in the education process over recent years, mainly in the surgical field. It has been applied to various training levels and is equipped with a large range of artificial environments where trainees can safely practice and gain experience. Types of simulation include the following:

- *Physical Simulation*: Provides realistic, tactile feedback to the trainee and may be animate or inanimate.
  - *Animate Simulators*: Include live or cadaveric models of animals or humans. Although human cadavers provide suitable surgical anatomic models, they lack dynamic properties, such as bleeding, pulsation, or physiological reactions to surgical insult that a trainee is required to learn to manage during his or her training. Live animal models provide a more sophisticated tool for dynamic feedback and response in the event of surgical error but differ in anatomy.
  - Both cadaveric and live animate simulators offer three-dimensional displays of anatomy and tactile feedback by manipulation. However, the fiscal, ethical, and biological restrictions weighted against limited realism (tissue rigidity for human cadavers, not perfectly reliable anatomy for animals) and use (not reusable for multiple similar approaches) confine its application.
  - *Inanimate Simulator*: Much more readily available for use than are inanimate simulators and include synthetic models and box trainers. These tools allow trainees to learn basic motor skills and to develop hand-eye coordination in a reproducible environment but generally have limited reliability, realism, recordable metrics, and tactile feedback and usually only address partial components of tasks.
- *Human Patient Simulation*: Sophisticated, computer-driven mannequins have been developed to teach normal physiological responses, rehearse critical situations, and test a trainee's managing capability. Some limitations of this training modality are cost and time constraints, as evidenced by the need for a dedicated and trained staff.
- *Web-Based Simulation*: With the right Internet and computer access, this form of simulation can be easily accessible, has limited cost, and allows the trainee to obtain standardized knowledge and decision-making assessments. Computer-generated surgical models now allow the trainee to practice a variety of procedures with different degrees of visual feedback. However, haptic cues are still missing.
- *Three-Dimensional Technology Simulation*: Three-dimensional reproduction of neurosurgical instruments and pathology with multimaterial printers allow high-fidelity stereoscopic and haptic reproduction. Additionally, this information can be recorded and reviewed in three-dimensional videos. This is particularly helpful for preoperative planning and improves anatomical understanding of a patient's specific pathology. However, it is currently an expensive and time-consuming technology and less suitable for training for emergency settings.
- *Virtual Reality Simulation*: Based on computer-generated graphics, virtual reality simulation offers recreation of human anatomy and surgical models obtained from radiologic images in a virtual space. This provides a more accurate representation of reality and adds the option to broaden the scope of trainable models [1, 7].

Virtual Reality (VR) Simulation

VR simulation has improved operating room performance in laparoscopic and endovascular surgery and recently gained a critical role in residency training, becoming a required part of core curricula [8, 9, 10]. VR simulation in neurosurgical training programs is emerging as a possible answer to the question of how to teach sophisticated techniques in a safe environment, but further trials are needed to test the impact on in vivo neurosurgical skills [7, 11]. Interest in neurosurgical VR simulation has increased over time due to the introduction of newly enhanced technologies. Three different virtual systems exist thus far [1]:

- *Simplified*: Three-dimensional anatomic representations offer the user only a passive visual interface without any other sensory interaction. It is the most basic form of VR and image reconstruction which utilizes cadaveric dissection images that are integrated into a simulated intraoperative environment to provide volumetric representations of generic surgical procedures (e.g., virtual dissector) [12, 13]. Volumetric representation may also be reconstructed from a patient-specific imaging study (e.g., Dextroscope) to aid in preoperative surgical planning [14].
- *Augmented*: Three-dimensional reconstruction can be manipulated by the user in this form of simulation, demonstrating real-time tissue deformation and providing an interactive experience. In addition to visual feedback from the manipulation performed, additional software may offer acoustic feedback during surgical task assessments (e.g., audiovisual ventriculostomy simulators or Robo-Sim endoscopic neurosurgical simulator) [14].
- *Immersive*: Immersive simulation seems to be the most promising system among the current existing VR simulators. The simulator-user interaction provides both visual and haptic feedback, yielding a more realistic experience by the manipulation of virtual models. This VR system enables training of hand-eye coordination in inherent, metric models that facilitate the acquisition of sophisticated psychomotor skills.

Introduced for the first time in 2005, three different haptic VR systems have been produced:

ImmersiveTouch by the University of Illinois at Chicago (Illinois) [4, 8, 17, 18] ImmersiveTouch was the first system to provide seamless integration of haptic and stereoscopic visual rendering in VR. This system includes head and hand electromagnetic tracking to compute the viewer's perspective by his or her head and hand movements around the virtual anatomic reconstruction. The continuously evolving technology of ImmersiveTouch has allowed for practicing various neurosurgical procedures with the opportunity for skill level assessments (Fig. 14.1).

TempoSurg by the University of Hamburg (Germany) [15] TempoSurg provides an interactive computer-user interface to offer surgical practice on a three-dimensional, virtual temporal bone through a phantom arm that simulates the surgical drill and foot pedal. This system has different surgical corridors available for training but is limited

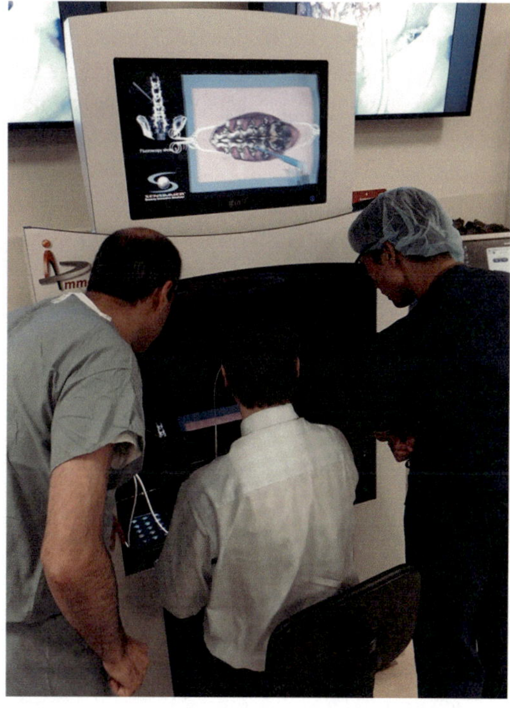

Fig. 14.1 Senior Neurosurgical Resident Boot Camp Training Course 2015. ImmersiveTouch platform is designed to introduce important principles of neurosurgical care to trainees under direct supervision (Used with permission of ImmersiveTouch)

to this specific anatomical area and provides a low graphic resolution of important structures, such as various vessels and nerves, whose avoidance is essential for neurosurgery [16].

NeuroTouch by Montreal University (Canada) [7] NeuroTouch focuses on training short, specific neurosurgical tasks with bilateral manipulation of three-dimensional anatomic models. The system has options to select different surgical tools, increase difficulty level, track metrics, and time the user. It is mainly oriented to simulate partial tasks of neurosurgical procedures in order to address basic skill requirements for a trainee: ventriculostomy, endoscopic nasal navigation, tumor debulking, hemostasis, and microdissection.

ImmersiveTouch

In recent years, the traditional "learning by observing" method has faced increasing pressures of new minimally invasive and percutaneous techniques along with legal/ethical concerns of patient safety. The need to address alternative methods of neurosurgical training has become imperative. ImmersiveTouch was the first system to add haptic and kinesthetic feedback to existing augmented virtual reality reconstructions (2005; Fig. 14.2).

It is equipped with four hardware components [18]:

- Three-dimensional stereodisplay with high resolution (1600 × 1200 pixels) and high visual acuity (20/24.74) that provides clear vision of small anatomical details, with more realistic and efficient operative learning.
- Head tracking through stereoscopic goggles equipped with an electromagnetic sensor that allows virtual reality scene adjustment according to viewer's perspective by means of real-time computation.
- Hand tracking through an electromagnetic sensor located inside the SpaceGrip that tracks the surgeon's hand. It defines the cutting plane

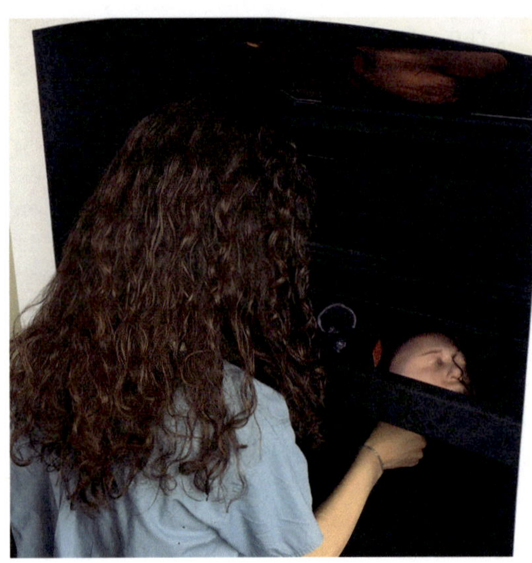

Fig. 14.2 ImmersiveTouch platform setup. The trainee looks into the screen that creates three-plane CT reconstruction (different modules available) wearing stereoscopic googles that track head positioning and adjust virtual reality scene to viewer's perspective. The nondominant hand controls the SpaceGrip that allows the model positioning adjustment, and the dominant hand holds the haptic stylus that simulates the surgical tool (Used with permission of ImmersiveTouch)

and the light source in order to integrate hand position in the virtual environment.
- A haptic stylus that simulates surgical tools, provides position and orientation information, computes collision forces with the virtual head, and generates tactile feedback.

ImmersiveTouch software uses four interconnected modules to acquire, process, and render seamless integration of graphic and haptic data [4, 18]:

- *Volume data pre-processing (VTK 4.5)*: two-dimensional images generated by MRI or CT are analyzed, segmented, and combined to create a virtual three-dimensional volume of the patient's head. The virtual head is made of polygonal isosurfaces corresponding to the different anatomic layers. Each isosurface is qualified by specific features to match real tissue behavior under defined haptic stimulations.
- *Head and hand tracking (pciBIRD)*: Dual sensors allow both computation of the viewer's

perspective according to his or her head movements and adjustment of both the cutting plane and light source according to his or her hand position.

- *Haptic rendering (Ghost 4.0)*: Each three-dimensional isosurface of the virtual volume is defined by four parameters: stiffness, viscosity, static friction, and dynamic friction. Through the haptic stylus and rapid refresh rate, the user can interact with three-dimensional multilayer surgical models and obtain realistic visual feedback of tissue deformation. The three-dimensional multilayer virtual volume also provides distinct tactile feedback according to the different textures of isosurfaces and generates various haptic forces computed from collisions with the stylus in virtual reality. Integration of visual and haptic feedback is the key feature of this virtual reality system and offers more effective training of hand-eye coordination.
- *Graphic rendering (Coin 2.3)*: The virtual three-dimensional model is displayed through a special camera node that depicts the stereo-scopic perspective in a frame-sequential fashion adjusted to the viewer's head position. The perspective is further adjusted in volumetric depth through SpaceGrip control.

This haptic-based, three-dimensional, and virtual system is a valuable tool to learn new skills and to improve surgical proficiency through repetition and practice; it combines the advantages of generic virtual reality simulation with the distinguished properties of immersive VR (Table 14.1).

The flexibility of virtual reality applied to ImmersiveTouch technology has brought on the development of a library of anatomical variations and training modules. Several neurosurgical skills are addressed and assessed by this platform, but proficiency, improvement, and transfer of these abilities on live neurosurgical fields have not been proven. In order to justify the high expense of this sophisticated technology, full validation of its usefulness in neurosurgical training is required. ImmersiveTouch modules should be evaluated along three main characteristics:

Table 14.1 Advantages of VR and ImmersiveTouch simulation systems

Virtual reality [7, 16, 17, 18]	ImmersiveTouch [4, 16, 18, 20]
Practice in a harmless environment, which addresses the ethical issues of patient safety	Perspective adjustment to viewer's head position through stereoscopic goggles equipped with electromagnetic sensor
Multiple and variable learning modules focusing on different surgical procedures and tasks	Three-dimensional volume depth adjustment through hand tracker electromagnetic sensor (SpaceGrip)
Repeatable and reusable modules, guaranteeing consistent skill training and maintenance with minimal financial burden	Real-time interaction with a three-dimensional simulated surgical field through a superimposed virtual tool (this feature is also present in other VR systems like TempoSurg or Dextroscope)
Proven results for laparoscopic surgery (not currently for neurosurgery)	Haptic rendering with kinesthetic and tactile feedback, providing real-time force generation according to both the user's hand position in the field and the virtual tool's collision with specific three-dimensional isosurface characteristics
Transfer of expertise and knowledge independently of the operating room	
Objective measurements and the ability to assess competency through scoring systems	Immediate stereoscopic feedback of "blinded" procedures, whose performance is based on correct detection of external landmarks (e.g., ventriculostomy), through a cutaway tool in which it is possible to look "inside" the three-dimensional model after the task is performed (direct trajectory control on "open head")
Unsupervised self-learning with immediate feedback	
Uniform and standardized educational learning	
Preoperative planning and rehearsal	

VR = Virtual reality

- Discrimination of surgical abilities already owned by the trainee
- Enhancement of personal skills through practice in simulated modules
- Realistic learning transferable in vivo

Ventriculostomy [4, 18, 19, 20]

The first generation of ImmersiveTouch ventriculostomy simulator showed limited usefulness for teaching and measuring neurosurgical expertise. Nevertheless, second-generation ameliorations were introduced including viewer-centered perspective and precise overlapping of the haptic device stylus with its virtual representation in the simulated field. Ventriculostomy is one of the most commonly performed procedures in neurosurgery, allowing for measurement of intracranial pressure and drainage of cerebrospinal fluid when needed. It is usually one of the first surgical procedures a neurosurgical resident performs. For this reason, and for its simplicity compared to other neurosurgical interventions, it is the most frequently reproduced technique by virtual simulators.

This module is aimed at improving trainee ability to place a ventricular catheter using external landmarks with as few attempts as possible. ImmersiveTouch helps in learning the psychomotor skills by use of hand-eye coordination in the three-dimensional environment with haptic feedback of the technical gesture performed. The haptic stylus works as a ventricular catheter with exact overlapping onto the virtual reproduction in the three-dimensional workspace; the user has the option to visualize the trajectory of the catheter by means of virtual lines traced through the virtual head. The trainee can choose among three burr-hole options and measure the distance from external landmarks to one of the selected burr hole to aid in correct catheter placement (Fig. 14.3a, b). The second-generation software is enriched with a bone drilling module that simulates the burr-hole performance in order to have step-by-step replication of the procedure (Fig. 14.3c, d). The user plans his or her trajectory with the help of a corresponding projection from a three-plane CT scan reconstruction displayed on screen, easing the stereo-tactical learning process. While introducing the catheter into the virtual head, the trainee perceives the haptic feedback corresponding to actual brain consistency. As the catheter enters the virtual ventricle, a giveaway "pop" sensation is felt over the haptic stylus. A chromatic code indicates the outcome of the procedure: in a successfully performed ventriculostomy, the catheter turns green (Fig. 14.3e). To enhance the stereo-tactical education, the trainee can directly verify final catheter position inside the virtual head by opening it with virtual scissors (Fig. 14.3f, g). The software has broadened its module library, including 15 different ventricular anatomies with normal, shift, and slit/compressed ventricles. Ventriculostomy is currently the only module that has been tested and verified as a realistic learning alternative to actual procedures. The discriminative power of a trainee's abilities is also accurate, as proven during the 3-day Top Gun competition at the 2006 annual meeting of the American Association of Neurological Surgeons (AANS). Seventy-eight neurosurgical fellows and residents were evaluated on an ImmersiveTouch module for ventricle cannulation and evaluated based on the distance from the virtual catheter tip to the foramen of Monro. The score generated from this module proved to be consistent with distances calculated retrospectively from postoperative CT scans of actual freehand ventriculostomies [20]. The enhancing capacity of this module on resident skills was verified through the demonstration of increased success after repeated practice of normal and abnormal ventricle catheterization on simulated modules [11, 19]. The practical learning potential was assessed by comparing in vivo procedural outcomes before and after practice on simulated modules on a group of 12 residents. A positive effect on the overall success on first-attempt cannulation after simulated practice was statistically significant [11].

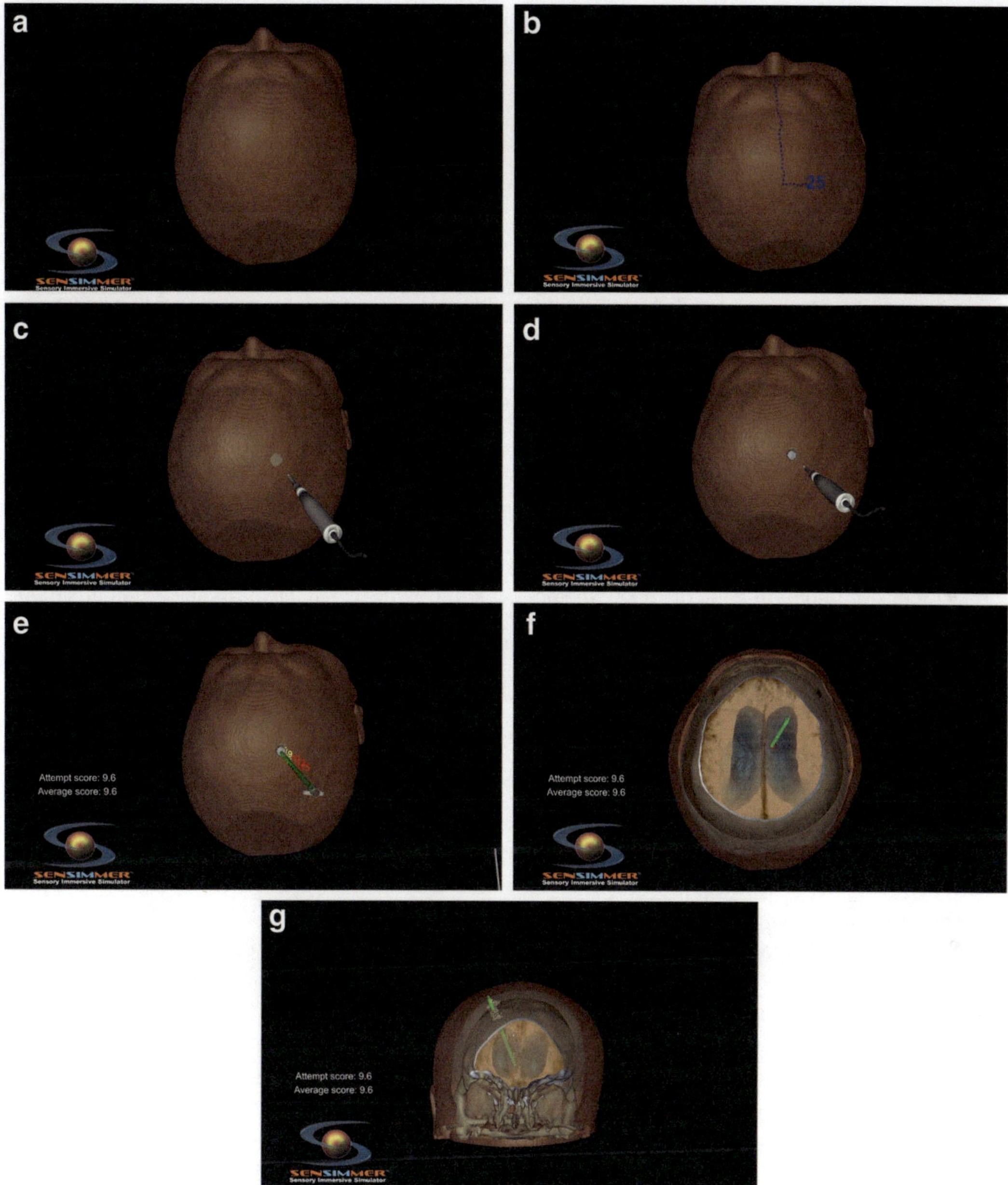

Fig. 14.3 (**a**) Virtual head reconstruction from three-plane CT. (**b**) The trainee can measure the distance from external landmarks to help him in choosing the correct burr-hole placement. (**c**, **d**) Bone drilling module that simulates the burr-hole performance. (**e**) At the end of the catheter positioning trial, the software computes the position accuracy providing a score. If the outcome of the performance is successful, the catheter turns *green*. (**f**, **g**) Direct verification of the final catheter position inside the virtual head: (**f**) axial projection, (**g**) coronal projection (Used with permission of ImmersiveTouch)

Bone Drilling [19]

This module was first introduced as a partial component of the ventriculostomy module (see Fig. 14.3c, d) and then was further developed and separately added to the library of virtual surgical interventions. Bone drilling is an essential skill common to all neurosurgical procedures and often requires certain dexterity to prevent damage of delicate structures located directly beneath the skull. Learning the tactile feedback of different bone components assumes vital importance. In the simulated drilling module, the bone is removed in a piecemeal fashion. Current options allow practicing different tasks within larger modules, such as burr holes for ventriculostomies or anterior clinoidectomies for aneurysm clippings, or stand-alone modules, such as occipital craniectomies or temporal bone drilling. No specific study has been developed to assess the educational efficacy of these simulated tasks.

Trigeminal Rhizotomy [19, 21]

This intervention is most often performed through a percutaneous approach (Fig. 14.4a). Exact recognition of external landmarks is crucial for a successful procedure. The simulation is aimed at providing familiarization with specific external points on the virtual head to practice the correct trajectory to reach the foramen ovale (Fig. 14.4b). The haptic stylus mimics the needle used in a real rhizotomy, offers tactile perception of tissues along the selected trajectory, and turns green when the trainee reaches the correct final location (Figs. 14.4c, d). The task can be eased by the use of simulated fluoroscopic guidance. After completion, the user can directly compare the tip of the needle to the ideal target by opening the head with virtual scissors (Fig. 14.4e).

Validation of this module as an assessment tool was demonstrated during the American Association of Neurological Surgeons' Top Gun 2014 competition. Ninety-two neurosurgery residents were tested for a simulated percutaneous trigeminal rhizotomy, and their performance was scored by evaluating the distance from the ideal entry point, ideal target, and number of fluoroscopy images acquired. Senior residents showed significantly more successful outcomes than junior residents, validating this module as a good predictor of surgical experience. However an overall suboptimal score for all the residents was found, regardless the year of training, highlighting the need for more practice of this sophisticated kind of surgical procedure. In regard to this specific procedure, data on effective learning and practical application are currently missing.

Hemostasis [22]

Three-dimensional representation of the virtual surgical cavity after evacuation of a hematoma is reproduced, and multiple bleeding vessels are randomly distributed over its surface in this module. It addresses the ability to utilize cautery appropriately and implements different task difficulties as time duration increases. The difficulty level can be tailored to the user's skill level. Cauterization is evaluated as successful when the user touches the bleeding vessel with both bipolar tips for 2 sec; excess of this time frame will cause injury to adjacent simulated tissue. The usefulness of this module as an educational tool was tested through an effectiveness self-assessment questionnaire; medical students perceived higher benefit compared to neurosurgical residents, most probably because surgically inexperienced trainees (such as medical students) are the ideal training target for this basic and low-fidelity task. This simple module is specifically directed to develop elementary surgical skills, such as binocular vision, and to assess personal orientation. In the future, multiple aspects of this task could also be validated: depth perception, precision of dexterity, optimal timing, and strategy.

Aneurysm Clipping [23]

The increased treatment of cerebral aneurysms with endovascular technique has decreased the surgical opportunities for trainees to par-

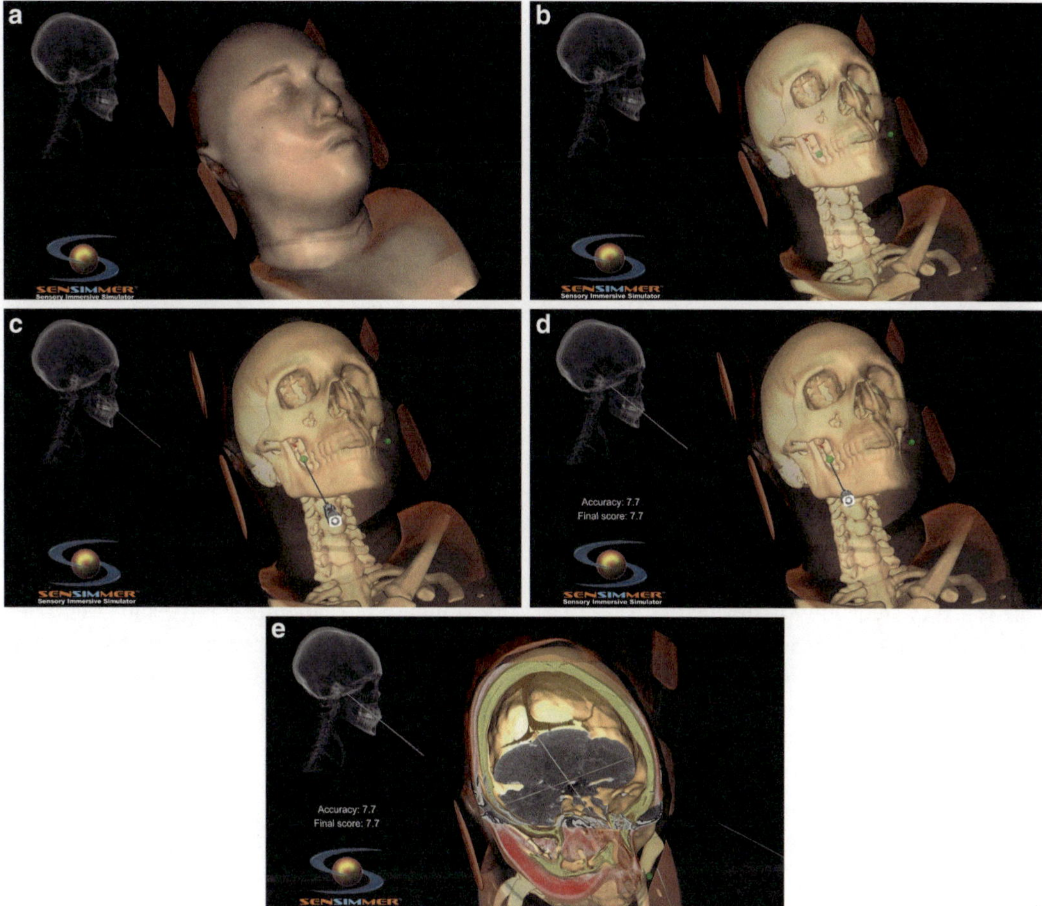

Fig. 14.4 (**a**) Virtual head reconstruction in rhizotomy module. (**b**) To enhance the optic feedback, the simulator provides on request different simulation planes: In the example the projection of the needle's ideal entry point on the skull is shown. (**c**) Virtual rhizotomy: the trainee attempts to reach the final target. The haptic stylus simu- lates the needle. (**d**) At the end of the task, the needle turns green if the attempt of the rhizotomy was successful. The software provides the accuracy score of the procedure. (**e**) Direct verification of the final needle position inside the virtual head. Simultaneous CT scan display is provided by the software (Used with permission of ImmersiveTouch)

ticipate in operative aneurysm clipping. A three-dimensional, immersive virtual reality environment has also been created for this complex surgical intervention, and development of virtual training seems to be the best suitable alternative to learn this demanding technique.

ImmersiveTouch created the first simulated prototype of middle cerebral artery aneurysm clipping. The complexity of this module stems specifically from the calculation burden in reproducing three-dimensional blood vessel wall deformations at multiple points simultaneously when the blades of the virtual clip contact the aneurysm. Two-handed practice is offered. The module also simulates intraoperative rupture, in case of excessive aneurysm manipulation or force of the clip, providing valuable kinesthetic and tactile feedback. The simulator allows the selection and placement of different virtual clips when the aneurysm neck is exposed sufficiently. Future development of this prototype could include score assessment according to patency of the parent vessel, strength of retraction, duration of retraction, complete neck obstruction, and proper clip selection. Currently, the validation of the above training module has been assessed only through a survey of residents who tested the simulator. It was positively rated as a helpful tool to improve anatomical understanding, surgical approach selection, and practical skills training. The highest score from this model was achieved by senior residents, who had more live operative expertise than junior residents in aneurysm clipping. The module might play a possible role in enhancing pre-existing skills rather than affecting the beginning of the learning curve. However, further improvements for more sensitive haptic feedback are required, and further trials are needed to validate the usefulness of this sophisticated module.

Lumbar Puncture [19]

This is a very frequently performed procedure – not only by neurosurgical residents but also by residents of other disciplines such as anesthesiology, neurology, or emergency medicine. Variation in size and anatomy between each patient may turn this basic procedure into a challenge; therefore, practice on a library of different anatomic models may assist the trainees in detecting the external anatomic landmarks, improve successful initial attempts, and reduce complications. ImmersiveTouch provides a three-dimensional model of the spine overlaid by soft tissue (Fig. 14.5a), providing tactile feedback on needle insertion (Fig. 14.5b). The final position is considered correct if the virtual needle tip is located within the thecal sac (Fig. 14.5c–f).

Pedicle Screw Implant [19, 24, 25]

This module utilizes thoracic and lumbar models (Fig. 14.6a). Referring to bony landmarks, the trainee practices cannulation of the pedicle with a virtual pedicle finder (Fig. 14.6b, c). Haptic feedback is once again added to simulate real, open surgery. Soft tissue retraction and virtual bone drilling tasks are simulated, the latter of which produce force feedback according to drill frequency and position. The drill is activated under the user's control.

Simulated image guidance helps beginners to select and monitor the correct trajectory of the screw in three directions (Fig. 14.6d). At the end of the procedure, the trainee can directly correlate the virtual experience with his or her technique by opening the spine model with virtual scissors and observing screw position (Fig. 14.6e). This module is focused on learning the internal spinal bone structures and utilizing fluoroscopy image references to assist in screw insertion. During the Top Gun competition held at the annual meetings of the American Association of Neurological Surgeons of 2006, 2009, and 2012, this module was tested for discrimination and enhancement abilities. Pedicle screw insertion scored by ImmersiveTouch correlated with retrospective evaluation of operating room screw placement, proving the discriminative capability of the module. Furthermore, greater screw placement accuracy and fewer fluoroscopy requests were achieved after practice with the partial task simulator during the competition.

Percutaneous Spinal Fixation [26]

Adopting partial tasks from previous modules, ImmersiveTouch also developed a percutaneous spinal fixation module (Fig. 14.7a). Learning this minimally invasive technique is a demanding task due to the need for surgical precision and exact detection of anatomical landmarks. Here, haptic perception assumes primary importance; it aims to improve anatomical understanding by force feedback recognition in order to minimize fluoroscopic guidance requests and reduce the amount of radiation exposure during pedicle screw placement (Fig. 14.7b, c). The amount of radiation exposure is measured by the duration of time the foot pedal is pressed to obtain the fluoroscopic images. The effectiveness of this module was tested at the 2010 AANS annual meeting and the 2011 Chicago Review Course in Neurological Surgery. These two trials showed that practice with these modules improves final percutaneous needle position accuracy and reduces fluoroscopic exposure.

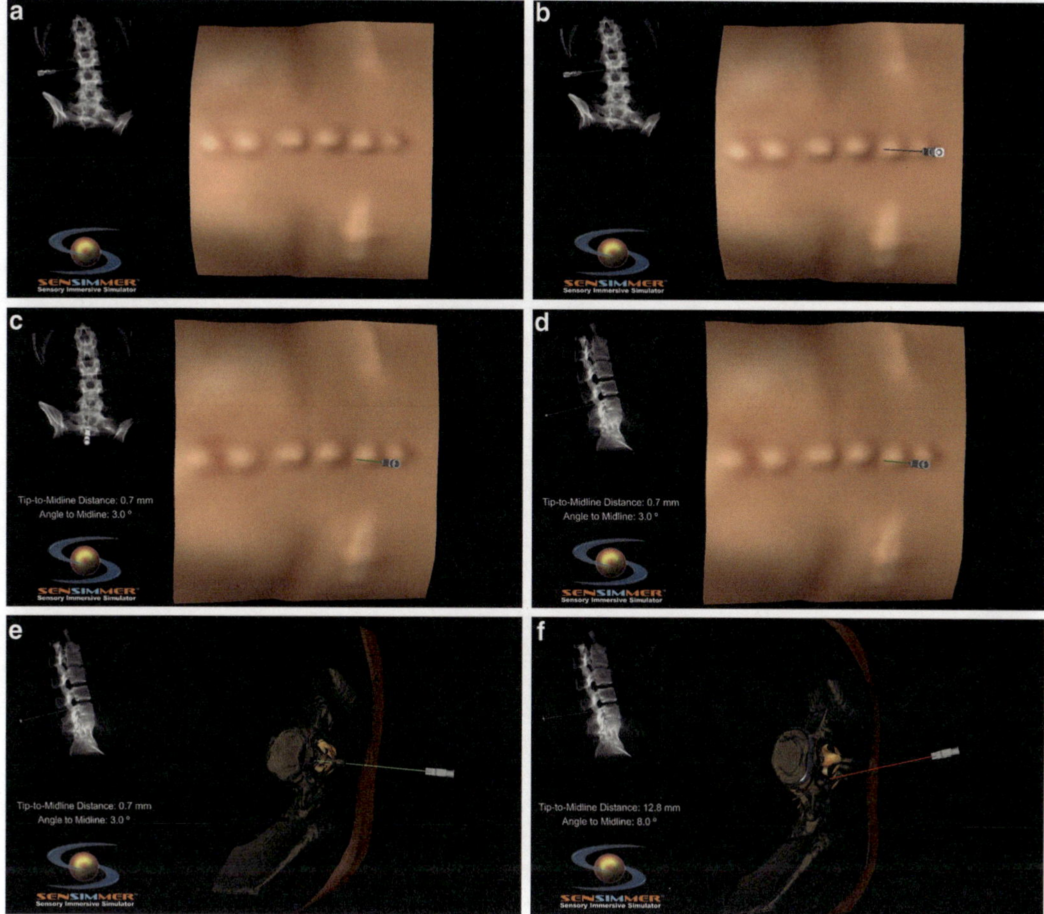

Fig. 14.5 (**a, b**) Three-dimensional model of the spine overlaid by soft tissue. The haptic stylus simulates the needle (**b**). (**c, d, e**) At the end of the task, the needle turns *green* if the attempt of the lumbar puncture was successful. The software provides also the needle projection on the CT scan view in coronal (**c**) and sagittal (**d**) sequences and on the axial 3D reconstruction (**e**). (**f**) At the end of the task, the needle turns *red* in failed attempt of lumbar puncture (Used with permission of ImmersiveTouch)

Vertebroplasty [19]

Combining the tasks of pedicle screw placement and percutaneous spinal fixation brought about the creation of the percutaneous vertebroplasty simulation module. This procedure also relies heavily on sight and touch for proper execution. While no trials have currently been conducted to verify its usefulness as an educational tool, previously published results for other spinal modules support the hypothesis that this module would minimize errors.

Limitation and Future Directions [1, 7, 8, 16, 19, 27]

Through the combination of existing partial task simulators, ImmersiveTouch has created multiple new modules reproducing several neurosurgical procedures to prepare for live neurosurgical interventions such as cerebral tumor resection, hematoma removal, and Jamshidi needle biopsy. In the near future, several of the following cranial and spinal modules will also be available:

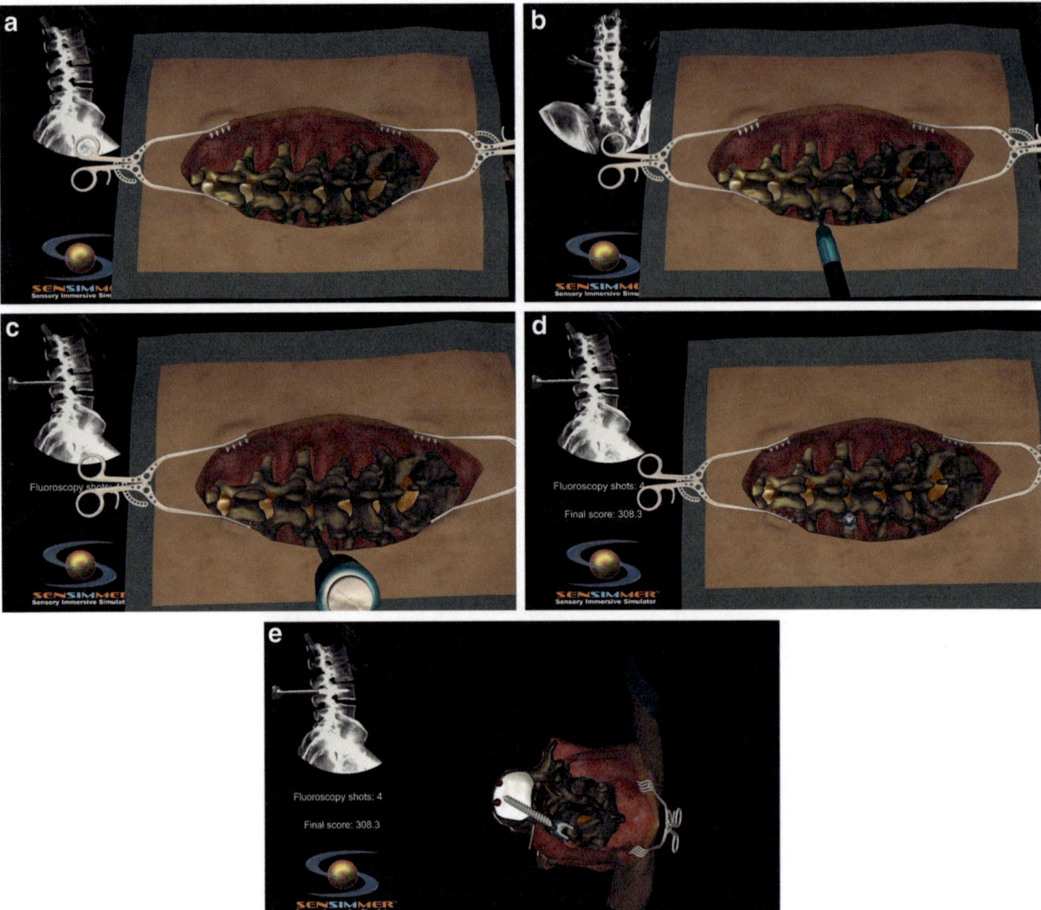

Fig. 14.6 (**a**) Lumbar model with soft tissue retraction and bone landmark exposure. (**b**, **c**) The haptic stylus simulates the surgical tools: the pedicle finder (**b**) and the pedicle probe (**c**). (**d**) Screw positioning and simulated sagittal image guidance that might help beginners to select the correct trajectory during the whole procedure. (**e**) At the end of the task, the trainee can verify the accuracy of his or her procedure by observing directly the screw trajectory on the virtual spine (Used with permission of ImmersiveTouch)

- Nasal cavity procedures
- Third ventriculostomy
- MicroDexterity
- Suturing
- Anterior cervical discectomy
- C1–C2 transarticular screw fixation
- Lumbar microdiscectomy
- Lumbar laminectomy
- Lateral mass fixation
- Minimally invasive DLIF

At the present time, further educational tools are needed to create standardized competency acquisition in neurosurgical training and address legal and ethical concerns regarding patient safety. Over recent years, haptic and computerized simulations have replaced older forms such as cadavers, animals, or physical models. Among all the existing haptic simulators, ImmersiveTouch technology seems to be the most versatile, reproducing all main neurosurgical procedures and addressing the progressive stages of training. Documenting a baseline level of competency within surgical curricula has only been evaluated in general and laparoscopic surgical training programs [7, 19]. Despite not having been systematically introduced in neurosurgical education programs, societal expectations of flawless

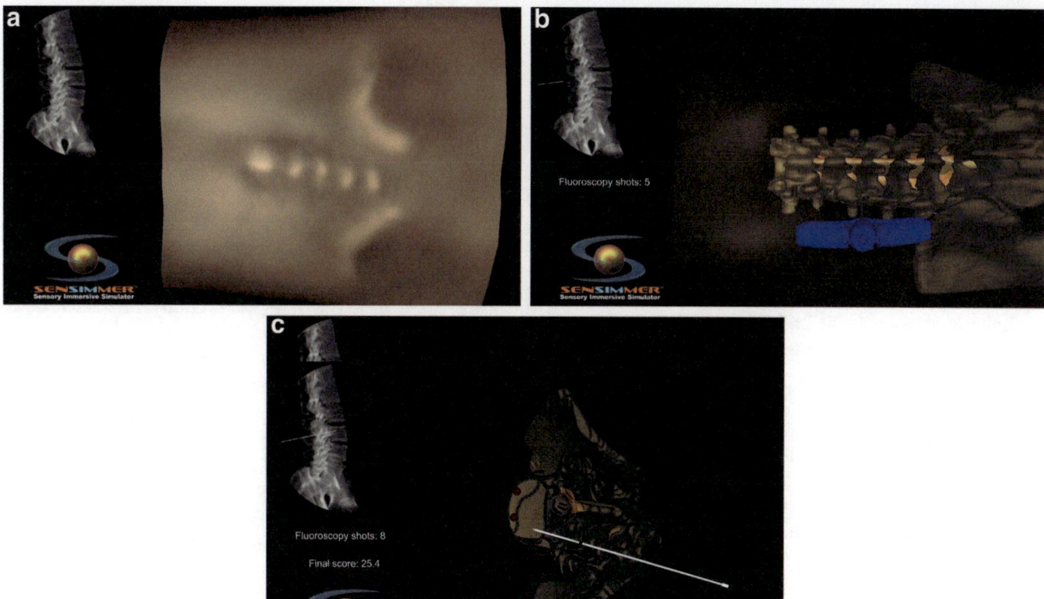

Fig. 14.7 (**a**) Lumbar percutaneous model overlaid by soft tissue. (**b**) Lumbar percutaneous model, bone view. The software provides on request the bone view during the needle positioning to verify the trajectory selected against the fluoroscopic image guidance (*top left* of the figure). (**c**): At the end of the task, the trainee can verify the accuracy of his or her procedure over the 3D reconstruction of the spine model. The software provides the final score based on the needle position accuracy and on the number and length of fluoroscopic shots used during the procedure (Used with permission of ImmersiveTouch)

outcomes and current work-hour limitations make virtual reality simulators an appealing teaching tool for educators. Virtual reality simulation modules also objectively document achievement of minimum standard skills and progress in surgical learning through scored assessments. Such modules have been proven to shorten the learning curve, especially for novice residents. Additionally, virtual reality modules may also play a potential role for experienced surgeons to maintain acquired skills, restore lapsed procedural skills, learn new techniques, or become acquainted to the specific anatomy of each patient prior to surgery. Due to their versatility, training modules can be tailored to the specific needs of a training program or physician.

In addition to their advantages, virtual reality simulations also possess limitations as a comprehensive learning tool. There is an innate learning curve associated with the virtual reality technology itself, and the difficulty of becoming familiar with the technical components of the virtual environment may not reflect the actual surgical difficulty. Also, simulated proficiency may not necessarily translate into operative dexterity; further randomized studies are needed to validate all of the existing simulation modules.

Virtual reality modules still need ameliorations in visual and haptic feedback for the most complicated surgical interventions, in which practice is essential; however, calculation burden may interfere with a close-reality rendering. More work is necessary before virtual reality simulation becomes a mainstay in neurosurgical training and formally approved for educational use in the neurosurgery residency curriculum.

References

1. Suri A, Patra DP, Meena RK. Simulation in neurosurgery: past, present and future. Neurol India. 2016;64(3):387–95.
2. Polavarapu HV, Kulaylat AN, Sun S, et al. 100 years of surgical education: the past, present, and future. Bull Am Coll Surg. 2013 Jul;98(7):22–7.
3. Leach DC. Simulation: it's about respect. ACGME Bull. 2005, December:2–3. http://www.acgme.org/Portals/0/PFAssets/bulletin/bulletin09_05.pdf
4. Lemole M, Banerjee P, Luciano C, et al. Virtual reality in neurosurgical education: part-task ventriculostomy simulation with dynamic visual and haptic feedback. Neurosurgery. 2007;61(1):142–9.
5. Bradley P. The history of simulation in medical education and possible future directions. Med Educ. 2006;40:254–62.
6. OED online (2006) http://dictionary.oed.com.
7. Choudhury N, Gèlinas-Phaneuf N, Delorme S, et al. Fundamentals of neurosurgery: virtual reality tasks for training and evaluation of technical skills. World Neurosurg. 2013;80(5):9–19.
8. Alaraj A, Lemole MG, Finkle JH, et al. Virtual reality training in neurosurgery: review of current status and future applications. Surg Neurol Int. 2011;2:52.
9. Aggarwal R, Black SA, Hance JR, et al. Virtual reality simulation training can improve inexperienced surgeons' endovascular skills. Eur J Vasc Endovasc Surg. 2006;31:588–93.
10. Lugana MP, de Reijke TM, Hessel W, et al. Training in laparoscopic urology. Curr Opin Urol. 2006;16:65–70.
11. Yudkowsky R, Luciano C, Banerjee P, et al. Practice on an augmented reality/haptic simulator and library of virtual brains improves residents' ability to perform a ventriculostomy. Society for Simulation in Healthcare. 2013;8(1):25–31.
12. Balogh AA, Preul MC, Laszlo K, et al. Multilayer image grid technology: four-dimensional interactive image reconstruction of microsurgical neuroanatomic dissection. Neurosurgery. 2006;58(1):157–65.
13. Bernardo A, Preul MC, , Zabramsky JM et al. A three-dimensional interactive virtual dissection model to simulate transpetrous surgical avenues. Neurosurgery 2003; 52:499–505.
14. Kockro RA, Serra L, Tseng-Tsai Y, et al. Planning and simulation of neurosurgery in a virtual reality environment. Neurosurgery. 2000;46:118–35.
15. Kockro RA, Hwang PY. Virtual temporal bone: an interactive 3-dimensional learning aid for cranial base surgery. Neurosurgery. 2009;64(Suppl 2):216–29.
16. Malone HR, Syed ON, Downes MS, et al. Simulation in neurosurgery: a review of computer-based simulation environments and their surgical applications. Neurosurgery. 2010;67:1105–16.
17. Banerjee P, Luciano C, Rizzi S. Virtual reality simulations. Anesthesiology Clin. 2007;25:337–48.
18. Luciano C, Banerjee P, Lemole GM Jr, et al. Second generation haptic ventriculostomy simulator using the ImmersiveTouch system. Stud Health Technol Inform. 2006;119:343–8.
19. Alaraj A, Charbel T, Birk D, et al. Role of cranial and spinal virtual and augmented reality simulation using ImmersiveTouch modules in neurosurgical training. Neurosurgery. 2013;72(Suppl 1):115–23.
20. Banerjee P, Luciano C, Lemole M, et al. Accuracy of ventriculostomy catheter placement using a head- and hand-tracked high-resolution virtual reality simulator with haptic feedback. J Neurosurg. 2007;107:515–21.
21. Shakur S, Luciano C, Kania P, et al. Usefulness of a virtual reality percutaneous trigeminal rhizotomy simulator in neurosurgical training. Operative Neurosurgery. 2015;11(3):420–5.
22. Gasco J, Patel A, Luciano C, et al. A novel virtual reality simulation for hemostasis in a brain surgical cavity: perceived utility for visuomotor skills in current and aspiring neurosurgery resident. World Neurosurg. 2013;80(96):732–7.
23. Alaraj A, Luciano C, Bailey D, et al. Virtual reality cerebral aneurysm clipping simulation with real-time haptic feedback. Neurosurgery. 2015;11(2):52–8.
24. Gasco J, Patel A, Ortega-Barnett J, et al. Virtual reality spine surgery simulation: an empirical study of its usefulness. Neurol Res. 2014;36(11):968–73.
25. Luciano C, Banerjee P, Bellotte B, et al. *Learning retention of thoracic pedicle screw placement using a high-resolution augmented reality simulator with haptic feedback*. Operative. Neurosurgery. 2011;69(1):14–9.
26. Luciano C, Banerjee P, Sorenson J, et al. Percutaneous spinal fixation simulation with virtual reality and haptics. Neurosurgery. 2013;72(suppl 1):89–96.
27. Gasco J, Holbrook TJ, Patel A, et al. Neurosurgery simulation in residency traininig: feasibility, cost, and educational benefit. Neurosurgery. 2013;73(4):39–45.

Connie Ju, Jonathan R. Pace,
and Nicholas C. Bambakidis

Introduction

Recent reforms in neurosurgical training requirements set forth by the Accreditation Council for Graduate Medical Education (ACGME) have changed the way education is delivered to residents, as well as what information should be disseminated and what milestones need to be met. Limiting workweek hours firstly creates implications for patient-volume-dependent training in fields such as neurosurgery, where patient exposure traditionally provides opportunities for residents to enhance their surgical skills [1, 2]. Additionally, the changing landscape of the healthcare economy set forth by legislative reforms has largely emphasized patient outcomes and more efficient delivery.

Electronic supplementary material: The online version of this chapter https://doi.org/10.1007/978-3-319-75583-0_15 contains supplementary material, which is available to authorized users.

C. Ju (✉)
Department of Neurological Surgery, Case Western Reserve University, Cleveland, OH, USA
e-mail: connie.ju@case.edu

J. R. Pace · N. C. Bambakidis
Department of Neurological Surgery,
University Hospitals Case Medical Center,
Cleveland, OH, USA
e-mail: jonathan.pace@uhhospitals.org;
nicholas.bambakidis2@uhhospitals.org

Less tolerance from both healthcare institutions and consumers for surgical errors and postoperative complications has resulted in increasing pressures on providers to establish more efficient care practices [3, 4]. These reforms create an ideal environment for highlighting and implementing surgical simulation to not only enhance the educational experience for trainees but also to improve patient outcomes in the field of neurological surgery.

Simulators have been used with great success in other fields, including the military and oft-quoted area of aviation. War game simulations were used in the 1900s by German and Prussian armies, with the Prussian *Kriegspiel* being credited for the French victory in the Franco-Prussian war [5]. Flight simulation has also been very successful in the training of armed forces pilots as well as commercial aircraft pilots. Indeed, mandatory simulated water landings prescribed for commercial pilots are partially credited for the successful landing of the US Airways craft on the Hudson River in 2009 [6–9]. The benefits of rehearsal prior to action within these fields have been recognized and adopted by the medical community to reduce errors, which in the field of healthcare can have profound consequences on quality of life.

Though the concept of simulation has been integrated into medical education and planning as far into the past as 600 BC with the use of clay models [9], its application to surgical

A. Alaraj (ed.), *Comprehensive Healthcare Simulation: Neurosurgery*,
Comprehensive Healthcare Simulation, https://doi.org/10.1007/978-3-319-75583-0_15

specialties including neurosurgical training in recent years has shifted from tactical modules toward virtual simulation. Simulators have already been adopted for specialized training in laparoscopy, basic life support, and advanced trauma life support courses where hands-on education and simulation allow for development and refinement of skills in a controlled setting, prior to applying these skills in an actual patient care scenario [9–11]. Like other surgical fields, neurosurgery has embraced modern technology in the form of virtual and augmented reality in order to increase procedural exposure and planning [6]. These simulation platforms provide rehearsal opportunities that promote the best operative experience and patient outcomes via acquisition of competency in critical aspects of procedures. Physicians have a duty to their patients to be able to perform tasks with competence and skill, and implementation of simulation into training will allow for more rapid development of proficiency [12]. It has also been demonstrated that early implementation of tactile, or haptic, feedback in simulator use is associated with increased learning, and a study by Seymour and colleagues demonstrated increased psychomotor skill and hand-eye coordination when simulators were used by trainees compared to a cohort without simulator training [13].

The immense variation in cerebral aneurysm presentation is one particular area in which the use of simulation is readily applicable. Clinical presentation, location, size, and morphology of a particular aneurysm all factor into treatment approaches and render this disease entity more complex and intricate. With the recent emergence of, and rapid advancements in, endovascular techniques for the treatment of aneurysms, opportunities to perform intracranial clip ligation has greatly decreased due to the larger risk of morbidity relative to endovascular treatments such as coiling [14, 15]. Though much debate remains on which treatment modality is superior when comparing microsurgical approaches with endovascular therapies, treatment planning often considers both aneurysm characteristics and patient anatomy and has not eliminated the neces-

sity of clip ligation. Additionally, the ability to perform aneurysm clipping remains a level 3 milestone as indicated by the ACGME, which suggests that new methods of educational delivery are required to ensure appropriate acquisition of skills [16, 17]. The role of simulation platforms for surgical clipping therefore has a role in skills training for neurosurgical residents and for optimizing patient outcomes through rehearsal.

Historical Progression of Surgical Training

Surgical training has remained largely unchanged since its inception. The Halstedian technique, described by Dr. William S. Halsted of Johns Hopkins University in 1889, set the foundation for the apprenticeship model of surgical training and highlighted experiential learning based on exposure, practice, and close supervision (Fig. 15.1). Eventually, the realization that basic

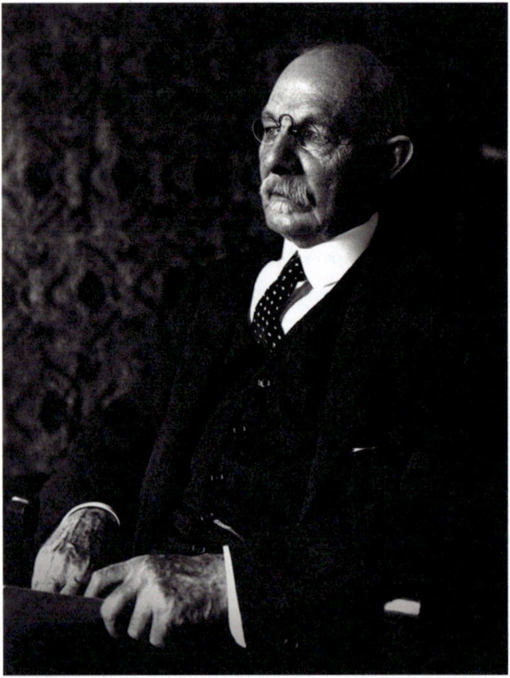

Fig. 15.1 Portrait of William Stewart Halsted, the surgeon responsible for advances in early medical education as well as pioneering the first surgical residency in America (With permission from Alan Mason Chesney Medical Archives, Johns Hopkins Medical Institutions)

surgical skills could be fragmented into modules in the absence of patient exposure led to a gradual transition away from a pure Halstedian approach [18]. Ensuing development of surgical skills labs allowed the substitution of specific skill development in place of pure operative exposure by providing patient-independent rehearsal opportunities in simple techniques such as knot-tying, suturing, and basic laparoscopic technique. The use of instructional materials and textbooks in conjunction with these skills labs remains common practice in modern institutions. Given the tangible nature of surgery, further advances included the use of porcine and human cadavers in anatomical labs. Cadaveric use has played a large role in simulation and continues to provide trainees with opportunities to rehearse with tissue feedback near real-life situations, which has been shown to aid resident training and improved anatomic understanding and technical skills intraoperatively [19–21]. Resource and space limitations, however, create substantial obstacles against the standardized use of cadavers [22]. Further, anatomical variation among different cadaveric models makes this type of educational module an imperfect simulation of actual cases. These restrictions, compounded by the dawn of computer and imaging technology in the past three decades, have promoted simulation to the forefront of a continually evolving neurosurgical training agenda.

Explosive advancements in robotics and imaging within the past century continue to challenge modern methods of surgical training with introduction of minimally invasive and robot-assisted techniques. The rising popularity and demand of such procedures greatly decreased patient volume for cases requiring more invasive approaches and hold implications for burgeoning surgeons that rely on patient exposure for mastery of complex procedures. As the demand for training in these areas has risen, virtual reality and the use of technological simulation have concomitantly risen to fill such demands [20, 23, 24]. Simulation technology has made great advancements in the endoscopic, laparoscopic, and endovascular realms particularly because many of the procedures involve similar technological equipment

and rely on video monitor guidance [6]. Studies in these fields have demonstrated that the effects of pre-procedural simulation are readily appreciable through enhanced operative prowess and reduced error rates [25–28].

Use and Evolution of Simulation in Neurosurgery

At the 2011 Congress of Neurological Surgeons national meeting, the first simulation course was initiated and included elements of vascular, spinal, and cranial simulation, primarily incorporating virtual reality and physical simulators. After initial review of the course and feedback from attendees of the course, a standardized educational curriculum was established in 2012. The course included a pretest, short didactics, demonstration of the simulator, and hands-on use of the simulator followed by a posttest and debriefing. By far, the majority of the time was spent utilizing the hands-on aspect of the simulator, with facilitators available to answer questions and give feedback on performance [22]. Specifically, a trauma module was developed to improve education and performance in a decompressive hemicraniectomy module. Lobel and colleagues demonstrated significant improvement in incision planning, burr hole placement, size of the decompressive craniotomy, and scores from pretest to posttest, with the most significant improvements made by the novice trainees [29]. This continues to reinforce the importance of simulation prior to application of surgical skills on real patients.

Simulation is highly applicable to the field of neurosurgery given the routine use of image guidance for navigation and planning as well as the inherent high-risk procedures involved. The advent and standardization of high-resolution imaging in the early 1980s with magnetic resonance imaging (MRI) and computed tomography (CT) paralleled the advent of simulation technology. Reconstructed scans provided an opportunity to create anatomically accurate, three-dimensional (3D) models of the human anatomy [20]. These initial endeavors offered visualization of anatomic structures without the use of human cadavers, but basic computer-mouse user interfaces were nonetheless limited in providing sensory and motor rehearsal valued by surgeons. Virtual dissection eventually transitioned from standardized patient images to individualized scans that were able to reflect case-specific pathology and provide more relevant simulation. One of the earliest entries into the market was Dextroscope and VizDexter software, which integrated patient-specific images and projected a 3D hologram in front of the user to allow for virtual visualization and surgical planning [30]. Secondary applications of the technology have since allowed users to recreate higher definition images of intracranial nerves and vessel and rehearse clip ligation for intracranial aneurysm management. Most simulation platforms now use this method of tissue segmentation to recreate patient-specific 3D anatomy [20].

The initial applications of virtual dissection targeted the visualization of important skull base structures, where the understanding of complex anatomical relationships in the region could be most readily augmented by 3D anatomical visualization. Modern technological applications have since grown to encompass nearly every facet of the neurosurgical field including cerebrovascular, spinal, and tumor resection procedures, as evidenced by the growth of literature on simulation applications in recent years [31]. Currently, the status of virtual reality simulation is now attempting to provide more realistic user interfaces by enhancing sensory and motor experience through features such as tissue deformation and haptic feedback [32].

The ImmersiveTouch platform (Chicago, Illinois), like Dextroscope, projects a volume-rendered image using patient-specific MRI or CT data, and 3D model parameters are further defined by stiffness, viscosity, and friction to project tactile feedback to the user during ventriculostomy rehearsal [33–35]. ImmersiveTouch has also been developed to simulate aneurysm clipping, which has demonstrated positive feedback from trainees that the haptics were realistic, and the simulator was

useful for preoperative planning and rehearsal [33]. More recent virtual reality simulators that also offer opportunities for preoperative rehearsal include NeuroSim (Germany) and NeuroTouch (Canada), which have developed platforms for microsurgical applications such as aneurysm clipping and tumor resection [36, 37]. NeuroTouch allows for a full procedure to take place skin-to-skin but may make sacrifices in the form of realism [32]. Even so, the ability to perform complete procedures, even with slightly less realism, may be of great benefit to trainees early in their career [38].

Use of Surgical Theater in Aneurysmal Clipping

Surgical rehearsal platforms that offer rehearsal of clip ligation are relatively novel developments in the field of surgical simulation. Intracranial aneurysm treatment is a particular area in which the rise of minimally invasive embolization and coiling procedures has diminished resident exposure to more invasive aneurysm clipping. This is further reflected in practice, where an increasing amount of aneurysms are continuing to be treated via endovascular means. The fewer aneurysms being treated in an open fashion have diminished the experience of younger neurosurgeons and residents in this crucial aspect of training. Given the variability in aneurysm morphology, coiling techniques cannot be readily universalized, and the ability to perform clip ligation remains a critical technique in which proficiency needs to be demonstrated in neurosurgical trainees [16].

The surgical rehearsal platform (SRP) developed by Surgical Theater LLC (Mayfield, Ohio) is a response to the increasing demand of simulation technology to minimize the burden of patient-volume-dependent exposure during training. Surgical Theater consists of the SRP for preoperative planning and the Surgical Navigation Advanced Platform (SNAP) for high-resolution 3D image reconstruction. The software, developed in part by ex-Israeli air force engineers, was inspired by aviation technology originally intended for flight simulation in air force pilot training. Since receiving FDA clearance in 2013, the platform has been used at institutions across the United States to plan for intracranial tumor resection, AVM embolization, intracranial aneurysm treatment, and spinal procedures. These centers include University Hospitals Case Medical Center, University Hospitals Rainbow Babies and Children's Hospital, Ronald Reagan UCLA Medical Center, Mount Sinai Hospital, Mayo Clinic, and NYU Langone Medical Center, among other nonacademic institutions [39].

The technology requires a personal computer, two liquid-crystal/light-emitting diode monitors, two 3D controllers, and 3D stereoscopic goggles, which work synergistically to provide a realistic surgical theater environment for users. Software used by SRP uses quad-buffering technology for enhanced graphics resolution. Visual reconstruction involves a 20-minute segmentation of patient-specific DICOM images that produces volume-rendered images of the aneurysm and relevant surrounding tissue. Haptic feedback on the platform is incorporated through the use of a pair of SensAble Technologies PHANTOM Omni haptic devices, which allows users to navigate the virtual reality environment and receive sensory feedback during simulation. Surgeons are able to modify tissue segmentation and virtually handle any surgical instruments used in the operative setting. Additionally, the program allows for a 360-degree field of view rotation within the operative field, which provides visualization of adjacent neurovascular structures otherwise inaccessible to the surgeon (Fig. 15.2). Tissue deformation also offers users a more responsive virtual model that simulates the mechanical and sensory feedback experienced during an actual procedure. Further customizable options include scaling, color, and tissue window adjustments for soft tissue, bones, or vessels. These enhanced visual features allow for surgeons to practice and review their clip application for complete occlusion by viewing the aneurysm from an otherwise inaccessible angle [15] (Video 15.1).

While the patient-specific image rendering allows for more realistic case preparation for the surgeon, it does not include the ability to rehearse bony removal aspects of the procedure and is intended specifically for the rehearsal of aneurysmal clipping. Surgeons are able to choose the appropriate clips for the specific patient and plan for an optimal surgical approach prior to the scheduled procedure (Fig. 15.3). Partial aneurysm occlusion results in an aneurysm remnant, which can lead to rebleeding and secondary rupture, both intraoperatively and perioperatively, and an increase in morbidity and mortality. The primary intent of the SRP is to provide neurological surgeons an avenue for rehearsal in order to minimize such post-procedural complications. Other secondary benefits of this software include minimizing clip attempts, clip removals, and time under anesthesia, which may impact patient outcome.

Surgical Theater in Preoperative Planning and Rehearsal: How It Works

Let us consider a theoretical patient who presents after spontaneous subarachnoid hemorrhage, with the CT angiogram demonstrating an anterior communicating (ACom) aneurysm. The patient is stabilized, and the decision is made that this particular aneurysm is more favorably treated utilizing open microsurgical techniques. The patient's DICOM image datasets are loaded into the SRP, and processing of the data occurs. The datasets undergo segmentation and can be defined by volumes of interest. Once this processing is complete, tissue quality may be altered based on Hounsfield units by tailoring unique threshold values. Defining proper threshold values allows for future tailoring of the image during rehearsal, when different tissue layers can be subtracted to reveal the underlying cerebrovasculature. SNAP is preloaded with default tissue segmentation values based on preloaded DICOM scans from over 100 cases from various hospitals. While rendering the two-dimensional image, the user can employ these threshold windows as a starting point and later manually fine-tune the segmentation. At this point, the user may choose to alter the color palate, thus highlighting areas of pathol-

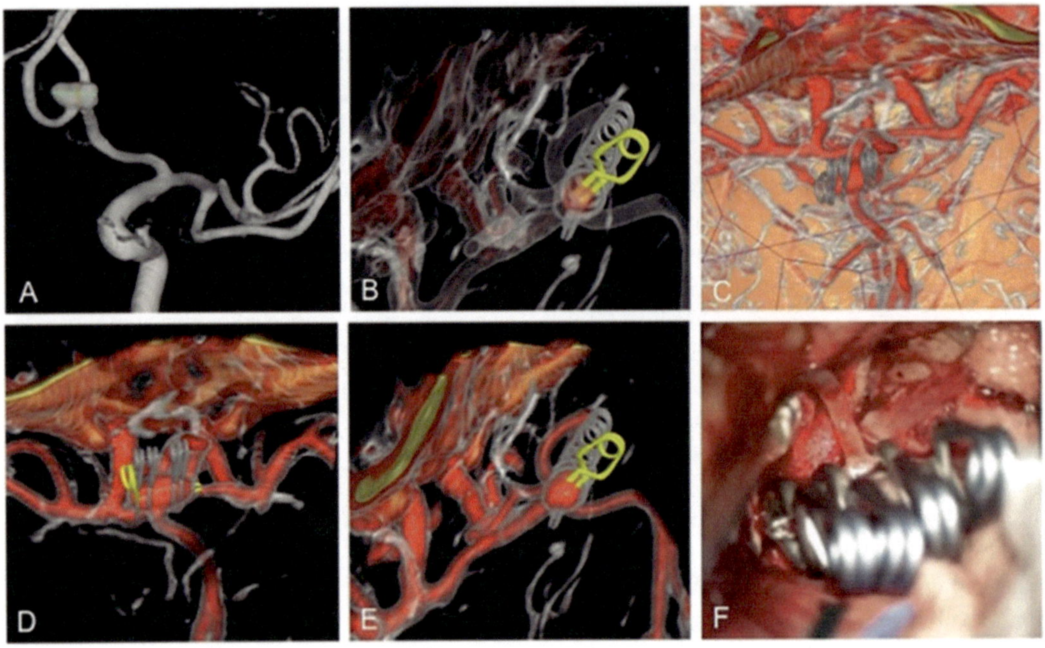

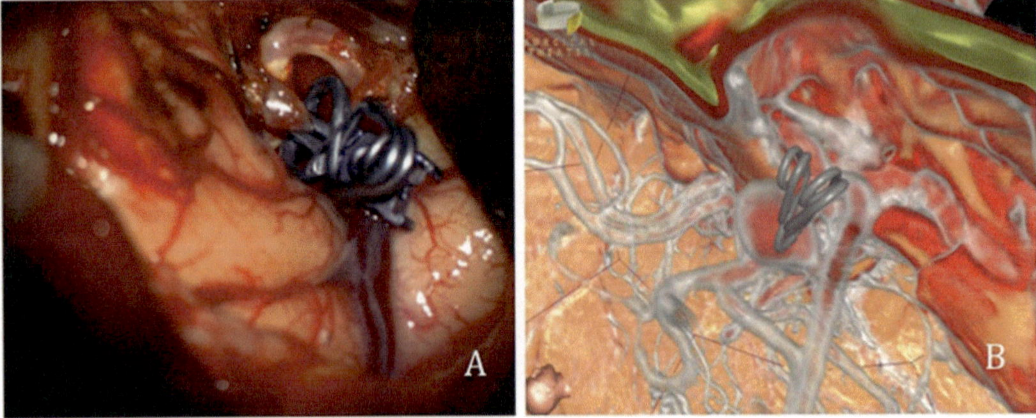

Fig. 15.2 (**a**) Preoperative CT angiogram depicting a pericallosal artery aneurysm. (**b–e**) Varying views demonstrating application of clips during preoperative surgical planning with surgical rehearsal platform. (**f**) Intraoperative view demonstrating clip reconstruction based on preoperative planning (With permission from Journal of Neurosurgery Publishing Group. Ref. [40])

Fig. 15.3 (**a**) Intraoperative view and (**b**) surgical rehearsal platform comparison demonstrating usefulness of the surgical rehearsal platform (With permission from Journal of Neurosurgery Publishing Group. Ref. [40])

ogy and allowing for visualization of the bone, brain, and vessel, hollow vessel view, or any combination therein. Multiple DICOM datasets may also be fused to enhance visualization of the anatomical relationships between structures. For instance, the CT angiogram of the aforementioned ACom aneurysm can be added to a secondary MRI dataset to gain a better appreciation for the tissue environment surrounding the target vessels. Adjusting transparency levels of tissue segments can enhance vascular definition, and further altering clipping planes allows the user to traverse different layers of anatomy. This allows users to subtract irrelevant tissue layers, as defined by their threshold values, to isolate relevant vasculature. For convenience, different threshold and intensity settings can be saved and toggled during the planning session.

Once the patient data has been manipulated to give the best approximation of the pertinent anatomy to be encountered intraoperatively, the treatment planning session may proceed, which allows the operator to plan trajectories and perform measurements. Users can interact with the image by rotating, customizing corridor parameters, and linking to a 3D controller (Figs. 15.4 and 15.5).

To plan the craniotomy for aneurysm treatment, surgeons must decide on optimal approaches for skull entry. In the theoretical patient with a ruptured ACom aneurysm, the surgeon may consider performing a supraorbital keyhole approach and would prefer to evaluate the corridor placement. Though the simulation platform was intended for rehearsal of the clip application, users have the ability to plan for the bony removal procedure by employing a virtual drill tool and visualizing what cerebrovascular structures are revealed with different craniotomies. After measuring and planning for laterality

and angle of entry based on the imaging dataset, the surgeon may link the 3D controller to the drill tool and proceed with visualization of bony removal on the desired skull region most appropriate to reveal the target aneurysm. With supraorbital or keyhole craniotomies, for instance, the surgeon is able to create a corridor with the drill and rehearse clip ligation within a limited working angle (Fig. 15.6). Should the simulated entry result in a suboptimal field of view of the aneurysm, the user can alter the degree of anatomy removed or simply change the boundaries of the corridor by repositioning it on the monitor until an optimal placement is found. The surgeon then has the ability to assess the corridor placement and working view by altering the camera angle or zooming into the image. As the image is rotated, the extent of anatomy removed can be preserved allowing the user to evaluate corridor placements in different skull regions and determine how large the bony opening will need to be for an optimal approach. Multiple trajectory markers leading toward the area of pathology can also be mapped into the 3D scene, and the previously designed corridors can be snapped onto these markers for the surgeon to review. A virtual reality headset further immerses the user into the anatomical environment of the patient case by

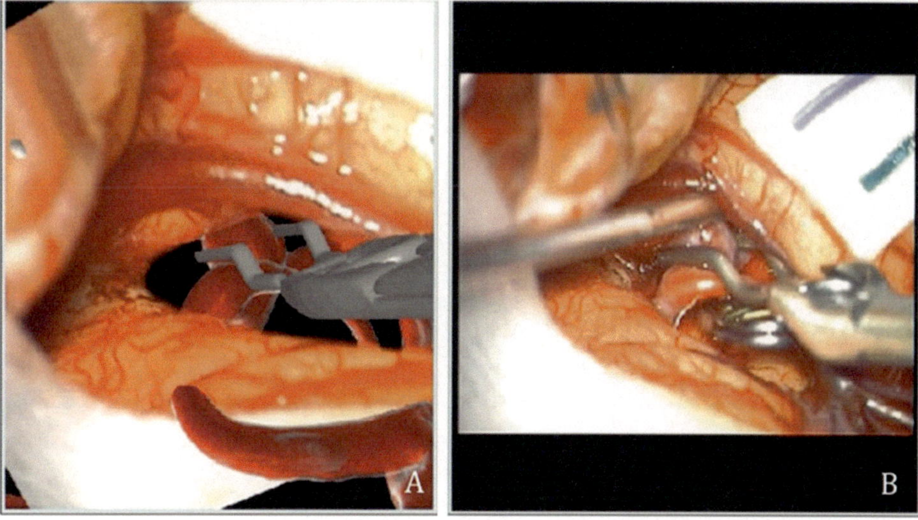

Fig. 15.4 (**a**) Surgical rehearsal platform and (**b**) intraoperative view demonstrating how preoperative planning is used for clip selection and rehearsal (With permission from Journal of Neurosurgery Publishing Group. Ref. [40])

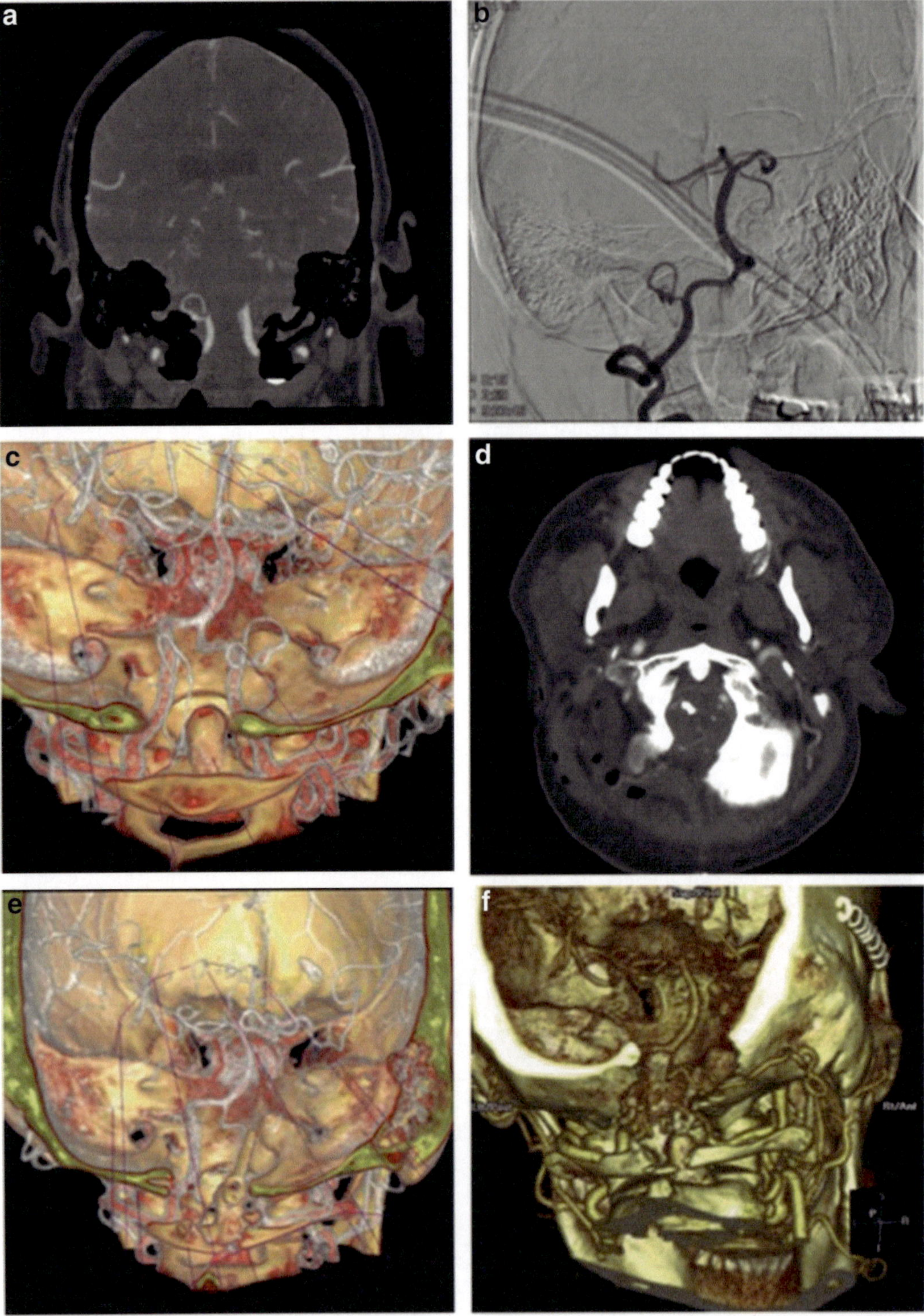

Fig. 15.5 Patient presented with subarachnoid hemorrhage and was found to have a right PICA dissecting aneurysm. He underwent right far lateral craniotomy for occipital artery (OA)-PICA trapping and bypass. (**a**) Coronal CT angiogram demonstrating the aneurysm. (**b**) Right vertebral injection oblique view conventional angiogram demonstrating the PICA aneurysm. (**c**) Preoperative viewing utilizing Surgical Theater, with *arrow* depicting the aneurysm. Cone represents surgical view. (**d**) Postoperative axial CT angiogram with *arrow* depicting the occipital artery en route to its anastomosis with the right PICA. (**e**) Postoperative Surgical Theater depiction of the OA-PICA bypass with *arrow* highlighting the surgical clip; the bypass is also visualized. (**f**) CT angiogram reconstruction with *arrow* highlighting the occipital artery and PICA anastomosis

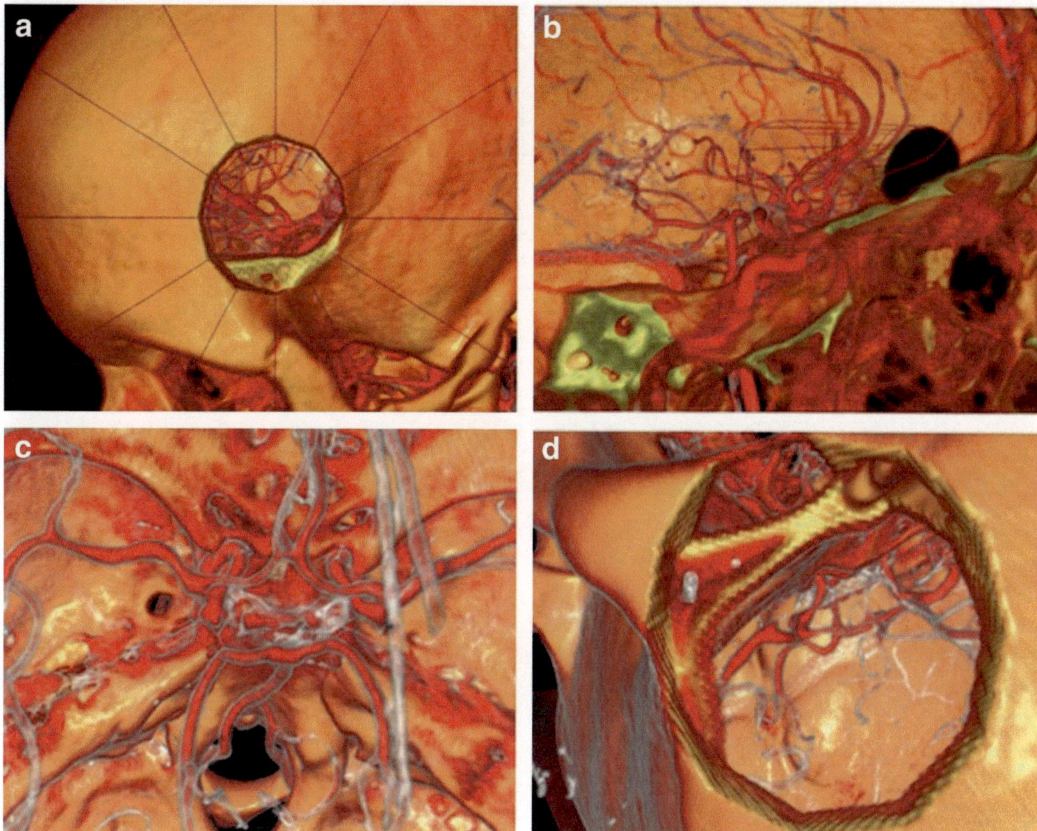

Fig. 15.6 Surgical Theater in action. (**a**) Surgical view through a supraorbital craniotomy viewing an anterior communicating artery aneurysm. (**b**) Rotated view examining the surgical corridor from the contralateral side. (**c**) View from above of a left posterior communicating aneurysm (*arrow*). (**d**) Surgeon's-eye view of the surgical corridor through the supraorbital craniotomy

providing an opportunity to "fly in" through the corridor and alter camera angles for maximal understanding of the aneurysm's feeding arteries and proximity to surrounding vasculature. A reverse view projects vascular structures deep to the target aneurysm that would have otherwise been hidden from view intraoperatively. Thus, even prior to rehearsal, the surgeon is provided a wealth of visual information to develop the optimal approach and treatment plan.

In practice, surgeons must choose from hundreds of clips with unique curvatures and lengths, and selection of the appropriate clip is crucial to the outcomes of the procedure. With the SRP, surgeons are able to link the clipping tool to the 3D controller and rehearse aneurysm treatment with a selected clip through the designed corridor. As the clip approaches the target aneurysm, the surrounding vessels undergo visible deformation to simulate the interaction between tools and tissue. The user can then zoom in or rotate the image to review the clip application in its entirety, identify any residual aneurysm neck, and change the clip used or the approach if necessary.

Once the procedure has been rehearsed to surgeon satisfaction, the navigation session may proceed intraoperatively. SNAP can be brought into the operative suite where it is linked with external navigation systems such as BrainLab (Munich, Germany) or the Medtronic Stealth Station (Dublin, Ireland) to allow for accurate intraoperative navigation and visualization of the previously defined anatomy utilizing the 3D

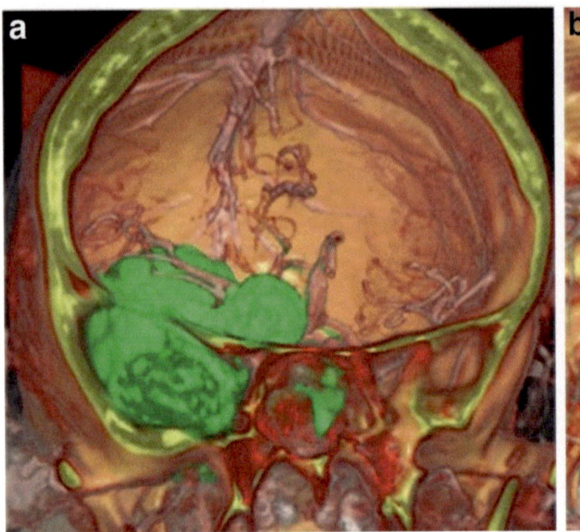

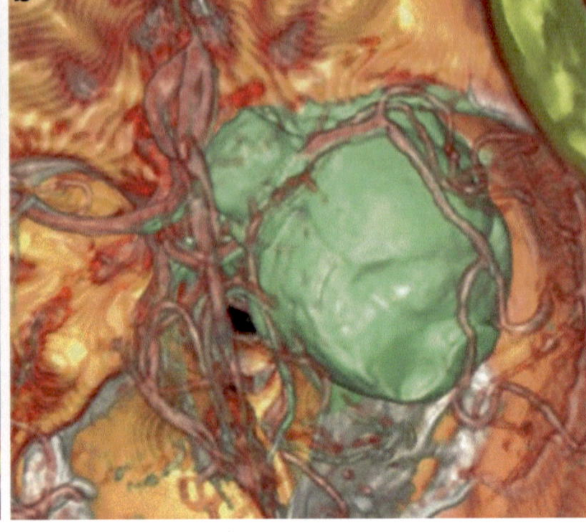

Fig. 15.7 Surgical Theater depicting a meningioma (**a**) from the front and (**b**) from above. Note the detail and contrast of tumor compared with vasculature. Also note how the right middle cerebral artery origin is encased in tumor proximally and draped over the tumor distally

model generated above for real-time navigation and feedback. Data from the rehearsed procedure including tools and measurements can be saved and exported into SNAP to provide "guided drilling" and subsequent intraoperative navigation.

Technological Validation

A recent blinded, prospective, randomized study looked at the improvement of aneurysmal clipping measures with and without prior rehearsal on the SRP [40]. Metrics assessed in the study included the total amount of microsurgical time, number of clip attempts, and total number of clips used. Patients were randomized to a treatment or control group that determined whether the surgical team would be exposed to preoperative rehearsal on the SRP. Video recordings of the surgeries were then analyzed for the metrics delineated above. The results demonstrated a significant improvement in the time spent and number of clip attempts per clip, which alludes to an overall improvement in operative efficiency and increased comfort with the surgical instruments involved. This reinforces the power this tool has in its utilization to help improve patient care.

Further studies validating the use of SRP for aneurysm clipping rehearsal should investigate the effects on patient outcomes in a larger trial. The promising results of rehearsing aneurysm clip placement has encouraged Surgical Theater LLC to expand the technology for rehearsing transnasal pituitary tumor resection, microvascular decompression, and skull base procedures. These expansions have already impacted patient care and surgical planning, allowing for 3D visualization of individual patient anatomy and critical relationships between pathology and various neurovascular structures of interest (Fig. 15.7).

Conclusion

Surgical Theater and similar platforms have seen increased utility in the field of healthcare due to dramatic advancements in imaging and computer technology within recent decades. The platform gives trainees the opportunity to rehearse aneurysm clipping with minimal risk by providing virtual tools to interact with patient-specific, radiological data. Construction of a 3D tissue model allows the surgeon to design and visualize optimal treatment trajectories and paths, while the rehearsal platform and 3D controllers preexpose surgeons to the procedure. Reduced opportunities to perform clip ligation as a consequence of rising minimally invasive, endovascular treatments encourage simulation platforms like Surgical Theater to provide surgical trainees an alternative avenue for hands-on, low-risk exposure to aneurysmal clipping. There is evidence that rehearsing procedures prior to a case promotes greater intraoperative efficiency, but further studies are necessary to correlate rehearsal with improved patient outcomes. The next step for Surgical Theater will be to expand its planning and rehearsal capabilities to a greater variety of neurosurgical procedures outside of aneurysm clipping and provide both surgeons and trainees a platform for developing skills and technical understanding.

References

1. Carlin AM, Gasevic E, Shepard AD. Effect of the 80-hour work week on resident operative experience in general surgery. Am J Surg. 2007;193(3):326–30.
2. Bina RW, Lemole GM, Dumont TM. On resident duty hour restrictions and neurosurgical training: review of the literature. J Neurosurg. 2015;124(March):1–7.
3. Stain SC, Hoyt DB, Hunter JG, Joyce G, Hiatt JR. American surgery and the affordable care act. JAMA Surg. 2014;149(9):984–5.
4. Papaspyros SC, Kar A, O'Regan D. Surgical ergonomics. Analysis of technical skills, simulation models and assessment methods. Int J Surg. 2015;18:83–7.
5. Caffrey M Jr. Toward a history-based doctrine for wargaming: Technical report, Defense Technical Information Center Document. Available from: http://www.airpower.maxwell. af.mil/airchronicles/cc/caffrey.html. Accessed Aug 2013.
6. Singh H, Kalani M, Acosta-Torres S, El Ahmadieh TY, Loya J, Ganju A. History of simulation in medicine: from resusci annie to the ann myers medical center. Neurosurgery. 2013;73(suppl. 4):9–14.
7. Mitha AP, Almekhlafi MA, Janjua MJJ, Albuquerque FC, McDougall CG. Simulation and augmented reality in endovascular neurosurgery: lessons from aviation. Neurosurgery. 2012;72(suppl. 1):107–14.
8. Wald ML. Plane crew is credited for nimble reaction. New York Times. 15 Jan 2009:A25.
9. Agha RA, Fowler AJ. The role and validity of surgical simulation. Int Surg. 2015;100(2):350–7.
10. Parson BA, Blencowe NS, Hollowood AD, Grant JR. Surgical training: the impact of changes in curriculum and experience. J Surg Educ. 2011;68(1):44–51.
11. Walter AJ. Surgical education for the twenty-first century: beyond the apprentice model. Obstet Gynecol Clin N Am. 2006;33(2):233–6.
12. Ziv A, Erez D, Munz Y, Vardi A. The Israel Centre for Medical Simulation: a paradigm for cultural change in medical education. Acad Med. 2006;81(12):1091–7.
13. Seymour NE, Gallagher AG, Roman SA. Virtual reality training improves operating room performance. Ann Surg. 2002;236(4):458–64.
14. Molyneux AJ, Birks J, Clarke A, Sneade M, Kerr RSC. The durability of endovascular coiling versus neurosurgical clipping of ruptured cerebral aneurysms: 18 year follow-up of the UK cohort of the international subarachnoid aneurysm trial (ISAT). Lancet. 2015;385(9969):691–7.
15. Bambakidis NC, Selman WR, Sloan AE. Surgical rehearsal platform: potential uses in microsurgery. Neurosurgery. 2013;73(suppl. 4):122–6.
16. Education AC for GM. ACGME Program Requirements for Graduate Medical Education in Emergency Medicine. 2013;2015(August 3).
17. Initiative J. The Neurological Surgery Milestone Project. 2015;(July).
18. Barnes RW, Lang NP, Whiteside MF. Halstedian technique revisited. Innovations in teaching surgical skills. Ann Surg. 1989;210(1):118–21.
19. Liu JKC, Kshettry VR, Recinos PF, Kamian K, Schlenk RP, Benzel EC. Establishing a surgical skills laboratory and dissection curriculum for neurosurgical residency training. J Neurosurg. 2015;123(November):1–8.
20. Robison RA, Liu CY, Apuzzo MLJ. Man, mind, and machine: the past and future of virtual reality simulation in neurologic surgery. World Neurosurg. 2011;76(5):419–30.
21. Castillo R, Buckel E, Leon F, Varas J, Alvarado J, Achurra P, et al. Effectiveness of learning advanced laparoscopic skills in a brief intensive laparoscopy training program. J Surg Educ. 2015;72(4):648–53.
22. Harrop J, Lobel DA, Bendok B, Sharan A, Rezai AR. Developing a neurosurgical simulation-based educational curriculum: an overview. Neurosurgery. 2013;73(suppl. 4):25–9.
23. Satava RM. Emerging medical applications of virtual reality: a surgeon's perspective. Artif Intell Med. 1994;6(4):281–8.
24. Malone HR, Syed ON, Downes MS, D'ambrosio AL, Quest DO, Kaiser MG. Simulation in neurosurgery: a review of computer-based simulation environments and their surgical applications. Neurosurgery. 2010;67(4):1105–16.
25. Sedlack RE, Baron TH, Downing SM, Schwartz AJ. Validation of a colonoscopy simulation model for skills assessment. Am J Gastroenterol. 2007;102(1):64–74.
26. Gallagher AG, Seymour NE, Jordan-Black J-A, Bunting BP, McGlade K, Satava RM. Prospective, randomized assessment of transfer of training (ToT) and transfer effectiveness ratio (TER) of virtual reality simulation training for laparoscopic skill acquisition. Ann Surg. 2013;257(6):1025–31.
27. O'Leary JD, O'Sullivan O, Barach P, Shorten GD. Improving clinical performance using rehearsal or warm-up. Acad Med. 2014;89(10):1416–22.

28. Zheng B, Fu B, Al-Tayeb TA, Hao YF, Qayumi AK. Mastering instruments before operating on a patient: the role of simulation training in tool use skills. Surg Innov. 2014;21(6):637–42.

29. Lobel DA, Elder JB, Schirmer CM, Bowyer MW, Rezai ARA. Novel craniotomy simulator provides a validated method to enhance education in the management of traumatic brain injury. Neurosurgery. 2013;73(suppl. 1):57–65.

30. Kockro RA, Serra L, Tseng-Tsai Y, Chan C, Yih-Yian S, Gim-Guan C, et al. Planning and simulation of neurosurgery in a virtual reality environment. Neurosurgery. 2000;46(1):117–8.

31. Schirmer CM, Mocco J, Elder JB. Evolving virtual reality simulation in neurosurgery. Neurosurgery. 2013;73(suppl. 1):127–37.

32. Chan S, Conti F, Salisbury K, Blevins NH. Virtual reality simulation in neurosurgery: technologies and evolution. Neurosurgery. 2012;72(suppl. 1):154–64.

33. Alaraj A, Luciano CJ, Bailey DP, Elsenousi A, Roitberg BZ, Bernardo A, et al. Virtual reality cerebral aneurysm clipping simulation with real-time haptic feedback. Neurosurgery. 2015;11(1):52–8.

34. Luciano C, Banerjee P, Lemole GM, Charbel F. Second generation haptic ventriculostomy simulator using the ImmersiveTouch system. Stud Health Technol Inform. 2006;119:343–8.

35. Banerjee PP, Luciano CJ, Lemole GM, Charbel FT, Oh MY. Accuracy of ventriculostomy catheter placement using a head- and hand-tracked high-resolution virtual reality simulator with haptic feedback. J Neurosurg. 2007;107(3):515–21.

36. Alotaibi FE, AlZhrani GA, Mullah MAS, Sabbagh AJ, Azarnoush H, Winkler-Schwartz A, et al. Assessing bimanual performance in brain tumor resection with NeuroTouch, a virtual reality simulator. Neurosurgery. 2015;11(1):89–98.

37. Beier F, Sismanidis E, Stadie A, Schmieder K, Männer R. An aneurysm clipping training module for the neurosurgical training simulator NeuroSim. Stud Health Technol Inform. 2012;173:42–7.

38. Dunkin B, Adrales GL, Apelgren K, Mellinger JD. Surgical simulation: a current review. Surg Endosc. 2007;21(3):357–66.

39. Surgical Theater. Press Releases [Internet]. Mayfield (OH): [cited 2016 June 9]. Available from: http://www.surgicaltheater.net/site/news-events/press-releases.

40. Chugh AJ, Pace JR, Singer J, Tatsuoka C, Hoffer A, Selman WR, et al. Use of a surgical rehearsal platform and improvement in aneurysm clipping measures: results of a prospective, randomized trial. J Neurosurg. 2017;126(3):838–44.

NeuroVR™ Simulator in Neurosurgical Training

Denise Brunozzi, Laura Stone McGuire, and Ali Alaraj

Introduction

Traditional neurosurgical training, mainly obtained in the operating room by assisting more experienced surgeons, may no longer meet the educational requirements of the current high-demanding standardized neurosurgical curriculum due to the expanding range of minimally invasive and highly sophisticated surgical techniques, cost of operating room utilization, concerns for patient safety, and trainee duty-hours restrictions [1–4]. Virtual reality (VR) simulators have been developed and utilized over the past decade in multiple surgical fields, which allow technical skills to be learned in a safe and controlled environment. Currently, several neurosurgical VR simulators have been created for cranial procedures, with training modules that range from simple tasks, such as ventricular catheter insertion or hemostasis, to complex procedures, including tumor resection, aneurysm clipping, and endoscopic approaches [1, 5].

Novel simulators have integrated haptic feedback to the virtual experience, achieving realistic model manipulation. Among the VR systems that incorporate visual and haptic feedback, NeuroVR™ simulator (CAE Healthcare, Canada) provides one of the most realistic interactions with 3D cranial model [1–6]. Created by the National Research Council of Canada, with the support of the Neurosurgical Simulation Research Centre at Montreal Neurological Institute and Hospital and also with the collaboration of an advisory pan-Canadian network of subject matter experts, NeuroVR™ underwent iterative validation through surveys, discussions, interviews, and collective semiannual meetings between the experts, in order to define the features to be developed in simulation, basic tasks, performance metrics, and levels of difficulty [1, 3].

NeuroVR™ simulator reproduces a three-dimensional neurosurgical field with a stereoscopic view and ergonomics of an operating room microscope. It allows bimanual manipulation of the 3D cranial model, and each simulated surgical tool on either side of the device provides the user with haptic feedback. A set of VR tasks are defined by different levels of difficulty, and feedback on the results of the procedure performed are provided. Additionally, NeuroVR™ assesses innovative metrics of the operator's performance, allowing objective measurements of the psychomotor skills [2, 5]. The training modules of NeuroVR™ are designed to meet the basic and advanced skill requirements of graduating neurosurgical residents into sequential acquisition, and their reli-

D. Brunozzi · L. S. McGuire · A. Alaraj (✉)
Department of Neurosurgery, University of Illinois
at Chicago, Chicago, IL, USA
e-mail: lmcguir1@uic.edu; alaraj@uic.edu

© Springer International Publishing AG, part of Springer Nature 2018
A. Alaraj (ed.), *Comprehensive Healthcare Simulation: Neurosurgery*,
Comprehensive Healthcare Simulation, https://doi.org/10.1007/978-3-319-75583-0_16

ability and validity have been assessed in multiple studies [5–13].

NeuroVR™ Platform [2, 3, 5, 11, 14]

The neurosurgical simulator includes a 3D graphic rendering system that dialogues with a bimanual haptic rendering system and with one or two computers that run the simulation software engine (Fig. 16.1).

The graphic rendering system consists of a binocular eyepiece, a large LCD screen, and an accompanying touch screen. The binocular eyepiece features ergonomics of an operating room microscope that generates stereoscopic view of the visual field (Fig. 16.2). Height and tilt angle

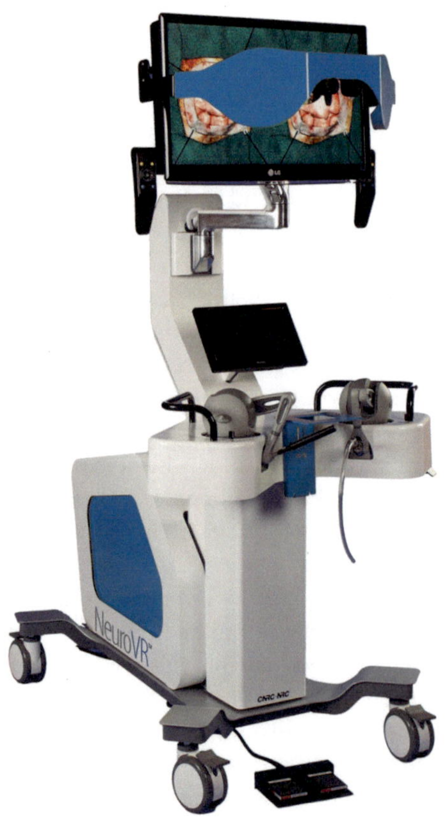

Fig. 16.1 Picture of NeuroVR™ simulator. It includes a 3D graphic rendering system connected to a bimanual haptic rendering system and with the computer that runs the simulation software engine (© 2017 Images courtesy of CAE Healthcare)

of the eyepiece are adjustable by the operator. A 24-inch LCD screen with 1280x1024 resolution as well as zoom and focus control shows the virtual surgical workspace in a high degree of visual realism with the haptic virtual tools displayed on it in real time. The size and distance of the LCD screen from the eyepiece provide a field of view of 30 degrees and focus that reduces eye strain; the height of the screen is adjustable to the operator standing position. A 25-inch touch screen for navigation through a graphical user interface displays task instructions and performance results. Additionally, it works as an auxiliary display for external observers that may follow the procedure sharing the operator's simulated view when the display is not used as graphical interface.

The haptic rendering system components combine two haptic tools with an open plastic head. The haptic apparatuses, one for each hand, simulate different neurosurgical instruments and allow for bimanual manipulation of the cranial model (Fig. 16.3). The haptic system tracks the position of the devices within the surgical field and renders the appropriate resistance of tissues with which the tools interact. Handles are crafted to the same dimension as actual surgical instruments. Their position may be adjusted with output knobs, and the framework includes adjustable wrist rests. Nine neurosurgical tools are available: bipolar forceps, microscissors, suction, neuroendoscope, neuronavigation pointer, microdebrider, microdrill, endoscope, and ultrasonic aspirator. Their function can be controlled with two floor pedals, one for each handle control. These two haptic tools are accompanied by an open plastic head, whose empty space simulates the craniotomy defect, which corresponds to the virtual surgical field as it appears on the screen.

The main computer has two quad-core processors (Intel, Santa Clara, California) that run the simulation software. By integrating graphics and haptics information, it computes collisions between haptic handles and virtual tissue surface, generates tissue deformation and topology changes through real-time image updating, and provides force feedback to the operator.

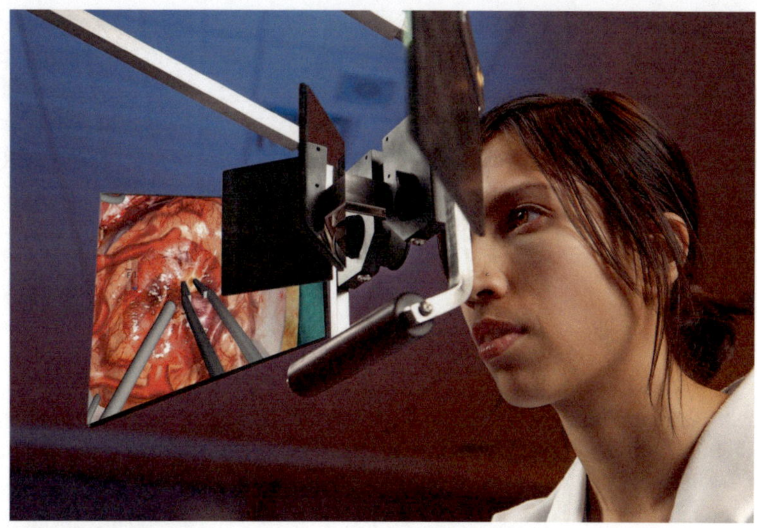

Fig. 16.2 The binocular eyepiece features ergonomics of an operating room microscope that generates stereoscopic view of the visual field (© 2017 Images courtesy of CAE Healthcare)

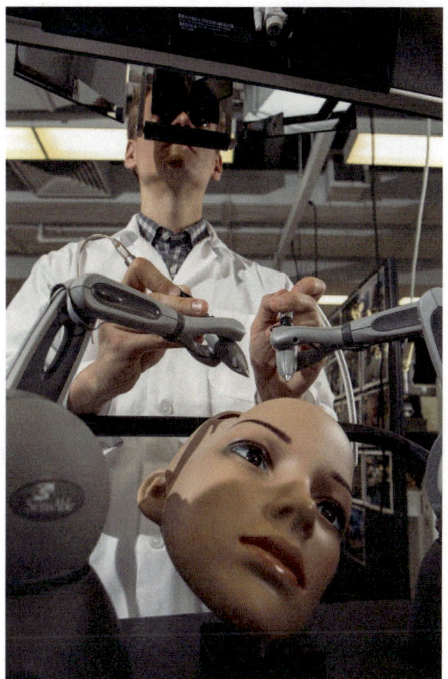

Fig. 16.3 The haptic rendering system components allow bimanual manipulation of the virtual surgical field projected in the cranial model, tracking of instruments position, and rendering of tissues resistance (© 2017 Images courtesy of CAE Healthcare)

In order to increase the accuracy of tissue-tool interactions, freshly excised brain tissue was studied, and different mechanic and thermal pro-prieties were explored to obtain a realistic model. Bleeding is triggered when vascularized tissue is dissected, and the bleeding rate is proportional to the vessel size that cross the surface and to the vascularization level of the dissected tissue. Cast shadows are computed and displayed on the surgical field, and an audible heartbeat synchronous to the image of pulsating brain tissue is integrated to enhance operative realism.

NeuroVR™ Modules [1, 3, 4, 14]

In an attempt to define standardized training modules for neurosurgical skill acquisition and to meet the new educational paradigms, appropriate tasks were identified and developed by the National Research Council of Canada, targeting different levels of practice. The main neurosurgical procedures were analyzed by cognitive tasks and subdivided into elemental technical subtasks that could be tailored for specific competencies (Table 16.1). Training modules were created using the different technical tasks, which then progress from simpler unilateral instrument handling to more complex bimanual procedures based on actual patient cases. Metrics specific for each module are computed to score the trainee performance, and visual feedback of the outcome is provided after the simulated procedure.

Table 16.1 Technical neurosurgical skills required for graduation in Neurosurgical Oncology set by the National Research Council of Canada. The items are listed in progression of postgraduate year, ranging from basic techniques to more complex procedures. 1,4,14

Technical skill requirements for graduation in neurosurgical oncology
1. Open and close scalp incisions
2. Perform ventriculostomies, place lumbar drains, and intracranial monitors
3. Position patients for craniotomy
4. Perform the opening and closing of craniotomies
5. Resect skull lesions
6. Perform image-guided biopsies
7. Demonstrate facility with the use of surgical instruments, including operating microscope and endoscope
8. Identify interface between tumor and the brain and use as an operating plane for tumor resection
9. Identify anatomic landmarks, functional regions, and major structures
10. Show how to minimize and control intraoperative bleeding
11. Perform resection of extra-axial and intra-axial brain tumors
12. Perform resection of supratentorial and infratentorial brain tumors
13. Perform resection of pituitary lesions
14. Perform basic skull base procedures
15. Detect and handle unexpected complications

Instrument Handling Modules

Instrument handling modules allow single-hand practice in maneuvering the most commonly used surgical instruments in neurosurgery. Four exercise modules include suction, ultrasonic aspirator, bipolar, and microscissors.

- *Suction*: allows practice in removing the blood from the surgical field and in retracting soft tissue, avoiding its accidental removal and damage due to excessive force application
- *Ultrasonic aspirator*: allows practice in removing spherical tumors of random stiffness embedded in healthy brain and in adjusting the aspirator amplitude to remove as much tumor as possible without damaging the surrounding healthy tissue
- *Bipolar forceps*: allows practice in coagulating vessels and bleeding sites of soft tissues, in grasping and retracting soft tissues, in blunt and sharp dissection, while avoiding excessive time and force applied
- *Microscissors*: allows practice in cutting fibers between two tissue layers avoiding to sever tiny blood vessels or surrounding tissues

Fundamental Skills Modules

Fundamental skills modules are designed to teach basic and advanced neurosurgical technical skills into a sequential acquisition, including microscopic and endoscopic procedures.

- *Anatomy*: these modules familiarize the user with the anatomical structures encountered during common neurosurgical procedures, including:
  - Burr-hole selection: allows practice in selecting the site of the burr hole for a free-hand ventriculostomy, looking at cranial surface landmarks of the mannequin head; performance metrics measure the insertion point, the angle, and the tip position of virtual catheter from the target point.
  - Ventriculostomy: allows practice in neuro-endoscope orientation and navigation with a pre-selected burr hole to either lateral ventricle along a straight path.
  - Endoscopic ventricular landmarks: allows practice in navigating the ventricular passages and in learning the anatomical structures encountered through labels displayed when contacting specific landmarks with the probe.
  - Endoscopic ventricular test: allows practice in navigating toward a fixed target landmark (e.g., clivus), avoiding potential damage to other anatomical structures.
  - Endoscopic nasal navigation: allows practice in navigating the nasal passages in

either nostril to reach the sphenoid ostium with the aim to learn the anatomy and the spatial orientation of the instruments; the foot pedal rinses the lens when it gets blurred due to bleeding or inadvertent contact with tissues.

- *Bimanual endoscopy*: addresses the nasal endoscopic procedure setup, with 2D view, optics with different orientations, and longer instruments. It includes a nasal debridement exercise to practice the coordinated use of the endoscope in one hand and the microdebrider in the other hand, activated by the foot pedal command, with the aim to remove nasal polyps within the nasal cavity while avoiding inadvertent damage to the underlying mucosa.

- *Tumor debulking*: permits practice debulking meningioma-like tumors with random stiffness, coordinating bimanual movements under the microscope, and controlling bleeding, until the user reaches underlying healthy brain tissue and avoids damage to it.

- *Tumor resection*: rehearses resection of glioma-like tumors located in four different sites (superficial gyrus, subcortical, transsulcal, and transfissural) with the aim of coordinating suction and bipolar forceps, discriminating tumor from health brain boundaries through visual and haptic feedback, and managing bleeding.

- *Hemostasis*: permits practice bleeding management through suction, cauterization, vascular clip application, suturing, packing with hemostatic agents, flushing, and cotton patties application. The bleeding site is sealed only if the appropriate technique is chosen and properly performed, and performance metrics include total blood loss, inadvertent healthy tissue removal, and time spent.

- *Exposure*: allows practice in grasping tissues through bipolar forceps and cutting connecting fibers through microscissors, abstaining from excessive tissue pulling; this exercise teaches tumor and aneurysm exposure (e.g., Sylvian fissure opening) and microdissection.

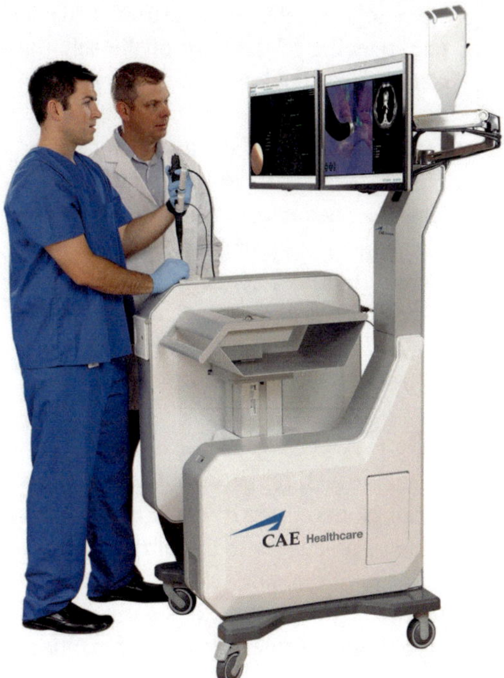

Fig. 16.4 NeuroVR™ includes endoscopic surgical training modules that allow practice of endonasal approaches and endoscopic third ventriculostomy procedures (© 2017 Images courtesy of CAE Healthcare)

Surgical Modules

Surgical modules simulate complete surgical procedures comprehensively, including several techniques and instruments.

- *Endoscopic surgery module* (Fig. 16.4): allows the practice of both endonasal approaches and endoscopic third ventriculostomy procedures. The endonasal approach includes:
  - Sphenoid ostium drilling: practices navigating toward the sphenoid ostium, enlarging it with the microdrill, approaching the sphenoid sinus, and avoiding trauma to the surrounding mucosa
  - Ethmoidectomy: simulates the nasopharynx to practice a complete ethmoidectomy and wide sphenoidotomy with the microdebrider
  - Pituitary adenoma removal: enables practicing a sphenoidotomy as well as

removing the sphenoid rostrum and septum, opening of the floor of the sella turcica, and suc.tioning the pituitary tumor

The third ventriculostomy module includes:
- Floor perforation and enlargement: simulates the anatomical landmarks to practice maintaining appropriate orientation to identify the floor of the third ventricle, to select the ideal perforation site, and to enlarge the perforation with Fogarty balloons or forceps

- *Microsurgery module*: rehearses the resection of the majority of primary brain tumors:
  - Meningioma convexity cases: allows tumor removal practice with the aim to remove as much tumor as possible while preserving functional integrity, including different levels of tumor stiffness and vascularization
  - Glioma cases: permits practice of soft subcortical glioma resection and avoidance of the removal of healthy tissue
- *Spine*: addresses specific skills for spine surgery, including a hemilaminectomy exercise, to remove lamina and to minimize bleeding and damage to adjacent structures, such as ligaments, muscles, or spinal cord

NeuroVR™ Validation

In order for NeuroVR™ to become formally incorporated into training, with assessing competencies and psychomotor skills, this technology must prove to be both valid and reliable. In general, validation should be demonstrated at four levels: the VR technology should present a realistic interface, close to the operating room experience (*face validity*); it should address fundamental aspects of the neurosurgical performance (*content validity*); it should discriminate and measure different levels of psychomotor skills (*construct validity*); it should provide learning skills that are applicable to the real surgical field (*concurrent validity*).

Face and Content Validity

Face and content validity have been tested at semiannual meetings by an advisory network of experts that made iterative updates to the modules, attempting to uphold the neurosurgical realism expectations and the educational requirements [1, 3]. Face and content validity were also reviewed by neurosurgical residents and medical students through subjective questionnaires and surveys [6, 10].

Construct Validity

In addition to providing a realistic experience to the user, NeuroVR™ also must demonstrate utility for educational purposes. Several studies examined the correlation of simulation performance with actual operative technical skills [5–11, 13]. The performance metrics provided by NeuroVR™ were analyzed and combined in tiers to assess the ability to measure the safety, quality, and efficiency of the simulated procedure and also to test the capacity to reflect the different levels of expertise.

NeuroVR™ must also address the goal of the neurosurgeon to apply forces to safely reach the target and perform the procedure while avoiding injury to surrounding normal brain tissue. For example, NeuroVR™ quantifies the percentage of tumor resection during the oncologic training module simulation, providing objective measurements about the quality of the surgeon performance. The measurements of the amount of blood loss, of the volume of health brain removed, and of the maximum, the sum, and the average of forces applied to instruments all provide quantification of procedure safety. Other metrics, such as total tip instruments length, tips average separation distance, pedal activation frequency, percentage of time of simultaneous use of bilateral instruments, percentage of time of active tumor resection, might be regarded as efficiency measures.

All these metrics were tested to assess the construct validity, and in multiple studies, NeuroVR™ proved to be a reliable tool to discriminate surgical skills proficiency: more experienced neurosurgeons presented higher score in safety, quality, and efficiency of the simulated performance than neurosurgical residents, who subsequently performed better in some metrics than medical students, suggesting that NeuroVR™ is able to differentiate operators based on their experience and personal level of competency and that proficiency benchmarks could be set to develop standardized training curricula [5–11, 13, 15].

Concurrent Validity

A pilot study was additionally conducted to assess the concurrent validity of NeuroVR™: by evaluating real endoscopic endonasal surgery procedures over 6 months by expert neurosurgeons, residents that trained on the simulated endoscopic module showed a higher performance score increase in the real intraoperative settings compared to untrained residents [12]. These data, even though preliminary, support the effectiveness of simulation training skills on the surgical performance in the real operating room; future work is still needed to prove these results on a larger scale.

NeuroVR™ Applications

In addition to providing a valid tool for training and assessment of neurosurgical technical skills to fulfill standardized competency-based education requirements, the objective measurements of neurosurgical bimanual psychomotor skills provided by NeuroVR™ may find additional applications intended to improve the neurosurgical proficiency also for skilled surgeons.

Metrics may allow a better understanding of psychomotor skill development and acquisition, guiding a tailored learning and a more efficient transfer of expertise from the neurosurgeon to the trainee. NeuroVR™ supports the "Fitts and Posner model of motor learning" that theorizes that motor learning progresses from stages of conscious performance to an automatic subconscious phase of motor ability: during a simulated neurosurgical procedure, expert neurosurgeons displayed higher consistency of force applications in the surgical field compared to residents, posing for automaticity of process [9].

With objective metrics provided, it is possible to explore the performance variation of operators under specific conditions. NeuroVR™ was experimentally used to assess the general impact of acute stress on the surgical performance, such as an expected severe bleeding in the surgical field during the neurosurgical simulation [16] or after sleep interruption during the night shift [17]. These results might help to select the best condition to perform surgery, and individual assessment of stress might guide specific cognitive training.

The spectrum of the potential applications of NeuroVR™ has not been completely explored. The possibility to create anatomical models from actual patients' imaging studies might provide a rehearsal of the surgical field, allowing practice and familiarization with the specific anatomy and exploration of different surgical corridors in a safe environment, prior to the actual surgery. NeuroVR™ might provide, in the near future, a valid tool for patient-oriented preoperative planning, especially in more complex cases, in an ultimate effort to reduce the rates of preventable errors and to improve the quality of surgical therapeutic options for the patient [2].

References

1. Choudhury N, Gèlinas-Phaneuf N, Delorme S, et al. Fundamentals of neurosurgery: virtual reality tasks for training and evaluation of technical skills. World Neurosurg. 2013;80(5):9–19.
2. Clark DB, D'Arcy RCN, Delorme S, et al. Virtual reality simulator: demonstrated use in neurosurgical oncology. Surg Innov. 2012;20(2):190–7.
3. Delorme S, Laroche D, DiRaddo R, et al. NeouroTouch: a physics-based virtual simulator for

cranial microneurosurgery training. Neurosurgery (1 Suppl Operative). 2012;71:32–42.

4. Rosseau G, Bailes J, Cabral A, et al. The development of a virtual simulator for training neurosurgeons to perform and perfect endoscopic endonasal transphenoidal surgery. Neurosurgery. 2013;73(Suppl 1):85–93.

5. Azarnoush H, Alzhrani G, Wnkler-Schwartz A, et al. Neurosurgical virtual reality simulation metrics to assess psychomotor skills during brain tumor resection. Int J CARS. 2015;10:603–18.

6. Alotaibi FE, Alzhrani GA, Mullah MAS, et al. Assessing bimanual performance in brain tumor resection with NeuroTouch, a virtual reality simulator. Neurosurgery (Suppl 2). 2015;11(1):89–98.

7. Alzhrani G, Alotaibi F, Azarnoush H, et al. Proficiency performance benchmarks for removal of simulated brain tumors using a virtual reality simulator NeuroTouch. J Surg Educ. 2015;72(4):685–96.

8. Azarnoush H, Siar S, Sawaya R, et al. The force pyramid: a spatial analysis of force application during virtual reality brain tumor resection. J Neurosurg. 2017;127:171–81.

9. Bugdadi A, Sawaya S, Olwi D, et al. Automaticity of force application during simulated brain tumor resection: testing the Fitts and Posner model. J Surg Educ. 2017 Jul 3. pii: S1931–7204(17)30114–9. doi: https://doi.org/10.1016/j.jsurg.2017.06.018. [Epub ahead of print].

10. Gelinas-Phaneuf N, Choudry N, Al-Habib AR, et al. Assessing performance in brain tumor resection using a novel virtual reality simulator. Int J CARS. 2014;9:1–9.

11. Holloway T, Lorsch ZS, Chary MA, et al. Operator experience determines performance in a simulated computer-based brain tumor resection task. Int J CARS. 2015;10:1853–62.

12. Thawani JP, Ramayya AG, Abdullah KG, et al. Resident simulation training in endoscopic endonasal surgery utilizing haptic feedback technology. J Clin Neurosci. 2016;34:112–6.

13. Winkler-Schwartz A, Bajunaid K, Mullah MAS, et al. Bimanual psychomotor performance in neurosurgical resident applicants assessed using NeuroTouch, a virtual reality simulator. J Surg Educ. 2016;73(6):942–53.

14. NeuroVR™ user guide, 7/8/2016, CAE Healthcare, 905K540052 v1.

15. Alotaibi FE, Alzhrani GA, Sabbagh AJ, et al. Neurosurgical assessment of metrics including judgment and dexterity using virtual reality simulator NeuroTouch (NAJD metrics). Surg Innov. 2015;22(6):636–42.

16. Bajunaid K, Mullah MAS, Winkler-Schwartz A, et al. Impact of acute stress on psychomotor bimanual performance during a simulated tumor resection task. J Neurosurg. 2017;126:71–80.

17. Micko A, Knopp K, Knosp E, et al. Microsurgical performance after sleep interruption: a NeuroTouch simulator study. World Neurosurg. 2017;106:92–101.

Neurosurgical Anatomy and Approaches to Simulation in Neurosurgical Training

Antonio Bernardo and Alexander I. Evins

Abbreviations and Acronyms

2D	Two-dimensional
3D	Three-dimensional
6D	6 Degrees
ADC	Apparent diffusion coefficient
AR	Augmented reality
ARAI	Augmented reality and artificial intelligence
CTA	Computed tomography angiography
FA	Fractional anisotropy
fMR	Functional magnetic resonance
HMDs	Head-mounted displays
MRA	Magnetic resonance angiography
OM	Operating microscope
OR	Operating room
RGB	Red green blue
SSML	Simulation markup language
VR	Virtual reality
VTK	Visualization tool kit

In the past two centuries, neurological dissections have moved from studying the nature of the nervous system to advancing our understanding of neuropathology, neurophysiology, and techniques in neurological surgery [1–3]. Advances in technology now allow neurosurgeons to pursue alternative, more complex surgical avenues to intracranial targets. The increasing popularity of minimally invasive techniques as a standard in the neurosurgical armamentarium demands more efficient and intensive methods of surgical education. However, while minimally invasive procedures are becoming common practice, the complex anatomy remains challenging to learn and manipulate. The historical record suggests that interactive information may provide advantages in learning or facilitating surgical skills [4–7].

Surgical training, whether it is in the form of observation or as practice in and out of the OR, is imperative to the development of a surgical resident's skills. Most neurosurgical approaches require dexterity with surgical instrumentation through restricted corridors, which contain vital structures in the surrounding area. This aspect of neurosurgery demands that the surgeon be adept not only with the tools but also with the complex anatomy to be negotiated. For example, the development of a sense of the anatomical relationships between neural and vascular structures encased by bone is critical and requires practice [5].

A well-developed understanding of the complex spatial relationships between brain structures, such as eloquent white matter, key

A. Bernardo (✉) · A. I. Evins
Weill Cornell Medicine, Neurological Surgery,
New York, NY, USA
e-mail: anb2029@med.cornell.edu;
ale2009@med.cornell.edu

© Springer International Publishing AG, part of Springer Nature 2018
A. Alaraj (ed.), *Comprehensive Healthcare Simulation: Neurosurgery*,
Comprehensive Healthcare Simulation, https://doi.org/10.1007/978-3-319-75583-0_17

functional areas, pathology, and vasculature, is a vital skill. The limitations imposed by the inherent perspective constraints of two-dimensional images, as well as of non-interactive 3D images, necessitate the development of neurosurgical educational systems that provide a convenient, satisfactory, simulated, and interactive 3D practice experience (Fig. 17.1). The ability to visualize and manipulate structures in three-dimensional (3D) space has proven to be important to both confidence and performance in identifying neuroanatomical structures [8]. Despite this, neurosurgeons are traditionally trained in two-dimensional (2D) space and commonly use disjointed 2D radiologic imaging clinically, which requires the mental translation of 2D images to a 3D understanding of the spatial relationship between the lesion and surrounding structures and landmarks. This requires the surgeon to create a mental representation based on 2D image slices while holding previous slices in working memory to complete their mental picture. This process corresponds to mentally rotating, translating, or scaling an entity to transform its spatial location and orientation from one frame of reference to another. Performing this spatial reconstruction requires mental resources that may cause cognitive overload and reduce performance if the capacity of the working memory is exceeded.

This high demand on working memory is detrimental to other cognitive processes and may lead to longer operation times and chance of error, especially for novices [9]. Junior residents, whose more limited experience affects their ability to quickly perform spatial reasoning, gradually acquire visual-spatial skills over several years throughout their residency by observ-

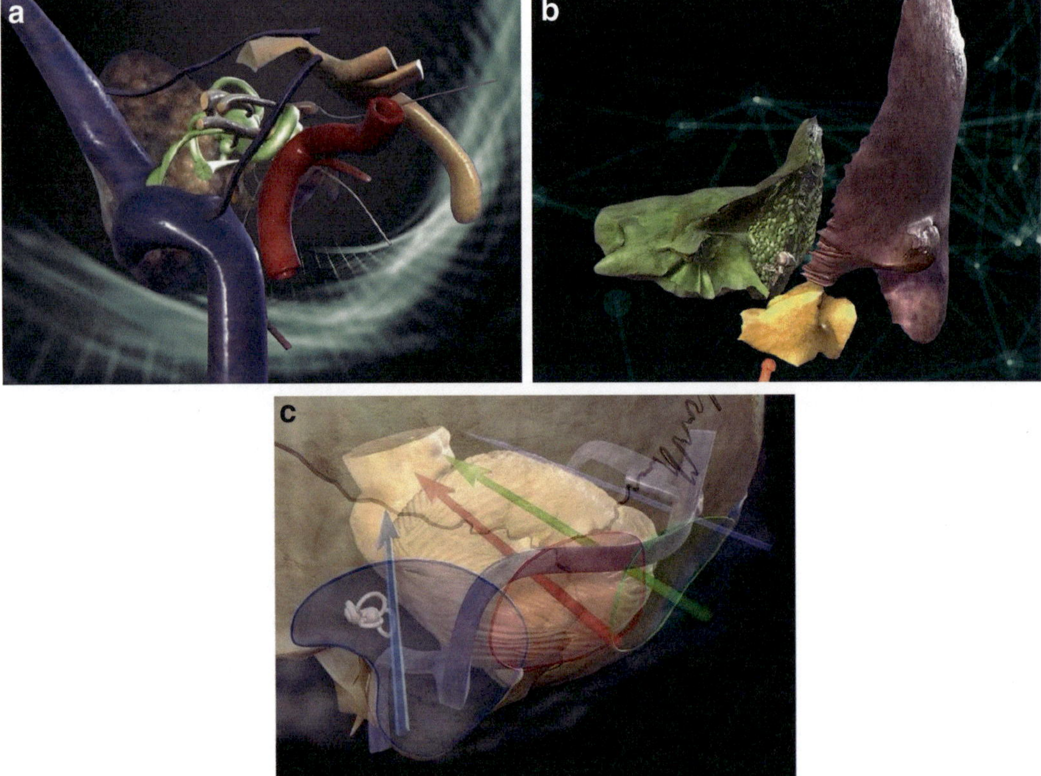

Fig. 17.1 (**a**) 3D virtual reality rendering of the anatomical structures located within the temporal bone. (**b**) 3D virtual reality rendering of the petrous, mastoid, and tympanic portions of the temporal bone. (**c**) 3D surgical planning aid for posterior and posterolateral approaches to the brainstem

ing expert neurosurgeons planning their approach. Meanwhile, residents rely heavily on neuronavigation systems, which may help them to decide the surgical approach but are not designed to improve their spatial reasoning abilities.

Visualization technology in the operating room has continued to change the surgical workflow and surgical training process. It has provided an opportunity for multimodal integration that allows surgeons to efficiently gather all the relevant information needed to create a complete mental picture. These visualization modalities include digital stereomicroscopy, surgical planning, augmented reality, and virtual reality. Surgical planning and augmented reality are becoming a critical and useful tool in the operating room [10]. Medical image data are manipulated to accurately plan surgery in a computer environment and then transferring that virtual plan to the patient using customized instruments. Surgeons can also use holographic displays like Microsoft's HoloLens or Magic Leap for localizing tumors and highlighting specific anatomy to help guide trainees, as well as for other uses that are still being discussed or that have yet to be explored [5].

Unlike VR, where the entire scene is computationally generated, AR is often described as an environment in which the view of the real world is enhanced by overlaying computer-generated information. A practical application of this technology is to complement the available information with computer-generated images, providing a rich view of the operative field and facilitating the performance of a surgical task. The integration of these modalities is beneficial in both the training and performance of surgical procedures and when combined with tactile simulation, can translate to a reduced learning curve, improved conceptual understanding of complex anatomy, and enhanced visuospatial skills for the developing neurosurgeon. This review highlights the technology that is used in modern surgical training for enriched visualization of the surgical field and the opportunity to apply and strengthen the integration of this data in neurosurgery.

As modern technological advances in neurosurgery—including 3D microscopy and endoscopy, virtual reality, surgical simulation, surgical robotics, and advanced neuroimaging—become more widespread and surgeons begin to rely more on their use, the need for integrated and specified training in their clinical utilization is imperative. Simulation-based neurosurgical training is now essential for the development and refinement of technical skills prior to their use on a living patient [2].

Cadaveric Surgical Simulation

While the apprenticeship model is the basis for surgical education, and intraoperative experience forms the irreplaceable foundation for surgical knowledge, the inability to alter or repeat surgical steps in order to satisfy or expand educational objectives, combined with the limits of performing only that which is clinically warranted and the inherent stress of live surgery render the operating room an imperfect classroom for learning or refining surgical skills [11]. In surgery, education always takes a backseat to the surgeon's primary responsibility to the patient [12, 13]. The current medicolegal climate suggests that patients should not be subjected to the learning curve of the surgeon. As such, laboratory-based surgical training is an essential component of residency and post-residency training [14, 15].

A thorough understanding of anatomical structures and their three-dimensional spatial relationships is essential in order to define an armamentarium of safe and effective surgical corridors to intracranial targets. Unfortunately, the anatomical knowledge possessed by even fully qualified neurosurgeons is often inadequate as most surgeons limit their anatomical knowledge to well-established surgical corridors.

As opposed to 2D "flat" anatomy depicted in textbook illustration and didactic lectures—which is often completely unrelated to surgically encountered anatomy—a surgically relevant approach to understanding structures in terms of their relationships, potential for complication, surgical manipulation, and importance in diagnosis and management is paramount. A curriculum that allows for trainees to take a self-guided tour of the skull base in an environment, where the trainee is encouraged to take their time as they progress through each anatomical region, should be highly sought after. An extremely slow and meticulous pace of dissection is essential for gaining a complete understanding of each tissue layer as well as learning how to gently and safely manipulate structures in order to avoid inadvertent iatrogenic complications. Entire weeks could be dedicated to extradural anatomical structures wherein trainees learn the concept of "unlocking" anatomical structures to enhance restricted surgical corridors. This progression would be designed to train surgeons to spend adequate time preparing the surgical corridors extradurally before opening the dura in order to benefit from enhanced exposure.

A key factor in maximizing the surgical value of cadaveric specimens is proper preservation so that they mimic living patients as closely as possible. While some techniques aim to achieve the long-term preservation of tissue using stiffening agents, our aim is to keep them as lifelike as possible in a way that preserves the tissue integrity, density, color, and consistency among other properties [16].

Unfortunately, anatomy is often approached by students as a task for rote memorization rather than conceptual understanding, and important points are easily forgotten. Retaining of anatomical knowledge requires constant practical application [17]. Our philosophy of anatomosurgical education is that the cadaver is the ultimate resource and no textbook can be considered a valid substitute for the abundance of information contained within a human specimen. During the initial period of training, we encourage trainees not to rely or follow surgical textbooks but rather to concentrate on learning the anatomy solely from studying the specimen in order to build an accurate intra- and extracranial road map that is essential for subsequent understanding of surgical corridors. Additionally, surgical trainees are mainly taught anatomy in the operating room through the "surgical window." This window of anatomical learning should be deplored as it limits understanding to only areas that can be seen at

that moment rather than what is in, around, and underneath that surgical window—areas that if incorrectly accessed or manipulated can cause significant complications [15].

Supervision from experienced faculty who teach from a clinical perspective is fundamental for comprehensive learning. However, in today's academic environment, professional survival depends on research and grant funding, which often takes precedent over teaching. Many accomplished surgeons who are best suited to teach these topics in many cases do not receive adequate support, and there are very limited grant opportunities for surgical education. This support is especially important to fund technologically based educational adjuncts that are becoming increasingly valuable and sought after, specifically virtual reality models.

In 2003, after the imposition of the 80-h workweek, residents spend a third less time in the operating room [18, 19]. There has been some evidence of possible adverse patient outcomes as a result of this change [20]. Along with a shift in emphasis on patient safety and the development of newer technologies, there has been increasing pressure to include virtual reality and other forms of simulation as teaching tools for residents as an adjuvant for cadaveric dissection and intraoperative training [21–24] (Figs. 17.2, 17.3). It has been shown that virtual reality and other simulations reduce operative time, error, and wasted movements and increase clinical confidence [25, 26]. In addition, the majority of surveyed residents and directors alike believe that surgical simulation is a useful tool to complement and enhance, without reducing or replacing, traditional avenues of training [27–30]. In the present climate of curricula reform, existing problem-based and systems-oriented studies, together with gross anatomy, should be open to technological enhancement and innovation. In a future where surgical robotics will in all likelihood replace surgeons as we know them, knowledge of topographical anatomy will remain indispensable for the human-machine interaction and essential for completion of a defined surgical task.

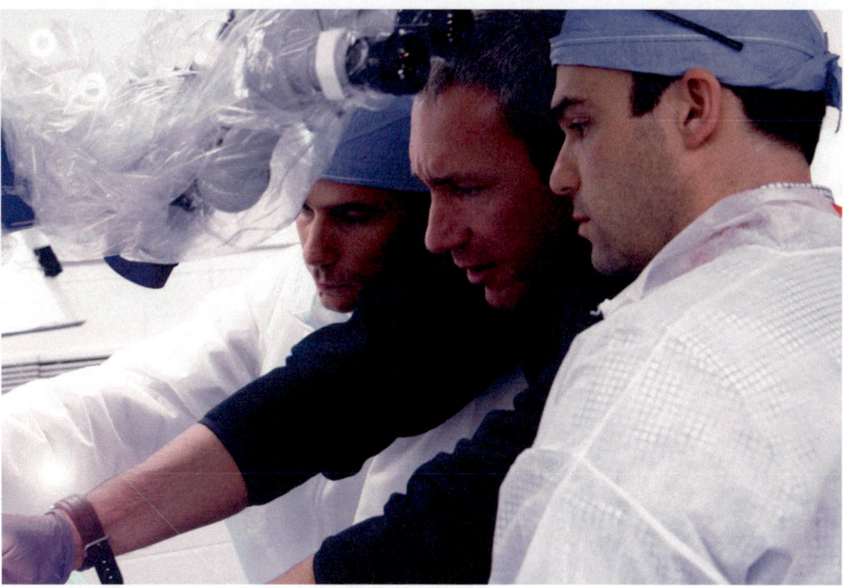

Fig. 17.2 Technologically integrated surgical training. Faculty-driven skills-based cadaveric surgical simulation

Synthetic Surgical Simulation

Also, *synthetic simulation* is becoming increasingly popular and capable of substituting for cadaver models (Fig. 17.4). Synthetic simulation is created using physical materials that represent the fidelity of the target being imitated, rather than in a virtual space of a computer-based simulation. Many models are made with realistic, artificial skin and muscles highly accurate in replicating the consistency of live tissue. An area of neurosurgery where synthetic simulators are commonly developed for is spine surgery, perhaps because the spine is mainly composed of solid bony material, rather than the hard-to-replicate brain tissue in the cranium [31, 32]. Creaplast (http://www.creaplast.eu/products.php. Accessed December 2, 2016) and SynDaver (http://syndaver.com/. Accessed December 2, 2016) are two companies that produce mannequins that serve as simulation for spine surgery. In comparison, SynDaver mainly produces lifelike full mannequins that can replace deceased bodies, as opposed to the more task-focused skeletal models or torsos created by Creaplast.

The recent development of 3D printing has accelerated the production of spine simulators. In addition, companies such as Synaptive Medical (https://www.synaptivemedical.com/products/simulate/. Accessed December 2, 2016) have utilized 3D printing to create anatomically accurate brain models with tactile properties that imitate that of a real brain (Fig. 17.5). 3D printing has also given hospitals the tools to create patient-specific cranial models for preoperative training. For example, the Hospital for Sick Children in Toronto has designed a synthetic brain simulator for endoscopic third ventriculostomy by converting CT and MRI data of a 4-month old into a 3D model that was then printed using silicone. This synthetic model was reusable, portable, and low cost, and surveys showed that the model represented the real anatomy well.

Additionally, a recent study out of the Oregon Health & Science University (OHSU) proposed a novel synthetic model for training neurosurgeons in completing basic routine operative tasks on an anatomically accurate digital model [33]. The model included a physical component involving a mannequin head to be operated on, as well as a

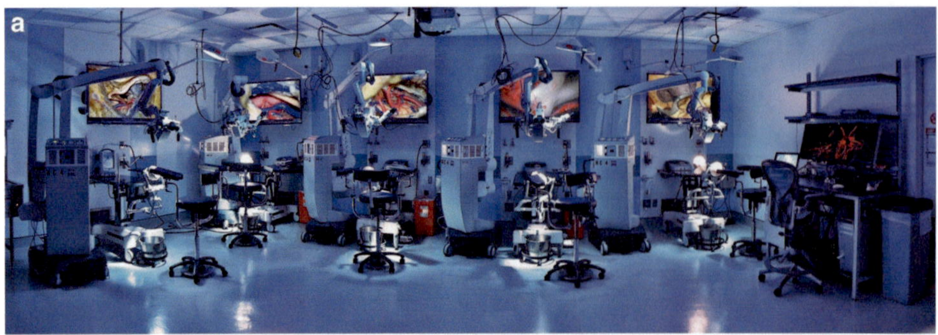

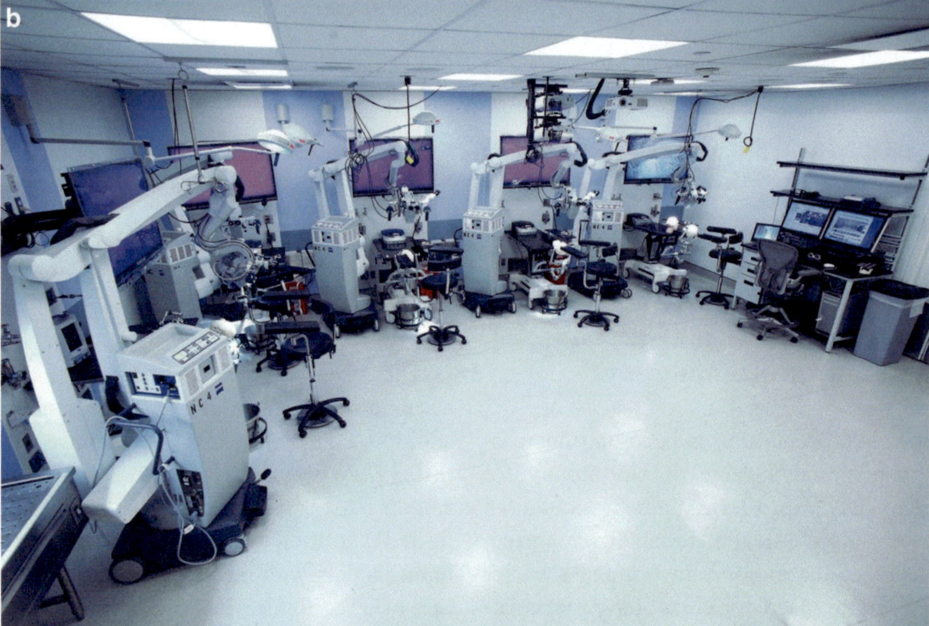

Fig. 17.3 (**a–d**) Surgical workstations in the Weill Cornell Microneurosurgery Skull Base and Surgical Innovations Lab. Five adjacent workstations that are designed to closely recreate the setting of a working operating room

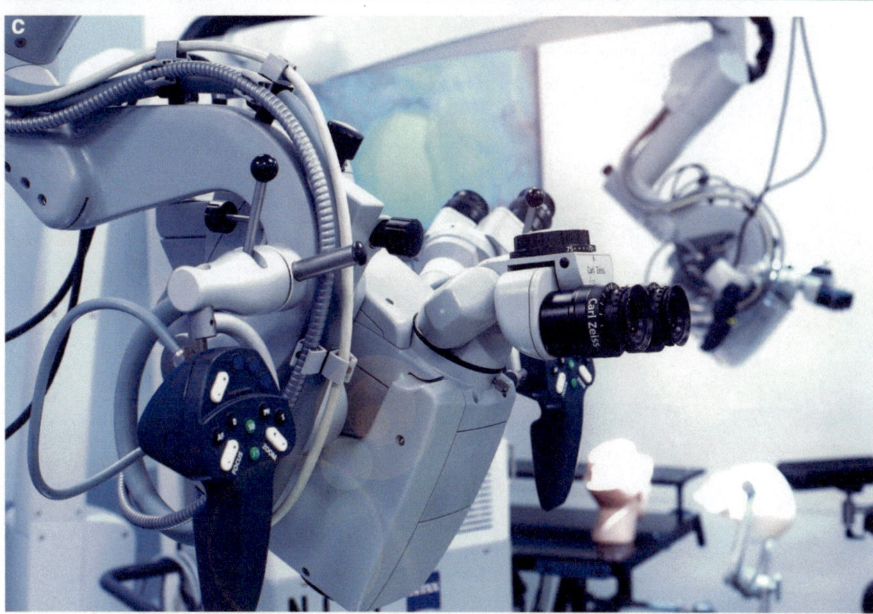

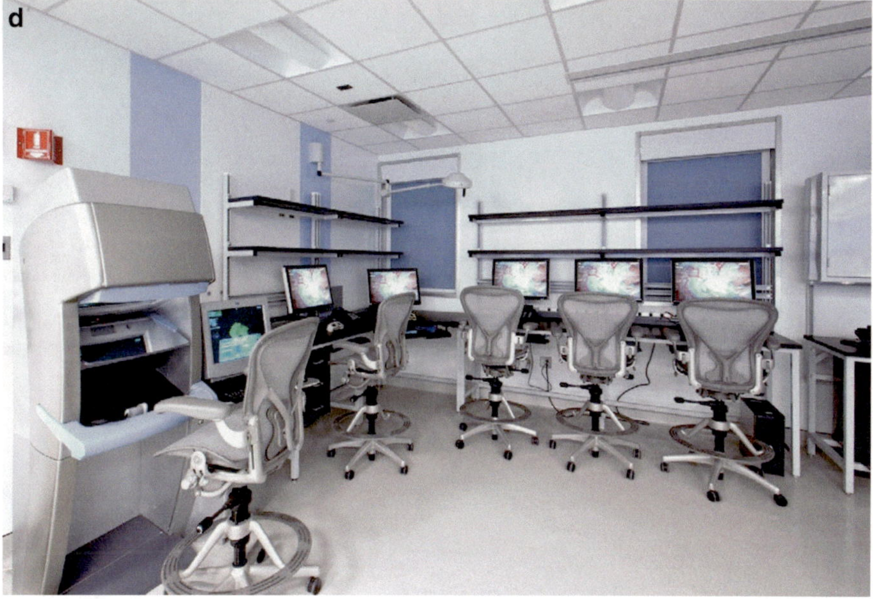

Fig. 17.3 (continued)

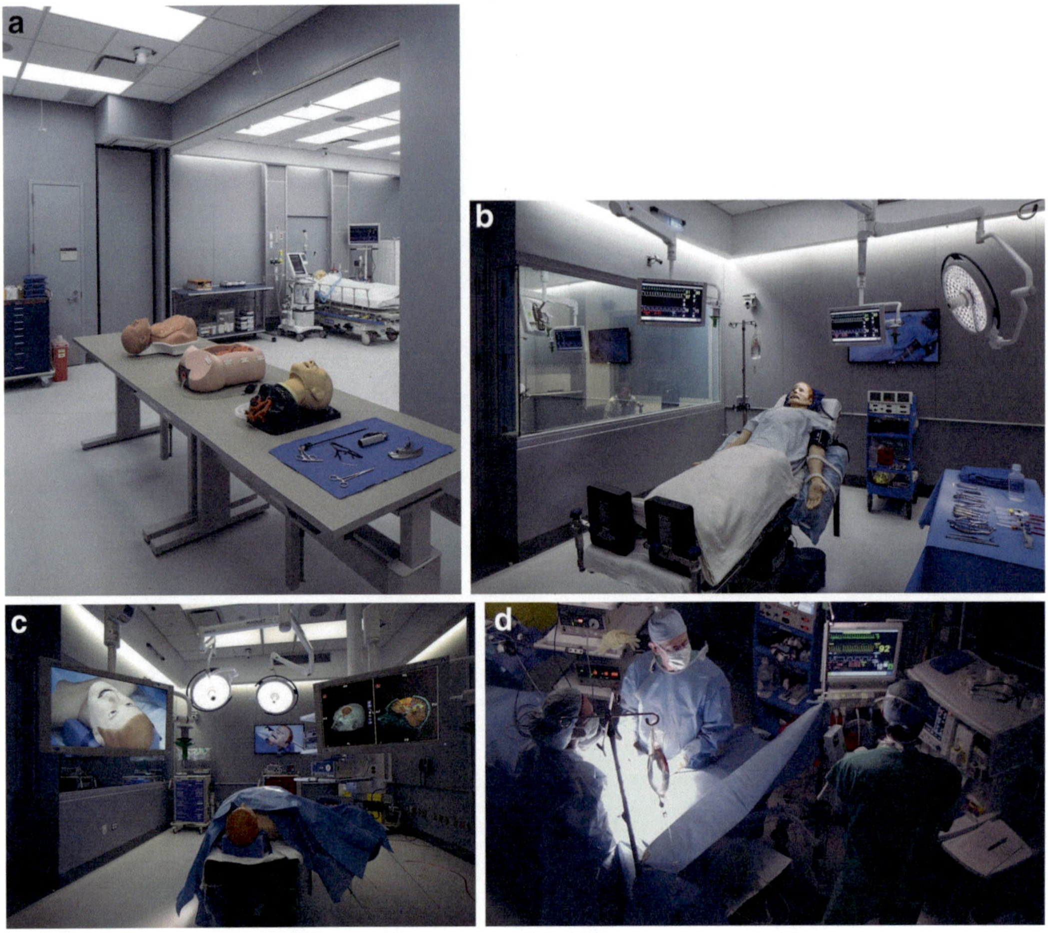

Fig. 17.4 (**a–d**) The Weill Cornell Skills Acquisition and Innovation Laboratory (SAIL) utilizes the most advanced simulation equipment within realistic physical environments to provide complete immersion training

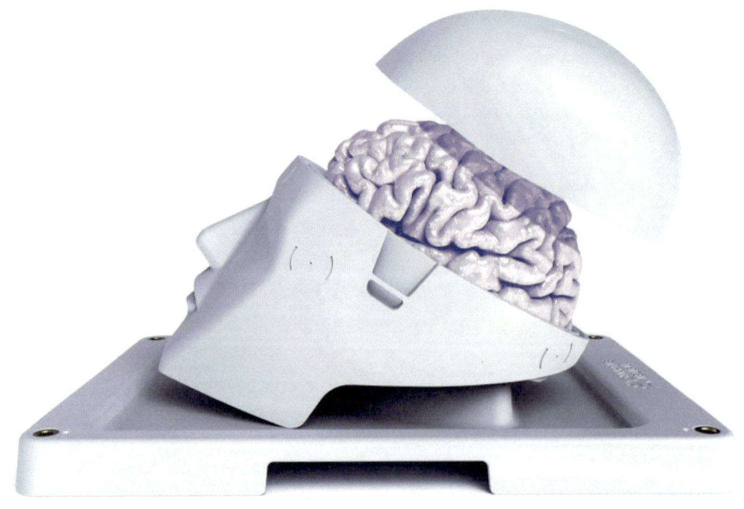

Fig. 17.5 The Synaptive BrightMatter™ simulator, a remarkably lifelike training tool that enables surgeons to practice minimally invasive neurosurgeries and those encompassing traditional craniotomies (Synaptive Medical Inc., Toronto, Canada)

digital aspect that displayed training objectives and simulated patient vital signs. Additionally, an OHSU pilot course designed to teach year 1 neurosurgery residents using the prototype model was conducted. It was found to be effective at inducing realistic surgical conditions, as well as successful at teaching the participants the relevant skills at a low cost and without the risks associated with live surgery.

Evaluation of Human Performance

A training environment that facilitates active learning, while providing a means for practical assessment and correction, is essential for preparing residents to care for patients. The incorporation of human performance monitoring serves to both evaluate the impact of intense surgical training on performance and assess the response to increased mental workload during different surgical procedures.

In order to evaluate surgical performance, physiological parameters—including brain waves, heart and respiratory rates, muscle activity, eye movement, galvanic skin response, and skin temperature—can be recorded during dissection along with video of the procedure and the participant's hands. These human factors can be assessed at different times during the training program and with varying real-life environmental distractors, to track the effect of additional training on these parameters [24, 34–36]). Surgical performance can be evaluated as a function of efficacy of exposure, time of the procedure, and appropriate selection and sequence of surgical steps among other criteria. The participant may also be surveyed at the end of the assessment to determine their perception of difficulty and the presence of any compounding factors including environmental distractors. Trainees can also undergo evaluation at different on-call and post-call periods to assess the effect of fatigue on task-specific performance. Such performance assessments can also help validate the efficacy of specific educational curriculums and reveal the individual learning curves. Areas of weakness can be identified and

used to determine when further instruction is required.

Stress is considered a key component of surgical performance, and the stressors that surgeons frequently encounter include insufficient knowledge, technical complications, time constraints, environmental and situational distractions, interruptions, and increased workload [37–40]. If intraoperative stress becomes excessive, it can compromise both technical and nontechnical skills. Mental workload and fatigue have been found to be among the greatest threats to patient safety in the operating room, and thus identifying contributing and mitigating factors can help reduce medical errors and identify which operative technologies assist versus those that unnecessarily increase workload [41–45].

Digital Surgical Simulation

The ideal surgical simulator should afford visual stereoscopic representation of the reality and an engaging haptic feedback to guarantee a realistic scenario for practice and rehearsing complex surgical procedures [46, 47]. The safety of simulation is particularly germane within neurosurgery, where anatomy is often so complex and complications catastrophic. The specialty recognizes this and has led the way in the development of simulators. An effort has already been made by various groups in different parts of the world in developing sophisticated virtual reality systems that elegantly simulate surgical procedures in a virtual environment. Initial work and results with virtual surgical simulators are encouraging, although problems still remain in faithfully reproducing a generalized anatomical haptic feedback. Although most of the simulators produce a 3D experience, these systems so far have proven costly because of their complex computer hardware and software and are not easily accessible or convenient. A diversity of applications is available: ventricular catheter placement, endoscopy, open cranial, transsphenoidal, skull base, spinal, and endovascular surgery.

In 2008, the National Research Council of Canada (NRC) initiated the *NeuroTouch* (now known as NeuroVR) research project to deliver simulation-based education for neurosurgery. Since then they have developed and validated new training modules that allow neurosurgery residents to practice in a risk-free environment [48]. This VR simulator with haptic feedback is being utilized to both train and assess technical skills in cranial microneurosurgery. The NeuroTouch platform features the surgical workspace of an open neurosurgical procedure by replicating the stereoscopic view and ergonomics of an operating room microscope. NeuroTouch houses two haptic devices permitting tactile interaction of virtual soft tissue with a surgical instrument in each hand. Neurosurgical tools are adapted and fixed on the handle on each haptic system. Foot pedals, tool handle sensors, dial knobs, and push buttons can be used for tool control and other on-the-fly settings and are connected to the main computer via a microcontroller. The software allows physics-based simulation of tissue properties and behavior, the interaction of surgical instruments with brain tissue, and bleeding dynamics using a high-end computer. To produce each image in the simulator, a high-resolution surface mesh is created from and updated by a lower resolution surface mesh used by the tissue mechanics process. The high-resolution mesh deforms to account for blood accumulation and local effects from surgical tools. Dissection of vascularized tissue triggers bleeding, and the bleeding rate depends on presence of large blood vessels going across the surface, the level of vascularization of tissues intersected by the surface, and time. Bleeding can be locally controlled by cauterization. Bleeding physics is efficiently computed on the graphic card to minimize CPU load. High-resolution textures are overlaid on the mesh to ensure realism. The resulting image is deformed and blurred to simulate the effects of lens distortion and depth of field. NeuroTouch allows simulating brain tumor removal using a craniotomy approach on three training tasks using the surgical aspirator, ultrasonic aspirator, bipolar electrocautery, and microscissors. Tissue stiffness can be adjusted independently at any time during the simulation using two dial knobs. In addition to the deformable tissues, the surgical workspace includes rigid and fixed representa-

tions of drapes, skin, cranium, dura, and hooks. Realistic tissue textures are displayed on all visible surfaces, including new surfaces appearing after tissue removal. Blood vessels are represented as textures at the surface and throughout the volume of the tissues. The brain and tumor surface pulsates at 60 beats per minute. Blood oozes on new surfaces at a rate proportional to the size of the blood vessels feeding the tissue. It flows on the tissue surface following gravity and accumulates in tissue valleys [49].

Founded in 2005, ImmersiveTouch provides simulators for neurosurgical training. These simulators are immersive pods that use virtual reality and haptic feedback to recreate surgical scenarios (http://www.immersivetouch.com/ ImmersiveTouch.html; 2016 Accessed 01.12.16). Each simulator has a high-resolution screen; 3D glasses with head-tracking, haptic devices; and a specialized foot pedal. The simulators reproduce visual, tactile, and audio sensations of a surgical procedure with realistic force feedback and head/ hand tracking. The user reaches in with both hands behind a half-silvered mirror to enter an interactive, immersive stereoscopic environment containing the patient's specific 3D imaging data, as well as various tools. Well-matched haptics and graphics volumes are realized, and high-resolution visualization and head and hand tracking are provided. Wearing the head-tracking device allows the operator to have a fully immersive experience of the macroscopic parts of the operation. Real-time haptics feedback is possible bimanually. Haptic feedback provides a tactile sensation in response to the user's actions. By holding two styli, called the Phantom Omni, the user's hand gestures can be tracked on screen using a coordinate system. When the hand or instrument on the screen comes into contact with the patient or tissue, the user will experience a vivid tactile response. Manipulation of the tissue with surgical instruments will also produce a variety of haptic sensations. The use of 3D technology allows for greater immersion within the virtual reality, as do the realistic sound effects of operating room noises (suction, drilling, etc.). There are two foot pedals at the base of the machine, and both styli have buttons which further add to the utility of the simulator. The function of these pedals can change depending on the procedure and may produce suction, cautery, drilling, etc. The presence of pedals is another addition that contributes to the wholly immersive nature of this virtual reality (Geomagic http://www.geomagic.com/en/products/haptic-applications/haptic-application-gallery/industrial-vr-immersive/; Accessed 01.12.16.).

The ImmersiveTouch device offers multiple training modules that have all been developed using real MRI and CT imaging of patient anatomy and pathology (Fig. 17.6). The availability of these modules depends on the package purchased; base, pro, and premium are all available. While most forms of surgical simulation focus on teaching anatomy, ImmersiveTouch offers a unique perspective by focusing on both anatomy and pathology simultaneously. It achieves this through clear visual depiction of the lesions presented in each case and allowing detailed manipulation of the 3D images. ImmersiveTouch also allows the operator to observe how an instructor would perform the procedure in a step-by-step format. This feature is beneficial if an instructor is not present and was one of the desirable elements raised at the American Society of Neurological Surgeons boot camp. Several surgical modules have been developed, including cerebral aneurysm clipping, spine surgery, hemostasis in a brain surgical cavity, percutaneous spinal fixation, and ventriculostomy [50].

Procedicus Vascular Intervention Simulation Trainer (VIST) is a simulator developed in Gothenburg, Sweden, and consists in a mechanical unit within a mannequin cover, a desktop computer, and two screens [51]. By using a simulated fluoroscopic screen, the surgeon inserts modified instruments through an access port using a haptic interface device. VIST contains simulation modules for cardiovascular diseases, neuro-interventions, and caval filters. After each procedure a report containing performance results is automatically generated. The system measures the performance of the surgeon using

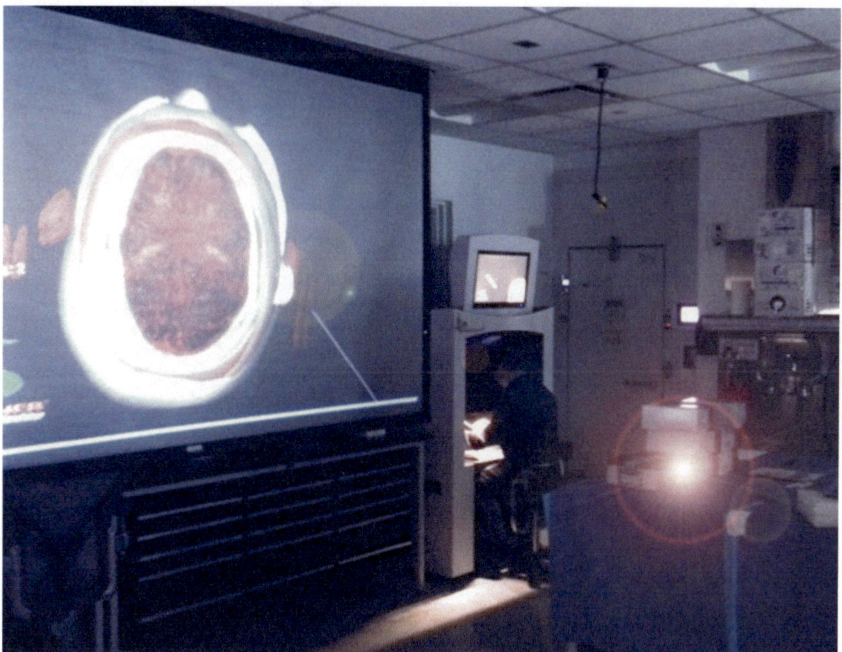

Fig. 17.6 ImmersiveTouch provides a high-performance haptic and augmented reality system that combines haptics, human tracking, and 3D visualization to simulate surgical procedures. The simulation platform is able to create a virtual tridimensional model of a patient's anatomy, so surgeons can learn and practice on a hologram-like virtual patient (ImmersiveTouch, Inc., Chicago, Illinois)

the following parameters: contrast fluid used, total time, fluoroscopy time, endovascular tools used, stent placement accuracy, and errors.

Surgical Planning, Augmented Reality, and Computer Simulation

Advanced imaging modalities and algorithms have provided neurosurgeons with the tools to quantify meaningful patient-specific data that has changed the way neurosurgery is conducted. These modalities are used for preoperative planning and diagnosis, intraoperative guidance, and postoperative surveillance. Multimodal imaging allows for visualization of the surgical target within the brain [52], as well as the structure and function of the surrounding brain with modalities such as diffusion tractography, used to infer the structure of white matter; functional MRI (fMRI) to quantify the functional properties of the brain; and MR angiography (MRA) and computed tomography angiography (CTA) to visualize the vasculature. These enriched data can be visualized in tandem with stereoscopic digital microscopy, augmented reality,

and virtual reality to elevate the surgeon's mental reconstruction of the surgical target and the surrounding anatomy (Figs. 17.7, 17.8). Commercially available surgical computer-assisted navigation and robotic systems (e.g., Medtronic Stealth Station, Stryker NAV3, BrainLab Curve, Medtech ROSA) provide intraoperative image guidance to facilitate percutaneous cranial and spinal neurosurgical procedures. These navigation systems utilize optical and/or electromagnetic tracking to follow the surgical instruments and the patient in real time while displaying multiple coronal, sagittal, and axial views of patient anatomy obtained by presurgical and/or intraoperative CT and MRI. The literature shows considerable evidence that surgical accuracy has been significantly improved by current surgical navigation systems compared to those procedures performed without computer assistance [53]. However, this literature also presents the following limitations:

(a) Surgeons are forced to continuously look up at the navigation 2D monitor located across the operation room and look down at the operative field to manipulate the surgical instruments

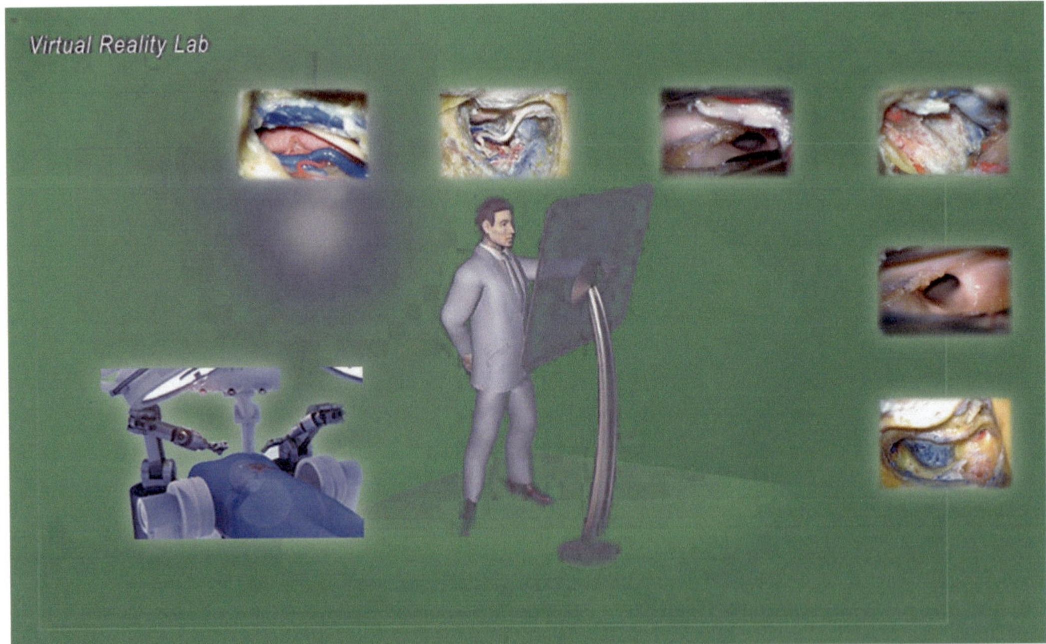

Fig. 17.7 Artistic rendering of a future integrated virtual reality workstation

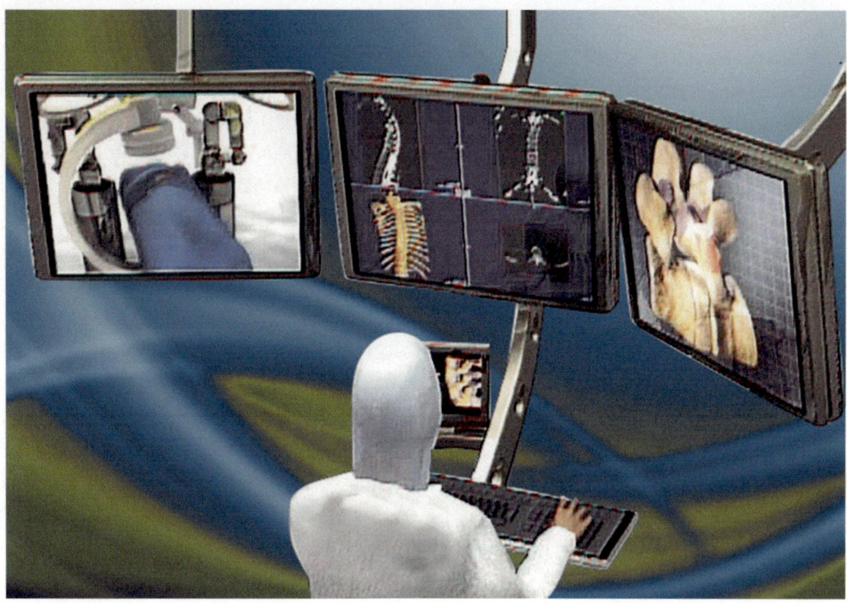

Fig. 17.8 Artistic rendering of a combined operative planning, robotic, and imaging station

based on the information provided by the navigation system. The cumbersome process of focusing their attention back and forth between the navigation system monitor, and the operative field requires surgeons to develop complex and unnatural hand-eye coordination. The highly inefficient process of stopping surgery to see the screen causes a disruptive surgical workflow, unnecessarily prolonging surgical time and, therefore, substantially incrementing the operational cost for hospitals, health insurance companies, and, ultimately, patients themselves.

(b) Surgeons need to mentally interpret the multiple 2D coronal, sagittal, and axial views, and imagine the relationship between the highly complex 3D patient anatomy and the surgical instruments in the operative workspace according to the 2D information provided by the surgical navigation system. The tedious and unintuitive mental process increases the risk of human errors as well as the surgeon's level of stress, negatively affecting surgical outcomes.

Advanced intraoperative overlay, or fusion imaging, may be used with the same effect as external navigations systems and has the potential to solve the critical limitations associated with current surgical navigation and robotic systems [54]. Preoperative radiologic images can be registered to the intraoperative 3D digital images that are acquired in the actual surgical position, and can subsequently be overlaid to provide a visible underlying architecture. The fusion of these two volumes can be overlaid consecutively onto live digital microscopy. This 3D/3D fusion and overlay in live imaging helps the surgeon to guide his or her instruments, visualize the pathology, select optimal trajectories, and avoid crucial anatomy such as vessels or nerves.

Augmented reality (AR) allows a surgeon to visualize the live surgical field with an enriched virtual data overlay, including different sets of data deriving from different imaging modalities, such as tractography, angiography, or ultrasound imaging [5, 9, 10]. This allows the surgeon to interact with the tissue while simultaneously considering the white matter fibers or the vascular architecture that they want to avoid damaging. In the case of neurovascular surgery, AR can be used to allow surgeons to visualize the vascular architecture below the visible brain surface and determine whether they are veins or arteries, which may aid decision-making, reduce operative time, and increase accuracy. The combination of preoperative patient-specific-enriched medical imaging with the live surgical field allows both the experienced and novice surgeon to improve their spatial understanding of the anatomy to determine the most atraumatic approach [30, 55].

Dextroscope (Bracco) was one of the first and most elegant implementations of surgical planning and augmented reality in a purely stereoscopic environment. The system is no longer commercially available, but its engineers pioneered a concept which has been adopted by subsequent groups of researchers [56]. The system integrates tomographic images from CT, CTA, MRI, and MRA into true 3D volumetric objects that can be viewed stereoscopically and interacted with easily and intuitively. Multiple data sets and segmented volumes are automatically co-registered for individual or simultaneous visualization. Surfaces and selected volumes are accurately segmented to isolate critical structures to determine anatomic relationships. An intuitive virtual control allows users to adjust the display of individual objects for optimal visualization. The system utilizes a 6D controller and stylus in place of keyboard and mouse, giving the ability to interact with and manipulate the volumetric images with precision and dexterity. The visual interface displays complex anatomic relationships and pathology in stereoscopic 3D and co-register multimodal images to combine data for better appreciation of anatomical structures. Dextroscope also created the first true stereoscopic augmented reality by overlaying the rendered stereoscopic diagnostic images from the simulator onto the actual visual information from a stereoscopic camera aimed at the patient. Accurate placement of skin and bone flap was achieved with the capability of locating the lesion in transparency [57, 58].

HoloSurgical is currently developing an augmented reality and artificial intelligence (ARAI) surgical navigation system that has the potential to solve the critical limitations associated with current surgical navigation and robotic systems (Fig. 17.9). The ARAI system utilizes state-of-the-art augmented reality technology to overlay a 3D holographic-like virtual image of the patient's internal anatomy directly onto the surgical field. The system enables surgeons to visualize the complex 3D anatomical structure through the patient's skin in percutaneous procedures by simply and intuitively without looking up from the surgical field. ARAI also simultaneously tracks the patient's anatomy, surgical implants, and instruments in real time with an optical tracking system that maintains the equivalent accuracy of commercially available systems. However, unlike traditional surgical navigation systems, the innovative ARAI system enhances the process by tracking the surgeon's head to display the correct 3D perspective of patient anatomy based the surgeon's perspective. In addition to the orthogonal 2D views surgeons are accustomed to seeing in traditional systems, ARAI displays a highly detailed stereoscopic 3D volumetric rendering of patient-specific internal anatomical structures perfectly collocated with the patient's anatomy, without occluding the surgeon's hands or surgical instruments, and substantially simplifying the surgical procedure.

VPI Reveal is a 3D visualization suite for medical imaging data. VPI Reveal (VPI BV, Eindhoven, The Netherlands; Vpi-reveal. http://www.vpireveal.com/; 2016 Accessed 09.12.16) offers state-of-the-art real-time volumetric rendering for CT and MRI data with interactive 3D display on high-end and mainstream desktop and mobile platforms (Fig. 17.10). The user has full control over selection of regions of interest (ROIs) and tissue types through intuitive controls. VPI Reveal supports different paradigms for navigating through a 3D body scan using an input device of your choice, including keyboard and mouse, touch screen, six-degrees-of-freedom controllers, head tracking, and gesture recognition. 3D stereoscopic display is supported on multiple display systems (3D monitor/beamer, head-mounted display) offering a holographic

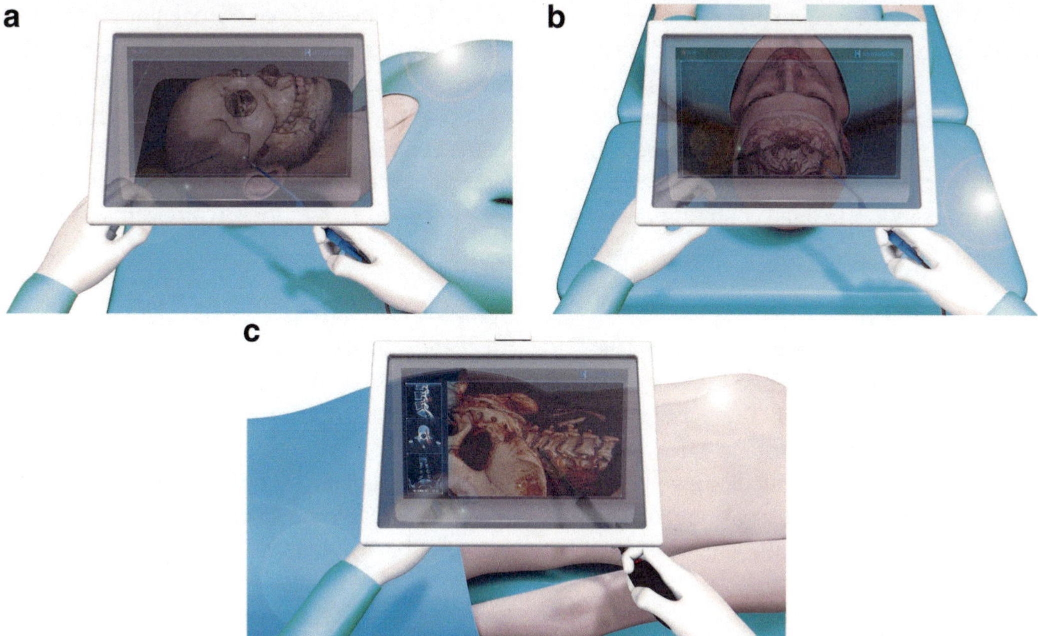

Fig. 17.9 (**a–c**) Real-time 3D projection of internal anatomical structures onto the live surgical field using HoloSurgical (Screenshots, HoloSurgical, Chicago, United States)

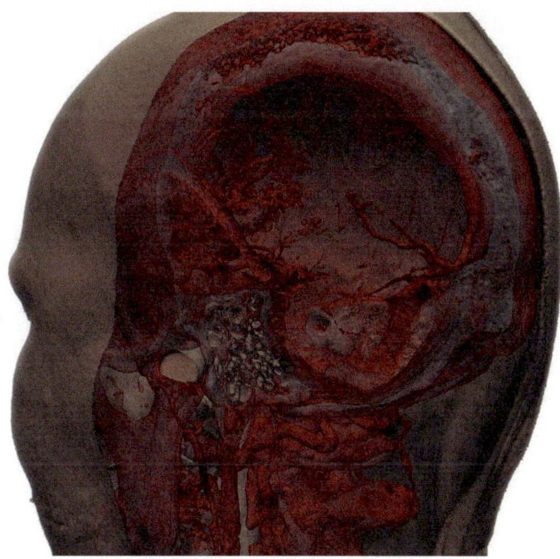

Fig. 17.10 Real-time holographic 3D volumetric rendering of CT and MRI data of the skull using VPI reveal. The user has full control over selection of regions of interest (ROIs) and tissue types through intuitive controls (Virtual Proteins International BV, Eindhoven, the Netherlands)

view of the patient. The holographic view creates a lifelike perception of location and proportion of viewed tissues, which cannot be offered by traditional 2D viewers.

Development of VPI Reveal started in 2008. At that time, the huge power of graphical hardware pushed by the game industry was largely untapped for medical imaging. Common 3D visualization solutions such as VTK relied mostly on CPU computations for volumetric rendering. VPI saw the potential of GPUs for medical imaging and was one of the first companies to offer a solution for high-quality volumetric rendering on the GPU. Apart from its high performance, enabling real-time full-HD rendering, VPI Reveal's state-of-the-art volumetric renderer offers a number of unique features: It allows volumetric scan data and polygonal CAD models to be combined in a single image allowing for quick validation of planned interventions or prosthetic placement. It supports view-camera placement inside the volume, giving the user a perspective of a camera navigating through the body similar to using Google Street View. The renderer supports proper lighting and shadow casting both for volumetric and polygonal data. Shadows offer an important clue about the relative distance between objects in a 3D scene. Similarly, the light source can be placed and moved interactively anywhere in the 3D scene, helping to place focus on a body feature and assess its proportions. Intuitive controls for navigation and ROI selection are crucial for opening up all this graphical power to a user that is not trained to use 3D software. This is especially important in an OR setting where, during an intervention, manual control of the system using keyboard and mouse is not possible or less convenient.

Surgical Theater has developed a patented technology which can import and fuse any DICOM files with volumetric data. The system can fuse patient-specific two-dimensional DICOM images from multiple imaging modalities (CT, MRI, DTI, angiography) to create volumetric models in VR. The software digitally stacks the layers of the scan in space, accurate to the slice thickness of the scan. The model is then volume rendered from the scans. The color and opacity can be adjusted for any structure that exists within that range. DTI data are integrated within the technology by either using DICOM scans that have the tracks burnt onto the scan itself by a radiologist or by importing as a VTK or OBJ object that appears in the model independent of the volume rendering. To create physical 3D-printed models of anatomy and pathology, the volume-rendered portion of the model can be saved as a polygon mesh and exported if the physician chooses (How Surgical Theatre Changes The Way Neurosurgeons Operate. http://uploadvr.com/surgical-theater-neurosurgeons/; 2016 Accessed 11.12.16.).

The system registers scans of a patient to the corresponding anatomy in the operating room intraoperatively, allowing the visualization of tools to be seen on 2D DICOM slices. Surgical Theater's 3DVR technology connects to these systems and significantly enhances this visualization by displaying 3D representations of the surgical tools within the 3DVR environment of the anatomy and pathology. Examples of surgical tools the software has the ability localize in the 3DVR scene are the microscope's focal point, a shunt, an endoscope and suction for tissue removal. During navigation, it can provide a view of the 3DVR model from the point of view of the tip of the probe as it is moving throughout the patient's brain. The software also has the ability to clip away or make transparent any tissue of interest to allow visualization of "hidden" structures (Surgical Theater, where surgeons & virtual reality connect. http://www.surgicaltheater.net/; 2016 Accessed 11.12.16.).

Synaptive Medical is a multi-solution platform for integrated neurosurgical applications. Synaptive's BrightMatter™ provides the surgeon with augmented clarity when visualizing, evaluating, and modifying possible trajectories for the creation of preoperative neurosurgical approaches (Fig. 17.11). Multiple trajectories can be explored through the hands-free fusion of high-fidelity, structural MR images in real time. Featuring tools that simplify the surgeon's complex spatial reasoning tasks by emphasizing 3D visualization, the workflow-driven user interface, automatic data processing, and world-class 3D tractographic rendering aids the intricate process of creating a surgical plan.

Virtual Reality and Computer Simulation

Virtual reality and computer simulation refer to a human-computer interface that facilitates highly interactive visualization and control of computer-generated 3D scenes and their related components with sufficient details and speed so as to evoke sensorial experience similar to that of reality. In aviation and military, virtual reality training is an attractive alternative to live training with expensive equipment, dangerous situations, or sensitive technology [59]. Commercial pilots can use realistic cockpits with VR technology in holistic training programs that incorporate virtual flight and live instruction, while police and soldiers are able to conduct virtual raids that avoid putting lives at risk.

Similarly in medicine, the mini-worlds of test tubes and Petri dishes are translated into mini-worlds contained within silicon chips. On a different scale, simulations of biological systems

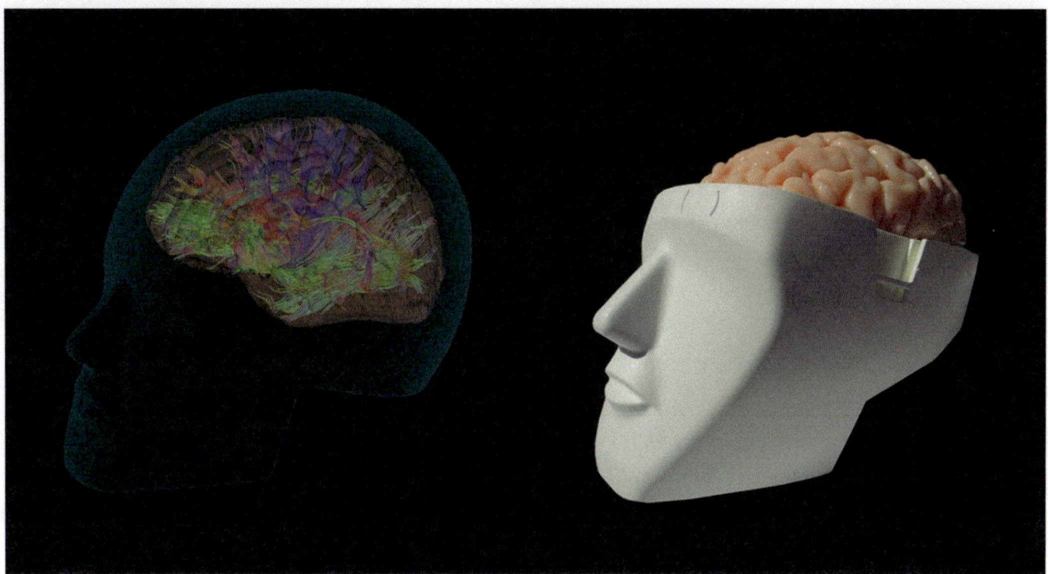

Fig. 17.11 Synaptive BrightMatter™ planning provides the surgeon with augmented clarity when visualizing, evaluating, and modifying possible trajectories for the creation of preoperative neurosurgical approaches. The workflow-driven user interface, automatic data processing, and world-class 3D tractographic rendering aid the intricate process of creating a surgical plan (Synaptive Medical Inc., Toronto, Canada)

can serve as educational tools. In surgical training, knowledge of the human body is improved through intuition, repetition, and objective assessment. Now that computers are replacing patients, surgeons can train with virtual tools and simulated patients and transfer their virtual skills into the operating room. The ability to manipulate 3D models and to view the anatomy from different perspectives is especially useful in complex surgical specialties such as neurosurgery where preoperative planning and port placement often dictates and restricts the angle of approach. Many components have to be integrated and synchronized in order to generate the perception of the artificial reality of a virtual environment. Typical virtual reality-based surgical simulators consist of a physics simulation engine, as well as a visual and haptic interface; a simulator provides an environment which allows interactive surgical manipulation with vital organs via visual and haptic feedback. VR environment in the simulator represents physical object and phenomena. A surgical procedure has several major surgical scenes. In a scene, anatomical objects are located in three-dimensional environments, and surgical manipulation is conducted to the objects. Hence, anatomical objects and conducted manipulation are key pieces of information necessary to construct a virtual surgery environment.

Soft tissue modeling is one of the most important components in surgical simulation. Many models have been proposed and applied to varying results (i.e., mass-spring model, finite element model, etc.). Cutting and ablation manipulations are destructive manipulations and are very different from the aspect of determination of destruction [60–62; see also About Vascular Simulations. http://www.vascularsimulations.com/About; 2016 Accessed 13.12.16].

Accuracy and interactivity are trade-off, because physics-based simulation requires high computational resources. Computational power and requirements of simulation modules are key factors in accurate tissue display, deformity, and destruction. Developing simulation modules takes much effort for developers, because the technical background of VR-based surgical simulators ranges extremely wide (computer graphics, physics, haptics, real-time simulation, etc.). Recently, open source and simulation libraries have been provided by several research groups, thus accelerating development [63]. SSML represents a surgical procedure, which consists of target anatomical structures, surgical manipulations, initial state of the scene, a goal of the manipulation, and pitfalls to be taken care of. Cutting, suturing, palpating, and other surgical manipulations are conducted to the tissues. Simulation programs can also be produced semiautomatically from surgical documents with good approximation of the surgical scenes in a specific operation [64].

Visual Displays

Display technology is often the single biggest difference between immersive virtual reality systems and traditional user interfaces. Head-mounted displays (HMDs) are the most engaging display devices associated with virtual reality. Most commonly, the display component of the HMD is an LCD panel, although OLED (organic light-emitting diode) technology, with a refresh rate as high as 120 Hz and a latency (time between input and output) of 20 ms or less, is becoming more popular. Some newer technologies, such as Microsoft HoloLens and Google's project Tango, can use multiple sensors, in addition to accelerometers for head tracking and positional calculation, to provide a full immersion experience [65, 66].

Recent development has focused on adding eye tracking [67]. With this technology, the HMDs could potentially change the depth of field of the visuals on-screen to simulate natural vision much more closely. Audio plays a key role in a virtual world, and HMDs with an advanced level of immersion have to incorporate sophisticated hearing impression in the design. Hearing is arguably more relevant than vision to a person's sense of space, and human beings react more quickly to audio cues than to visual cues. In order to create a truly immersive virtual reality experience, accurate environmental sounds and spatial characteristics are a must. These lend a powerful sense of presence to a virtual world.

Consumer and industrial wearables are more popular than more sophisticated display systems that can be only used in universities and big labs. For instance, CAVE automatic virtual environments actively display virtual content onto room-sized screens [68]. They consist of three walls upon which stereoscopic images are displayed. An observer standing in the enclosed space perceives the illusion of being immersed in a 3D environment. In the simpler setting, stereoscopic images are displayed using a pair of DLP projectors. Passive stereo projection is utilized, and users wear lightweight polarized glasses to view the scene. In order to handle very complex scenes, a scalable hardware configuration is adopted.

Haptic Feedback

The study of haptics has closely paralleled the rise and evolution of automation. Many scientists have actively studied how humans experience touch and how this sense incredibly relates humans to the environment. A branch of science became known as human haptics and revealed that the human hand, the primary structure associated with the sense of touch, was extraordinarily complex. With 27 bones and 40 muscles, including muscles located in the forearm, the hand offers tremendous dexterity. Scientists quantify this dexterity using a concept known as degrees of freedom. A degree of freedom is movement afforded by a single joint. Because the human hand contains 22 joints, it allows movement with 22 degrees of freedom. When we use our hands to explore the world around us, we receive haptic feedback, which is generally divided into two different classes—tactile and kinesthetic [69].

Kinesthetic feedback provides the brain with information deriving from peripheral proprioceptors. The proprioceptors, embedded in muscles, tendons, and joints, generate a unique set of data points describing joint angle, muscle length, and tension. These receptors carry these unique signals to the brain, where they are processed by the somatosensory region of the cerebral cortex. The brain processes this kinesthetic information to provide a sense of an object's gross size and shape, as well as its position relative to the hand, arm, and body.

Tactile feedback feeds the brain information deriving from cutaneous receptors. The data coming collectively from these receptors helps the brain understand subtle tactile details such as light touch, heavy touch, pressure, vibration, and pain. Also, thermal input is sensed through tactile receptors. Thus, haptic feedback in a virtual environment is a combination of both tactile and kinesthetic feedback.

Force feedback is also a term often used to describe tactile and/or kinesthetic feedback. Computer scientists began working on haptic interface devices that would allow users to feel virtual objects via force feedback. Early attempts were not successful, but a new generation of haptic interface devices is now delivering an unsurpassed level of performance, fidelity, and ease of use (the PHANTOM interface from SensAble Technologies, CyberGrasp from Immersion Corporation) [53, 70–72]. Haptic systems have two important things in common— software to determine the forces that result when a user's virtual identity interacts with an object and a device through which those forces can be applied to the user. The actual process used by the software to perform its calculations is called haptic rendering. A common rendering method uses polyhedral models to represent objects in the virtual world. These 3D models can accurately portray a variety of shapes and can calculate touch data by evaluating how force lines interact with the various faces of the object. Such 3D objects can be made to feel solid and can have surface texture. The job of conveying haptic images to the user falls to the interface device. The most sophisticated touch technology is found in industrial, military, and medical applications. Medical students can now perfect delicate surgical techniques on the computer, feeling what it's like to suture blood vessels in an anastomosis. In training and other applications, haptic interfaces are vital because the sense of touch conveys rich and detailed information about an object. When it's combined with other senses, especially sight, touch dramatically increases the amount of information that is sent to the brain

for processing. The increase in information reduces user error, as well as the time it takes to complete a task. It also reduces the energy consumption.

Metrics

There have been many studies conducted to assess the value and real-world properties of neurosurgical simulation, many concluding that benefits can be gained during simulation training [73, 74]. Ideal learning has been suggested to occur under the following conditions: feedback during training, repetitive practice, curriculum integration, range of difficulty level, multiple learning strategies, capturing of clinical variation, a controlled environment, individualized learning, defined outcomes, and validity [73]. Many of these factors are achieved with simulation training. At a basic level, simulation fidelity is less important with no significant difference in endoscopic skills acquisition between box trainers and virtual reality simulation. Box training is, however, more cost-effective, while virtual reality training is more efficient.

Operatively, simulation may occur in many locations including dedicated wet or dry labs in specialist simulation laboratories, within working theaters, and even in the trainee's home either using cheap, basic jigs, or increasingly sophisticated computer equipment. Optimally, such VR systems should include measures to track the user's performance and the ability to provide feedback without requiring the presence of an instructor. One of the most important advantages of computer simulators for surgical training is the opportunity they afford for independent learning. Unlike the anatomy lab or operating room, a simulator allows a student to practice at his/her convenience, regardless of the availability of cadavers or patients. If the simulator does not provide useful instructional feedback to the user, its educational value is significantly reduced, requiring an instructor to supervise and tutor the trainee while using the simulator. The incorporation of relevant metrics is essential to the development of efficient simulators that provide convenience for trainees while minimizing the costs associated with instructors directly supervising training. Also, the metrics should provide the users with constructive feedback that facilitates independent learning and improvement. Within a skills-based system, proficiency is determined by sequential mastery of skills. With the improvement of the surgical simulators, competency is assessed not only by the subjective assessment of the surgeons that are responsible for training but also by objective and standardized assessment tools.

Thus, there has been an increasing interest in incorporating objective metrics into surgical simulators. Several basic metrics, such as the number of collisions between a user's tool and simulated anatomy, task completion time, and efficiency of movement, have been reported by several existing endoscopy simulators. Other systems have incorporated metrics for percentage of surface area visualized, number of wall collisions, path length, motion smoothness, depth perception, and response orientation [75]. Force and torque sensors have been applied to dissectors and spatulas, and the continuous data stream consisting of forces, rotational torques, and grip force has been translated via a vector quantization algorithm to analyze surgical gestures. Many important elements of good surgical technique have not yet been explored, including proper exposure and identification of anatomic structures, maintenance of proper visibility of the surgical field, and proper drilling and suctioning technique. Real-time visual feedback and/or haptic feedback have recently been applied to the teaching of surgical gestures.

There are some areas of neurosurgery where research has identified consistent parameters to be used as metrics. For instance, metrics are particularly useful in the simulation of temporal bone surgery, which is surgically challenging. Analytical models of bone erosion have been developed as a function of applied drilling force and rotational velocity [76]. Other studies have modeled a drilling instrument as a point cloud, and used a modified version of the Voxman-Pointshell algorithm to sample the surface of the drill and generate appropriate forces at each sampled point [77–80]. Bernardo et al. [80] have also integrated a simple tutor into the first instance of their simulator for temporal bone surgery, helping the user to identify relevant anatomy (Fig. 17.12). Most of these projects have incorporated haptic feedback into volumetric simulation environments that make use of CT and MR data and use volume-rendering techniques for graphical display. By incorporating a large number of metrics and feedback mechanisms, simulators may soon be able to serve as virtual instructors that may be adequate substitutes for the real instructor throughout much of the learning process.

With the increasing emphasis on incorporating patient-specific data into simulators, the value

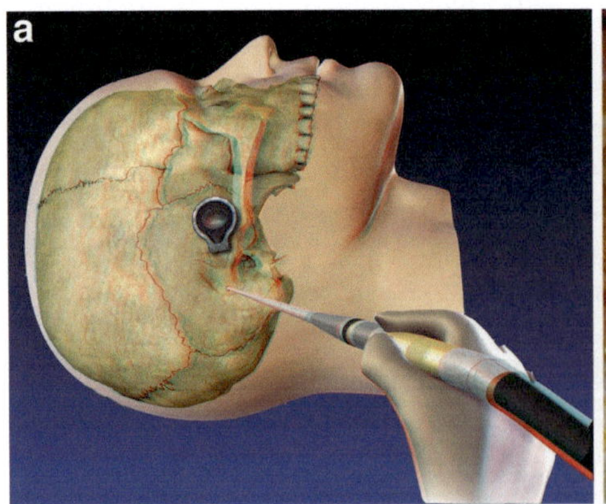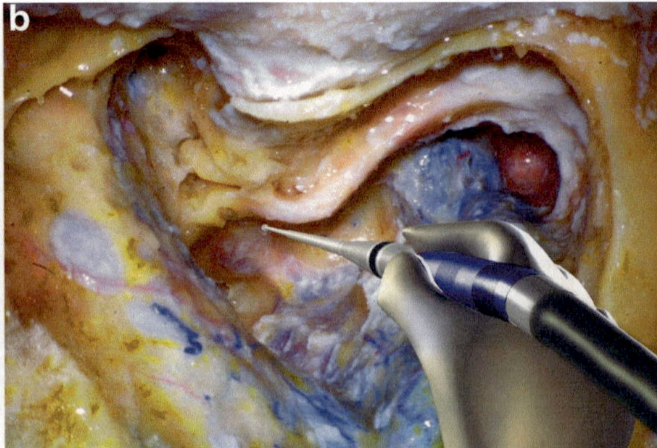

Fig. 17.12 Interactive virtual dissection. (**a–b**) A 3D interactive virtual dissection surgical simulation program designed to teach surgeons the visuospatial skills required to navigate through a transpetrosal approach

of such simulators may be extended not only to young surgical residents but also to experienced surgeons in the context of patient-specific rehearsal for upcoming procedures. The simulation system has to be the essential component of a structured curriculum where the trainee can benefit from a sequential and constructive learning process.

The skull base fellowship at our institution has been structured to create a fully immersive stereoscopic environment where exercises take place under conditions that closely simulate the actual operation. In order to provide adequate preoperative training and rehearsal of complex approaches to the skull base, we have fragmented the neurosurgical curriculum into blocks or modules. Each module affords the surgeon a thorough understanding of a surgical approach to intracranial regions and is preceded by a detailed map of intracerebral topographical anatomy. The modules are self-contained and can be used either as freestanding learning activities or in a stepwise fashion as part of the entire curriculum. Modules can be implemented either in a proctored small or large group setting or individually. Features of the modules include the following: 3D lectures on anatomy, 3D lectures on surgical technique, interaction with 3D computer animations, computer simulation, and, ultimately, cadaveric dissection.

The process is divided in three stages: learning, practice, and performance testing. Trainees are first presented with 3D lecturers and 3D instructional videos describing the target procedure on the anatomy indicating the desired appearance of the model at various stages in the procedure. They are then encouraged to interact with 3D animation models to become familiar with the anatomical spatial relationships. After a tutorial of the simulator, trainees are allowed to practice using the haptic devices and the simulator's user interface. Finally, the trainees are asked to perform the same procedure twice to test performance. Each participant's hand movements, haptic forces, and surgical interactions are recorded and then later rendered to video. Videos are assigned a global score on a scale of 1 to 7 by two experienced surgical instructors, wherein the highest score, 7 points, corresponds to experienced surgeons while the 1-point lowest score corresponds to the novice. The instructors are not aware of which video comes from which subjects, and videos are viewed in randomized order. Several of the cited parameters are utilized to assess performance.

Skills-Based Medicine

The increasing number of hands-on surgical courses underscores the increasing need for more comprehensive skills training. However, these brief courses cannot provide the in-depth teaching and lack the time and stepwise instruction required for trainees to actually gain proficiency at a given procedure. Frequently, a course must be taken several times before the surgeon is confident enough to perform a new procedure in the operating room. For this particular reason, the number of cadaver dissection laboratories has increased in the last few years in order to provide better opportunities for surgeons to refine their skills and to gain working knowledge of surgical anatomy. However, dissection laboratories also have limitations, especially in terms of supporting complex visual learning objectives, conveying or teaching 3D relationships via 2D images and flat representation poses a significant challenge. Use of spatially inaccurate representation can lead to inaccurate and spatially oversimplified conceptions of anatomical relationships. Both virtual reality and stereoscopic technology, especially when used together, provide a way of accurately depicting the spatial 3D nature of anatomical structures and understanding the corridors in which visuospatial tasks will need to be performed. The ability to visualize and understand spatial anatomical relationships is crucial in surgical planning, and stereoscopic projection is invaluable for this purpose [15, 81, 82].

In the past several years, there has been a huge emphasis in the medical community on evidence-based medicine. While evidence- and science-based medicines are no doubt an important mainstay of modern practice, that evidence is of little value in surgery if it is derived from inadequate surgical skills or anatomical knowledge. How can we be certain that one therapeutic intervention is superior to another if the outcomes are subject to significant heterogeneity in surgical skills and armamentarium? Neuropathology—something for which trainees will never be directly responsible—is given equal weight academically as neuroanatomy and surgical skills. If we continue down this path of deemphasizing the surgical component of neurosurgery and do not sufficiently educate residents in surgical skills and anatomy, we are doing our successors a terrible disservice and will inhibit their ability to independently practice the full scope of our specialty.

Conclusion

There are several reasons why simulators are becoming more and more common in medicine: hospitals can evaluate the performance of their doctors, physicians can learn and improve their skills faster, and the risk of the treatment can be reduced for patients. In 2003, after the imposition of the 80-h workweek, residents began to spend approximately one third less time than before in operating rooms, and there has been some evidence to suggest possible adverse patient outcomes as a result of this change. Along with a shift in emphasis on patient safety, as well as development of newer technologies, there has been increasing pressure to include virtual reality and other forms of simulation as teaching tools for residents in addition to the traditional "see one, do one" approach to training on cadavers and actual patients.

Studies generally show that virtual reality and other simulations reduce operative time and error by increasing confidence and wasted movements of the surgeon. In addition, the majority of surveyed residents and directors alike believe that surgical simulation is a useful tool to complement traditional forms of training on patients and cadavers. Cadaveric studies allow the user to apply their training and understanding in an extremely realistic, tactile environment. This physical feedback is important for the user to

develop their skills. Cadaveric simulation has been reported to have the highest benefit when compared to physical simulators and computerized models. The ability of the user to visualize their target in 3D is achieved with these cadaveric models. However, the most common disadvantages of this method are high cost and the limitation to one-time use. Despite these barriers, cadavers are often the preferred methods of simulation, if available.

Synthetic physical simulators are an alternative to cadaveric training, as they can provide the same physical environment with tactile feedback but are generally more cost-effective and readily available. Physical simulators have been reported as the second preferred method of simulation after cadavers [83]. Initial work and results with virtual surgical simulators are encouraging, although problems still remain in faithfully reproducing a generalized anatomical haptic feedback. Although most of the simulators produce a 3D experience, these systems so far have proven costly because of their complex computer hardware and software and are not easily accessible or convenient. One of the most important advantages of computer simulators for surgical training is the opportunity they afford for independent learning. Unlike the anatomy lab or operating room, a simulator allows a student to practice at his/her convenience, regardless of the availability of cadavers or patients.

For simulators to be of value, they must provide realistic feedback that allows the user to apply this training in a real procedure. Beyond these ideal conditions, the integration of enriched data with simulation has the potential to further improve surgical training.

The value of VR in the context of training is that it provides an environment that is as similar as possible to a real-life scenario. In the case of medical imaging, a surgeon can visualize a patient's white matter tractography or their vascular anatomy, for example. This can be used as a surgical planning or navigation tool, as it allows the user to immerse themselves in a 3D, patient-specific environment to gain a better appreciation for the anatomy and to create the ideal surgical plan to avoid eloquent tissue. VR can be used as a training tool, either to visualize anatomy in 3D, as mentioned above, or to practice procedural skills. The translation between VR simulation and real-life has been debated, as the user does not get the physical feedback or interaction that is imperative in training. VR has been rated as having a lower impact on proficiency improvements when compared to tactile simulation such as cadaveric and physical models. However, senior users reported higher improvement when compared to junior users [83, 84]. VR has been used most robustly in endovascular surgery largely because the real-world procedure involves catheter and wire-based instruments that provide limited haptic feedback, meaning that the limitations of VR are less relevant [85]. This suggests that VR can be valuable at different stages of training and skill development and for specific applications.

Neurosurgeons require a fine-tuned understanding of the complex spatial relationship between eloquent tissue and a surgical target. Recent biotechnological advancements can facilitate this understanding to optimize training and performance. This comes in the form of intraoperative stereoscopic visualization and enriched imaging modalities that can be integrated into the OR on the fly or used to create an immersive 3D environment for surgical planning. These modalities can contribute to neurosurgical training both in the OR and beyond in the form of tactile simulation training.

It is important to note that any one of these modalities or enriched datasets used in isolation will not provide the same value as when a multimodal approach to both surgery and surgical training is taken. The combined use of this technology is synergistic, as it allows the neurosurgeon to create a mental 3D model that is a key to learning and surgical success. For instance, with the combination of fMRI and tractography, surgeons are able to pinpoint key functional areas and determine their connectivity to improve their anatomical view and increase resection without damaging eloquent tissue [86, 87]. When the combination of tractography and multimodal vessel imaging was studied, prediction of nerve location was found to be improved in vestibular schwannoma cases when compared to either

modality in isolation [87]. When combined, the surgeon can create a more complete, 3D mental image of the surgical target and the structure and function of the surrounding tissue than with any one modality alone.

Using a tactile learning environment to apply this 3D, understanding is important to consolidate learning. Whether it may be in a cadaveric environment or using a physical simulator, clinicians can gain technical skills and apply them in the OR. This allows surgeons to bridge and strengthen their training knowledge. This review highlights the value of multimodal integration, specifically of digital stereomicroscopy, surgical planning, augmented reality, and virtual reality, in surgical training and performance. The greatest potential for revolutionary innovation in the teaching and practice of the art of surgery lies in dynamic, fully immersive, multisensory fusion of real and virtual information data streams. However, we stress that such a system will not replace the realism of actual painstaking cadaver dissection experience. Neither is VR yet able to create the stress associated with actual surgery or the concomitant physiological sequelae and necessary treatment intervention that accompany, for example, major hemorrhage or dangerous brain swelling. While the training of neurosurgeons should not transform them into computerized surgeons, VR technology can be used to significantly augment the educational process.

References

1. Cappabianca P, Magro F. The lesson of anatomy. Surg Neurol. 2009;71:597–89.
2. Moon K, Filis AK, Cohen AR. The birth and evolution of neuroscience through cadaveric dissection. Neurosurgery. 2010;67:799–810.
3. Aboud E, Al-Mefty O, Yaşargil MG. New laboratory model for neurosurgical training that simulates live surgery. J Neurosurg. 2002;97:1367–72.
4. Kockro RA, Stadie A, Schwandt E, et al. A collaborative virtual reality environment for neurosurgical planning and training. Neurosurgery. 2007;61:379–91.
5. Kin T, Nakatomi H, Shojima M, et al. A new strategic neurosurgical planning tool for brainstem cavernous malformations using interactive computer graphics with multimodal fusion images. J Neurosurg. 2012;117(1):78–88.

6. Abhari K, Baxter JSH, Chen ECS, et al. Training for planning tumour resection: augmented reality and human factors. IEEE Trans Biomed Eng. 2015;62(6):1466–77.

7. Moisi M, Tubbs RS, Page J, et al. Training medical novices in spinal microsurgery: does the modality matter? A pilot study comparing traditional microscopic surgery and a novel robotic optoelectronic visualization tool. Cureus. 2016;8(1):e469.

8. Ruisoto P, Juanes JA, Contador I, Mayoral P, Prats-Galino A. Experimental evidence for improved neuroimaging interpretation using three-dimensional graphic models. Anat Sci Educ. 2012;5(3):132–7.

9. Weigl M, Stefan P, Abhari K. Intra-operative disruptions, surgeon's mental workload, and technical performance in a full-scale simulated procedure. Surg Endosc. 2015;30(2):559–66.

10. Valdés PA, Roberts DW, Lu F-K, Golby A. Optical technologies for intraoperative neurosurgical guidance. Neurosurg Focus. 2016;40(3):E8.

11. Healey AN, Sevdalis N, Vincent CA. Measuring intraoperative interference from distraction and interruption observed in the operating theatre. Ergonomics. 2006;49:589–604.

12. Christian CK, Gustafson ML, Roth EM, et al. A prospective study of patient safety in the operating room. Surgery. 2006;139:159–73.

13. Etchells E, O'Neill C, Bernstein M. Patient safety in surgery: error detection and prevention. World J Surg. 2003;27:936–42.

14. Schreuder HW, Wolswijk R, Zweemer RP, Schijven MP, Verheijen RH. Training and learning robotic surgery, time for a more structured approach: a systematic review. BJOG. 2012;119:137–49.

15. Maertens H, Madani A, Landry T, Vermassen F, Van Herzeele I, Aggarwal R. Systematic review of e-learning for surgical training. Br J Surg. 2016;103:1428–37.

16. Urgun K, Toktas ZO, Akakin A, Yilmaz B, Sahin S, Kilic TA. Very quickly prepared, colored silicone material for injecting into cerebral vasculature for anatomical dissection: a novel and suitable material for both fresh and non-fresh cadavers. Turk Neurosurg. 2016;26(4):568–73.

17. O'Donnell RD, Eggemeier FT. Workload assessment methodology. In: Handbook of perception and human performance. Cognitive processes and performance, vol. 2. New York: Wiley; 1986. p. 42.1–4.

18. Selye H. The evolution of the stress concept. Am Sci. 1973;61:692–9.

19. Satava RM. Historical review of surgical simulation-a personal prospective. World J Surg. 2008;32:141.

20. Hohl BL, Neal DW, Kleinhenz DT, Hoh DJ, Mocco J, Barker FGII. Higher complications and no improvement in mortality in the ACGME resident duty-hour restriction era: an analysis of more than 107.000 neurosurgical trauma patients in Nationwide inpatient sample database. Neurosurgery. 2012;70:1369–82.

21. Selden NR, Barbaro N, Origitano TC, Burchiel KJ. Fundamental skills for entering neurosurgery residents: report of a Pacific region "boot camp" pilot course, 2009. Neurosurgery. 2011;68:759–64.

22. Bohnen HG, Gaillard AW. The effects of sleep loss in a combined tracking and time estimation task. Ergonomics. 1994;37:1021–30.

23. Mascord DJ, Heath RA. Behavioral and physiological indices of fatigue in a visual tracking task. J Saf Res. 1992;23:19–25.

24. Borghini G, Astolfi L, Vecchiato G, Mattia D, Babiloni F. Measuring neurophysiological signals in aircraft pilots and car drivers for the assessment of mental workload, fatigue and drowsiness. Neurosci Biobehav Rev. 2014;44:58–75.

25. Muns A, Meixensberger J, Lindner D. Evaluation of a novel phantom-based neurosurgical training system. Surg Neurol Int. 2014;5:173.

26. Patel A, Koshy N, Ortega-Barnett J, Chan HC, Kuo Y, Luciano C, et al. Neurological tactile discrimination training with haptic-based virtual reality simulation. Neurol Res. 2014;36:1035–9.

27. Ofek E, Pizov R, Bitterman N. From a radial operating theatre to a self-contained operating table. Anaesthesia. 2006;61:548–52.

28. Ganju A, Aoun SG, Daou MR, Ahmadieh TY, Chang Wang L, et al. The role of simulation in neurosurgical education: a survey of 99 United States neurosurgery program directors. World Neurosurg. 2013;80:e1–8.

29. Kshettry VR, Mullin JP, Schlenk R, Recinos PF, Benzel EC. The role of laboratory dissection training in neurosurgical residency: results of a national survey. World Neurosurg. 2014;82:554–9.

30. Wehbe-Janek H, Colbert CY, Govednik-Horny C, White BAA, Thomas S, Shabahang M. Residents' perspectives of the value of a simulation curriculum in a general surgery residency program: a multimethod study of stakeholder feedback. Surgery. 2012;151(6):815–21.

31. Breimer GE, Bodani V, Looi T, Drake JM. Design and evaluation of a new synthetic brain simulator for endoscopic third ventriculostomy. J Neurosurg. 2015;15(1):82–8.

32. Congress of Neurological Surgeons. Congress Quarterly. https://www.cns.org/news-advocacy/congress-quarterly; 2016 Accessed 1 Dec 2016.

33. Cleary DR, Siler DA, Whitney N, Selden NR. A microcontroller-based simulation of dural venous sinus injury for neurosurgical training. J Neurosurg. 2017:1–7.

34. Grandjean E. Fatigue in industry. Br J Ind Med. 1979;36:175–86.

35. Grandjean E. Fitting the task to the man: a textbook of occupational ergonomics. 4th ed: Taylor & Francis; 1988. philadelphia, PA

36. Johns MW, Chapman R, Crowley K, Tucker A. A new method for assessing the risks of drowsiness while driving. Somnologie. 2008;12:66–74.

37. Hull L, Arora S, Kassab E, Kneebone R, Sevdalis N. Assessment of stress and teamwork in the operating room: an exploratory study. Am J Surg. 2011;201:24–30.

38. Arora S, Sevdalis N, Nestel D, Woloshynowych M, Darzi A, Kneebone R. The impact of stress on surgical performance: a systematic review of the literature. Surgery. 2010;147:318–30. e1-e6
39. Wetzel CM, Kneebone RL, Woloshynowych M, et al. The effects of stress on surgical performance. Am J Surg. 2006;191:5–10.
40. Cinaz B, La Marca R, Arnrich B, Tröster G Monitoring of mental workload levels. Proceedings of the IADIS International Conference e-Healt. pp. 189–193. 2010.
41. Yurko YY, Scerbo MW, Prabhu AS, Acker CE, Stefanidis D. Higher mental workload is associated with poorer laparoscopic performance as measured by the NASA-TLX tool. Sim Healthcare. 2010;5:267–71.
42. Zheng B, Cassera MA, Martinec DV, Spaun GO, Swanstrom LL. Measuring mental workload during the performance of advanced laparoscopic tasks. Surg Endosc. 2010;24:45–50.
43. Hart SG, Staveland LE. Development of NASA-TLX: results of empirical and theoretical research. In: Human Mental Workload. Amsterdam: Elsevier; 1988. p. 139–83.
44. Montero PN, Acker CE, Heniford BT, et al. Single incision laparoscopic surgery (SILS) is associated with poorer performance and increased surgeon workload compared with standard laparoscopy. Am Surg. 2011;77:73–7.
45. Carswell C, Clarke D, Seales W. Assessing mental workload during laparoscopic surgery. Surg Innov. 2005;12:80–90.
46. Carter FJ, Schijven MP, Aggarwal R, et al. Consensus guidelines for validation of virtual reality surgical simulators. Surg Endosc. 2005;19(12):1523–32.
47. Das P, Goyal T, Xue A, Kalatoor S, Guillaume D. Simulation training in neurological surgery. Austin Neurosurg Open Access. 2014;1(1):1004–10.
48. Anichini G, Evins AI, Boeris D, Stieg PE, Bernardo A. Three-dimensional endoscope-assisted surgical approach to the foramen magnum and craniovertebral junction: minimizing bone resection with the aid of the endoscope. World Neurosurg. 2014;82(6):e797–805.
49. Raspelli S, Pallavicini F, Carelli L, et al. Validating the neuro VR-based virtual version of the multiple errands test: preliminary results. Presence Teleop Virt. 2012;21(1):31–42.
50. UIC BVIS Students. Surgical simulation and augmented reality. https://uicbvisstudents.wordpress.com/tag/immersive-touch/; 2016 Accessed 1 Dec 2016.
51. Willaert WIM, Aggarwal R, Van Herzeele I, Cheshire NJ, Vermassen FE. Recent advancements in medical simulation: patient-specific virtual reality simulation. World J Surg. 2012;36(7):1703–12.
52. Kockro RA, Reisch R, Serra L, Goh LC, Lee E, Stadie AT. Image-guided neurosurgery with 3-dimensional multimodal imaging data on a stereoscopic monitor. Neurosurgery. 2013;72:A78–88.
53. Barsom EZ, Graafland M, Schijven MP. Systematic review on the effectiveness of augmented reality applications in medical training. Surg Endosc. 2016;30:4174–83.
54. Doulgeris JD, Gonzalez-Blohm SA, Filis AK, Shea Thomas M, Aghayev K, Vrionis FD. Robotics in neurosurgery: evolution, current challenges, and compromises. Cancer Control. 2015;22(3):352–9.
55. Goetz J, Engineering. New technology may help surgeons save lives. https://uanews.arizona.edu/story/new-technology-may-help-surgeons-save-lives. Accessed 1 Dec 2016.
56. Espadaler JM, Conesa G. (2011) Navigated repetitive transcranial magnetic stimulation (TMS) for language mapping: a new tool for surgical planning. In: Duffau H. (eds) Brain Mapp. Springer, Vienna.
57. De Notaris M, Palma K, Serra L, et al. A three-dimensional computer-based perspective of the skull base. World Neurosurg. 2014;82(6):S41–8.
58. Christian E, Yu C, Apuzzo MLJ. Focused ultrasound: relevant history and prospects for the addition of mechanical energy to the neurosurgical armamentarium. World Neurosurg. 2014;82(3–4):354–65.
59. Robison RA, Liu CY, Apuzzo MLJ. Man, mind, and machine: the past and future of virtual reality simulation in neurologic surgery. World Neurosurg. 2011;76(5):419–30.
60. Hochman JB, Kraut J, Kazmerik K, Unger BJ. Generation of a 3D printed temporal bone model with internal fidelity and validation of the mechanical construct. Otolaryngol Head Neck Surg. 2013;150(3):448–54.
61. Lobel DA, Elder JB, Schirmer CM, Bowyer MW, Rezai AR. A novel craniotomy simulator provides a validated method to enhance education in the management of traumatic brain injury. Neurosurgery. 2013;73(Suppl 1):57–65.
62. Hooten KG, Lister JR, Lombard G, et al. Mixed reality ventriculostomy simulation. Neurosurgery. 2014;10:576–81.
63. Ramaswamy A, Monsuez B, Tapus A. Saferobots: a model-driven approach for designing robotic software architectures. Collab Technolog Syst. 2014:131–4.
64. Dharmendra, La G, Saxena K. AUC based software defect prediction for object-oriented systems. e-Learning. 2016;64(57)
65. Lee B, Liu CY, Apuzzo MLJ. Quantum computing: a prime modality in Neurosurgery's future. World Neurosurg. 2012;78(5):404–8. 3
66. Sabbadin M. Interaction and rendering with harvested 3D data. 2016.
67. Kurzhals K, Burch M, Pfeiffer T, Weiskopf D. Eye tracking in computer-based visualization. Comput Sci Eng. 2015;17(5):64–71.
68. DeFanti TA, Sandin DJ, Cruz-Neira CA. "Room" with a "view". IEEE Spectr. 1993;30(10):30–3.
69. Lemole GM, Banerjee PP, Luciano C, Neckrysh S, Charbel FT. Virtual reality in neurosurgical education. Neurosurgery. 2007;61(1):142–9.
70. Besharati Tabrizi L, Mahvash M. Augmented reality–guided neurosurgery: accuracy and intraoperative

application of an image projection technique. J Neurosurg. 2015;123(1):206–11.

71. Pun T, Roth P, Bologna G, Moustakas K, Tzovaras D. Image and video processing for visually handicapped people. EURASIP J Image Video Process. 2007;2007:1–12.

72. Kersten-Oertel M, Gerard I, Drouin S, et al. Augmented reality in neurovascular surgery: feasibility and first uses in the operating room. Int J Comput Assist Radiol Surg. 2015;10(11):1823–36.

73. Barry Issenberg S, Mcgaghie WC, Petrusa ER, Lee Gordon D, Features SRJ. Uses of high-fidelity medical simulations that lead to effective learning: a BEME systematic review. Med Teach. 2005;27(1):10–28.

74. Kirkman MA, Ahmed M, Albert AF, Wilson MH, Nandi D, Sevdalis N. The use of simulation in neurosurgical education and training. J Neurosurg. 2014;121(2):228–46. 6

75. Choudhury N, Gélinas-Phaneuf N, Delorme S, Del Maestro R. Fundamentals of neurosurgery: virtual reality tasks for training and evaluation of technical skills. World Neurosurg. 2013;80(5):e9–e19.

76. Bajka M, Tuchschmid S, Bachofen D, Fink D, Szekely G, Harders M. Hysteroskopie: Operations training in der Virtuellen Realität. Geburtshilfe Frauenheilkd. 2008;68(S 01). S43.

77. Morris D, Sewell C, Barbagli F, Salisbury K, Blevins NH, Girod S. Visuohaptic simulation of bone surgery for training and evaluation. IEEE Comput Graph Appl. 2006;26(6):48–57.

78. Steuer J. Defining virtual reality: dimensions determining telepresence. J Commun. 1992;42(4):73–93.

79. Burdea GC, Lin MC, Ribarsky W, Watson B. Guest editorial: special issue on Haptics, virtual, and augmented reality. IEEE Trans Vis Comput Graph. 2005;11(6):611–3.

80. Bernardo A, Preul MC, Zabramski JM, Spetzler RF. A three-dimensional interactive virtual dissection model to simulate Transpetrous surgical avenues. Neurosurgery. 2003;52:499–505.

81. Evans CH, Schenarts KD. Evolving educational techniques in surgical training. Surg Clin North Am. 2016;96:71–88.

82. Willis RE, Van Sickle KR. Current status of simulation-based training in graduate medical education. Surg Clin North Am. 2015;95:767–79.

83. Gasco J, Holbrook TJ, Patel A, et al. Neurosurgery simulation in residency training. Neurosurgery. 2013;73:S39–45.

84. Schirmer CM, Mocco J, Elder JB. Evolving virtual reality simulation in neurosurgery. Neurosurgery. 2013;73:S127–37.

85. Dimou S, Battisti RA, Hermens DF, Lagopoulos JA. Systematic review of functional magnetic resonance imaging and diffusion tensor imaging modalities used in presurgical planning of brain tumour resection. Neurosurg Rev. 2012;36(2):205–14.

86. Romano A, D'Andrea G, Minniti G, et al. Pre-surgical planning and MR-tractography utility in brain tumour resection. Eur Radiol. 2009;19(12):2798–808.

87. Yoshino M, Kin T, Ito A, et al. Combined use of diffusion tensor tractography and multifused contrast-enhanced FIESTA for predicting facial and cochlear nerve positions in relation to vestibular schwannoma. J Neurosurg. 2015;123(6):1480–8.

Virtual Reality Simulation for the Spine

Ben Roitberg

The need to train surgeons how to perform operations before trying them on patients is not new, but the option of learning basic surgical skills by operating on patients appears less palatable to the public now than ever before. Beyond the acquisition of basic skills, learning all the difficult complex anatomical or pathological situations a surgeon may encounter in practice arguably cannot be accomplished during a typical residency using just the old apprenticeship model. Limited duty hours without extension of the duration of training provide further challenge to clinical learning. As such, more formal training is needed. Program directors, faculty, and residents are aware of the educational needs. Cadaver dissection labs have been popular and remain so, as demonstrated by a recent study by Kshettry et al. [1], employing a questionnaire of residency programs. Response rate was 65%; most of the responding programs (93.8%) incorporate laboratory dissection into resident training. Most programs have 1–3 (36.1%) or 4–6 (39.3%) sessions annually. Residents in

postgraduate years of 2–6 (85.2%–93.4%) most commonly participate. Although many of the labs consist of classical cadaver dissection, technological advances over the past few decades created a new environment and new opportunities for formal surgical training in a laboratory-based, preclinical setting.

The term "simulation" has been used loosely, to include everything from discussion of clinical scenarios, work with manikins, animals, animal parts, cadavers, artificial tissues and organs (like "sawbones"), and various degrees of computer-assisted simulations. The latter range from integration of 3D navigation into a cadaver dissection session and combined artificial object with sensors and computer-based additional visualization – all the way to fully 3D computerized models with virtual tools and haptic feedback – setups approaching true virtual reality. The popularity of the term "simulation" may be due to the extensive and successful use of computerized, fully immersive simulation in both military and civilian pilot training. The simulation of surgical procedures offers many tough challenges for engineers in comparison with flight simulators – large variety of procedures and scenarios, difficulty in modeling anatomy in dynamic situations, true tissue responses and interaction with various tissues, large degree of freedom needed of surgical instruments (compared to airplane controls), and rather limited training budgets. Moreover, it is very difficult to assess the value of any available

Electronic supplementary material: The online version of this chapter https://doi.org/10.1007/978-3-319-75583-0_18 contains supplementary material, which is available to authorized users.

B. Roitberg (✉)
Department of Neurological Surgery, Case Western Reserve University School of Medicine, MetroHealth Campus, Cleveland, OH, USA
e-mail: broitberg@metrohealth.org

© Springer International Publishing AG, part of Springer Nature 2018
A. Alaraj (ed.), *Comprehensive Healthcare Simulation: Neurosurgery*,
Comprehensive Healthcare Simulation, https://doi.org/10.1007/978-3-319-75583-0_18

training tool in the context of surgical training. The ultimate goal of any new or additional training method is to accelerate correct learning and increase patient safety. Proof of increased patient safety would require a randomized study where some patients are assigned to be treated by physicians who had the training and some who did not. Such a study is rather difficult to design, since in all residency training programs, the trainees are not supposed to operate without direct supervision until they are deemed ready and safe. Thus, if we see the patient as the subject in such a study, it is hard to see how it could show a change in patient outcomes even if learning occurred and proficiency increased faster than without the simulation. In neurosurgery in general, and spine surgery in particular, we have largely been limited to demonstrating the face validity and measures of efficacy of learning in simulated environments. That is, it has been possible to demonstrate improvement and learning in trainees in several studies. Accumulating data measures of improved performance and accelerated learning provides important evidence of efficacy of training. Despite the notable technical, budgetary, and other difficulties, the enthusiasm for advancing the field of simulation remains high.

This chapter will focus on simulation for spine surgery – progressing from a variety of more traditional training tools which have been called "simulation" by their users to the most recent advances toward true virtual reality training.

What Should Be Simulated and Who Would Benefit from Simulation Training?

Surgical procedures can be conceived as consisting of multiple phases and steps. Most of them are routine and repetitive. Many components do not constitute a particular challenge and are rarely the cause of technical difficulty for the surgeon. The focus of surgical laboratory training and of any simulation approach is on procedures and critical components of procedures, where anatomical, conceptual, or manual skill challenges exist.

Examples specific to spine surgery include anatomical challenges – especially correct placement of hardware such as pedicle screws; open and percutaneous approaches, with X-ray or simulated navigation guidance; proper alignment of the spine and correction of deformity; correct extent of decompression or tumor resection; dealing with complications such as neural and vascular injury and unintentional durotomy.

Surgical labs as such can be used at any level of training, but most simulations, in our experience, are used for the training of novice and early learners.

Enhanced Variants of Cadaver Dissection as a Basic Form of Simulation

The classic cadaveric dissections have not lost their place, prevalence, or relevance. Mostly, our laboratory and many others use fresh human cadaver parts for spine surgery training – the head and neck or torso. Human cadavers are hard to beat for realistic anatomy and haptic feedback. Real operative tools and hardware are used, as well as regular radiographic equipment when possible. Cadaver-based labs are good for simulation of a routine surgical approach, proper steps, and correct anatomical view. The problem is the cost and difficulty of obtaining cadavers, potential risk of infection of operating personnel, which requires meticulous use of protective gear, and the rather short time the fresh specimen can be kept even if refrigeration is available. Cadaveric dissection requires a specialized laboratory and is generally limited to a few organized courses or training sessions. It is difficult and costly to make cadaveric dissections a routine part of the resident training curriculum. Moreover, the paucity and cost of fresh cadavers make it difficult to do repeated training, or to expose and then cover the anatomy several times. The anatomy and condition of the spine are determined by available cadavers, so training to deal with complications, correction of deformity, or dealing with unusual anatomy cannot be covered by cadaver-based training.

Preserved cadavers can help deal with some of the issues of cost and spoilage. Tomlinson et al. reported trying to optimize the type of embalmment by evaluating which method provides better haptic feel [2]. The issue of realism in visuals and haptic feel is often discussed in the context of simulation. Optimizing the cadaver model for better haptic feel may be important. However, the role of perfect haptic realism for meaningful learning remains unproven. Most of the safety and cost issues mentioned above remain problematic for cadaveric dissections even if embalmed specimens are used.

Training on animals is an alternative, not rare in fields like general surgery, where training in laparoscopic surgery on pigs has been practiced [3]. It is difficult to use animal models to train for human spine surgery, as human spine anatomy is unique. Nevertheless, animal models and even cadaveric animal tissues have been used for training. Goat spines are a common model for biomechanics, and use for training was reported by Suslu et al. [4]. An interesting approach was reported in 2009 by Walker et al. [5], where a complex physical setup of tubes and frames was affixed to deer skulls and spines in order to teach residents minimally invasive spine surgery. Laminectomy and instrumentation were attempted, although lack of human-like spine configuration made the instrumentation training very limited.

The classic cadaveric tissue dissections remain a mainstay of training, but the desire for a more tractable, safer, and less costly model, something that can be used outside of a specialized lab, prompted the development of artificial physical models. In such models, not only the instruments or frames but the tissue itself is artificial.

development was needed [6]. Advantage of a synthetic model over the cadaver is not only the cleaner and easier use but also the ability to reuse the model except for a certain expendable component that is used up in training. The models are standard and can be constructed to offer progressive levels of difficulty, as well as built-in systems of feedback for better and more uniform assessment [7]. Physical models can also help train for pediatric spine procedures, where cadaveric specimens are (fortunately) rare [8].

Although the current main use of simulation, including physical models, is for resident training, ultimately the great advantage over cadaveric dissections is the ability to perform "mission rehearsal" using the patient's imaging data. Stereolithography was used to generate a 3D model of a very complex case for rehearsal and preoperative planning [9]. Such "rapid prototyping"/physical models for training and preoperative rehearsal are currently costly and time consuming, likely to be useful only for selected extreme cases, although cheap 3D printing easily accessible to the surgeon can help accelerate the process. The constructed case-specific model cannot be reused – for those concerned about garbage accumulation and this aspect of environmental protection, repeated and extensive 3D printing of single use items is not an optimal solution. In general, good surgical models for spine surgery rapidly become complex, expensive, and challenging to develop [6]; Physical models have inherent limits, as ultimately building materials that will have very precise "biological feeling" tissues, and electronics for feedback are not cheap, especially in the case of spine surgery where the size and complexity of a good model are an issue.

Artificial Physical Model

Synthetic tissues or organs – like the common "sawbones" spine models or synthetic tubes model for training in micro-suturing techniques – provide great convenience advantage over the cadaver or the live animal. In order to make the physical model a more realistic simulation, much

Hybrid Physical Model/Mixed Reality

The next logical step-up of the simulation ladder from a purely physical model is to use a hardware-based model, with artificial spine and soft tissues, combined with a variety of sensors and imaging and with varying degrees of computerization.

The physical component provides the real object on which to operate, and the computer with the sensors provides feedback about the performance, visualization of deeper structures, richer detail, and the ability to perform objective evaluation of performance.

A recent mixed reality model for posterior cervical surgery – foraminotomy and laminectomy were developed under the auspices of the Congress of Neurological Surgeons (CNS) simulation committee. Harrop et al. reported its use in nine participants at the course at a CNS meeting. Most of the participants were international visitors, and learning was demonstrated by increasing scores on a technical and a didactic assessment [10]. A model for ACDF training was also developed by the same group and used in a small number of participants at the CNS simulation course [11]. A synthetic model can be designed to help train for a specific critical skill, which would not be doable using a cadaver. Ghobrial et al. used a synthetic model of the spine with membranes mimicking the dura, designed to teach repair of a cerebrospinal fluid leak at the CNS course; the experience of six participants was reported [12]. The experience at the CNS simulation course demonstrated the hard work and dedication of the neurosurgeons and engineers developing novel simulations but also the difficulty inherent in the physical model approach. High cost, limited number of participants and difficulty exporting and expanding the experience to every residency program have been evident. However, the CNS courses faced these challenges and served as a necessary testing bed for simulation methods as well as for the development of curricula and objective evaluation of the performance of trainees. The lessons learned and the development that occurred, especially in curriculum design, are immensely important for the future of simulation. National and regional simulation-based courses are certain to become more common, and in the opinion of Ghobrial et al., national development of simulation modules can be translated to individual residency programs [13].

Mixed reality models share many of the advantages and weaknesses of physical models. Each procedure requires dedicated hardware with unique design, which is used up either completely or partially during training. Models that include electronics add related costs, which depend on the degree of computer integration into the simulation. The main advantage over purely computer-based simulation is the availability of more realistic haptic feedback and interaction with a real 3D object, while the electronic component provides visualization aids and uniform scoring and additional feedback. The persistent high cost of this approach makes it difficult to fund without an external source of support. The courses and the devices are sometimes developed jointly with and are supported by hardware companies [10, 11], who have a marketing goal. Resident education is a cost for institutions and programs. Current system provides for payment of resident salaries by the institutions; some or most of the resident positions are funded by the government. However, payment is indeed limited to salary support – education budgets are very limited at most residency programs. Lack of funding for education or income from education is a central problem when we consider an increase in formal and laboratory training. Thus, several mixed reality simulation constructs were developed with cost control in mind.

The use of 3D printing in combination with image guidance using existing equipment [14] can make combined physical-computerized spine surgery simulation models accessible without the need for capital equipment dedicated only to simulation. The combined system also had the flexibility needed to generate training. However, 3D printers' capabilities are limited when the construct has to include multiple layers and textures – like a simulator for a complete spine with bone and various soft tissues.

Two recent studies demonstrated the potential benefit of a rather straightforward mixed reality approach that does not require a sophisticated specially designed model. An orthopedic residency program [15] compared training in the placement of lateral mass cervical spine screws with and without navigation. The pre-test was performed on cadavers, without feedback, and then some of the trainees performed training on a cadaver or on sawbones model, with 3D navigation feedback as to their trajectory. A significant benefit to the training was shown, about equal for sawbones vs cadaver model. The results are intriguing because they support the idea that learning with feedback is important, whereas the exact model may be less important, as learning occurred in an artificial model – sawbones, just like it did in the cadaver. A more recent study by Sundar et al. [16] generally reproduced these results in a single-program study in neurosurgical residents and students. Again, navigation-assisted cadaver and sawbones training session in spinal screw placement was performed, this time including pedicle screws as well. No comparison was made between cadaver and sawbones, but trainees who experiences the practical sessions demonstrated better performance than those who received only theoretical instruction. Although the result is intuitively expected, such validation of construct is important in order to justify the notable investment in simulation [16].

These studies suggest that using sawbones and existing 3D navigation can be a reasonable and inexpensive approach to simulation, though the approach is limited to basic training in spinal screw placement. More sophisticated procedures (percutaneous placement, soft tissue, anatomical variants) require more complex simulation. Moreover, optimal training must extend beyond initial exposure to the anatomy and the technique, into scenario-based training [17]. None of the mixed reality models above can accommodate such training. Thus, a rather sophisticated system to integrate physical models with sensors and capability for evaluation were developed and described by Aderman et al. [17] – the simulator consists of synthetic bone structures, synthetic soft tissue, and an advanced bleeding system. The simulator includes sensors for pressure and traction on the artificial nerve roots and dura. The article mentions good satisfaction with realism, as well as acceptance of the objective scoring and correction [17]. Intensive development of mixed reality models promises good realism and haptic feedback; but they require extensive development or soft and hard tissue-simulating materials [6, 17]. However, more sophisticated systems will tend to increase in price, and thus the cost of repeated practice will be high, although such repetitions are central to acquisition of surgical skill. Moreover, the cost of development of each training module is high when new hardware needs to be designed and manufactured. The advantage of highly sophisticated models with optimal haptic feedback over simpler ones has not been proven in comparative studies.

Computerized Simulations

If the goal of the training session is only visualization and learning of surgical anatomy without the expectation of haptic feedback or complex interactions with the tissues – a simpler computerized approach may be adequate. Indeed, a lot can be accomplished using game-like software and available high-resolution imaging files. An early attempt at this approach was desktop-based software to provide visualization of insertion of pedicle screws as part of training. It used predefined images and demonstration of insertion, without haptic feedback and not yet based on real scans of the patients [18]. Podolsky et al. integrated a three-dimensional computer-based simulation for pedicle screw insertion into a cadaveric spine surgery instructional course. The tool was positively regarded by the participants, but "the limited training with the simulator did not translate into widespread comfort with its operation or into improvement in physical screw placement" [19].

Simulation and Visualization Research Group [20] performed a relatively sophisticated simulation without haptics for residents in an orthopedic program. As a step toward virtual reality (VR), it generates images from a CT scan and guides the trainee to learn to use virtually generated 2D fluoroscopy to correctly guide the pedicle screw. It basically teaches how to use the 2D fluoro guidance. The single-center experience was reported as "positive" [20]. Indeed, such simulation can potentially teach the key skill required for correct adjustment of pedicle screw trajectory based on the 2D fluoro image. For those surgeons who rely on such images for surgery, this is an adequate training platform. The system offers no 3D visuals, no ability to remove tissue, and model or pre-do complex cases, and it provides no haptic feedback from the interaction with the bone or other tissues. The great advantage is the very low cost of repetitions. For some, this will be adequate adjunct to training, though the benefit still needs to be demonstrated.

Toward True Virtual Reality: Immersive Simulation

We have reviewed a variety of training and teaching methods and even ways to prepare for specific operations, which were called "simulation." However, the final frontier of simulation is the full VR operative experience. As is often the case, terminology has not been uniform or clear. Fully computerized surgical experience has been called "virtual reality" [21], or sometimes "augmented reality." I feel that current technological capabilities fall short of complete virtual reality, because of limited realism. Nevertheless, simulation that includes 3D visuals, haptic feedback, and the ability to interact with the tissue by cutting, drilling, etc. exists already. It may be called "immersive simulation," or partial/imperfect virtual reality. This technology provides the best if not the only opportunity to reach progressively improved realism and true virtual reality. Rather than trying to find a system of software or hardware to solve a particular training problem or prepare for a particular operation, a fully computerized virtual reality system allows us to define a complete set of general curricular goals for simulation, for spine surgery as well as other surgical procedures, and for open as well as endoscopic and microsurgical approaches. VR allows us to think of a complete set of requirements for the ideal surgical simulation program. We can try to define our goals and then see whether VR is really moving toward these goals or is just the great future promise that will always remain in the future.

The ideal simulation for surgery – and by extension for spine surgery – will play the same role in surgical training and certification that simulation plays in pilot training and certification. It will have adequate realism in terms of visualization and haptic feedback, large variety of simulated procedures, and a large library of anatomical and pathological variants. There will be interaction with tissue – cutting, drilling, placement of screws, with tissue removal and retraction – to enable simulation of procedures such as a laminectomy or a tumor removal, as well as instrumentation. The device will be able to measure and record performance and guide the trainee up an ascending ladder of performance levels. A library of cases and anatomical variants will be integrated. The device will be able to present scenarios and crisis situations and will have stored set of scenarios and the ability to integrate guidance and evaluation by an instructor. Naturally, there will be the capacity for unlimited number of attempts/unlimited rehearsal without additional cost except for time.

Virtual reality faces challenges related to precision, natural feeling, feedback, and evaluation. The barriers are technological, but there is no theoretical limit to quality of VR. As such, with the improvement in immersive simulation on the way to true virtual reality, other methods of simulated surgery – artificial tissues, partly computerized systems, and eventually even cadaver-based surgical laboratories, are likely to become obsolete. We are far from this point, but over the past decade, significant strides were made in the direction of real virtual reality simulation for spine surgery.

An early example was a spine needle biopsy simulator, based on visual and force feedback [22]. The simulation remained limited and did not produce a more versatile simulation device, because serious technological issues had to be overcome. The creation of the 3D model in the computer, with rich and realistic coloration, and smooth continuous surfaces for haptic interaction proved difficult. The available data – such as DICOM files, even when acquired at a high resolution typical of surgical navigation cases, is not sufficient in raw form. The surface will appear discontinuous to the haptic device. Movement of the spine, and other interactions, requires additional processing and data analysis. Moving virtual surgical tools within that space, interacting with the tissue, and co-localizing the perceived position of the virtual tool with the location of the tissue in the virtual space all require extensive computer science research. So did generation of surface mesh and segmentation of the image into vertebrae [23] [24].

Our group started working on spine simulation in 2009–2010, basing the development on an immersive surgical simulation system already in use at the University of Illinois at Chicago (UIC). The system consists of a computer with advanced video card, proprietary software, one or two robotic arms for performance of procedures and haptic feedback, and a high-resolution inverted computer screen, viewed by the operator or trainee through a semitransparent glass surface which provides a reflection of a 3D model. The image is viewed through 3D glasses, which have a position sensor and can track the motion of the head of the operator, so that it is possible to look at the virtual model from different directions (Fig. 18.1). The system was developed at UIC, for a variety of educational applications – neurosurgical, ophthalmological, and others, and the spine modules were developed with the assis-

tance of the author, at the University of Chicago and UIC. The earliest immersive spine simulation was that of thoracic pedicle screw placement – a relatively common and anatomically challenging component of spine surgery and a good target for simulation-based training. A preliminary idea was discussed among the surgeons and the engineers, a prototype developed using images of a real spine, without gross pathology. The procedure was refined by an iterative process involving the surgeons and the engineers. Then the teaching module was validated using local residents and then a national sample, in this case – the Top Gun competition at the AANS [25]. Fifty-one fellows and residents performed thoracic pedicle screw placement on the simulator. The virtual screws were drilled into a virtual patient's thoracic spine derived from a computed tomography data set of a real patient. The full-color 3D image could be rotated and viewed from different directions. The trainee would drive a virtual drill into the pedicle, and then the system placed a screw in the same trajectory and to the same depth. With a 12.5% failure rate, the performance accuracy on the simulator was comparable to the accuracy reported in literature on recent retrospective evaluation of such placements. The failure rates indicated a minor drop from practice to test sessions and also indicated a trend ($P = 0.08$) toward learning retention resulting in improvement from practice to test sessions. The performance accuracy showed a 15% mean score improvement and more than a 50% reduction in standard deviation from practice to test. It showed evidence ($P = 0.04$) of performance accuracy improvement from practice to test session. This study demonstrated the face validity of our simulation – trainees were able to perform pedicle cannulation at a success rate similar to that for thoracic pedicle screw placement reported in the literature. Preliminary construct validity – that learning was occurring – was also demonstrated. However, since the learning pertains to the model – transfer to real life is not proven. The realism was also not complete in the early simulation – as in reality a pedicle finder is the most common initial tool that defines the trajectory of the placement of the screw.

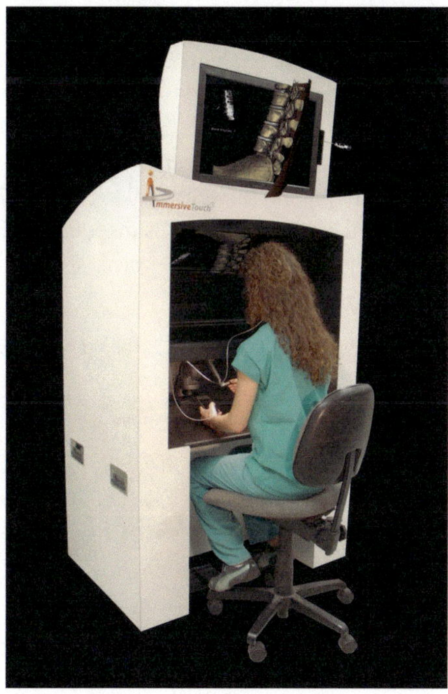

Fig. 18.1 The immersive simulation device. Seen are the box that contains the screen and robotic arms, as well as the foot pedal controllers, a 3D screen on top for additional viewers (Used with permission of ImmersiveTouch)

The next phase was to establish training modules for percutaneous pedicle cannulation with a virtual Jamshidi needle. The percutaneous simulation used a more realistic setup compared to the initial thoracic screw module. It included penetration of the skin and then the bone with the heavy needle, virtual fluoroscopy, and the ability to change transparency of the tissues for changing the level of difficulty of the procedure (Fig. 18.2) [26]. Sixty-three fellows and residents performed needle placement on the simulator in our study. A virtual needle was percutaneously inserted into a virtual patient's spine derived from an actual patient computed tomography data set. Ten of 126 needle placement attempts by 63 participants ended in failure for a failure rate of 7.93%. From all 126 needle insertions, the average error (15.69 vs 13.91), average fluoroscopy exposure (4.6 vs 3.92), and average individual performance score (32.39 vs 30.71) improved from the first to the second attempt. The experiments showed evidence ($P = 0.04$) of performance accuracy improvement from the first to the second percutaneous needle placement attempt. This result, combined with previous learning retention and/or face validity results of using the simulator for open thoracic pedicle screw placement, supports the efficacy of immersive simulation with haptics as a learning tool.

A key advantage of the fully computerized simulation is the ability to add modules and answer curricular challenges without building a new device or adding new hardware. Only new images need to be loaded and new software written. The key component becomes preparation of curriculum and the iterative process of development – surgeons and engineers together. In response to the inclusion of lumbar pedicle screw placement in the SNS Bootcamp2, and the proposal to include the computerized simulation in the program, an open pedicle screw placement module for the lumbar spine was developed (Fig. 18.3, Video 18.1). It included the use of a virtual pedicle finder for greater realism, but otherwise was similar to the thoracic model. Additional upgrades included a screen with greater resolution. Part of the development of the new module was its validation in a group of trainees. This time, rather than a national neurosurgical course, a group of medical student volunteers was chosen by Gasco et al. [27]. Twenty-six senior medical students anonymously participated and were randomized into two groups (A = no simulation; B = simulation). Both groups were given 15 min to place two pedicle screws in a sawbones model. Students in Group A underwent traditional visual/verbal instruction, whereas students in Group B underwent training on pedicle screw placement in the simulator. The students in both groups then placed two pedicle screws each in a lumbar sawbones models that underwent triplanar thin slice computerized tomography and subsequent analysis based on coronal entry point, axial and

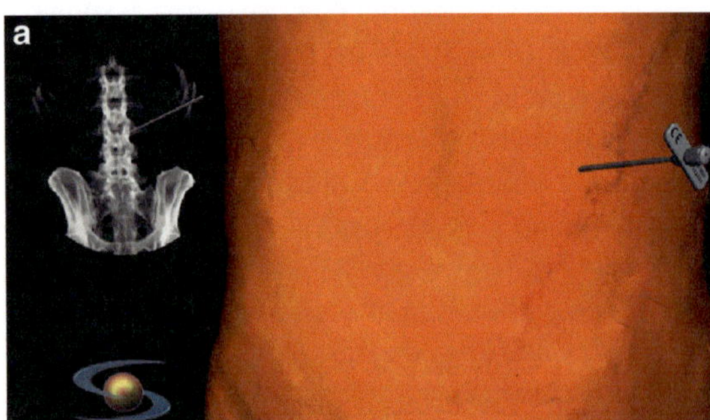
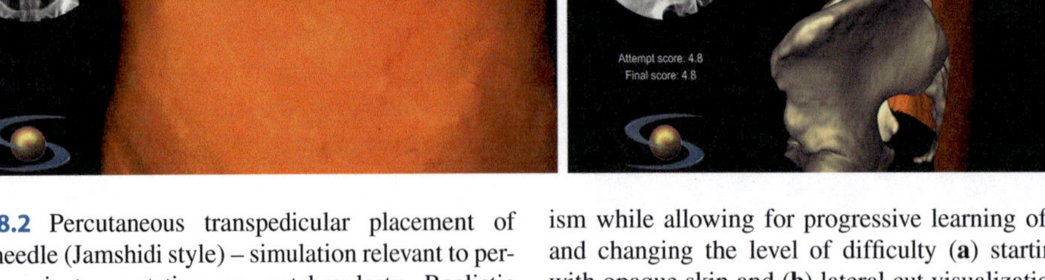

Fig. 18.2 Percutaneous transpedicular placement of heavy needle (Jamshidi style) – simulation relevant to percutaneous instrumentation or vertebroplasty. Realistic anatomy based on real patients and ability to vary tissue resistance, coloration, and transparency to optimize realism while allowing for progressive learning of anatomy and changing the level of difficulty (**a**) starting screen with opaque skin and (**b**) lateral cut visualization for orientation and feedback (Used with permission of ImmersiveTouch)

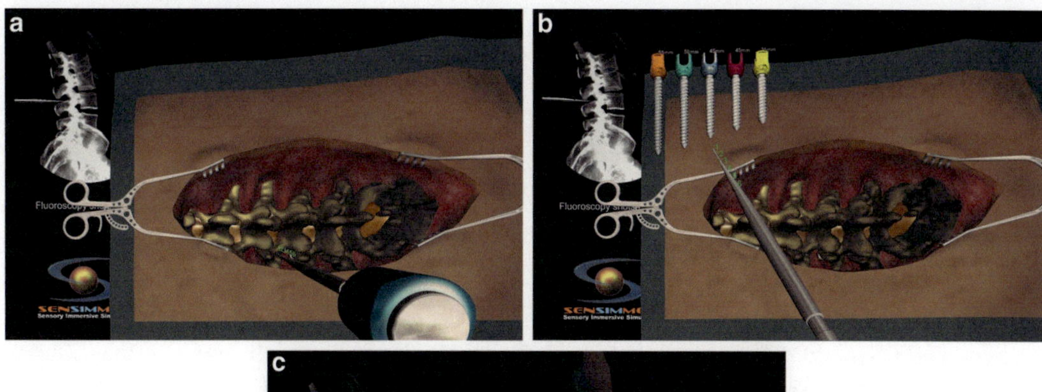

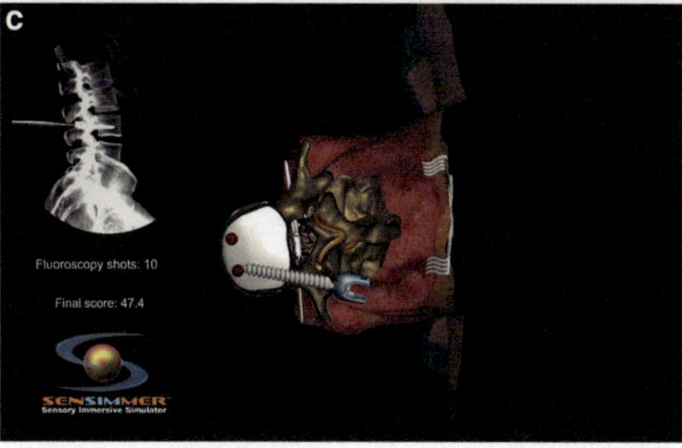

Fig. 18.3 The lumbar screw placement module, in the configuration used at the SNS course (**a**) using a pedicle finder, (**b**) selecting a screw, (**c**) feedback with virtual X-ray and cross cut – virtual dissection for feedback and orientation (Used with permission of ImmersiveTouch)

sagittal deviations, length error, and pedicle breach. The average number of errors per screw was calculated for each group. A total of 52 pedicle screws were analyzed. The reduction in the average number of errors per screw after a single session of simulation training was 53.7% ($P = 0.0067$). The average number of errors per screw in the simulation group was 0.96 versus 2.08 in the non-simulation group. The simulation group outperformed the non-simulation group in all variables measured. The three most benefited measured variables were length error (86.7%), coronal error (71.4%), and pedicle breach (66.7%). Computer-based simulation appeared to be a valuable teaching tool for non-experts in a highly technical procedural task such as pedicle screw placement that involves sequential learning, depth perception, and understanding triplanar anatomy.

Current immersive computerized simulation already meets some of the requirements for an ideal training system: unlimited repetition, objective scoring, game-like environment and engagement, progressive acquisition of skills, and the ability to run a library of cases of various degrees of difficulty enabling progressive training. Inherent to the fully computerized immersive simulation is the ability to "gamify" training. Each module, each procedure can be designed with adjustable levels of difficulty and gradual progression of learning. Even before moving to a more difficult case in a library, training can be made progressive by varying the use of virtual X-ray, changing the transparency of tissues, showing landmarks and other guiding instructions on the screen, etc. All these are already part of the immersive simulations. Multiple scenarios with background history and complications can be programed. Current immersive simulation allows for bone-drilling simulation with bone removal. The fully computerized platform generates its virtual patients from high-resolution medical imaging like MRI or CT of the same type used for operative navigation. This offers the potential for integration and preoperative planning.

However, current immersive simulation only qualifies as partial VR. It is still difficult to achieve good realism; many surgical steps are hard to simulate on a computer. Haptic feedback has value in VR simulation, making it a true VR, yet it is very difficult because of the very high-quality source images required, and the limitations of the robotic arms – the less expensive lack freedom of movement and realism of tissue resistance, and the more advanced robotic arms are very expensive. In spine, the problem is exacerbated by the varying nature of the tissues – ranging from soft fat, fluid to bone. The haptic interaction and visual deformation are very different, with sharp transitions from soft to hard that are difficult to simulate with electronic equipment. Current limited virtual reality simulation has demonstrated feasibility, face validity, and construct validity. Ongoing work by us and other groups includes realistic bone milling with 6 degrees of freedom of movement for the virtual drill [28] and varying tactile response and visual texture for bone drilling [29]. Notable progress has been made even since the latest. The current version of the lumbar laminectomy and pedicle screw placement meets the curricular criteria established by the Society of Neurological Surgeons for this simulation at Bootcamp2.

General Lessons and Future Directions

Over the years of development, simulation has made great inroads into surgical training. It has not yet replaced cadaver dissections, but a greater realization of the advantages of using a variety of methods for surgical education is evident [1]. The importance of a structured curriculum has been emphasized [13, 30]. We also learned that junior residents benefit most from simulation [30], which is expected, and this has been our experience as well. Cadaveric sessions will not remain the "golden standard," as they do not meet most of the criteria for ideal simulation. They represent authentic human anatomy but fail on other aspects. However, despite the recent progress and new publications, if we exclude cadaver-based surgical labs, the field of simulation for neurosurgical training is still in its infancy. This is particularly true for spine surgery. Much progress is needed, and I believe much of it will come from advances in fully computerized simulation. Key future directions can already be discerned from the technological perspective:

- One promise of computerized VR is the ability to rapidly create a VR model of the difficult case and perform the operation in virtual reality before the actual procedure. Ideally, the rehearsal images and pre-done case will someday be seamlessly integrated into the intraoperative navigation.
- There is a trajectory of improving performance and realism of computerized models. Increased realism of interactions with the bone is already in development. This will be followed by increasing realism in interaction with soft tissues.
- The utility of immersive computerized simulation training is cumulative, with expansion of user/training libraries of various anatomical deformations and variants and the generation of detailed curricula for a wide range of spinal procedures.

References

1. Kshettry VR, Mullin JP, Schlenk R, Recinos PF, Benzel EC. The role of laboratory dissection training in neurosurgical residency: results of a national survey. World Neurosurg. 2014;82(5):554–9.
2. Tomlinson JE, Yiasemidou M, Watts AL, Roberts DJ, Timothy J. Cadaveric spinal surgery simulation: a comparison of cadaver types. Global Spine J. 2016;6(4):357–61.
3. Lucas SM, Zeltser IS, Bensalah K, Tuncel A, Jenkins A, Pearle MS, Cadeddu JA. Training on a virtual reality laparoscopic simulator improves performance of an unfamiliar live laparoscopic procedure. J Urol. 2008;180(6):2588–91. discussion 2591
4. Suslu HT, Tatarli N, Karaaslan A, Demirel NA. Practical laboratory study simulating the lumbar microdiscectomy: training model in fresh cadaveric sheep spine. J Neurol Surg A Cent Eur Neurosurg. 2014;75(3):167–9.

5. Walker JB, Perkins E, Harkey HLA. Novel simulation model for minimally invasive spine surgery. Neurosurgery. 2009;65(6 Suppl):188–95.

6. Hollensteiner M, Fuerst D, Schrempf A. Artificial muscles for a novel simulator in minimally invasive spine surgery. Conf Proc IEEE Eng Med Biol Soc. 2014;2014:506–9.

7. Woodrow SI, Dubrowski A, Khokhotva M, Backstein D, Rampersaud YR, Massicotte EM. Training and evaluating spinal surgeons: the development of novel performance measures. Spine (Phila Pa 1976). 2007;32(25):2921–5.

8. Mattei TA, Frank C, Bailey J, Lesle E, Macuk A, Lesniak M, Patel A, Morris MJ, Nair K, Lin JJ. Design of a synthetic simulator for pediatric lumbar spine pathologies. J Neurosurg Pediatr. 2013;12(2):192–201.

9. Paiva WS, Amorim R, Bezerra DA, Masini M. Application of the stereolithography technique in complex spine surgery. Arq Neuropsiquiatr. 2007;65(2B):443–5.

10. Harrop J, Rezai AR, Hoh DJ, Ghobrial GM, Sharan A. Neurosurgical training with a novel cervical spine simulator: posterior foraminotomy and laminectomy. Neurosurgery. 2013;73(Suppl 1):94–9.

11. Ray WZ, Ganju A, Harrop JS, Hoh DJ. Developing an anterior cervical diskectomy and fusion simulator for neurosurgical resident training. Neurosurgery. 2013;73(Suppl 1):100–6.

12. Ghobrial GM, Anderson PA, Chitale R, Campbell PG, Lobel DA, Harrop J. Simulated spinal cerebrospinal fluid leak repair: an educational model with didactic and technical components. Neurosurgery. 2013;73(Suppl 1):111–5.

13. Ghobrial GM, Balsara K, Maulucci CM, Resnick DK, Selden NR, Sharan AD, Harrop JS. Simulation training curricula for neurosurgical residents: cervical Foraminotomy and Durotomy repair modules. World Neurosurg. 2015;84(3):751–5. e1-7

14. Bova FJ, Rajon DA, Friedman WA, Murad GJ, Hoh DJ, Jacob RP, Lampotang S, Lizdas DE, Lombard G, Lister JR. Mixed-reality simulation for neurosurgical procedures. Neurosurgery. 2013;73(Suppl 1):138–45.

15. Gottschalk MB, Yoon ST, Park DK, Rhee JM, Mitchell PM. Surgical training using three-dimensional simulation in placement of cervical lateral mass screws: a blinded randomized control trial. Spine J. 2015;15(1):168–75. https://doi.org/10.1016/j.spinee.2014.08.444. Epub 2014 Sep 4

16. Sundar SJ, Healy AT, Kshettry VR, Mroz TE, Schlenk R, Benzel EC. A pilot study of the utility of a laboratory-based spinal fixation training program for neurosurgical residents. J Neurosurg Spine, 2016; 24(5)850–6.

17. Adermann J, Geissler N, Bernal LE, Kotzsch S, Korb W. Development and validation of an artificial wetlab training system for the lumbar discectomy. Eur Spine J. 2014;23(9):1978–83.

18. Podolsky DJ, Martin AR, Whyne CM, Massicotte EM, Hardisty MR, Ginsberg HJ. Exploring the role of 3-dimensional simulation in surgical training: feedback from a pilot study. J Spinal Disord Tech. 2010;23(8):e70–4.

19. Eftekhar B, Ghodsi M, Ketabchi E, Rasaee S. Surgical simulation software for insertion of pedicle screws. Neurosurgery. 2002;50(1):222–3. discussion 223–4

20. Rambani R, Ward J, Viant W. Desktop-based computer-assisted orthopedic training system for spinal surgery. J Surg Educ. 2014;71(6):805–9.

21. Halic T, Kockara S, Bayrak C, Rowe R. Mixed reality simulation of rasping procedure in artificial cervical disc replacement (ACDR) surgery. BMC Bioinformatics. 2010;11(Suppl 6):S11.

22. Ra JB, Kwon SM, Kim JK, Yi J, Kim KH, Park HW, Kyung KU, Kwon DS, Kang HS, Kwon ST, Jiang L, Zeng J, Cleary K, Mun SK. Spine needle biopsy simulator using visual and force feedback. Comput Aided Surg. 2002;7(6):353–63.

23. Ghebreab S, Smeulders AW. Combining strings and necklaces for interactive three-dimensional segmentation of spinal images using an integral deformable spine model. IEEE Trans Biomed Eng. 2004;51(10):1821–9.

24. Teo JC, Chui CK, Wang ZL, Ong SH, Yan CH, Wang SC, Wong HK, Teoh SH. Heterogeneous meshing and biomechanical modeling of human spine. Med Eng Phys. 2007;29(2):277–90.

25. Luciano CJ, Banerjee PP, Bellotte B, Oh GM, Lemole M Jr, Charbel FT, Roitberg B. Learning retention of thoracic pedicle screw placement using a high-resolution augmented reality simulator with haptic feedback. Neurosurgery. 2011;69(1 Suppl Operative):ons14–9.

26. Luciano CJ, Banerjee PP, Sorenson JM, Foley KT, Ansari SA, Rizzi S, Germanwala AV, Kranzler L, Chittiboina P, Roitberg BZ. Percutaneous spinal fixation simulation with virtual reality and haptics. Neurosurgery. 2013;72(Suppl 1):89–96.

27. Gasco J, Patel A, Ortega-Barnett J, Branch D, Desai S, Kuo YF, Luciano C, Rizzi S, Kania P, Matuyauskas M, Banerjee P, Roitberg BZ. Virtual reality spine surgery simulation: an empirical study of its usefulness. Neurol Res. 2014;36(11):968–73.

28. Eriksson M, Wikander J. A 6 degrees-of-freedom haptic milling simulator for surgical training of vertebral operations. Stud Health Technol Inform. 2012;173:126–8.

29. Tsai MD, Hsieh MS. Accurate visual and haptic burring surgery simulation based on a volumetric model. J Xray Sci Technol. 2010;18(1):69–85.

30. Gasco J, Holbrook TJ, Patel A, Smith A, Paulson D, Muns A, Desai S, Moisi M, Kuo YF, Macdonald B, Ortega-Barnett J, Patterson JT. Neurosurgery simulation in residency training: feasibility, cost, and educational benefit. Neurosurgery. 2013;73(Suppl 1):39–45.

The Use of Simulation in the Training for Laser Interstitial Thermal Therapy for Amygdalo-hippocampectomy for Mesial Temporal Lobe Epilepsy

19

Dali Yin, Aviva Abosch, Steven Ojemann, and Konstantin V. Slavin

Introduction

Epilepsy is one of the most common, chronic, serious neurological disorders with the prevalence estimated at 0.5–1% [1, 2]. It affects approximately 3 million people in the United States [3] and more than 65 million people in the world [4]. Antiepileptic drugs are the mainstay of epilepsy treatment; however, one-third of patients with epilepsy become medically intractable [5–8] requiring neurosurgical evaluation and possible intervention. Epilepsy is associated with considerable morbidity and mortality [9]. The incidence of sudden unexplained death in patients with epilepsy is reported to be 2–5 per 1000 person-years in chronic epilepsy and up to 9 per 1000 among candidates for epilepsy surgery [10]. Surgical treatments of epilepsy include open resection or lesionectomy, open destruction or disconnection of epileptic brain tissue, laser interstitial thermal

therapy, and neuromodulation including deep brain stimulation, responsive neurostimulation, and vagus nerve stimulation. Epilepsy surgery is now widely accepted as an effective therapeutic option in carefully selected patients [11–15] and should be considered for patients with drug-resistant epilepsy and disabling seizures [16] in the hope of achieving seizure control. Therefore, there is an obvious need for neurosurgeon to learn these surgical techniques for the treatment of patients with epilepsy.

The surgical approach for epilepsy depends on many considerations, including focal or generalized seizures, localization and extent of the epileptogenic zone, MRI findings, preoperative monitoring, and balance of risk and benefit of procedures [17]. For appropriately chosen patients, anterior temporal lobectomy is gold standard in the treatment of temporal lobe epilepsy caused by hippocampal sclerosis [18–20]. However, 5–11% of epilepsy surgery is associated with complications, including dysphasia, memory decline, and hemiparesis [16]. Moreover, it has been reported that seizure recurred in approximately one-third of these seizure-free patients after temporal lobectomy during a 5-year follow-up [21].

The field of epilepsy has undergone remarkable transformation in the recent years due to advancement in science technology and development of novel devices. Magnetic resonance-guided laser

D. Yin · K. V. Slavin (✉)
Department of Neurosurgery, University of Illinois at Chicago, Chicago, IL, USA
e-mail: daliyin@uic.edu; kslavin@uic.edu

A. Abosch · S. Ojemann
Department of Neurosurgery, University of Colorado, Denver, CO, USA
e-mail: aviva.abosch@ucdenver.edu; steven.ojemann@ucdenver.edu

interstitial thermal therapy (MRgLITT) with Visualase technique (Medtronic, Minneapolis, MN) has been developed as a minimally invasive therapy for selected patients with mesial temporal lobe epilepsy. It potentially decreases the risks and complications associated with an open surgical procedure [22, 23]. It has been reported that stereotactic laser ablation of the amygdala and hippocampus resulted in meaningful seizure reduction in 77% and freedom from disabling seizures in 54% of patients [23]. Clinical study also suggests that MRgLITT provides outcomes comparable to resection in patients older than 50 [22]. Laser ablation of an epileptogenic focus has its advantages as compared to open surgery, such as less invasive procedure, precise targeting of the seizure-producing focus, least damage to and minimal disruption of healthy brain tissue, and reduction of hospital stays and costs [24, 25]. MRgLITT may offer a valuable therapeutic option to reduce the frequency and severity of seizures and improve the quality of life of the patients [26]. Moreover, as the indications for MRgLITT rise, the opportunity to do traditional temporal lobectomy is decreased.

However, MRgLITT is a technically sophisticated procedure that requires thoughtful judgment, technical expertise, meticulous focus, and fellowship training to minimize risks to patients. Moreover, high level of functioning in patients with temporal lobe epilepsy and esoteric interventions of laser ablation procedure performed in fewer medical centers has prevented hands-on training for neurosurgery residents. Therefore, improvement in such training and education is very important for both neurosurgery residents and ultimately patient safety. Working-hour restrictions of residents make it necessary to deliver high-quality training to surgeons in less time while ensuring optimal patient outcomes.

Simulation involves the use of models as a means to practice difficult procedures. It has been reported that simulation can provide appropriate training for neurosurgeons and allow them to obtain surgical skills and knowledge in a safe environment. This chapter focuses on the simulation of laser ablation of amygdalo-hippocampectomy for treatment of mesial tem-

poral epilepsy, which may be able to provide residents with realistic learning environment for improved performance of this procedure.

It has been clear that the ideal place for the initial acquisition and refinement of surgical skills, including MRgLITT, is not in the operating room. Moreover, it is required that neurosurgeons master fundamental technical skills in order to provide safe patient care. Simulation-based training enables surgeon to reproduce the MRgLITT techniques in a safe and protected environment. Simulation is diverse as a concept, including virtual reality (such as computer simulators), physical models (such as cadaveric models and synthetic models), and mixed-reality stimulator concerning on technical and nontechnical skills and knowledges. Simulation can serve as a useful platform for neurosurgeon training and provides surgeons with opportunities to refine techniques and enhance the safety and efficacy of surgical procedures before the actual clinical practice. The deliberate study with simulation would be an efficient learning strategy for MRgLITT procedure. The effectiveness of simulation training can be evaluated by the trainee and facility members at the site. One of the advantages of simulation is that surgeons can go back to simulation training repeatedly until they feel comfortable to perform laser ablation of epileptogenic focus to treat patients with epilepsy. Importantly, simulation training may help surgeons to avoid technical mistakes or failure, which may result in devastating consequences. Moreover, feedback from participants can also improve the simulation training course.

Laser Catheter Trajectory Planning with Brainlab Software

Surgeons can be trained using virtual reality for surgical planning of MRgLITT. The details are described as the following.

Laser ablation amygdalo-hippocampectomy requires high-level accuracy for accessing small and deep-seated target structures, the amygdala and hippocampus. We use the iPlan® Stereotaxy for target and trajectory planning (Software User

Guide Rev. 1.3 iPlan Stereotaxy Ver 3.0) for laser ablation amygdalo-hippocampectomy. The functional planning workflow is recommended for this complex treatment, which requires careful and time-intensive preoperative planning. The advantage of the functional planning workflow is that the patients only wear the head frame for stereotactic localization and during the final treatment. Treatment planning includes loading and importing image data; registration of patient data including stereotactic localization, image fusion, anterior commissure (AC), and posterior commissure (PC) localization; planning trajectories; and checking and modifying arc setting.

Stereotactic Localization

With the **localization** planning task, you can assign the localizer to the selected image set and perform stereotactic localization. Head CT and MR images can be used; we prefer to choose CT images. Stereotactic localization provides a specific coordinate system for Leksell or CRW frame in which it is possible to calculate the arc settings for a planned trajectory. Stereotactic localization should be performed prior to image fusion and planning trajectories.

To perform localization with head CT, you need to (1) select an image set from the "Image Sets" box in the functions area; (2) select a Leksell or CRW localizer from "Localizer" dialog, making sure to select the same head frame that is used during CT scanning; (3) localize the image set using "Assign Localizer"; and (4) carefully verify each slice in the main view to ensure that localization has been successful. The software localizes the available slices and displays a status report of the localization. This provides a frame of reference for the slice set. Depending on the localization result, the color of the slices varies in the catalog overview. Green indicates slices are successfully localized; yellow indicates slices have been localized, but precision is low due to one or more misplaced rod markers, poor image quality, or an inaccurate localizer geometry; and red indicates slices could not be localized. Localization depends on reliable hardware. If the localizer hardware is defective due to, for example, bubbles in the rods, localization will not be possible. If the rod geometry of head frame is not correct, this can either cause localization to fail or lead to incorrect results. If slices are located beyond the localizer rod geometry and could not be successfully localized, select the relevant slices and click "Ignore." The "Ignore" function allows you to localize slices with insufficient rod marker definition but does not delete slices from the localization. For failed localization, check the assigned localizer and if head CT is done in a correct way. If the wrong localizer has been selected, assign the correct localizer and repeat localization.

Image Fusion

Image fusion allows you to fuse together two or more image sets with CT and MRI with automatic fusion method. To do image fusion, first choose fusion pairs, and then activate automatic fusion. The software fuses the selected image sets together by shifting and rotating the images based on anatomical structures common to both image sets. Once the images are fused, you can visually verify the accuracy of the image fusion by dragging the spyglass area over important anatomical landmarks and comparing them at the two image sets. Usually the image fusion is very satisfactory. Once two image sets are fused, all targets and trajectories planned in one image set are visible in the other image set.

AC and PC Localization

In AC and PC localization, the AC/PC system can be determined in midsagittal plane of T1 MR images. To define the AC/PC system, by clicking "Set AC/PC system" in the functions area, the default AC/PC system is displayed in the image views. To modify the AC/PC system, enable "Set AC/PC system," place the mouse pointer onto the AC/PC system in the image views, click the mouse pointer and drag the AC/PC system to reposition it, or adjust planes by rotating image.

AC and PC localization is required for patient orientation, alignment of the reconstructed views, trajectory planning based on definable AC/PC coordinates, and matching of Schaltenbrand-Wahren atlas images to patient images. For laser ablation amygdalo-hippocampectomy, AC and PC localization is not necessary because targets can be visualized clearly.

Stereotactic Planning

You need to know the anatomy of the amygdala and hippocampus well for stereotactic panning. To create trajectory, by clicking "New Trajectory," you can name the trajectory, define a diameter for the trajectory in millimeters, and select a color for the trajectory.

It is better to give each trajectory a name so it can be clearly identified. To position trajectory, by clicking the "Target" button, click the amygdala on the image to place the target point, and by clicking the "Entry" button, click the occipital scalp on the image to place the entry point. Once a trajectory is added, it can be viewed and verified in the image views. To get arc setting, just click "Arc Setting." To adjust values for the target coordinates in millimeters and the angle parameter in degrees, enter the values in the fields provided, X, Y, Z, ring angle, and arc angle. Trajectories and depth position along the track can be viewed and verified with the probe view to make sure sulci and blood are avoided by surgical trajectory. Lastly, save treatment plan and exit iPlan.

Surgical Techniques of Laser Ablation Amygdalo-Hippocampectomy

Surgeons can be trained using physical models for MRgLITT technique. The details are described as the following.

Laser ablation amygdalo-hippocampectomy is often used to treat mesial temporal lobe epilepsy. In brief, the patient presented on the morning of surgery, and the Leksell stereotactic head frame is applied under local anesthesia in the preoperative area. Patients undergo a stereotactic head CT scan and MRI with the Leksell frame in place. These images are inspected for adequacy, exported to the Brainlab navigation system, and merged with one another. The accuracy of image fusion is confirmed by navigation to common anatomical landmarks. The surgical planning regarding the target for amygdala and hippocampus and trajectory of laser probe are manually performed in three planes (Fig. 19.1). The Brainlab planning software provides us with the ability of optimizing the occipital entry point and linear trajectory through the long axis of the hippocampal body and into the amygdala while avoiding vasculature in the sulcus and the choroid plexus in the ventricle if possible. This produces an X, Y, and Z coordinates and arc and ring angle for the Leksell frame.

Patient is taken to the operating room, and fiber-optic intubation is performed. Patient is given a dose of intravenous antibiotics for surgical wound infection prophylaxis. Under general anesthesia, patient is placed in the semi-sitting position. Care is taken to pad all pressure points, and the left occipital region is prepped and draped in the usual sterile fashion. The Leksell frame is assembled according to preplanned coordinates, and the entry point is defined on the scalp surface. This area is infiltrated with local anesthesia, and a small incision is made with a #15 blade. Then the arc and ring angles are reset and the Stryker drill guide is advanced to the bone surface. The drill is introduced with a depth stop placed 1 cm beyond the edge of the cannula, and then a small twist drill craniostomy is performed. When the loss of resistance is encountered, a sharp stylet is placed through the appropriate reducing tube and the dura is coagulated and traversed with this instrument. Next, the Visualase bolt is applied through the appropriate bushing and T wrench. Under fluoroscopic guidance, stylet is introduced through the Visualase bolt and slowly to the arc center. The Visualase laser fiber (Fig. 19.2) is introduced and monitored under real-time fluoroscopy until it is at the target and secured at the bolt with the screw tip.

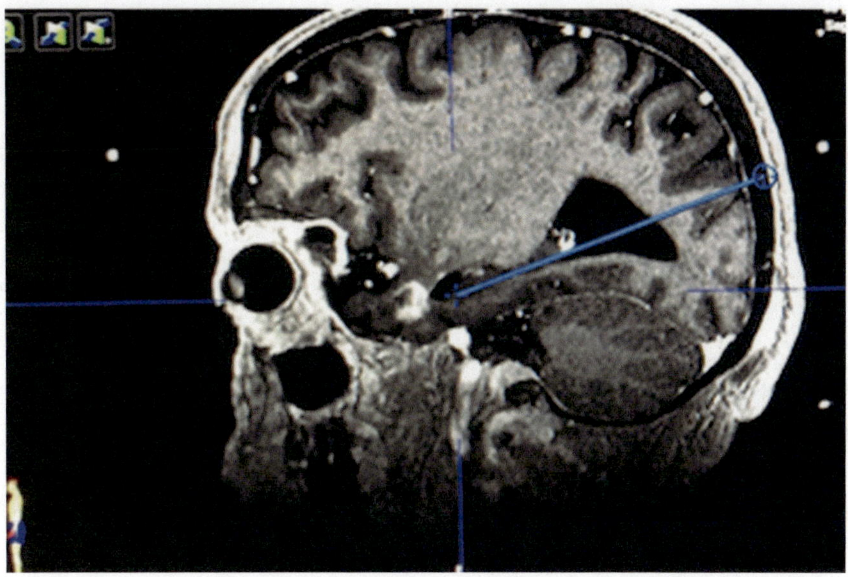

Fig. 19.1 Trajectory planning using Brainlab software for laser ablation amygdalo-hippocampectomy

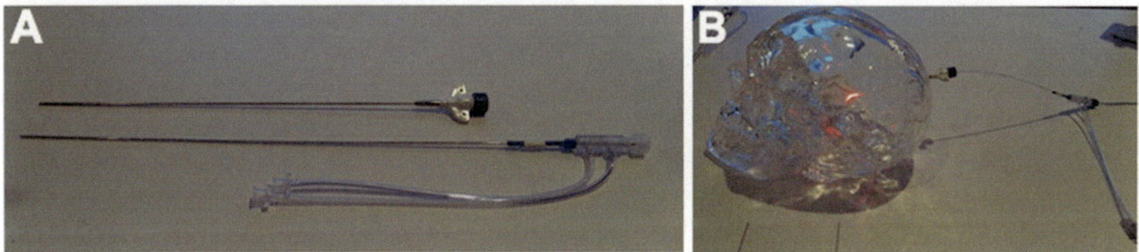

Fig. 19.2 (**a**) laser cooling catheter and stylets; (**b**) simulation of laser ablation amygdalo-hippocampectomy

Patient is then taken down to MRI scanner, taking great care to avoid disruption of the laser fiber. Patient is carefully positioned within the transmit-receive coil, with head turned to the right side and care taken to pad all pressure points. In the MRI scanner, localizing and planning scans are obtained. The cooling system and laser were connected to the workstation. The safety regions in adjacent thalamus and cerebral peduncles were designated with temperature limits to minimize off-target thermal damage to surrounding normal tissue. A test dose with 30% laser power is undertaken to confirm MR images are set right and heating appears at both the right target and the tip of the cooling catheter. The 70% laser power is then used for thermal ablation. Using the Visualase software, laser is tested with a test dose and then an initial lesion is made in the first position. Estimate of the ablated tissue is provided by the software as shown by MRI thermography (Fig. 19.3), and based on the initial lesion, a second lesion is performed then after withdrawing the laser 10 mm. A total of four to six ablations need to be performed with sequential withdrawals, and some interval imaging is performed using FLAIR sequences to assess the lesion as it is partially completed. The lesions usually involve the amygdala, hippocampus, and parahippocampal gyrus. The ablation power and time may be different case by case. A T1-weighted image with gadolinium, FLAIR image, and diffusion-weighted images are performed to assess the full extent of the lesions prior to removal (Fig. 19.4). Following this, laser fiber is completely withdrawn, bolt removed, and skin incision closed with a suture. Patient is extubated and admitted to the intensive care unit for observation.

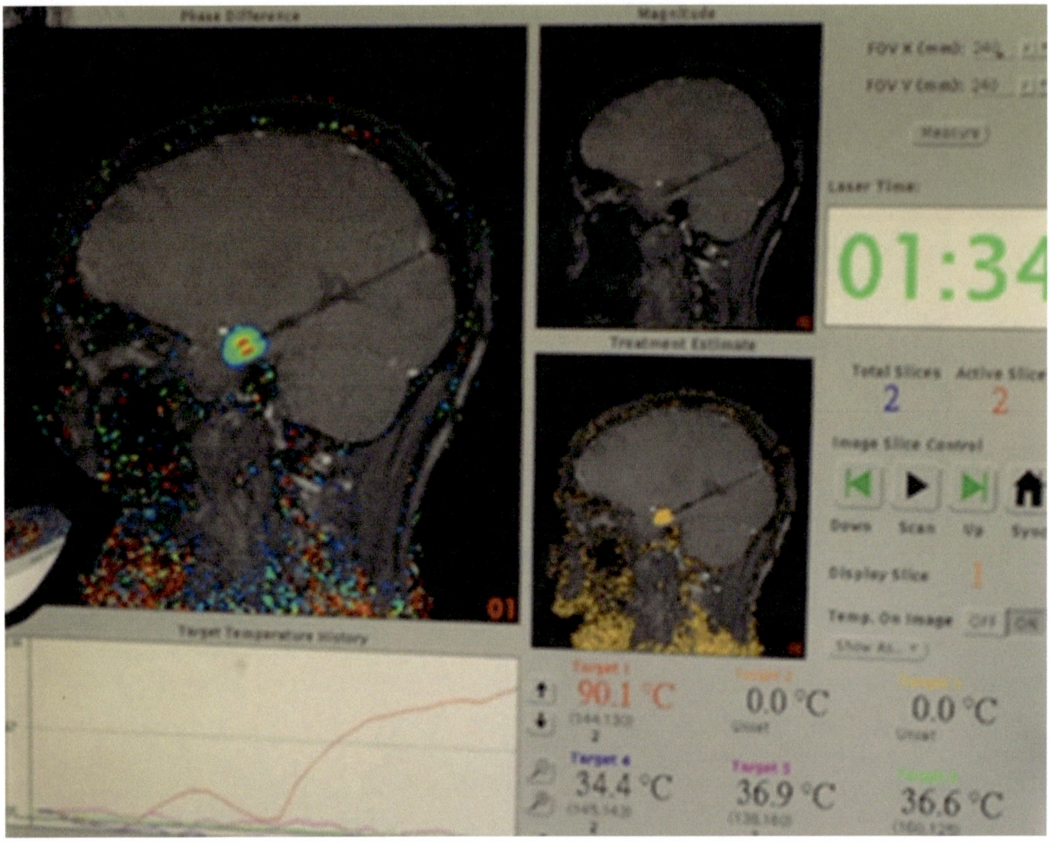

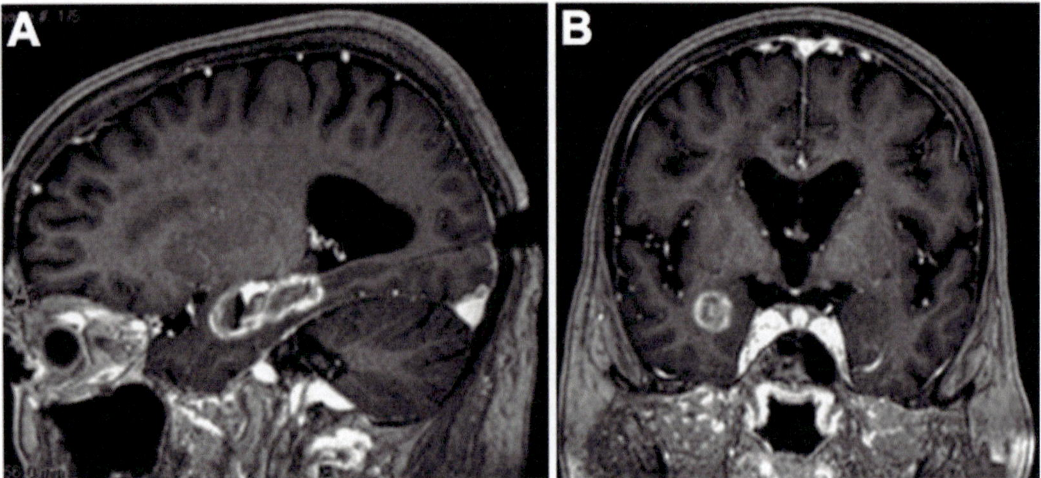

Fig. 19.3 MRI thermography during laser ablation amygdalo-hippocampectomy

Fig. 19.4 Post-gadolinium MRI scan (**a**, sagittal; **b**, coronal) at the completion of laser ablation disclosed enhancement surrounding inferior amygdala and hippocampus, back to the level of the tectal plate

In summary, this book chapter provides information about simulation of laser ablation amygdalo-hippocampectomy for treatment of mesial temporal epilepsy, which may allow residents to acquire the knowledge and surgical skills in this regard in a safe environment.

References

1. Wu CY, Sharan AD. Neurostimulation for the treatment of epilepsy: a review of current surgical interventions. Neuromodulation. 2013;16:10–24.
2. Hirtz D, Thurman DJ, Gwinn-Hardy K, Mohamed M, Chaudhuri AR, Zalutsky R. How common are the common neurologic disorders? Neurology. 2007;68:326–37.
3. Salanova V, Witt T, Worth R, Henry TR, Gross RE, Nazzaro JM, Labar D, Sperling MR, Sharan A, Sandok E, Handforth A, Stern JM, Chung S, Henderson JM, French J, Baltuch G, Rosenfeld WE, Garcia P, Barbaro NM, Fountain NB, Elias WJ, Goodman RR, Pollard JR, Troster AI, Irwin CP, Lambrecht K, Graves N, Fisher R. Long-term efficacy and safety of thalamic stimulation for drug-resistant partial epilepsy. Neurology. 2015;84:1017–25.
4. Thurman DJ, Beghi E, Begley CE, et al. And the ILAE commission on epidemiology. Standards for epidemiologic studies and surveillance of epilepsy. Epilepsia. 2011;52(suppl 7):2–26.
5. Kwan P, Brodie MJ. Early identification of refractory epilepsy. N Engl J Med. 2000;342:314–9.
6. Devinsky O, Pacia S. Epilepsy surgery. Neurol Clin. 1993;11:951–71.
7. Engel J Jr. Surgery for seizures. N Engl J Med. 1996;334:647–52.
8. Connor DE Jr, Nixon M, Nanda A, Guthikonda B. Vagal nerve stimulation for the treatment of medically refractory epilepsy: a review of the current literature. Neurosurg Focus. 2012;32(3):E12.
9. World Health Organization. The world health report 2001 – mental health: new understanding, new hope. Geneva: World Health Organization; 2001. Available from: http://www.who.int/whr/2001/en/whr01_en.pdf?ua=1. Accessed 18 Sept 2014
10. Tomson T, Nashef L, Ryvlin P. Sudden unexpected death in epilepsy: current knowledge and future directions. Lancet Neurol. 2008;7:1021–31.
11. Engel J, Wiebe S, French J, et al. Practice parameter: temporal lobe and localized neocortical resection for epilepsy. Epilepsia. 2003;44:741–51.
12. Spencer SS, Berg AT, Vickrey BG, et al. For the multicenter study of epilepsy surgery. Initial outcomes in the multicenter study of epilepsy surgery. Neurology. 2003;61:1680–5.
13. McIntosh AM, Kalnins RM, Mitchell LA, Fabinyi GC, Briellman RS, Berkovic SF. Temporal lobectomy: long term seizure outcome, late recurrence, and risks for seizure recurrence. Brain. 2004;127:2018–30.
14. Wallace SJ, Farrell K, editors. Epilepsy in children. 2nd ed. London: Arnold Publishers; 2004.
15. Berg A, Shinnar s, Levy SR, Testa FM, Smith-Rapaport S, Beckerman B. Early development of intractable epilepsy in children. Neurology. 2001;56:1445–52.
16. Jette N, Reid AY, Wiebe S. Surgical management of epilepsy. CMAJ. 2014;186:997–1003.
17. Elger CE, Schmidt D. Modern management of epilepsy: a practical approach. Epilepsy Behav. 2008;12:501–39.
18. Chang EF, Englot DJ, Vadera S. Minimally invasive surgical approaches for temporal lobe epilepsy. Epilepsy Behav. 2015;47:24–33.
19. Wiebe S, Blume WT, Girvin JP, Eliasziw M. Effectiveness and efficiency of surgery for temporal lobe epilepsy study group. A randomized, controlled trial of surgery for temporal-lobe epilepsy. N Engl J Med. 2001;345:311–8.
20. Duncan JS. Epilepsy surgery. Clin Med. 2007;7:137–42.
21. Schmidt D, Baumgartner C, LoÅNscher W. Seizure recurrence after planned discontinuation of antiepileptic drugs in seizure-free patients after epilepsy surgery: a review of current clinical experience. Epilepsia. 2004;45:179–86.
22. Waseem H, Osborn KE, Schoenberg MR, Kelley V, Bozorg A, Cabello D, Benbadis SR, Vale FL. Laser ablation therapy: an alternative treatment for medically resistant mesial temporal lobe epilepsy after age 50. Epilepsy Behav. 2015;51:152–7.
23. Willie JT, Laxpati NG, Drane DL, Gowda A, Appin C, Hao C, Brat DJ, Helmers SL, Saindane A, Nour SG, Gross RE. Real-time magnetic resonance-guided stereotactic laser amygdalohippocampotomy for mesial temporal lobe epilepsy. Neurosurgery. 2014;74:569–85.
24. Hawasli AH, Bandt SK, Hogan RE, Werner N, Leuthardt EC. Laser ablation as treatment strategy for medically refractory dominant insular epilepsy: therapeutic and functional considerations. Stereotact Funct Neurosurg. 2014;92:397–404.
25. Hawasli AH, Bagade S, Shimony JS, Miller-Thomas M, Leuthardt EC. Magnetic resonance imaging-guided focused laser interstitial thermal therapy for intracranial lesions: single-institution series. Neurosurgery. 2013;73:1007–17.
26. Salanova V, Witt T, Worth R, Henry TR, Gross RE, Nazzaro JM, Labar D, Sperling MR, Sharan A, Sandok E, Handforth A, Stern JM, Chung S, Henderson JM, French J, Baltuch G, Rosenfeld WE, Garcia P, Barbaro NM, Fountain NB, Elias WJ, Goodman RR, Pollard JR, Troster AI, Irwin CP, Lambrecht K, Graves N, Fisher R. Long-term efficacy and safety of thalamic stimulation for drug-resistant partial epilepsy. Neurology. 2015;84:1017–25.

Future of Visualization and Simulation in Neurosurgery

Laura Stone McGuire, Amanda Kwasnicki,
Rahim Ismail, Talia Weiss, Fady T. Charbel,
and Ali Alaraj

Introduction

Technological advancement defines the practice of neurosurgery, perhaps more than any medical specialty. The advent of computed tomography in the 1972 revolutionized how we visualize the nervous system [1], and similarly, the development of three-dimensional image reconstruction has allowed for dramatic changes in neurosurgical education, surgical precision, and even synthetic implantation.

Perhaps the most fundamental change in neurosurgical imaging of recent history has been the invention of the computed tomography scan, prior to which physicians were limited to plain films and crude angiography. The initial version of the scanner was utilized in South London in hopes of better characterizing a potential frontal lobe tumor. The voxel dimension at the time was 3 mm × 3 mm × 13 mm [1]. Since its installation in the United States in 1973, the use of this technology has grown dramatically, with 82 million procedures reported in 2016 and a spatial resolution of up to 0.24 mm [2, 3].

Inception of magnetic resonance imaging (MRI) for clinical use occurred in a similar timeframe, initially focused on the differentiation of tumors. In 1977, report of the first MRI scan was published [4]. This scan of the thorax utilized two magnets at 0.1 tesla each and produced a resolution of approximately 0.25 inches. In 2013, over 33 million MRIs were performed in the United States [5]. The newest MRI technology boasts a 7 T magnetic field and 0.2 mm spatial resolution and is utilized heavily for the brain [6, 7].

The natural consequence of these increasingly high definition two-dimensional images was their three-dimensional reconstructions. Mathematical algorithms are utilized in order to create reconstruction techniques that allow rendering of a three-dimensional image. Common algorithms for three-dimensional rendering include maximum intensity projections, minimum intensity projections, shaded surface virtual rendering, and multiplanar reconstructions [8].

Virtual and augmented reality now enhances both neurosurgical education and operative technique, specifically in their ability to simulate neurosurgical cases and surgical planning. Arguably, through the use of simulation, the quality of care and patient safety subsequently improve as well. Virtual simulators, such as ImmersiveTouch ®, have been developed for a

L. S. McGuire · A. Kwasnicki · F. T. Charbel
A. Alaraj (✉)
Department of Neurosurgery, University of Illinois at Chicago, Chicago, IL, USA
e-mail: Alaraj@uic.edu

R. Ismail
Department of Neurosurgery, University of Rochester Medical Center, Rochester, NY, USA

T. Weiss
College of Applied Health Sciences, University of Illinois at Chicago, Chicago, IL, USA

© Springer International Publishing AG, part of Springer Nature 2018
A. Alaraj (ed.), *Comprehensive Healthcare Simulation: Neurosurgery*,
Comprehensive Healthcare Simulation, https://doi.org/10.1007/978-3-319-75583-0_20

variety of procedures, such as ventriculostomy, bone drilling, hemostasis, trigeminal rhizotomy, aneurysm clipping, lumbar punctures, vertebroplasty, and percutaneous spinal fixation [9–19]. Studies conducted in which residents used this learning aid have shown positive effects on first time cannulation, improved percutaneous needle accuracy, and decreased fluoroscopy time. While ImmersiveTouch ® involves a cubicle-style workstation for training purposes, even more recent developments of virtual reality have utilized more mobile structures, such as the Microsoft HoloLens ®, to aid in placement of extraventricular drains at the bedside [20]. The rapid progress in this arena is making such integration of technology into both training and practice a soon-to-be reality.

As the field of neurosurgery has advanced, so have the visualization techniques that are implemented. In neurosurgery, a variety of new technologies have been introduced, which will be reviewed in this chapter. A sampling of these forms of visualization of operative anatomy and surgical simulation will be discussed, including three-dimensional visualization, stereoscopy, virtual reality, augmented reality, and mixed reality platforms. Often, these technologies overlap and integrate multiple visualization modalities.

Three-Dimensional Visualization

Two-dimensional formatting of imaging is the traditional viewing of studies. Magnetic resonance imaging, computed tomography scans, conventional angiography, and ultrasound all present the acquired images in a two-dimensional format on a computer screen. While the technological advances in visualization of the human nervous system expanded capabilities of neurosurgeons, severe limitations remain. Specifically, depth perception was an absent feature, and it has been this recreation of depth in imaging modalities that has led to three-dimensional reconstructions.

In computed tomography, several algorithms for post-processing segmentation and three-dimensional rendering for CT imaging have been developed: multiplanar reformations with maximum intensity projections or post-processing reconstructions, such as surface rendering, volume rendering, and cinematic rendering. MRI has similar post-processing techniques for generating three-dimensional reconstructions. Three-dimensional rendering enhances viewing of pathology for physicians and surgeons; however, despite these advances, these reconstructions remain three-dimensional projections on a two-dimensional workstation.

Various advances have attempted to circumvent this limitation: three-dimensional stereoscopy, virtual reality, augmented reality, and mixed reality. These different modalities also incorporate varying degrees of immersion and interactivity. Several examples of these technologies will be explored in the next sections.

Image Processing Software: Conventional Angiography and MRI

An example of software that provides automatized, interactive, and editable three-dimensional reconstructions includes the Siemens ® syngo ® with DynaCT ® (Siemens, Erlangen, Germany) for conventional cerebral angiography [21]. This software provides an almost instantaneous three-dimensional reconstruction of the two-dimensional images captured. Because this software is based on defined user presets, no manual post-processing is necessary. This system synchronizes with the biplane angiography suite for endovascular procedures and allows for selected dimensions of the three-dimensional reconstruction to project to each C-arm for optimal positioning. The literature describes several uses of syngo ® in neurointerventional cases, such as hypotensive balloon occlusion testing [22], the use of stent retrievers in acute stroke [23], cerebral aneurysm treatment with flow-diverter devices [24], and indirect measurement of arteriovenous malformation hemodynamics [25] (Fig. 20.1).

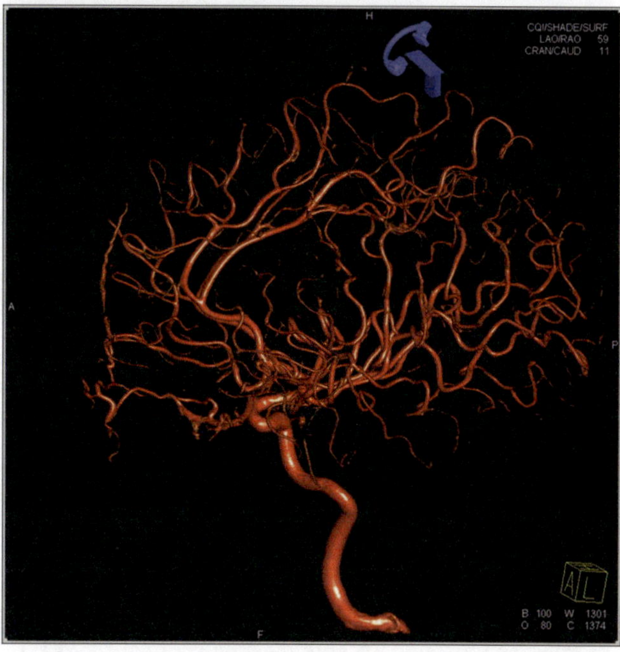

Fig. 20.1 © Courtesy of Siemens® syngo®

Analogous to the image processing of syngo ® for conventional angiography, BrainSuite (UCLA and USC, Los Angeles, CA) is a collection of open-source software tools that enable interactive and mostly automated image processing of data from human brain MRI [26]. This program extracts and segments layers of the cerebral cortex from standard DICOM files, processes this data, and uses joint surface and volume rendering for further analysis. An easy-to-use interface allows users to process, visualize, manipulate, and study imaging data. BrainSuite also contains a statistical toolbox, which supports additional analyses for research purposes. Multiple applications of BrainSuite have been published, particularly in magnetoencephalography and stereoelectroencephalography in epilepsy and focal cortical dysplasia and also in atlasing neurological disease processes, such as Huntington, Alzheimer, and Rasmussen diseases [27–33]. More recently, a visualization technique for intracranial tumors and vasculature using BrainSuite software has also been described to generate interactive three-dimensional reconstructions, utilizing standard MRI T1-weighted sequences with MR angiography and venography [34]. However, BrainSuite has not yet been integrated into surgical planning or navigational usages.

Three-Dimensional Stereoscopy

Stereoscopy creates an illusion of depth and three-dimensional structure within an image through binocular vision. This technique originated in the early nineteenth century with the invention of the Wheatstone stereoscope, and it has been developed over time for various industries, from entertainment to healthcare. Multiple virtual reality systems integrate stereoscopy to provide the desired depth perception. This visualization form capitalizes on one feature of the complexity of human vision, called stereopsis, that uses horizontal disparities seen between two eyes to generate a perception of depth and relative distance. Stereoscopy produces this perceived three-dimensional image through the presentation of dual, slightly different, two-dimensional images to each eye, subsequently processed in the visual cortex. However, this visualization modality imperfectly generates depth perception for several reasons, among which: first, the image focus may not be adjusted appropriately among different items of varying distances from the viewer and, second, a mismatch between convergence and accommodation to light for the viewer's eyes due to disparity among the perceived object position and the actual light source creating the image.

Surgical Microscope Applications: TrueVision ® and Trenion ®

TrueVision ® (Santa Barbara, CA) is a stereoscopic, three-dimensional high-definition visualization system that displays the surgical field of view in real time on a flat-panel display in the operating room [35]. TrueVision ® has developed a digital surgery platform more recently utilized in neurological microsurgery, which integrates applications for both existing surgical microscopes and a digital surgical microscope to replace the traditional optical surgical microscopes. TrueVision ® software goes beyond the existing optical microscope software and creates digital surgical platforms, allowing the surgeon to integrate patient data with robotics, precise visualization, and intraoperative navigation. This software translates the existing surgical field seen through the microscope onto a three-dimensional-capable screen, which has twice the depth of the field over the optics. Small movements with this software translate to the wide image screen, enhancing deliberate instrument control. The surgeon then may record and edit three-dimensional videos of surgical procedures and integrate the images with patient data including CT, MRI, and cerebral angiography images (Fig. 20.2).

Zeiss Trenion ® (Dublin, CA) is a similar stereoscopic, high-definition video system that integrates with the OPMI ® PENTERO ® 800 or 900 microscope to translate the existing surgical field viewed through the eyepiece of the microscope to a three-dimensional viewing screen [36]. This software enables surgeons to share three-dimensional images in real time with all members of the operative team within the operating room, enhancing the educational experience overall. Three-dimensional visualization of the surgical field grants viewers with a more comprehensive and detailed understanding of complex surgical anatomy and surgical techniques.

Stereoscopic Virtual Reality Simulators: Dextroscope and Dextrobeam

The Dextroscope ®, developed by Volume Interactions LTD (Bracco Group, Princeton, NJ), is a stereoscopic, virtual reality environment in which the user's hands are immersed into patient data, allowing for more precise preoperative planning and practice of surgical technique [37]. The virtual patient is composed of computer-generated, three-dimensional multimodal images obtained from DICOM tomographic data, including CT, CTA, CTV, MRI, MRA, MRV, PET, SPECT, functional MRI, and tractography. Using stereoscopic visualizations displayed via a mirror, the user sees the patient floating behind the mirror within reach and is able to manipulate and rotate the patient using hand movements. One hand of the user holds a handle, which allows the three-dimensional image to be moved in space, and in the other hand, the user holds a pencil-shaped stylus, which is used to select a variety of instruments from a virtual control panel to perform detailed manipulations and operations on the three-dimensional patient image. Also designed by Bracco Imaging, the Dextrobeam ® replaces the mirror display of the Dextroscope ® with a different stereoscopic display, either a large monitor or projector, allowing for more interactivity and collaboration among both large and small groups [38]

The application of the Dextroscope ® in perioperative planning in neurosurgery has been explored extensively since its release. The Dextroscope ® employs an interactive, three-dimensional interface, called virtual intracranial visualization and navigation (VIVIAN), for coregistration of patient data and selective segmentation of imaging studies into the bone and soft tissue [39]. The anatomy of the virtual reality productions has been compared to human cadavers in several studies to validate the simulations

Fig. 20.2 © Courtesy
of TrueVision ®

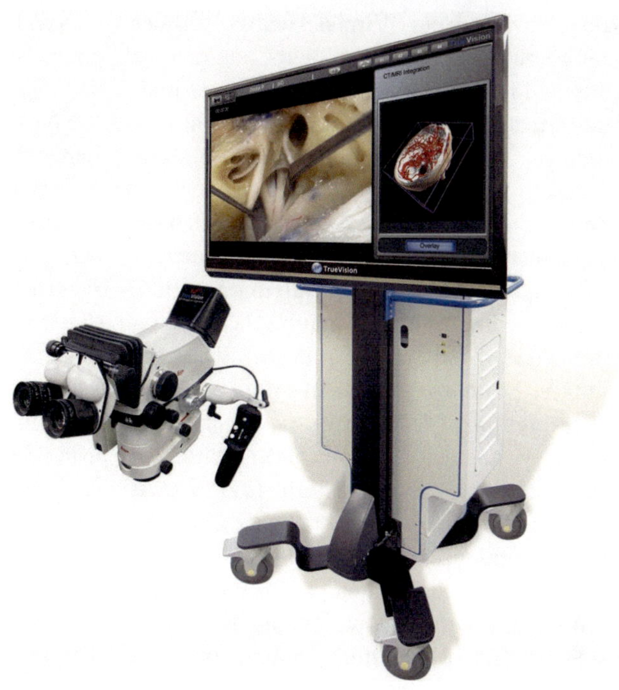

and to demonstrate its utility as an adjunct in education and preoperative planning. For instance, the anatomy of the temporal bridging veins of 25 patients in planning tumor resections across the petrosal crest were accurately simulated by this stereoscopic, virtual reality device when compared to the 20 human cadavers [40]. Dextroscope ® simulations have been investigated in a variety of neurosurgical scenarios, including operative management of sellar and skull base tumors [41–44], gliomas within eloquent cortex [45], arteriovenous malformations [46, 47], cerebral aneurysms [48–51], epilepsy [52], cranial nerve decompression [53, 54], spinal lesions [55, 56], and more.

Virtual Reality

Virtual reality technology generates realistic images and sounds as well as other sensations, such as haptic feedback, to simulate three-dimensional, real, or imaginary, physical environments to the user. Over the past decade especially, virtual reality has become increasingly popular with both mainstream and specialty use and a plethora of applications. In addition, virtual reality head-mounted displays have been produced by multiple companies, and examples include Oculus Rift ®, Samsung Gear VR ®, and HTC Vive ®, among others. These headsets enable the user to observe and explore the virtual world, and more advanced technology involves interactive elements, including games and Internet connectivity.

Virtual reality may be visualized in multiple modalities: immersive, semi-immersive, or non-immersive configurations and interactive or non-interactive formats. *Immersive* technology stimulates the senses to create perceptually real sensations, including not only visual and audio cues but also tactile and olfactory information, whereas non-immersive modalities only allow the user to view the virtual world through a portal or window. Importantly, immersion differentiates from another term commonly used in this setting, *presence*. Presence refers to the subjective sensation of immersion of the user within the virtual environment, equating the virtual experience to a real one; it's the "magic" of virtual reality to suspend disbelief. Within *interactive* platforms, users manipulate and engage the virtual environment. Virtual reality further encompasses two emerging fields, augmented reality and mixed reality, which layer and integrate virtual elements with the user's real surroundings and will be discussed in later sections.

In healthcare, virtual reality simulators have become incorporated in medical school curriculums, residency training, and patient education. Specifically, neurosurgical training is evolving with the use of virtual reality, especially as the field faces challenges in patient safety and duty hour restrictions. The literature on virtual simulators in graduate medical education focuses on basic procedural skill acquisition [57]; virtual simulations allow residents to learn anatomy, practice techniques, develop skills, and receive feedback, prior to introduction into the operating room [58]. Furthermore, it could accommodate preoperative planning, which may be integrated into intraoperative navigational systems. Virtual simulator modules have also been issued to teach the "fundamentals of neurosurgery," including ventriculostomy, endoscopic nasal navigation, tumor debulking, hemostasis, and microdissection using the NeuroTouch ® device [59].

Virtual Reality and Surgical Planning: Surgical Theater ®

Current virtual reality simulation software enables surgical training for both the novice and expert as well as preoperative planning and intraoperative navigation by combining registered patient data with anatomical information from an atlas for a case-by-case visualization of known structures. Various virtual reality platforms have been described in the literature for surgical planning, including neurosurgical craniotomy localization [60]. In neurosurgery, although numerous programs have been introduced, a well-known example of these simulators includes Surgical Theater ® (Mayfield, OH). The Dextroscope ® and Dextrobeam ® employ virtual reality visualization for use in surgical planning and were discussed in the previous section.

Surgical Theater ® offers planning and navigation software, called Surgical Planner (SRP) and Surgical Navigation Advanced Platform (SNAP), respectively, which generate interactive, immersive virtual reality reconstructions of patient-specific imaging data [61]. Surgical Theater ® integrates its own virtual reality medical visualization platform into these programs, Precision VR ™, which generates three-dimensional renderings from conventional two-dimensional imaging data, including CT, MRI, DTI, and more. Surgeons can both explore complex anatomy and test techniques preoperatively using SRP and also apply patient-specific surgical plans during actual surgeries with SNAP. These reconstructions can be viewed through tablet, wall-mounted, or virtual reality head-mounted displays, like the Oculus Rift ® or HTC Vive ®. An additional platform for Surgical Theater ® has been developed and evaluated for microsurgery, such as aneurysm clipping, called the Selman Surgical Rehearsal Platform [62]

Immersive Virtual Reality Environment: The CAVE ™

Now in its second iteration, the original CAVE became the world's first room-sized virtual immersive environment [63]. The first CAVE was a high-resolution three-dimensional video and audio environment invented at the Electronic Visualization Laboratory at the University of Illinois at Chicago in 1991. Graphics were projected onto three walls and the floor and were viewed with active stereo glasses equipped with a location sensor. As the user would move within the display boundaries, the correct perspective would be displayed in real time to achieve a fully immersive experience. This system used the Intersense IS-900 ultrasonic−/accelerometer-based tracking system and was powered by a single Windows machine with a fast Intel CPU and an NVIDIA Quadro Plex graphics engine.

Launched in 2012, CAVE2 Hybrid Reality Environment, also referred to as Next-Generation CAVE, expanded the capabilities of the original CAVE significantly [64, 65]. CAVE2 features tiled LCD display walls, in contrast to the projection technology used in the original CAVE. The three-walled original CAVE grew to a 24-foot diameter and nearly 8-foot tall panoramic circular room with 18 columns of four 46-inch LCD screens, powered by a 36-node computer cluster connected to high-speed networks and surrounded by 20 speakers. Furthermore, the wall of CAVE2 can operate as a single screen or multiple smaller partitioned windows through the Scalable Adaptive Graphics Environment, which allows viewing of 2D and 3D information simultaneously.

The CAVE and CAVE-based systems have been introduced into the field of medicine over the past decade, and although it has not been implemented significantly in neurosurgery, there have been several breakthroughs within the neurosciences in general. The CAVE2 has shown potential as a new visualization method for the prevention and treatment of stroke at the University of Illinois at Chicago [66]. Further work at this institute includes neural network mapping to identify connections responsible for depression [67]. A CAVE-based system has been applied in electron microscopy to study cellular compartments of neural tissues, which identified nonrandom distribution of glycogen and led to the further development of tools to analyze glycogen clustering [68]. Additionally, the CAVE has been studied alongside a walking virtual reality system for use in neurorehabilitation [69]. Recent work combining the CAVE with electrocorticography recordings evaluated electrocortical signatures of brain monitoring of errors using first-person virtual avatars, specifically goal-directed behavior with fine-tuning of motor skill learning; this research could potentially be applied to the future development of brain-computer interfaces [70] (Fig. 20.3).

Tangible User Interface for Virtual Reality Simulation: The Props-Based Interface and ANGIO Mentor ®

The props-based interface, first described by the University of Virginia in 1995, represents a

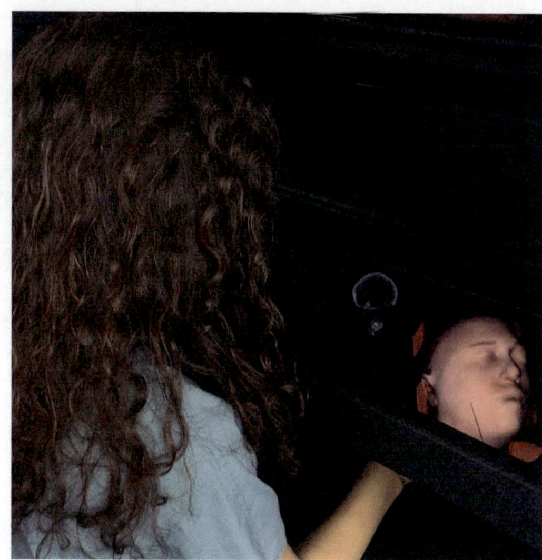

Fig. 20.3 © Courtesy of ImmersiveTouch ®

tangible user interface (TUI) and relies on physical manipulation of handheld objects, or "props," in free space, which are then synchronized to virtual reality elements. The original visualization technique juxtapositioned human interaction with physical tools and computer-based software, called Netra, for surgical planning [71]. Within the props interface, the user holds a miniature head in one hand and selects a tool, like a stylus, for the other hand to interact with and cross-section the head to view the sample imaging study; thus, the computer software integrates hand-coupled motion cues and relates them to the relative position on the miniature head [72]. This particular model grants six degrees of freedom of movement, allowing inspection of complex anatomy from multiple vantage points for the neurosurgeon (Fig. 20.4).

Other tangible user systems have been released since then. 3D Systems ® (Cleveland, OH), formerly Simbionix ®, has a variety of surgical simulators; in particular, ANGIO Mentor ™ replicates the angiography suite with numerous endovascular procedures available for practice [73]. The ANGIO Mentor ™ simulator utilizes actual catheters and wires introduced through a port similar to the diaphragm of an arterial sheath. These catheters and wires then engage internal rollers that mimic force vectors expected from

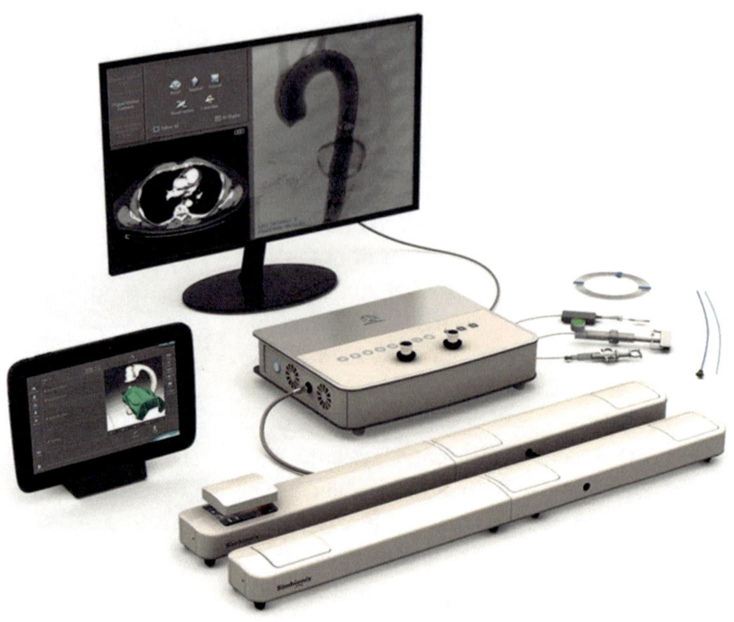

Fig. 20.4 © Courtesy of ANGIO Mentor ®

the endovascular procedure and allow the user to practice the fine movement required to advance and navigate them. Joysticks and foot petals then recreate the control panel of the angiography suite to change bed position and to control the simulated fluoroscopy. ANGIO Mentor ™ provides hands-on training with more than 23 modules and 158 clinical case scenarios. With the addition of the PROcedure Rehearsal Studio ™, which visualizes patient-specific imaging studies and utilizes them for pre-procedure preparation, the number of training modules expands immensely. A recent study demonstrated improvement in skills of participants in conducting diagnostic cerebral angiograms, aneurysm coil embolization, and mechanical thrombectomy [74]

Immersive Virtual Reality Simulation with Haptic Feedback: ImmersiveTouch ® and NeuroTouch ®

ImmersiveTouch ® (Chicago, IL) was the first system to add haptic and kinesthetic feedback to existing augmented virtual reality in 2005 and provides a host of neurosurgical simulators with which the user can engage. Several unique features, such as stereoscopic goggles, electromagnetic hand tracking, and a haptic stylus, are part of this teaching modality that allows for an interactive, three-dimensional training program. Unlike surgery, students are able to use objective metrics to track their progress. Color indicators, numerical scores, and postoperative anatomical dissections allow the trainee to gauge accuracy, reliability, and progress. Simulations that have been published include ventriculostomy, bone drilling, hemostasis, trigeminal rhizotomy, aneurysm clipping, lumbar punctures, vertebroplasty, and percutaneous spinal fixation [9–19] ,and the capacity to discriminate skill level has been proven in multiple different simulations.

NeuroTouch ® is a virtual reality medical simulation platform developed by the National Research Council Canada, currently under license to CAE Inc. and called CAE NeuroVR ™ (Quebec, Canada) [75, 76]. NeuroVR ™ enables neurosurgeons and residents to practice a variety of open cranial and endoscopic procedures. Modules on tumor debulking, soft tissue dissection, bipolar hemostasis, and transnasal transsphenoidal approaches replicate instruments, imaging, and neurosurgical techniques. The system consists of two monitors placed side by side for stereoscopic visualization, and two haptic feedback devices mimic a variety of surgical instruments. NeuroVR ™ records objective operator metrics, such as anatomical landmarks, so that participants can track and improve their skills. Two studies assessing bimanual surgical performance and evaluating proficiency measures in tumor debulking accurately discriminated level of training [77, 78]

Virtual Reality Head-Mounted Displays: Oculus Rift ®, HTC Vive ®, Samsung Gear VR ®, and More

Virtual reality head-mounted displays (HMDs) consist of either a helmet containing or a strap securing a screen in front of one eye, referred to as a monocular display, or both eyes, a binocular display. Binocular HMDs afford stereoscopic, three-dimensional presentations of the computer-generated visual data. HMDs have become increasingly popular with mainstream use in a variety of forums, from gaming and engineering to medicine. Several companies have generated their own devices for distribution, including now Facebook-owned Oculus Rift ®, HTC Vive ®, Samsung Gear VR ®, and Sony PlayStation VR ®. HMDs offer both visual and audio components, creating an immersive virtual reality, and often include interactive components, managed with a remote control. Newer HMDs connect with users' smartphones, making them even more accessible to the general public. HMDs typically provide an individual user-driven experience, but future iterations for collaborative viewing and interaction among groups are currently under way. Both an advantage and limitation of these devices, HMDs often completely barricade the immersive, virtual environment from the physical world, which produces unparalleled presence but consequentially generally prevents their application in augmented reality.

The development of medical applications for these devices remains in its infancy, especially within neurosurgery. A computer-based system has been introduced to produce an immersive learning experience for surgical education by recording the procedure with multiple depth cameras, generating a three-dimensional reconstruction, and annotating the scene in spacetime with more information, all of which viewed through virtual reality headsets [79]. Surgical Theater ® implemented its program for surgical planning, which transforms traditional CT or MRI data into patient-specific three-dimensional renderings, such that the interactive reconstructions may be viewed on a touchscreen device or through a virtual reality headset, such as the Oculus Rift ® or HTV Vive ®. BRAINtrinsic, an open-source virtual reality visualization system, explores connectivity of the central nervous system, and a novel system to explore the human connectome has been designed to be compatible with the Oculus Rift ® [80]. A pilot observational cohort study investigated the use of Samsung Gear VR ® in hospitalized patients to reduce pain and anxiety [81]. Additionally, researchers have designed an immersive, user-centered wheelchair training system using Oculus Rift ® for patients with spinal cord injury [82].

Augmented Reality

Augmented reality incorporates both a live view of the physical environment with computer-generated content, including video, graphics, sound, and more. Essentially, augmented reality takes the user's view of the real world and layers digital information onto it, which may be through a projector or screen; however, in principle, the real-world and computer-generated content do not interact with one another. Medical uses of augmented reality range from vein finding for intravenous access to optical biopsy mapping for minimally invasive cancer screening [83, 84]. Siemens designed an early integration of augmented reality into the medical field with a stereoscopic video system for an interactive in situ visualization of three-dimensional medical imaging data [85]. In neurosurgery, augmented reality has been used in intraoperative neuronavigation as well as remote viewing of procedures, practitioner skills training, and patient education

[86–88]. In clinical practice, augmented reality has been incorporated into postoperative interactions with patients [89] ,and it has also been introduced within a platform, called virtual interactive presence and augmented reality (VIPAR), for providing remote surgical assistance in real time yet virtual interaction between a local resident and with a remote attending surgeon [90]

Augmented Reality Head-Mounted Display: Google Glass ®

Google Glass ® is arguably one of the most well-known augmented reality head-mounted displays that has been introduced to the medical field and specifically neurosurgery [91]. Google Glass ® is an optical head-mounted display, developed by X (formerly Google X), that provides users with a lightweight, smartphone-like, hands-free, voice-activated system, resembling a set of eyeglasses. The original Google Glass ® prototype was released on April 15, 2013; however, due to several concerns regarding privacy and safety, the product was discontinued. It is currently set to re-release in 2017. It allows the user to access a wide network of information, including Internet material, images, and videos via WiFi or Bluetooth connections, and then overlays this information upon the physical, real world in the right upper corner of the user's visual field. It also includes a touchscreen, which allows for swiping through a timeline-oriented display.

Google Glass ® has been tested in a variety of neurosurgical clinical settings and has demonstrated several clinical, educational, and surgical applications, granting hands-free photo and video documentation with access to the electronic medical record and diagnostic laboratory results and test analyses [92]. In addition, it has been used as a teaching tool with live video broadcasting and with video recordings of surgical and angiographic procedures used for viewing both during and after the procedure, enhancing residents' and students' educational experience [93, 94]. In one study, Google Glass ® significantly improved neurosurgery residents' comfort level and understanding of surgical procedures following a thorough debriefing session reviewing the live video recording acquired through the HMD [93]. Google Glass ® also provides the surgeon with the opportunity to access neuronavigation throughout the procedure without turning their head away from the patient to view the navigation monitors [95, 96]

Neuronavigation with Augmented Reality

Similar to standard image-guidance neuronavigation, augmented reality systems register patient-specific anatomical landmarks or fiducials but then project the information over the physical structure, whether it is the actual patient head or a phantom skull. It is important to note that the augmented reality technology utilized in neuronavigation is similar to mixed reality, which will be discussed in the next section, in that it can anchor computer-generated information to the physical environment through the device registration of the patient. However, it lacks real-time reaction to and interaction between the virtual materials itself to the real world, which stands as a necessary distinction.

Operations that utilize augmented reality require highly accurate integration of imaging data with the real patient. Investigators have developed a variety of augmented reality image-guidance systems. In one report, researchers designed an augmented reality system for image-guided neurosurgery using direct image projection onto a phantom head with a video projector, and in a follow-up study, this technique was used intraoperatively in five patients with tumors and found a mean projection error of 1.2 +/− 0.54 mm [97, 98]. Recently, the Intraoperative Brain Imaging System (IBIS) was introduced, which is a novel open-source image-guided platform using an optical tracking device attached to a video camera, intraoperative ultrasound for brain shift calculation, and augmented reality to facilitate the visualization of neuronavigation information [99]. Augmented reality-based image guidance has further been integrated into tablets and mobile devices to increase accessibility and ease of use in the operating room [100–105]

The utility of augmented reality in neuronavigation has been examined within specific neurosurgical subspecialties, and studies have applied this technology within vascular procedures, tumor resections, endoscopic or skull base approaches, spinal fusions, and more.

Vascular An early system-generated three-dimensional vascular models, which were reconstructed from CT or MR angiography and then overlaid those reconstructions on motion pictures from X-ray fluoroscopy by 2D/3D registration using fiducial markers [106]. A more recent iteration and proof-of-concept study in rats augmented the neurovascular procedure with a real-time overlay of fluorescence videoangiography within the white light field of view of conventional operative microscopy [107]. Further studies have developed systems to integrate augmented reality in surgery for arteriovenous malformation resection [108–110] ,extracranial-intracranial bypass [111, 112] ,and aneurysm treatment [113]

Tumors An augmented reality-based neuronavigation system using web cameras connected to infrared optical tracking sensors has been trialed in situ on one patient with glioblastoma and two with convexity meningiomas [114]. Another platform with the DEX-Ray handheld video probes that overlaid transparent patient-specific MRI and MRV reconstructed on a Dextroscope ® workstation were successfully implemented in the resection of parasagittal, falcine, and convexity meningiomas in five patients [115, 116]. Smartphone apps have been devised for the localization of intracranial masses with a high level of accuracy for superficial supratentorial lesions, which could provide potentially low-cost, image-based augmented reality alternatives for frameless neuronavigation [101, 103]. Further, a tablet-based platform, called the Trans-Visible Navigator, has also been developed; it has achieved volumetric navigation, as opposed to standard point-to-point navigation, and has been tested in six patients for tumor resection [105]

Skull Base and Endoscopic Approaches Endoscopic augmented reality navigation has been described in the literature. An early system projected patient-specific, three-dimensional virtual images from MRI or CT of the tumor and surrounding structures over the real-time, operative endoscopic view and was verified in 12 cases of endoscopic transnasal transsphenoidal pituitary tumor resection [117]. Another more recent augmented navigation display has been developed for endoscopic and skull base surgery, fusing endoscopic images with three-dimensional virtual images, such as superimposition of vascular structures through the endoscope, and when validated in cadavers, target registration error was 1.28 +/− 0.45 mm [118]. In addition, augmented reality-based neuronavigation has also been reported for the use for clival chordoma resection [119]. Augmented reality-navigated neuroendoscopy was further tested for intraventricular pathologies, whereby operative planning included defining the entry points, regions of interests and trajectories, superimposed as augmented reality on the endoscopic video screen during the intervention [120]. As an additional example of this technology in practice, researchers used an Android ® app, called Sina neurosurgical assist, for endoscopic evacuation of spontaneous supratentorial intracranial hematomas in 25 patients [121]; another study similarly used an iPhone ® app for localization of basal ganglia hemorrhages for subsequent endoscopic evacuation [102]

Spine The literature on augmented reality neuronavigation in spinal procedures is currently sparse. Only one cadaveric laboratory study was identified at present, which employed intraprocedural three-dimensional reconstructions and examined augmented reality with optical camera-based navigation for free-hand thoracic pedicle screw placement [122]

Mixed Reality

Similar to augmented reality, mixed reality merges virtual elements with those in the real world; however, mixed reality technologies anchor virtual objects to a point in real space from the perspective of the user. However, as an important distinction, mixed reality produces a visualization where physical and digital objects interact with one another in real time; virtual elements receive feedback and respond according to their programmed purpose. For instance, some systems track the user's eye movement, and those virtual objects not directly in field of view may appear blurred. Certain virtual elements may also layer with the real environment, such that a hologram placed in the corner of the room will appear to be behind furniture as the user moves and the viewpoint changes. The goal of mixed reality is to establish a seamless integration between the virtual and physical environment, creating the most realistic experience possible. The most recently released device that utilizes mixed reality is the Microsoft HoloLens ®, which will be discussed in this section. Other head-mounted displays will be released soon, including Acer ® and HP ® devices, which will hit the market in the summer of 2017.

Holographic Mixed Reality Head-Mounted Displays: Microsoft HoloLens® and Beyond

The recent release of the Microsoft HoloLens ® in January 2015 presents a new and unexplored opportunity to the field of neurosurgery for technological advancement. This mixed reality holographic computing system allows the user to explore and manipulate interactive holograms. The Microsoft HoloLens ® incorporates virtual elements generated by the user within the surrounding physical environment. It features an augmented reality operating system in which any Universal Windows Platform application may function (Fig. 20.5).

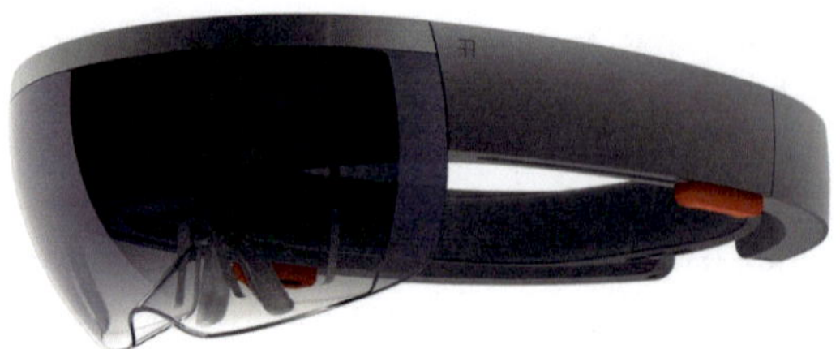

Fig. 20.5 © Courtesy of Microsoft HoloLense ® (Attribution: https://news.microsoft.com/imageGallery/?filter_cats%5B%5D=2843#72QKI9r2kgsigYLo.97)

The medical application of this technology is in its early stages of development. Case Western Reserve University has pioneered the first use of the HoloLens ® in this setting. Their medical school integrated this technology into their anatomy course and small group presentations. Stryker Communications uses the HoloLens to custom design operating rooms with its clients and to build the "operating room of the future." [123] Duke University became the first known institution to apply the HoloLens to neurosurgical practice by using a holographic projection of the ventricular system on a patient model for ventriculostomy training [20]. The HoloLens ® has also been recently implemented as a new image-guidance system for pedicle screw placement [124].

The Microsoft HoloLens ® carries immense potential for applicability in neurosurgery. Interactive holograms could be utilized in resident educational programs for the study of radiology, anatomy, and surgical approaches; in patient care for case planning and decision-making; and in the operating room for image guidance.

Additional companies have soon-to-be released head-mounted displays for mixed reality, including HP, Acer, and Lenovo, among others. These models will be available at significantly lower cost compared to the Microsoft HoloLens ®. These devices in particular will be priced around $300 to $400 for the developer editions, in contrast to the $3000 expense of the HoloLens ® and will be built with the Microsoft reference design for mixed reality software [125]

Future Directions

Future iterations of three-dimensional visualization and virtual, augmented, and mixed reality will expand current applications to improve patient safety, resident education, operative planning, and surgical techniques and will further develop new uses. Like aviation training, programs will evolve to include simulations that not only allow the user to plot and practice surgical trajectories but also train in the management of emergencies, for instance, venous sinus injury with air embolism or intraoperative aneurysm rupture. Furthermore, virtual and augmented reality may become an integral part of research publications and presentations, comparable to the recent integration of operative videos in journals.

Additionally, these visualization strategies will likely become incorporated into the rapidly growing field of telemedicine. Using virtual reality to enhance telemedicine and remote conferencing could improve stroke diagnosis and treatment by connecting emergency medical services to stroke neurologists and then by routing to appropriate stroke comprehensive centers, and devices that provide three-dimensional viewing of the patient's exam or imaging completed in the field could further complement the physician sign-out process. Telemedicine could bring remote audiences into the operating room to learn about a rare disease or new technique, as live video courses could be broadcasted in real time or as recordings to global audiences. Furthermore, as virtual interactive presence brought live surgical assistance remotely into the operating room [90] ,theoretically, teleoperation could even be possible with integrated robotics.

As the interactivity of this technology improves, gesture-based navigation of these platforms, through XBox Kinect ® or similar products, could be incorporated in the operating room as well, allowing for sterile manipulation of the augmented or mixed reality devices. This type of touchless interface has been introduced already in navigating radiological studies [126–129]. Combining all these technological advances provides a wealth of potential to generate seamless integration between multiple devices in the operating room to view and interact with surgical plans, imaging studies, vital signs, and more simultaneously.

Robotics within neurosurgery is an additional emerging area in the field and ripe with potential and represents another possible technology in which to infuse augmented reality. A recent review on this topic discussed the literature available to date on robotic neurosurgery; spinal applications include pedicle screw placement and cranial procedures consist of deep brain stimulator placement, laser thermal ablation, tumors, and endoscopic navigation [130]. The field can anticipate that as visualization technologies advance so will that of robotics.

The horizon is the limit for the future of visualization and simulation in neurosurgery. Not only did this chapter review the multitude of visualization modalities available to date, but also the discovery and development of new technologies remain unseen. Although this review was comprehensive, a variety of devices and software currently in development were not discussed but may present opportunities for advancement within neurosurgery in the future. Several challenges persist within the field, however, to make the virtual or augmented reality both realistic and accurate, to improve depth perception, to enhance interactivity and ease of use, to advance the ergonomics of the hardware, to streamline the automatization of the three-dimensional reconstruction, to decrease costs in the development and distribution of this technology, and more. The goal to address and overcome all these challenges endures, and the ultimate outcome will produce an immersive, real-time rendering of patient information with intuitive, interactive features within an affordable, accessible device.

References

1. Beckmann EC. CT scanning the early days. Br J Radiol. 2006;79(937):5–8.
2. CT market outlook report. In: IMVinfo. http://www.imvinfo.com/index.aspx?sec=ct&sub=dis&itemid=200081. 2016. Accessed 3 Jul 2017.
3. SOMATOM Force. In: Siemens. https://www.healthcare.siemens.com/computed-tomography/dual-source-ct/somatom-force/use. Accessed 25 Jan 2017.
4. Damadian R, Goldsmith M, Minkoff L. NMR in cancer: XVI. FONAR image of the live human body. Physiol Chem Phys. 1977;9(1):97–100, 108.
5. Magnetic resonance imaging (MRI) exams (indicator). In: OECD-iLibrary. https://doi.org/10.1787/1d89353f-en. Accessed 5 Jan 2017.
6. MAGNETOM Terra. In: Siemens. https://usa.healthcare.siemens.com/magnetic-resonance-imaging/7t-mri-scanner/magnetom-terra/features. Accessed 25 Jan 2017.
7. Van der Kolk AG, Hendrikse J, Zwanenburg JJ, Visser F, Luijten PR. Clinical applications of 7T MRI in the brain. Eur J Radiol. 2013;82(5):708–18.
8. Perandini S, Faccioli N, Zaccarella A, Re T, Mucelli RP. The diagnostic contribution of CT volumetric rendering techniques in routine practice. Indian J Radiol Imaging. 2010;20(2):92–7.
9. Alaraj A, Charbel FT, Birk D, Tobin M, Luciano C, Banerjee PP, Rizzi S, Sorenson J, Foley K, Slavin K, Roitberg B. Role of cranial and spinal virtual and augmented reality simulation using ImmersiveTouch modules in neurosurgical training. Neurosurgery. 2013;72(Suppl 1):115–23.
10. Alaraj A, Luciano CJ, Bailey DP, Elsenousi A, Roitberg BZ, Bernardo A, Banerjee PP, Charbel FT. Virtual reality cerebral aneurysm clipping simulation with real-time haptic feedback. Neurosurgery. 2015;11(Suppl 2):52–8.
11. Banerjee PP, Luciano CJ, Lemole GM, Charbel FT, Oh MY. Accuracy of ventriculostomy catheter placement using a head – and hand-tracked high-resolution virtual reality simulator with haptic feedback. J Neurosurg. 2007;107(3):515–21.
12. Gasco J, Holbrook TJ, Patel A, Smith A, Paulson D, Muns A, Desai S, Moisi M, Kuo YF, Macdonald B, Ortega-Barnett J, Patterson JT. Neurosurgery simulation in residency training: feasibility, cost, and educational benefit. Neurosurgery. 2013;73(Suppl 1):39–45.
13. Gasco J, Patel A, Luciano C, Holbrook T, Ortega-Barnett J, Kuo YF, Rizzi S, Kania P, Banerjee P, Roitberg BZ. A novel virtual reality simulation for hemostasis in a brain surgical cavity: perceived utility for visuomotor skills in current and aspiring neurosurgery resident. World Neurosurg. 2013;80(6):732–7.
14. Gasco J, Patel A, Ortega-Barnett J, Branch D, Desai S, Kuo YF, Luciano C, Rizzi S, Kania P, Matuyauskas M, Banerjee P, Roitberg BZ. Virtual reality spine surgery simulation: an empirical study of its usefulness. Neurol Res. 2014;36(11):968–73.
15. Lemole GM, Banerjee PP, Luciano C, Neckrysh S, Charbel FT. Virtual reality in neurosurgical education: part-task ventriculostomy simulation with dynamic visual and haptic feedback. Neurosurgery 2007;61(1):142–8; discussion 148–9.
16. Luciano CJ, Banerjee PP, Bellotte B, Oh GM, Lemole M, Charbel FT, Roitberg B. Learning retention of thoracic pedicle screw placement using a high-resolution augmented reality simulator with haptic feedback. Neurosurgery 2011;69(1 Suppl Operative):ons14–9; discussion ons19.
17. Luciano C, Banerjee P, Lemole GM, Charbel F. Second generation haptic ventriculostomy simulator using the ImmersiveTouch system. Stud Health Technol Inform. 2006;119:343–8.
18. Luciano CJ, Banerjee PP, Sorenson JM, Foley KT, Ansari SA, Rizzi S, Germanwala AV, Kranzler L, Chittiboina P, Roitberg BZ. Percutaneous spinal fixation simulation with virtual reality and haptics. Neurosurgery. 2013;72(Suppl 1):89–96.
19. Shakur SF, Luciano CJ, Kania P, Roitberg BZ, Banerjee PP, Slavin KV, Sorenson J, Charbel FT, Alaraj A. Usefulness of a virtual reality percutaneous trigeminal rhizotomy simulator in neurosurgical training. Neurosurgery 2015;11(Suppl 3):420–5; discussion 425.
20. Manke K (2016). Brain surgery may get a bit easier, with augmented reality. In: Duke Today. https://today.duke.edu/2016/10/brain-surgery-may-get-bit-easier-augmented-reality. Accessed 3 Jul 2017.
21. Syngo Dyna3D. In: Siemens. https://www.healthcare.siemens.com/angio/options-and-upgrades/clinical-software-applications/syngo-inspace-3d/features. Accessed 3 Jul 2017.
22. Yang M, Wu J, Ma L, Pan L, Li J, Chen G, Struffert T, Sun Q, Beilner J, Deuerling-Zheng Y. The value of syngo DynaPBV neuro during neuro-interventional hypotensive balloon occlusion test. Clin Neuroradiol. 2015;25(4):387–95.
23. Wenger KJ, Berkefeld J, Wagner M. Flat panel detector computed tomography for the interaction between contrast-enhanced thrombi and stent retrievers in stroke therapy: a pilot study. Clin Neuroradiol. 2014;24(3):251–4.
24. Faragò G, Caldiera V, Tempra G, Ciceri E. Advanced digital subtraction angiography and MR fusion imaging protocol applied to accurate placement of flow diverter device. J Neurointerv Surg. 2016;8(2):e5. https://doi.org/10.1136/neurintsurg-2014-011428.
25. Shakur SF, Brunozzi D, Hussein AE, Linninger A, Hsu CY, Charbel FT, Alaraj A. Validation of cerebral arteriovenous malformation hemodynamics assessed by DSA using quantitative magnetic resonance angiography: preliminary study. J Neurointerv Surg 2017. pii: neurintsurg-2017-012991.
26. BrainSuite. In: BrainSuite. http://brainsuite.org/. Accessed 3 Jul 2017.
27. Phillips OR, Joshi SH, Piras F, Orfei MD, Iorio M, Narr KL, Shattuck DW, Caltagirone C, Spalletta G, Di

Paola M. The superficial white matter in Alzheimer's disease. Hum Brain Mapp. 2016;37(4):1321–34.

28. Phillips OR, Joshi SH, Squitieri F, Sanchez-Castaneda C, Narr K, Shattuck DW, Caltagirone C, Sabatini U, Di Paola M. Major superficial white matter abnormalities in Huntington's disease. Front Neurosci. 2016;10:197.

29. Wang ZI, Jones SE, Ristic AJ, Wong C, Kakisaka Y, Jin K, Schneider F, Gonzalez-Martinez JA, Mosher JC, Nair D, Burgess RC, Najm IM, Alexopoulos AV. Voxel-based morphometric MRI post-processing in MRI-negative focal cortical dysplasia followed by simultaneously recorded MEG and stereo-EEG. Epilepsy Res. 2012;100(1–2):188–93.

30. Wang ZI, Krishnan B, Shattuck DW, Leahy RM, Moosa AN, Wyllie E, Burgess RC, Al-Sharif NB, Joshi AA, Alexopoulos AV, Mosher JC, Udayasankar U, Pediatric Imaging, Neurocognition and Genetics Study, Jones SE. Automated MRI volumetric analysis in patients with Rasmussen syndrome. AJNR Am J Neuroradiol. 2016;37(12):2348–55.

31. Wang ZI, Ristic AJ, Wong CH, Jones SE, Najm IM, Schneider F, Wang S, Gonzalez-Martinez JA, Bingaman W, Alexopoulos AV. Neuroimaging characteristics of MRI-negative orbitofrontal epilepsy with focus on voxel-based morphometric MRI post-processing. Epilepsia. 2013;54(12):2195–203.

32. Wang ZI, Suwanpakdee P, Jones SE, Jaisani Z, Moosa AN, Najm IM, von Podewils F, Burgess RC, Krishnan B, Prayson RA, Gonzalez-Martinez JA, Bingaman W, Alexopoulos AV. Re-review of MRI with post-processing in nonlesional patients in whom epilepsy surgery has failed. J Neurol. 2016;263(9):1736–45.

33. Kakisaka Y, Alkawadri R, Wang ZI, Enatsu R, Mosher JC, Dubarry AS, Alexopoulos AV, Burgess RC. Sensitivity of scalp 10-20 EEG and magnetoencephalography. Epileptic Disord. 2013;15(1):27–31.

34. Neyaz Z, Phadke RV, Singh V, Godbole C. Three-dimensional visualization of intracranial tumors with cortical surface and vasculature from routine MR sequences. Neurol India. 2017;65(2):333–40.

35. TrueVision is 3D HD visualization for microsurgery. In: TrueVision. http://www.truevisionsys.com/visualization-neuro.html. Accessed 3 Jul 2017.

36. Trenion SD HD from Zeiss. In: Zeiss. https://www.zeiss.com/meditec/us/products/spine-surgery/visualization-systems/trenion-3d-hd.html. Accessed 3 Jul 2017.

37. Gerweck K. Dextroscope changes the neurosurgical planning paradigm 3D virtual reality system. In: Bracco Imaging Inc. http://www.braccoimaging.com/us-en/dextroscope-changes-neurosurgical-planning-paradigm-3d-virtual-reality-system. 2006. Published August 16, 2006. Accessed 3 Jul 2017.

38. Gerweck K. Interactive virtual reality environment transforms surgical group collaboration and education. In: Bracco Imaging Inc. http://www.braccoimaging.com/us-en/interactive-virtual-reality-environment-transforms-surgical-group-collaboration-and-education. 2006. Accessed 3 Jul 2017.

39. Kockro RA, Serra L, Tseng-Tsai Y, Chan C, Yih-Yian S, Gim-Guan C, Lee E, Hoe LY, Hern N, Nowinski WL. Planning and simulation of neurosurgery in a virtual reality environment. Neurosurgery 2000;46(1):118–35; discussion 135–7.

40. Gu SX, Yang DL, Cui DM, Xu QW, Che XM, Wu JS, Li WS. Anatomical studies on the temporal bridging veins with Dextroscope and its application in tumor surgery across the middle and posterior fossa. Clin Neurol Neurosurg. 2011;113(10):889–94.

41. Stadie AT, Reisch R, Kockro RA, Fischer G, Schwandt E, Boor S, Stoeter P. Minimally invasive cerebral cavernoma surgery using keyhole approaches – solutions for technique-related limitations. Minim Invasive Neurosurg. 2009;52(1):9–16.

42. Wang SS, Li JF, Zhang SM, Jing JJ, Xue LA. Virtual reality model of the clivus and surgical simulation via transoral or transnasal route. Int J Clin Exp Med. 2014;7(10):3270–9.

43. Wang SS, Zhang SM, Jing JJ. Stereoscopic virtual reality models for planning tumor resection in the sellar region. BMC Neurol. 2012;12:146.

44. Yang DL, Xu QW, Che XM, Wu JS, Sun B. Clinical evaluation and follow-up outcome of presurgical plan by Dextroscope: a prospective controlled study in patients with skull base tumors. Surg Neurol 2009;72(6):682–9; discussion 689.

45. Qiu TM, Zhang Y, Wu JS, Tang WJ, Zhao Y, Pan ZG, Mao Y, Zhou LF. Virtual reality presurgical planning for cerebral gliomas adjacent to motor pathways in an integrated 3-D stereoscopic visualization of structural MRI and DTI tractography. Acta Neurochir. 2010;152(11):1847–57.

46. Ng I, Hwang PY, Kumar D, Lee CK, Kockro RA, Sitoh YY. Surgical planning for microsurgical excision of cerebral arterio-venous malformations using virtual reality technology. Acta Neurochir 2009;151(5):453–63; discussion 463.

47. Wong GK, Zhu CX, Ahuja AT, Poon WS. Stereoscopic virtual reality simulation for microsurgical excision of cerebral arteriovenous malformation: case illustrations. Surg Neurol 2009;72(1):69–72; discussion 72–3.

48. Di Somma A, de Notaris M, Stagno V, Serra L, Enseñat J, Alobid I, San Molina J, Berenguer J, Cappabianca P, Prats-Galino A. Extended endoscopic endonasal approaches for cerebral aneurysms: anatomical, virtual reality and morphometric study. Biomed Res Int. 2014;2014:703792.

49. Guo YW, Ke YQ, Zhang SZ, Wang QJ, Duan CZ, Jia HS, Zhou L, Xu RX. Combined application of virtual imaging techniques and three-dimensional computed tomographic angiography in diagnosing intracranial aneurysms. Chin Med J. 2008;121(24):2521–4.

50. Kockro RA, Killeen T, Ayyad A, Glaser M, Stadie A, Reisch R, Giese A, Schwandt E. Aneurysm surgery with preoperative three-dimensional planning in a virtual reality environment: technique and outcome analysis. World Neurosurg. 2016 Dec;96:489–99.

51. Wong GK, Zhu CX, Ahuja AT, Poon WS. Craniotomy and clipping of intracranial aneurysm in a stereoscopic virtual reality environment. Neurosurgery 2007;61(3):564–8; discussion 568–9.

52. Serra C, Huppertz HJ, Kockro RA, Grunwald T, Bozinov O, Krayenbühl N, Bernays RL. Rapid and Accurate anatomical localization of implanted subdural electrodes in a virtual reality environment. J Neurol Surg A Cent Eur Neurosurg. 2013;74(3):175–82.

53. Du ZY, Gao X, Zhang XL, Wang ZQ, Tang WJ. Preoperative evaluation of neurovascular relationships for microvascular decompression in the cerebellopontine angle in a virtual reality environment. J Neurosurg. 2010;113(3):479–85.

54. González Sánchez JJ, Enseñat Nora J, Candela Canto S, Rumià Arboix J, Caral Pons LA, Oliver D, Ferrer Rodríguez E. New stereoscopic virtual reality system application to cranial nerve microvascular decompression. Acta Neurochir. 2010;152(2):355–60.

55. Archavlis E, Schwandt E, Kosterhon M, Gutenberg A, Ulrich P, Nimer A, Giese A, Kantelhardt SR. A modified microsurgical endoscopic-assisted Transpedicular Corpectomy of the thoracic spine based on virtual 3-dimensional planning. World Neurosurg. 2016;91:424–33.

56. Stadie AT, Kockro RA, Reisch R, Tropine A, Boor S, Stoeter P, Perneczky A. Virtual reality system for planning minimally invasive neurosurgery. Technical note. J Neurosurg. 2008;108(2):382–94.

57. Schirmer CM, Mocco J, Elder JB. Evolving virtual reality simulation in neurosurgery. Neurosurgery. 2013;73(Suppl 1):127–37.

58. Alaraj A, Lemole MG, Finkle JH, Yudkowsky R, Wallace A, Luciano C, Banerjee PP, Rizzi SH, Charbel FT. Virtual reality training in neurosurgery: review of current status and future applications. Surg Neurol Int. 2011;2:52.

59. Choudhury N, Gélinas-Phaneuf N, Delorme S, Del Maestro R. Evolving virtual reality simulation in neurosurgery. Neurosurgery. 2013;73(Suppl 1):127–37.

60. Stadie AT, Kockro RA, Serra L, Fischer G, Schwandt E, Grunert P, Reisch R. Neurosurgical craniotomy localization using a virtual reality planning system versus intraoperative image-guided navigation. Int J Comput Assist Radiol Surg. 2011;6(5):565–72.

61. Surgical Theater: Precision virtual reality. In: Surgical Theater http://www.surgicaltheater.net/. Accessed 3 Jul 2017.

62. Bambakidis NC, Selman WR, Sloan AE. Surgical rehearsal platform: potential uses in microsurgery. Neurosurgery. 2013;73(Suppl 1):122–6.

63. The CAVE Virtual reality theater. In: Electronic Visualization Laboratory. https://www.evl.uic.edu/entry.php?id=1769. Accessed 3 Jul 2017.

64. Brown M. CAVE2: an advanced cyberworld for data exploration. In: Electronic Visualization Laboratory https://www.evl.uic.edu/entry.php?id=1078. Accessed 3 Jul 2017.

65. Brown M. University of Illinois at Chicago: virtual reality's CAVE pioneer. In: Electronic Visualization Laboratory. https://www.evl.uic.edu/entry.php?id=1093. Accessed 3 Jul 2017.

66. State-of-the-art virtual reality system is key to medical discovery. In: National Science Foundation. https://www.nsf.gov/news/news_summ.jsp?cntn_id=126209. 2012. Accessed 3 Jul 2017.

67. Brown M. UIC/EVL's CAVE2 featured in discover magazine, July/Aug 2014 issue. In: Electronic Visualization Laboratory. https://www.evl.uic.edu/entry.php?id=1165. 2014. Accessed 3 Jul 2017.

68. Calì C, Baghabra J, Boges DJ, Holst GR, Kreshuk A, Hamprecht FA, Srinivasan M, Lehväslaiho H, Magistretti PJ. Three-dimensional immersive virtual reality for studying cellular compartments in 3D models from EM preparations of neural tissues. J Comp Neurol. 2016;524(1):23–38.

69. Borrego A, Latorre J, Llorens R, Alcañiz M, Noé E. Feasibility of a walking virtual reality system for rehabilitation: objective and subjective parameters. J Neuroeng Rehabil. 2016;13(1):68.

70. Pavone EF, Tieri G, Rizza G, Tidoni E, Grisoni L, Aglioti SM. Embodying others in immersive virtual reality: electro-cortical signatures of monitoring the errors in the actions of an avatar seen from a first-person perspective. J Neurosci. 2016;36(2):268–79.

71. Goble J, Hinckley K, Snell J, Pausch R, Kassell N. Two-handed spatial interface tools for neurosurgical planning. IEEE Comput. 1995:20–6.

72. Hinckley K, Pausch R, Downs JH, Proffitt D, Kassell NF. The props-based interface for neurosurgical visualization. Stud Health Technol Inform. 1997;39:552–62.

73. ANGIO Mentor: The most advanced endovascular training. In: Simbionix http://simbionix.com/simulators/angio-mentor/. Accessed 3 Jul 2017.

74. Pannell JS, Santiago-Dieppa DR, Wali AR, Hirshman BR, Steinberg JA, Cheung VJ, Oveisi D, Hallstrom J, Khalessi AA. Simulator-based angiography and endovascular neurosurgery curriculum: a longitudinal evaluation of performance following simulator-based angiography training. Cureus. 2016;8(8):e756.

75. CAE NeuroVR. In: CAE Healthcare Inc. https://caehealthcare.com/surgical-simulation/neurovr. Accessed 3 Jul 2017.

76. Delorme S, Laroche D, DiRaddo R, Del Maestro RF. NeuroTouch: a physics-based virtual simulator for cranial microneurosurgery training. Neurosurgery. 2012;71(1 Suppl Operative):32–42.

77. Alotaibi FE, AlZhrani GA, Mullah MA, Sabbagh AJ, Azarnoush H, Winkler-Schwartz A, Del Maestro RF. Assessing bimanual performance in brain tumor resection with NeuroTouch, a virtual reality simulator. Neurosurgery 2015;11(Suppl 2):89–98; discussion 98.

78. AlZhrani G, Alotaibi F, Azarnoush H, Winkler-Schwartz A, Sabbagh A, Bajunaid K, Lajoie SP, Del Maestro RF. Proficiency performance benchmarks for removal of simulated brain tumors using a virtual reality simulator NeuroTouch. J Surg Educ. 2015;72(4):685–96.

79. Cha YW, Dou M, Chabra R, Menozzi F, State A, Wallen E, Fuchs H. Immersive learning experiences for surgical procedures. Stud Health Technol Inform. 2016;220:55–62.

80. Ye AQ, Ajilore OA, Conte G, GadElkarim J, Thomas-Ramos G, Zhan L, Yang S, Kumar A, Magin RL, G Forbes A, Leow AD. The intrinsic geometry of the human brain connectome. Brain Inform. 2015;2:197–210.

81. Mosadeghi S, Reid MW, Martinez B, Rosen BT, Spiegel BM. Feasibility of an immersive virtual reality intervention for hospitalized patients: an observational cohort study. JMIR Ment Health. 2016;3(2):e28.

82. Nunnerley J, Gupta S, Snell D, King M. Training wheelchair navigation in immersive virtual environments for patients with spinal cord injury – end-user input to design an effective system. Disabil Rehabil Assist Technol. 2017;12(4):417–23.

83. Miyake RK, Zeman HD, Duarte FH, Kikuchi R, Ramacciotti E, Lovhoiden G, Vrancken C. Vein imaging: a new method of near infrared imaging, where a processed image is projected onto the skin for the enhancement of vein treatment. Dermatol Surg. 2006;32(8):1031–8.

84. Mountney P, Giannarou S, Elson D, Yang GZ. Optical biopsy mapping for minimally invasive cancer screening. Med Image Comput Comput Assist Interv. 2009;12(Pt 1):483–90.

85. Vogt S, Khamene A, Niemann H, Sauer F. An AR System with intuitive user interface for manipulation and visualization of 3D medical data. Stud Health Technol Inform. 2004;98:397–403.

86. Meola A, Cutolo F, Carbone M, Cagnazzo F, Ferrari M, Ferrari V. Augmented reality in neurosurgery: a systematic review. Neurosurg Rev 2016. [Epub ahead of print].

87. Barsom EZ, Graafland M, Schijven MP. Systematic review on the effectiveness of augmented reality applications in medical training. Surg Endosc. 2016;30(10):4174–83.

88. Pelargos PE, Nagasawa DT, Lagman C, Tenn S, Demos JV, Lee SJ, Bui TT, Barnette NE, Bhatt NS, Ung N, Bari A, Martin NA, Yang I. Utilizing virtual and augmented reality for educational and clinical enhancements in neurosurgery. J Clin Neurosci. 2017;35:1–4.

89. Ponce BA, Brabston EW, Shin Z, Watson SL, Baker D, Winn D, Guthrie BL, Shenai MB. Telemedicine with mobile devices and augmented reality for early postoperative care. Conf Proc IEEE Eng Med Biol Soc. 2016;2016:4411–4.

90. Shenai MB, Dillavou M, Shum C, Ross D, Tubbs RS, Shih A, Guthrie BL. Virtual interactive presence and augmented reality (VIPAR) for remote surgical assistance. Neurosurgery 2011;68(1 Suppl Operative):200–7; discussion 207.

91. Businesses have been getting hands-on with Glass Enterprise Edition. In: X Company. https://x.company/glass/. Accessed 3 Jul 2017.

92. Mitrasinovic S, Camacho E, Trivedi N, Logan J, Campbell C, Zilinyi R, Lieber B, Bruce E, Taylor B, Martineau D, Dumont EL, Appelboom G, Connolly ES Jr. Clinical and surgical applications of smart glasses. Technol Health Care. 2015;23(4):381–401.

93. Nakhla J, Kobets A, De la Garza Ramos R, Haranhalli N, Gelfand Y, Ammar A, Echt M, Scoco A, Kinon M, Yassari R. Use of Google glass to enhance surgical education of neurosurgery residents: "proof-of-concept" study. World Neurosurg. 2017;98:711–4.

94. Porras JL, Khalid S, Root BK, Khan IS, Singer RJ. Point-of-view recording devices for intraoperative neurosurgical video capture. Front Surg 2016;3:57. eCollection 2016.

95. Yoon JW, Chen RE, Han PK, Si P, Freeman WD, Pirris SM. Technical feasibility and safety of an intraoperative head-up display device during spine instrumentation. Int J Med Robot 2016. [Epub ahead of print].

96. Yoon JW, Chen RE, ReFaey K, Diaz RJ, Reimer R, Komotar RJ, Quinones-Hinojosa A, Brown BL, Wharen RE. Technical feasibility and safety of image-guided parieto-occipital ventricular catheter placement with the assistance of a wearable head-up display. Int J Med Robot 2017. [Epub ahead of print].

97. Besharati Tabrizi L, Mahvash M. Augmented reality-guided neurosurgery: accuracy and intraoperative application of an image projection technique. J Neurosurg. 2015;123(1):206–11.

98. Mahvash M, Besharati Tabrizi L. A novel augmented reality system of image projection for image-guided neurosurgery. Acta Neurochir. 2013;155(5):943–7.

99. Drouin S, Kochanowska A, Kersten-Oertel M, Gerard IJ, Zelmann R, De Nigris D, Bériault S, Arbel T, Sirhan D, Sadikot AF, Hall JA, Sinclair DS, Petrecca K, DelMaestro RF, Collins DL. IBIS: an OR ready open-source platform for image-guided neurosurgery. Int J Comput Assist Radiol Surg. 2017;12(3):363–78.

100. Deng W, Li F, Wang M, Song Z. Easy-to-use augmented reality neuronavigation using a wireless tablet PC. Stereotact Funct Neurosurg. 2014;92(1):17–24.

101. Eftekhar B. A smartphone app to assist scalp localization of superficial supratentorial lesions: technical note. World Neurosurg. 2016;85:359–63.

102. Hou Y, Ma L, Zhu R, Chen X. iPhone-assisted augmented reality localization of basal ganglia hypertensive hematoma. World Neurosurg. 2016;94:480–92.

103. Hou Y, Ma L, Zhu R, Chen X, Zhang JA. Low-cost iPhone-assisted augmented reality solution for the localization of intracranial lesions. PLoS One. 2016;11(7):e0159185.

104. Kramers M, Armstrong R, Bakhshmand SM, Fenster A, de Ribaupierre S, Eagleson R. Evaluation of a mobile augmented reality application for image guidance of neurosurgical interventions. Stud Health Technol Inform. 2014;196:204–8.

105. Watanabe E, Satoh M, Konno T, Hirai M, Yamaguchi T. The trans-visible navigator: a

see-through neuronavigation system using augmented reality. World Neurosurg. 2016;87:399–405.

106. Masutani Y, Dohi T, Yamane F, Iseki H, Takakura K. Augmented reality visualization system for intravascular neurosurgery. Comput Aided Surg. 1998;3(5):239–47.

107. Martirosyan NL, Skoch J, Watson JR, Lemole GM Jr, Romanowski M, Anton R. Integration of indocyanine green videoangiography with operative microscope: augmented reality for interactive assessment of vascular structures and blood flow. Neurosurgery 2015;11(Suppl 2):252–7; discussion 257–8.

108. Cabrilo I, Bijlenga P, Schaller K. Augmented reality in the surgery of cerebral arteriovenous malformations: technique assessment and considerations. Acta Neurochir. 2014;156(9):1769–74.

109. Kersten-Oertel M, Chen SS, Drouin S, Sinclair DS, Collins DL. Augmented reality visualization for guidance in neurovascular surgery. Stud Health Technol Inform. 2012;173:225–9.

110. Kersten-Oertel M, Gerard I, Drouin S, Mok K, Sirhan D, Sinclair DS, Collins DL. Augmented reality in neurovascular surgery: feasibility and first uses in the operating room. Int J Comput Assist Radiol Surg. 2015;10(11):1823–36.

111. Almefty RO, Nakaji P. Augmented reality-enhanced navigation for extracranial-intracranial bypass. World Neurosurg. 2015;84(1):15–7.

112. Cabrilo I, Schaller K, Bijlenga P. Augmented reality-assisted bypass surgery: embracing minimal invasiveness. World Neurosurg. 2015;83(4):596–602.

113. Cabrilo I, Bijlenga P, Schaller K. Augmented reality in the surgery of cerebral aneurysms: a technical report. Neurosurgery 2014;10(Suppl 2):252–60; discussion 260–1.

114. Inoue D, Cho B, Mori M, Kikkawa Y, Amano T, Nakamizo A, Yoshimoto K, Mizoguchi M, Tomikawa M, Hong J, Hashizume M, Sasaki T. Preliminary study on the clinical application of augmented reality neuronavigation. J Neurol Surg A Cent Eur Neurosurg. 2013;74(2):71–6.

115. Kockro RA, Tsai YT, Ng I, Hwang P, Zhu C, Agusanto K, Hong LX, Serra L. Dex-ray: augmented reality neurosurgical navigation with a handheld video probe. Neurosurgery 2009;65(4):795–807; discussion 807–8.

116. Low D, Lee CK, Dip LL, Ng WH, Ang BT, Ng I. Augmented reality neurosurgical planning and navigation for surgical excision of parasagittal, falcine and convexity meningiomas. Br J Neurosurg. 2010;24(1):69–74.

117. Kawamata T, Iseki H, Shibasaki T, Hori T. Endoscopic augmented reality navigation system for endonasal transsphenoidal surgery to treat pituitary tumors: technical note. Neurosurgery. 2002;50(6):1393–7.

118. Li L, Yang J, Chu Y, Wu W, Xue J, Liang P, Chen L. A novel augmented reality navigation system for endoscopic sinus and skull base surgery: a feasibility study. PLoS One. 2016;11(1):e0146996.

119. Cabrilo I, Sarrafzadeh A, Bijlenga P, Landis BN, Schaller K. Augmented reality-assisted skull base surgery. Neurochirurgie. 2014;60(6):304–6.

120. Finger T, Schaumann A, Schulz M, Thomale UW. Augmented reality in intraventricular neuroendoscopy. Acta Neurochir. 2017;159(6):1033–41.

121. Sun GC, Chen XL, Hou YZ, Yu XG, Ma XD, Liu G, Liu L, Zhang JS, Tang H, Zhu RY, Zhou DB, Xu BN. Image-guided endoscopic surgery for spontaneous supratentorial intracerebral hematoma. J Neurosurg. 2017:127(3):537–542. https://doi.org/10.3171/2016.7.JNS16932.

122. Elmi-Terander A, Skulason H, Söderman M, Racadio J, Homan R, Babic D, van der Vaart N, Nachabe R. Surgical navigation technology based on augmented reality and integrated 3D intraoperative imaging: a spine cadaveric feasibility and accuracy study. Spine (Phila Pa 1976). 2016;41(21):E1303–11.

123. Bardeen L. Stryker chooses Microsoft HoloLens to bring operating room design into the future with 3D. In: Microsoft Devices Blog. https://blogs.windows.com/devices/2017/02/21/stryker-chooses-microsoft-hololens-bring-operating-room-design-future-3d/#bO8jgYtmDfSqUyzf.97. 2017. Published February 21, 2017. Accessed 3 Jul 2017.

124. Robertson A. Microsoft HoloLens could help surgeons operate on your spine. In: The Verge. https://www.theverge.com/2017/5/5/15557790/scopis-medical-microsoft-hololens-ar-spine-surgery. 2017 Accessed 3 Jul 2017.

125. Ackerman D. HP's mixed reality headset gets ready for holiday wishlists. In: CNET. https://www.cnet.com/products/hp-windows-mixed-reality-headset/preview/. 2017. Accessed 25 Jul 2017.

126. Jacob MG, Wachs JP, Packer RA. Hand-gesture-based sterile interface for the operating room using contextual cues for the navigation of radiological images. J Am Med Inform Assoc. 2013;20(e1):e183–6.

127. Ma M, Fallavollita P, Habert S, Weidert S, Navab N. Device- and system-independent personal touchless user interface for operating rooms : one personal UI to control all displays in an operating room. Int J Comput Assist Radiol Surg. 2016;11(6):853–61.

128. Park BJ, Jang T, Choi JW, Kim N. Gesture-controlled interface for contactless control of various computer programs with a hooking-based keyboard and mouse-mapping technique in the operating room. Comput Math Methods Med. 2016;2016:5170379.

129. Wachs JP, Stern HI, Edan Y, Gillam M, Handler J, Feied C, Smith M. A gesture-based tool for sterile browsing of radiology images. J Am Med Inform Assoc. 2008;15(3):321–3.

130. Madhavan K, Kolcun JPG, Chieng LO, Wang MY. Augmented-reality integrated robotics in neurosurgery: are we there yet? Neurosurg Focus. 2017;42(5):E3.

Part V

Simulation Training Courses

The Role of the NREF Endovascular and Cerebrovascular Courses in Neurosurgical Residency and Fellowship Training and Future Directions

Jay Vachhani, Jaafar Basma, Erol Veznedaroglu, Michael Lawton, Emad Aboud, and Adam Arthur

Introduction

Simulation exercises have become an integral part of modern military and aviation training, where the cost of the smallest mistakes in judgment and technique can be costly and catastrophic. By comparison, surgical simulation training programs are not as well developed or validated but are gaining ground. Surgical simulation is particularly needed in areas where technical expertise is required, but it is difficult to gain significant practice without creating dangerous situations for patients. Technical skill requires practice to build motor skills and situational awareness in all procedural vascular neurosurgery. This includes both endovascular neurosurgery and open microneurosurgery.

Endovascular neurosurgery is a relatively young and technology-driven field. Early on in the growth of this field, dedicated efforts to provide learners with an introduction were much needed. As the field has developed, the dissemination of the knowledge regarding patient selection, proper planning, and techniques has become an ongoing necessity. The rapid pace of technological development has driven creative efforts to teach techniques via a number of different simulation models.

The other side effect of this rapid technological development is that as more patients are treated with endovascular techniques, there are fewer cases available for open microneurosurgery. Furthermore, these endovascular techniques usually are sufficient to deal with cases where anatomy is straightforward. This means that the preponderance of the open microneurosurgical cases is more technically difficult and today's learners do not have the luxury of developing their open neurosurgical skills by completing easier surgical cases.

In this chapter, we review the history of the Neurosurgery Research and Education Foundation simulation courses and their overall description, and we focus attention on the vascular courses held at the Medical Education Research Institute. We will also discuss the outcome of these courses as it relates to residents' satisfaction, improved technical skills, and transfer of surgical knowledge.

J. Vachhani (✉) · J. Basma · A. Arthur
University of Tennessee Health Sciences Center and Semmes-Murphey Neurologic and Spine Institute, Memphis, TN, USA

E. Veznedaroglu
Drexel Neurosciences Institute, Philadelphia, PA, USA

M. Lawton
Barrow Neurologic Institute, Phoenix, AZ, USA

E. Aboud
Arkansas Neurologic Institute, Little Rock, AR, USA

© Springer International Publishing AG, part of Springer Nature 2018
A. Alaraj (ed.), *Comprehensive Healthcare Simulation: Neurosurgery*,
Comprehensive Healthcare Simulation, https://doi.org/10.1007/978-3-319-75583-0_21

History of AANS/NREF Simulation Courses

The Neurosurgery Research and Education Foundation (NREF) was established by the American Association of the Neurological Surgeons (AANS) in 1980. Its mission has been to provide financial and academic resources for the promotion of research and training education in the field of neurosurgery. Since its foundation, the nonprofit organization has received over 18 million dollars in funding. It has provided 135 resident research grants and 76 post-residency clinical fellowships. It has organized 70 resident educational courses in different fields of neurosurgical subspecialties. These courses have covered the topics of spine (deformity and fundamentals), peripheral nerves, endovascular techniques, open vascular surgery, skull base surgery, stereotactic radiosurgery, pediatric resident review, exit strategies for chief residents, science of practice, and stereotactic and functional neurosurgery (Table 21.1). The courses were established in 2006 in cooperation with the AANS (Fig. 21.1). About 1700 residents have attended

Table 21.1 List of all the AANS Educational Residents and Fellows Courses

Course	Years
Endovascular techniques for residents	2006–2017
Minimally invasive spinal techniques	2006–2008
Socio-economic issues	2006–2008
Pediatric neurosurgery review	2007, 2008, 2011, 2013
Fundamentals in spine	2007–2017
Spinal deformity/PN	2008–2017
Peripheral nerves	2008
Cerebrovascular neurosurgery	2009–2017
Stereotactic radiosurgery	2009, 2010, 2012, 2014, 2017
Skull base	2010–2012, 2014–2017
Pain management	2010–2011
Endovascular techniques for fellows	2012–2017
Exit strategies	2013–2014
Science of practice	2014–2015
Stereotactic functional	2015–2016

these courses, and they have represented most of American neurosurgical training programs (Fig. 21.2). With the development of different surgical and training technologies, more simulation techniques have been incorporated into these courses. These techniques have significantly enhanced the interactive aspect of the courses, and the residents have expressed increasing enjoyment, satisfaction, and educational benefit. The AANS courses have demonstrated the possibility to integrate simulation techniques in neurosurgical training.

The first endovascular neurosurgery course was established by Dr. Robert Rosenwasser for midlevel and senior neurosurgical residents in 2006 (Fig. 21.2). This course has been held annually since then at the Medical Education and Research Institute in Memphis, TN. The original intent of the course was to provide neurosurgical residents with exposure to endovascular neurosurgery when most training programs did not provide this exposure. The faculty was composed of leaders in the field who worked with participating residents in both interactive-didactic sessions and hands-on laboratory exercises. The laboratory exercises included a range of simulation models which included live animals, silicon and glass models, and electronic simulators.

Endovascular techniques and technology have expanded terrifically, and this created a need for more simulation for open vascular neurosurgery. In 2011, Adam Arthur and Michael Lawton led the first open vascular neurosurgery course as an effort to meet this need. Neurosurgical residents were offered the opportunity to perform carotid endarterectomies on "living cadavers," microanastomosis of turkey wings under the guidance of experienced vascular neurosurgeons, and aneurysm clipping using the living cadaver model. The course was met with tremendous enthusiasm from participating residents, and demand for the course exceeded capacity.

Continuing assessment of the needs and desires of participating residents resulted in the merger of these two courses in 2013. This merger resulted in a course that included both open microsurgical and endovascular techniques over a 2-day period. While not a substitute for full

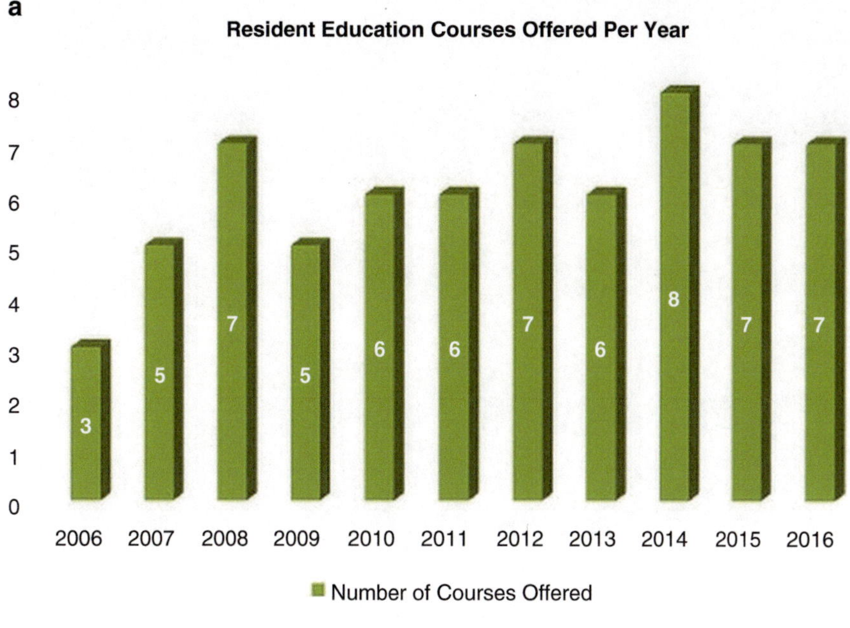

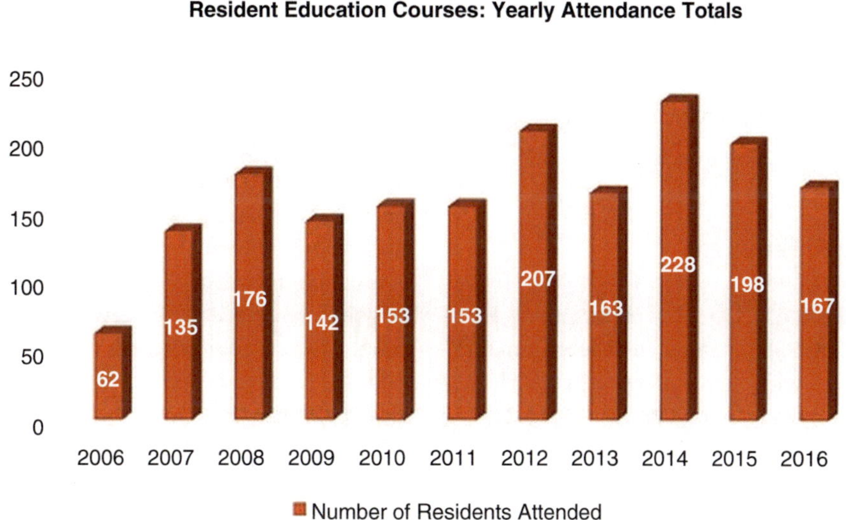

Fig. 21.1 (**a**) Resident Education Courses offered per year (*N* = 68) (**b**) Resident Education Courses: yearly attendance totals (*N* = 1700)

training, the intent of the course remains to expose residents to advanced techniques in an environment that fosters direct interaction with an expert faculty. The faculty is evaluated each year by the residents, and these evaluations are used to change the faculty, rewarding instructors who receive the best evaluations by inviting them to teach again the following year.

Erol Veznedaroglu and Adam Arthur established the NREF Endovascular Techniques Course for Fellows in 2012. This utilized a similar format and philosophy but included three parent specialties (neurology, neurosurgery, and radiology) both as course participants and faculty. The highest-rated instructor that first year was Alejandro Berenstein, who was invited to

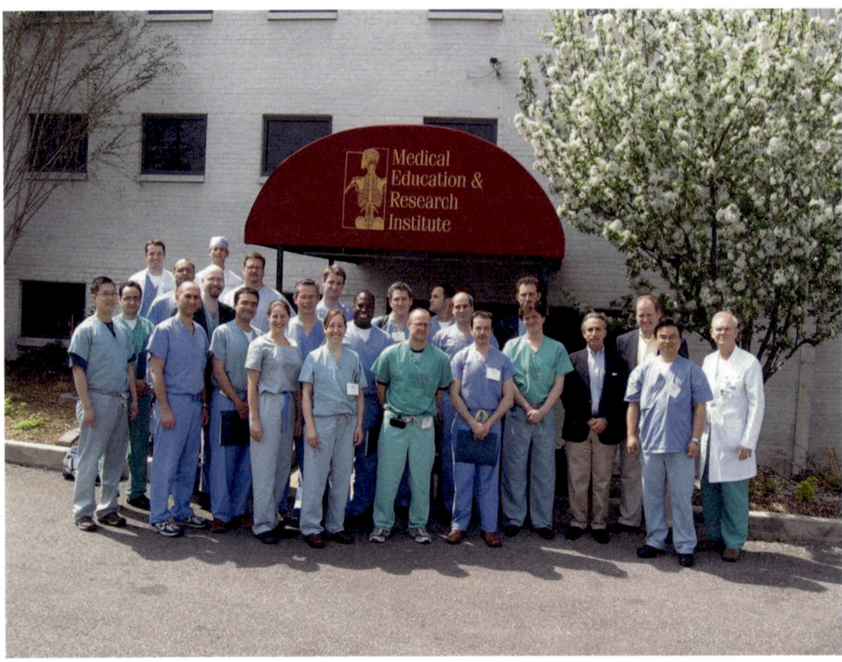

Fig. 21.2 Faculty and participants of the first AANS Endovascular Course in 2006

become a course director and has done so since that first year.

Role and Assessment

Since the birth of the field of neurosurgery, laboratory research and training have been intimately intertwined with clinical practice. Harvey Cushing directed the Hunterian neurosurgical laboratory at Johns Hopkins Hospital with the goals of student education, physiological research, and training in surgical techniques. The anatomic features of the pituitary gland were described, and the fields of endocrinology and neurosurgery were established. Alexis Carrel performed his first arteriovenous fistulas on dogs and promoted practice on animal models to refine vascular surgical techniques. Walter Dandy's work in the laboratory and his focus on hydrocephalus and cerebrospinal fluid circulation paved the way for the development of pneumoencephalography. Professor Yasargil devoted a year and countless hours for laboratory practice using animals and cadaver specimens as simulation

models to develop and practice microsurgical techniques. He created a school of modern neurosurgeons who frequently attend the lab to teach anatomy, microsurgical approaches, and microanastomosis through cadaveric dissections. Simulation has also expanded to the modern fields of endovascular surgery, stereotactic functional surgery, radiosurgery, and spine surgery. With the rapid development of specific technologies and nuances, modern neurosurgeons are faced with the need for continuous training, updating, and refining of their skills to accommodate the rapid change in technology. Trainees are faced with potentially decreased hands-on surgical experience due to work hour restrictions and the augmented vigilance of the medico-legal system. The development of simulation techniques provided excellent alternatives to prepare inexperienced residents with real-life surgical situations.

The NREF vascular courses provide a demonstrable and significant educational benefit to residents and fellows. As part of a pilot study, seven neurosurgery residents with no angiographic experience took part in a 2-day course beginning with didactic lectures, followed by multiple hands-on simulator training and practice sessions. The faculty noticed obvious improvement in the residents' skill and knowledge between the beginning and the end of the course. This positive role was observed not only by the teaching faculty but also by the residents themselves. The residents' reviews spoke very highly of simulation techniques, and many participants attest to the growth of their anatomical knowledge, technical skills, and confidence levels [1]. Due to the success of the pilot program, a 120-min. simulator-based training course was performed at two Congress of Neurological Surgeons Annual Meetings. Thirty-seven neurosurgery residents participated, and after the course, they showed a statistically significant increase in their posttest written and practical scores compared to the pretest scores ($p < 0.001$) [2].

Simulation-based boot camps have existed for some time within the field of general surgery. Participation in these boot camps has shown to significantly increase the clinical, anatomical, and technical performance of junior residents [3, 4]. In 2010, the Society of Neurological Surgeons Boot Camp Fundamental Skills Course was created to introduce important principles of neurosurgical care to postgraduate year 1 residents. Approximately 94% of residents attended the first course offered in 2010 and 99% of those residents believed the boot camp course benefited beginning neurosurgery residents and imparted skills and knowledge that would improve patient care. At 6 months, postcourse surveys completed by the attendees showed knowledge of items taught during the course were retained or slightly enhanced at a higher rate than items not taught in the course ($p < 0.001$) [5].

Spinal simulation has seen significant growth in the past few years. The University of Mississippi Neurosurgery Program created a minimally invasive spinal surgery simulator that was inexpensive and increased the confidence of neurosurgery residents performing a minimally invasive laminectomy [6]. In order to test the utility of simulation training in pedicle and lateral mass screw placement, Sundar et al. published the result of their a single blinded, prospective,

randomized pilot study on the subject. Eight junior residents and two medical students were given didactic training on spinal anatomy and screw placement techniques. Half of each group were randomized to receive additional training with navigation software combined with cadaveric specimen and accessibility to Sawbones models. They found a statistically significant reduction in the overall surgical error in the group that received additional training compared to the group that only received didactic training [7]. Similar studies with junior orthopedic surgery residents using didactic lectures, Sawbones teaching models, and cadaveric specimens showed improvement in the accuracy of thoracic pedicle screw placement on follow-up testing [8].

The "live cadaver" model (Fig. 21.3) was created to simulate aneurysm clipping and management of intraoperative rupture. Twenty-three cadaveric specimens harboring 59 aneurysms (57 artificial and 2 real) were used in 13 neurosurgical courses from 2009 to 2014. Ninety-one participants (faculty and residents) completed a questionnaire to assess their personal experience with the model. Most of them agreed or strongly agreed that the model provided a valid replication of live conditions surrounding cerebral aneurysm clipping and situations of intraoperative rupture. Over 90% believed that the model helps with the acquisition of microsurgical skills and offers benefits not available in other existing training models [9].

Future Directions

A surgical simulation training curriculum was implemented in June 2012 at the University of Texas Medical Branch Neurosurgery Program and was shown to significantly improve proficiency among residents, especially inexperienced junior residents. Cadaver simulations reported the highest benefit among resident surveys (72%), followed by physical simulators (64%), and haptic/computerized techniques (59%). The initial cost was estimated to be $342,000 with $27,900 annual expenses. Although the authors stated that their system worked well for their

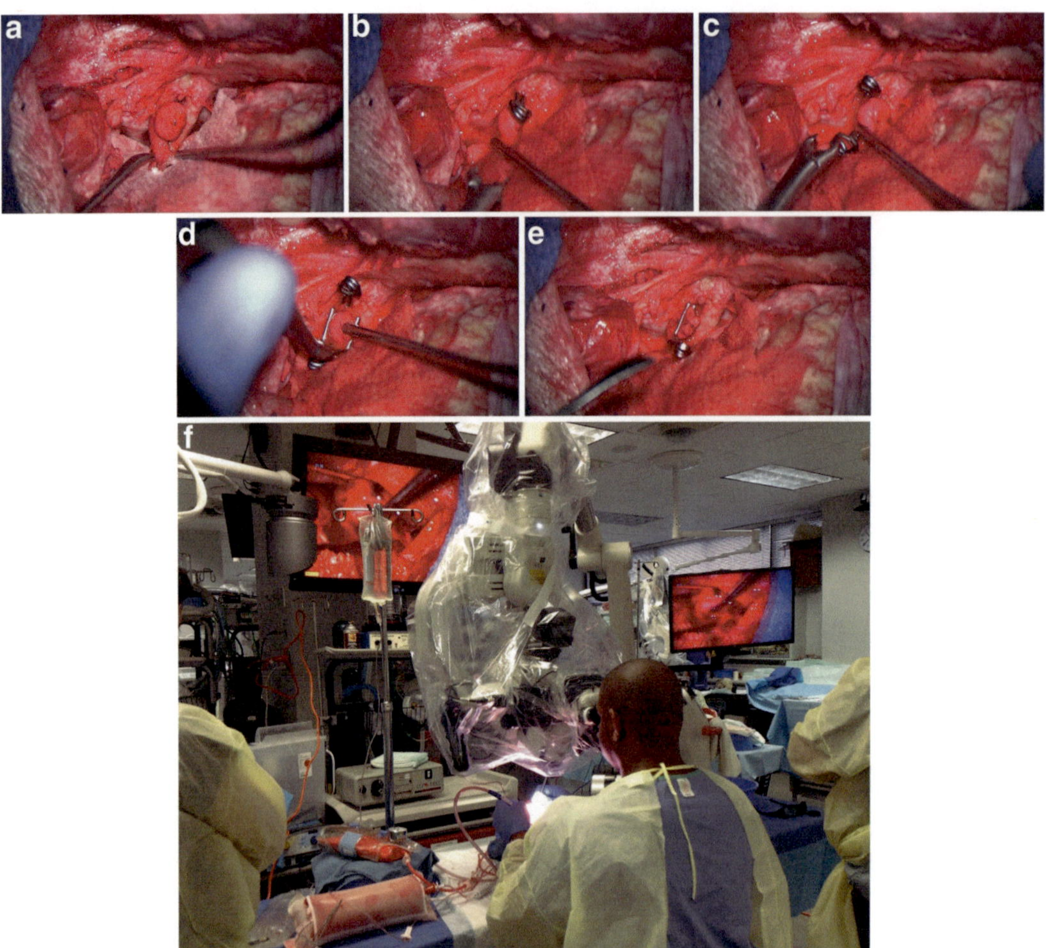

Fig. 21.3 (**a–f**) "Live Cadaver" with simulation of intraoperative "bleeding" and subsequent control with temporary clipping and aneurysm clipping

residents' training needs, they also acknowledge that developing a formal approved curriculum would be challenging given that every training environment is different [10].

In a national survey of neurosurgery residency program directors, the vast majority (94%) now incorporate laboratory dissection into resident training. The vast majority (95%) also believe laboratory dissection is an integral component of training, but no respondent believed simulation could currently provide greater educational benefit than laboratory dissection. However, approximately 48% of respondents do incorporate simulators into their residency program. Endoscopy was the most common (15.4%), followed by microvascular anastomosis (13.8%), and endovascular (10.8%). Most respondents (89%) would support a national "suggested" dissection curriculum and manual. According to the program directors surveyed, virtual reality and other forms of medical simulation, in their current form, are inadequate in replacing traditional forms of resident education. However, the field appears to be changing rapidly and still requires further investigation. [11] The NREF courses continue to provide a structured and cohesive program for study in both endovascular surgery and microneurosurgery as well as a range of other areas. It is clear that simulation is an important component of education on both new techniques and technologies and those that remain critical despite a lower case volume.

Acknowledgement The authors would like to acknowledge Joni Shulman who worked tirelessly and with great patience and humor to make the NREF educational courses possible. Many residents, fellows and faculty owe her a tremendous debt of gratitude.

References

1. Fargen KM, Siddiqui AH, Veznedaroglu E, Turner RD, Ringer AJ, Mocco J. Simulator based angiography education in neurosurgery: results of a pilot educational program. J Neurointerv Surg. 2012;4(6):438–41.
2. Fargen KM, Arthur AS, Bendok BR, Levy EI, Ringer A, Siddiqui AH, et al. Experience with a simulator-based angiography course for neurosurgical residents: beyond a pilot program. Neurosurgery. 2013;73(suppl_1):S46–50.
3. Fernandez GL, Page DW, Coe NP, Lee PC, Patterson LA, Skylizard L, et al. Boot camp: educational outcomes after 4 successive years of preparatory simulation-based training at onset of internship. J Surg Educ. 2012;69(2):242–8.
4. Fonseca AL, Evans LV, Gusberg RJ. Open surgical simulation in residency training: a review of its status and a case for its incorporation. J Surg Educ. 2013;70(1):129–37.
5. Selden NR, Anderson VC, McCartney S, Origitano TC, Burchiel KJ, Barbaro NM. Society of Neurological Surgeons boot camp courses: knowledge retention and relevance of hands-on learning after 6 months of postgraduate year 1 training. J Neurosurg. 2013;119(3):796–802.
6. Walker JB, Perkins E, Harkey HL. A novel simulation model for minimally invasive spine surgery. Neurosurgery 2009;65(6 Suppl):188–95; discussion 95.
7. Sundar SJ, Healy AT, Kshettry VR, Mroz TE, Schlenk R, Benzel EC. A pilot study of the utility of a laboratory-based spinal fixation training program for neurosurgical residents. J Neurosurg Spine. 2016;24(5):850–6.
8. Tortolani PJ, Moatz BW, Parks BG, Cunningham BW, Sefter J, Kretzer RM. Cadaver training module for teaching thoracic pedicle screw placement to residents. Orthopedics. 2013;36(9):e1128–33.
9. Aboud E, Aboud G, Al-Mefty O, Aboud T, Rammos S, Abolfotoh M, et al. "Live cadavers" for training in the management of intraoperative aneurysmal rupture. J Neurosurg. 2015;123(5):1339–46.
10. Gasco J, Holbrook TJ, Patel A, Smith A, Paulson D, Muns A, et al. Neurosurgery simulation in residency training: feasibility, cost, and educational benefit. Neurosurgery. 2013;73(suppl_1):S39–45.
11. Kshettry VR, Mullin JP, Schlenk R, Recinos PF, Benzel EC. The role of laboratory dissection training in neurosurgical residency: results of a National Survey. World Neurosurg. 2014;82(5):554–9.

Simulation Training Experience in Neurosurgical Training in Europe

Nabeel Saud Alshafai, Wafa Alduais, and Maksim Son

Introduction

The objective of this chapter is to encapsulate the past, current, and future contribution to neurosurgical training in simulation from a European prospective. This chapter does not touch advances related to outside the European continent.

Comprehensive Healthcare Simulation from European Prospective

The Value of Simulation in Medical Practice

As a medical professional committed to "first do no harm," some experts argue that it is an ethical imperative to develop and use simulators as a means to protect patients from being the "commodities to be used as conveniences of training" [1]. Neurosurgery ranks as the most liable specialty in all of medicine to malpractice, with 19.1% of neurosurgeons facing a claim a year [2]. A prospective study of 1108 elective neurosurgery cases showed that 78.5%

of errors were preventable and that the most frequent errors were technical in nature [3]. Yet, in a field such as neurosurgery that requires such high level of technical expertise, with large consequences for error, there are even fewer opportunities for younger trainees to practice on the most complicated cases, which may only be possible after finishing a neurosurgical residency at the independent attending level [4].

Historically, trainees have developed operative neurosurgical skills through the surgical apprenticeship model, following the old adage "see one, do one, and teach one" [5]. However, in recent years many factors have challenged this traditional apprenticeship model:

- Limitations on the working week hours of doctors were first started in the United States after the death of an 18-year-old female inpatient in 1984, determined by a grand jury to be partly a result of long hours worked by unsupervised interns and residents [6]. Similar changes occurred after the introduction of the European Working Time Directive, which limits the working week of junior doctors to 48 h [6].
- The development of assistant surgical nurse practitioners has reduced learning opportunities in the operating room [7].
- The introduction of modernizing medical careers and subspecialization has further

N. S. Alshafai (✉) · W. Alduais · M. Son
Alshafai Neurosurgical Academy A.N.A,
Toronto, ON, Canada

reduced the surgical caseload of neurosurgical trainees [5].

- There is a classical ethical dilemma inherent in training. The patients are best served when operated by a specialist rather than a trainee even if the trainee is supervised by the specialist [8].
- Improving patient safety is obviously a very important ultimate goal; however even with the most established advances, there are no enough studies that simulation would affect the patient outcome [9–11].

Some authors have described the European Working Time Directive as a bureaucratic constraint hindering high-quality postgraduate training [12]. It may seem impossible to educate neurosurgeons to an even better standard than previously, with reduced training time and at the same time exponentially increasing complexity created by our scientific endeavors [8].

In the book *Outliers*, Malcolm Gladwell evaluated experts across multiple disciplines and concluded that the common theme among them is the accumulation of 10,000 h of repeated practice at a specific task [13]. Residency training in Europe with the current working hour restriction of 48 h per week over 6-year residency program will result in approximately 13,824 h of training, excluding 1 month vacation every year. However, most of this time is spent devoted to evaluating and treating patients and doing administrative work outside of the operating room.

Simulation has been postulated as a potential solution to the challenge of providing appropriate training in less time and represents a useful proxy measure for expert surgical performance [14].

Simulation in Neurosurgery

The tides of postgraduate medical education in Europe are changing [8, 15]. The increasing complexity of neurosurgery has surpassed the ability for a single neurosurgeon to master all theoretical and practical aspects of this specialty and pushed trainees toward subspecialization [8]. At the same time, there is a reduction in the resident/trainee

working time to 48 h/week (including on calls) in the European Union [16], which contributes to a sense of need of additional training [12]. An additional challenge is that European residents in some countries have a less "hands-on" experience during residency than their counterparts in other European states [17]. In an international survey of neurosurgery program directors (PDs), only 15% European PDs felt confident that their senior residents could manage aneurysm by craniotomy and clipping, in contrast to 75% of their North American counterparts [17]. Adding to the fact that some studies estimated that classical surgical training in the operating room can cost an upward of $50,000 per graduating resident [18], simulation training presents an attractive alternative including Europe. A recent article mentioned that Russia currently has 50 simulation centers in medicine, with plans to increase that number to 80 centers by 2017 [19]. Since simulation training sessions can be standardized and reproduced, it may be effectively included in testing, licensing, and credentialing processes [20].

Surgeons Are Made and Not Born

To answer the continuous debate about whether some surgeons are born great and experts or is it the hard work and commitment to continuous practice, Sadideen et al. questioned Galton's innate talent theory. He mentioned that two studies conducted on novice medical students and surgical residents, respectively, have shown competency after repeated practice on a simulator [21, 22]. He also mentioned that testing the innate ability of an individual should be done to identify those who need extra training [23]. He concluded that although innate abilities play an important role in the development of surgical expertise, the literature suggests that the surgical experts are in fact "made," not born which is the same conclusion given by Jasper Halpenny 100 years ago [24].

As to surgery, surgeons are made, not born. The making process we call education. Education should commence when the child begins to use its hands. It should be taught to use both hands equally well, as nearly as possible. As it grows, it should have its reasoning power developed, its ability to observe and record its observations, and its mechanical ability should be encouraged.

Practice Made Perfect

No one could argue the fact that in order to develop neurosurgical expertise, one should continuously practice the same procedure repeatedly. This was called by Ericsson and colleagues [25] as "deliberate practice." The main characteristics of deliberate practice are motivation, detailed and immediate feedback, and the ability to perform the task repeatedly. Simulation provides the perfect learning tool for neurosurgical residents as it allows repeatedly performing the same task and also may provide immediate feedback using video recording and other tools such as the Imperial College Surgical Assessment Device which provide quantitative evaluation of the dexterity while performing core surgical skills [5, 26].

The Use of Simulation in Neurosurgical Residency Education

Medical educators have a very difficult task as medical knowledge is tremendously increasing in an exponential fast pattern and with the concern of patients being practiced upon by students [27]. A study which was conducted on 33 medical students in 2004 demonstrated that medical students value simulation-based learning highly and that they in particular value the opportunity to apply their theoretical knowledge in a safe and realistic setting [28]. Simulation has shown early success in helping junior residents learn the fundamentals of each operation, plan the approach, and rehearse the procedure [29]. However, for more senior residents, the advances in physical and virtual reality simulations were proved so far to be useful in training of intracranial endoscopy [30], tumor resection [31], and spine surgeries [32].

Europe's Contribution to Advancement in Neurosurgical Simulation

Preop Planning

As early as 1998, a German group (Hassfeld S et al.) published a paper about the value of stereolithographic models for preoperative diagnosis of craniofacial deformities and planning of surgical corrections and concluded that using computer-assisted simulation and navigation systems improves quality and reduces risk of more extensive and radical interventions [33].

In another study which compared the simulated 3D virtual endoscopy images to the intraoperative endoscopic anatomy in terms of distortion and angle of view, suggested that both were comparable. According to this study, virtual endoscopy was found to be particularly useful for the preoperative depiction of (1) the nasal anatomy and its variations for choosing the side of the approach, (2) the sphenoid sinus septa and chambers for improved intraoperative orientation, and (3) the transparent 3D simulated visualization of the pituitary gland, tumor, and adjacent anatomic structures in relation to the sphenoid sinus landmarks for planning the opening of the sellar floor. Finally, they concluded that virtual endoscopy has the potential to become a valuable tool in endoscopic pituitary surgery for training purposes and preoperative planning, and it may add to the safety of interventions in case of anatomic variations [34].

It is well known that all surgical approaches are tailored specifically for each patient depending on the anatomy and pathology in the neurosurgical practice. Having that in mind, precise preoperative planning for these procedures is necessary to achieve optimal therapeutic effect. Therefore, multiple radiological imaging modalities are used prior to surgery to delineate the patient's anatomy, neurological function, and metabolic processes. Beyer et al. from Vienna introduced an application that consists of three main modules which allow to (1) plan the optimal skin incision and opening of the skull tailored to the underlying pathology; (2) visualize superficial brain anatomy, function, and metabolism; and (3) plan the patient-specific approach for surgery of deep-seated lesions [35].

Stereolithographic Modeling

To the best of our knowledge one of the earliest papers about the stereolithographic modeling was published by a French group, Bouyssie JF et al., and it tested the accuracy of models derived from X-ray-computed tomography, which was found to be reliable enough to be used for surgical planning, for custom-made implants, and for surgical anatomy teaching [36].

Another study was conducted by a German group to assess the importance of stereolithographic models (SLMs) for preoperative diagnosis and planning in craniofacial surgery and to examine whether these models offer valuable additional information as compared to normal CT scans and 3D CT images [37].

Currently, 3D printing has been used primarily in neurosurgery for operative planning, teaching, practice, and prosthetics. Advances in 3D printing have enabled scientists, engineers, and physicians to create models for surgical planning and residency training based on patient-specific imaging studies [38]. High-fidelity 3D-printed models have the potential to assist clinical decision and allow surgeons to rehearse neurosurgical cases in a manner not previously possible [39].

Reality Training Applications

Virtual reality refers to the recreation of environments or objects as a complex, computer-generated image; haptic systems refer to those replicating the kinaesthetic and tactile perception (Fig. 22.1). Virtual reality and haptic systems are usually combined, and they are currently available to support vascular access training, endoscopy training, and laparoscopic surgical techniques [41].

Voxel-Man Group (Hamburg, Germany) developed virtual reality CT images, and the

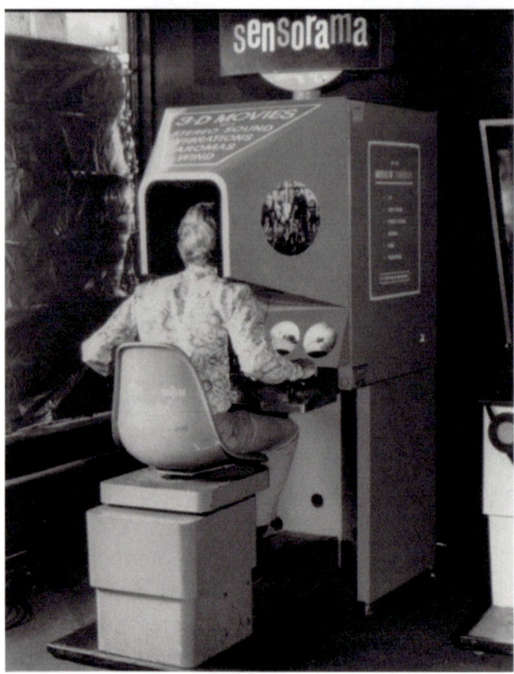

Fig. 22.1 The Sensorama was released in the 1950s (one of the earliest examples of immersive, multisensory multimodal technology) [40]

simulators were felt to improve the realism of surgical procedures in the middle ear and provided automatic skills assessment for each participant by the end of the procedure [42]. Kockro RA et al. from Germany have developed a highly interactive virtual environment that enabled collaborative examination of stereoscopic three-dimensional (3D) medical imaging data for planning, discussing, or teaching neurosurgical approaches and strategies. They found out that the system provides a highly effective way to work with 3D data in a group, and it significantly enhances teaching of neurosurgical anatomy and operative strategies [43].

The Human Brain Project

Decoding the human brain is perhaps the most fascinating scientific challenge in the twenty-first century. The Human Brain Project (HBP) is developing toward a European research infrastructure advancing brain research, medicine, and brain-inspired information technology [44].

Up to our knowledge, the earliest article written about the Human Brain Project was published in 1993, and it mentioned that an initiative of several NIH institutes and other US government agencies is being developed to provide a computer database that will allow neuroscientists' access to information at all levels of integration, from genes to behavior [45]. However, the core idea of the Human Brain Project was first developed by Henry Markram and was based on the research developed for the Blue Brain Project [46]. On May 2005 Blue Brain Project was founded by the Brain Mind Institute of the École Polytechnique Fédérale de Lausanne (EPFL) in Switzerland with an interesting mission of using biologically detailed digital reconstruction and simulation of the mammalian brain to identify the fundamental principles of brain structure and function in health and disease [47]. Markram, in 2006, published a paper, and he proposed that "the time is right to begin assimilating the wealth of data that has been accumulated over the past century and start building biologically accurate models of the brain from first principles to aid our understanding of brain function and dysfunction" [48].

Henry Markram is a professor of neuroscience at the Swiss Federal Institute for Technology (EPFL). He is the founder of the Brain Mind Institute, founder and director of the Blue Brain Project, and the founder of the Human Brain Project [49]. Starting in 2010, Markram created and coordinated the partnership of around 80 European and international partners that developed the original HBP proposal. HBP is one of the two 10-year one billion Euro Flagship Projects selected in January 2013 by the European Commission. The project began operations in October of the same year [50].

The HBP has the following main objectives:

- Create and operate a European scientific research infrastructure for brain research, cognitive neuroscience, and other brain-inspired sciences.
- Gather, organize, and disseminate data describing the brain and its diseases.
- Simulate the brain.
- Build multi-scale scaffold theory and models for the brain.
- Develop brain-inspired computing, data analytics, and robotics.
- Ensure that the HBP's work is undertaken responsibly and that it benefits society.

This project is exceptional in three respects: it is among the longest ever approved in the field of neuroscience (having a duration of 10 years), the most heavily financed (the HBP will receive about 1.1 billion euros), and the most transdisciplinary in nature [51].

The HBP has 12 subprojects (SP), and they are all interconnected (Table 22.1).

Our main concern in this chapter is related to subprojects 6 and 10 which will be discussed with further details below.

Brain Simulation Platform SP6

There are three main objectives for SP6 as stated by the Human Brain Project Framework Partnership Agreement (HBP FPA):

- Establish a generic strategy to reconstruct and simulate the multilevel organization of the brain for different brain areas and species.
- Use this strategy to build high-fidelity reconstructions, first of the mouse brain and ultimately of the human brain.
- Support community-driven reconstructions and simulations and to support comparisons between models based on different tools and approaches.

The platform will provide tools and services for the collaborative reconstruction and simulation of the brain, models of different brain areas and the whole brain (including models developed outside the HBP), and tools for in silico experimentation, supporting comparisons between different models

Table 22.1 The Human Brain Project subprojects [48, 52, 53]

Subproject No. (SP)	Name	Description
SP 1	Mouse brain organization	Understanding the structure of the mouse brain and its electrical and chemical functions
SP 2	Human brain organization	Understanding the structure of the human brain and its electrical and chemical functions
SP 3	Systems and cognitive neuroscience	Understanding how the brain performs its system-level and cognitive functional activities
SP 4	Theoretical neuroscience	Deriving high-level mathematical models to synthesis conclusions from research data
SP 5	Neuro-informatics platform	Gathering, organizing, and making available brain data
SP 6	Brain simulation platform	Developing data-driven reconstructions of brain tissue and simulation capabilities to explore these reconstructions
SP 7	High-performance analytics and computing platform	Providing the ICT capability to map the brain in unprecedented detail, construct complex models, run large simulations, and analyze large volumes of data
SP 8	Medical informatics platform	Developing the infrastructure to share hospital and medical research data for the purpose of understanding disease clusters and their respective disease signatures
SP 9	Neuromorphic computing platform	Developing and applying brain-inspired computing technology
SP 10	Neurorobotics	Developing virtual and real robots and environments for testing brain simulations
SP 11	Central services	Coordinating the scientific road map and supervision of the milestones and deliverables for the HBP's ICT platforms
SP 12	Ethics and society	Exploring the ethical and societal impact of the HBP's work

and approaches. A key goal is to collaborate with SP1–SP4, SP9, and SP10 to develop simplified versions of high-fidelity brain models, for cognitive, behavioral, and clinical studies, and to participate in research using these models [52].

Collaborations with Other National, European, and International Initiatives

In the article "Creating a European Research Infrastructure to Decode the Human Brain" by Amuntus K et al., the author concluded that there are a growing number of well-publicized brain research initiatives around the world which are mobilizing unprecedented levels of funding for neuroscience and that there is a strong interest to maximize cooperation and coordination between the various initiatives and that the Human Brain Project (HBP) is keen to help lay the foundations

for such interaction [44]. However, a particularly important collaboration is with the Allen Institute for Brain Science, Seattle, Washington, USA, on models of the visual and motor systems of the mouse ultimately leading to models of visuomotor behavior in mouse. Another collaboration with CENTER-TBI will provide data on specific traumatic brain injury lesions and multilevel data including electrophysiology, imaging, and cognitive measures that could be used to build models of brain injury [52].

Neurorobotics SP10

Neurorobotics can be defined as the science and technology of robots which are controlled by a simulated nervous system that reflects, at some level, the architecture and dynamics of the brain [54]. Probably the first researcher to develop a robot that fulfilled these criteria was Thomas

Ross, who in 1933 devised a mobile robot with a small electromechanical brain, which could navigate through a maze in real time [55]. Researchers have also developed a large number of robots, three of the most advanced are iCub (Fig. 22.2) (a humanoid robot "child") [57], Kojiro (a humanoid robot with about 100 "muscles") [58], and ECCE (a humanoid upper torso that attempts to replicate the inner structure and mechanisms of the human body) [59].

The overall objective of SP10 is to provide tools allowing researchers to test the cognitive and behavioral capabilities of the brain models developed in SP6 and the neuromorphic implementations of these models from SP9. The Neurorobotics Platform will provide researchers with access to detailed brain models on the Brain Simulation Platform running slower than real time [52] (Fig. 22.3).

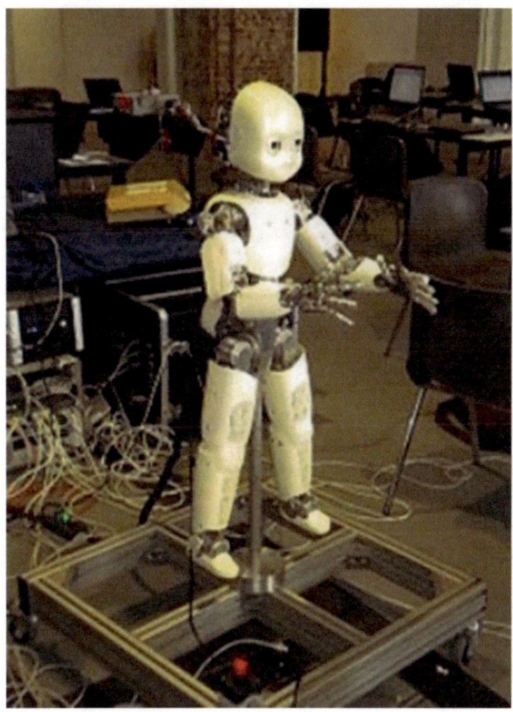

Fig. 22.2 An iCub robot mounted on a supporting frame. It was designed by the Robot Cub Consortium of several European universities and built by Italian Institute of Technology [56]

Recent European Contributions to Neurosurgical Simulators

European contribution to simulation training research is unfortunately somehow still limited. Limited operating room exposure to vascular neurosurgery for European trainees may be due to the consequences of reduced working week hours in the EU as well as a less "hands-on" approach as in the example of cerebral aneurysm clipping [8, 17]. This fact increases the need for training these valuable skills outside of the operating room. Practicing on animal tissue is an important aspect of neurosurgical training. Depending on the type of tissue, it offers trainees to practice on samples closely resembling realistic anatomy [61]. A recent article by the neurosurgeons from Turkey proposed a model of using fresh sheep cadavers to simulate microdiscectomy surgery [62]. Unfortunately, preservation of cadavers requires the use of harsh chemicals such as formaldehyde which alters tissue feel. To address the issue, British authors described embalming methods that realistically simulate the feel of the tissue or bone during pedicle placement [63]. Costs associated with setting up and maintaining animal labs present a general limitation to this teaching method. A Spanish team proposed a model of simulation of cerebral brain perfusion utilizing human brains instead of a more traditional use of decapitated heads [61]. For all the previous reasons, the development of alternative realistic training methods is vital (Fig. 22.4).

The Three Ways European Residents Can Access Simulators

In Europe, most of the simulation training that neurosurgery residents obtain comes from their respective residency site. The other sources include additional training at international simulation centers and participating in numerous training courses organized by national bodies or supranational organizations such as the European Association of Neurosurgical Societies (EANS).

The situation regarding the use of simulators in Europe is heterogeneous. Despite the rising

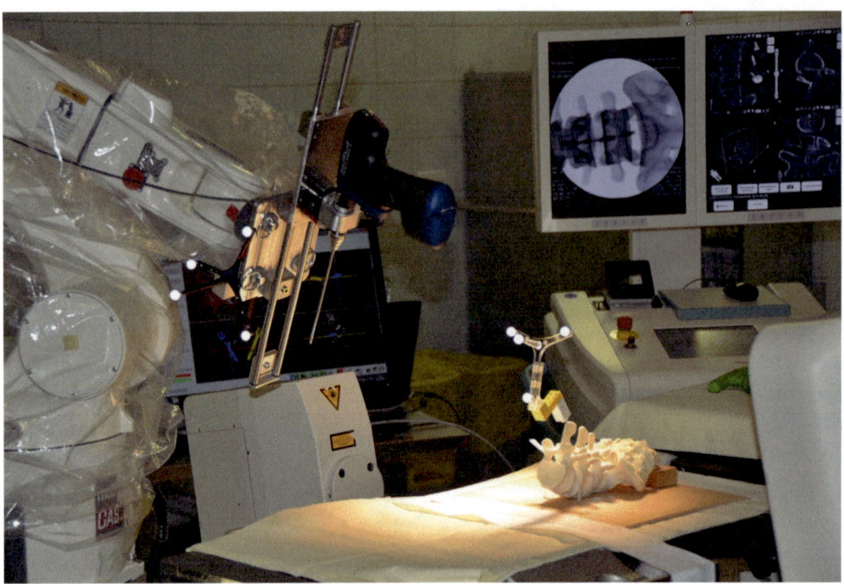

Fig. 22.3 An assistance system for minimally invasive spinal surgery: robot-assisted positioning of screws on a model of the lumbar vertebrae at the Research Project Centre for Sensor Systems (ZESS), University of Siegen and Neurosurgery Karlsruhe (Used with permission [60])

sentiment among the educators toward using more simulators [6], general trend suggests that simulation training continues to play only a minor role in the residency curriculum [65]. In a multinational study, PDs from 38 European countries (including Turkey and Israel) were surveyed on the state of neurosurgical education. Nine of the surveyed centers located in Western Europe and five surveyed centers in Eastern Europe had simulation facilities including either cadaveric labs, virtual labs, or phantoms (Fig. 22.5). Although the situation between different training sites within one country may vary, these preliminary results give an idea of the educational trends for the region as a whole. These findings corroborate results of a survey of 532 European neurosurgery residents, which indicated that less than half of European programs have simulation or cadaver labs [12]. Not surprisingly, only 13.4% of surveyed respondents were satisfied with their hands-on simulator training [12].

Besta NeuroSim Center is the only European training site that contains several advanced neurosimulators under one roof. Located in Milan, Italy, the center has the latest virtual

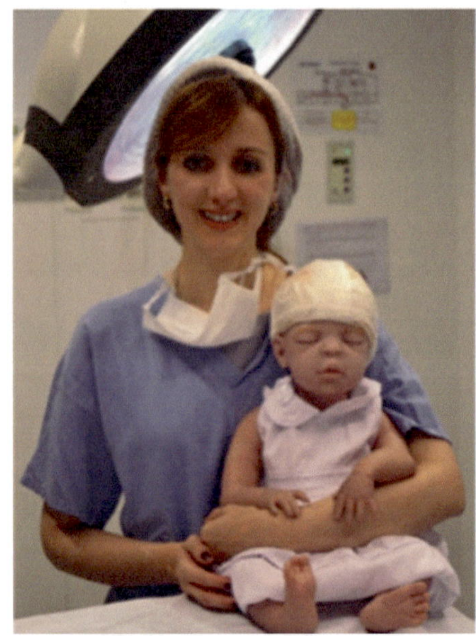

Fig. 22.4 Dr. Giselle Coelho and her realistic model, a mimic of an infant with craniosynostosis (Used with permission [64])

reality neurosimulators including NeuroTouch, ImmersiveTouch, Surgical Theater, and one 3D anatomical visualizer (Virtual Proteins) [66]. This training site has a close cooperation with

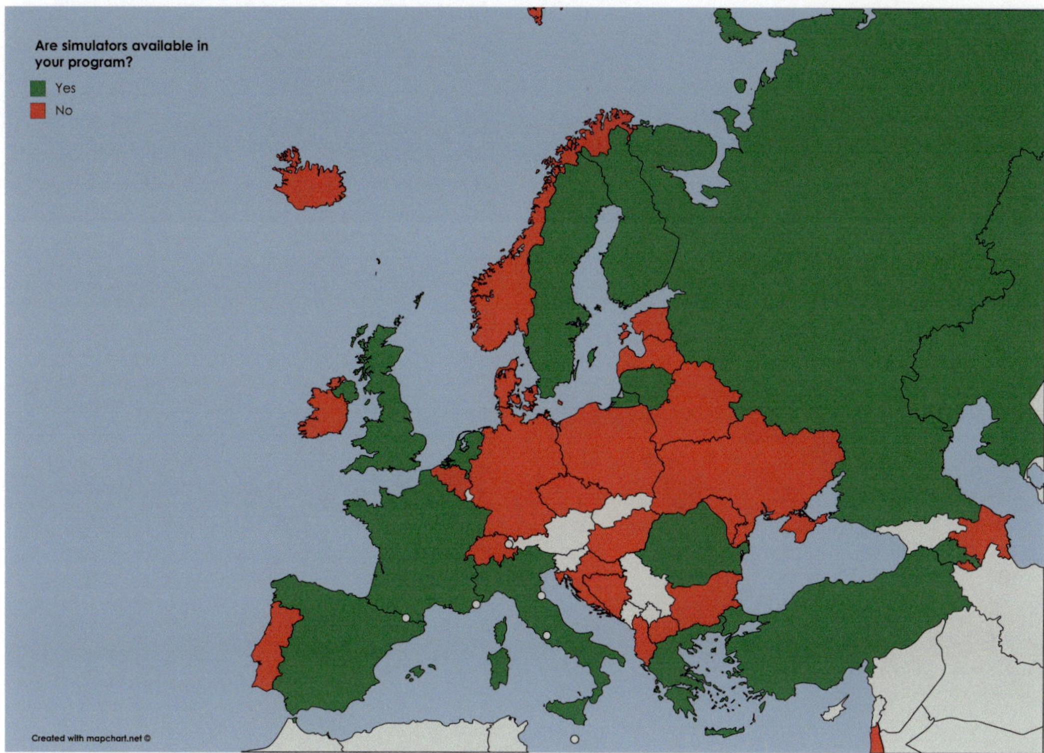

Fig. 22.5 The availability of simulators in European countries [65] (Obtained with permission from the European survey study conducted by the postgraduate education committee of the European Association of Neurosurgical Societies 2016)

McGill University (Canada). Besta NeuroSim Center offers postgraduate residency training, continuing medical education courses for practicing surgeons, and observerships for medical students in Europe [44].

The third source of simulation training for European residents comes from attending national and supranational courses – such as the EANS training courses. Founded in 2012, the EANS Hands-On Course is a 5-day biannual workshop. It offers trainees to practice cranial and spinal approaches and endoscopy techniques. Recently, there has been a push within EANS to include practical training aspects into courses that were previously exclusively theoretical [67]. For advanced trainees with interest in craniocervical junction, a special cadaveric workshop has been developed [68]. The course runs on an annual basis in Barcelona (Spain) and is taught by neurosurgical faculty from Europe and North America. This offers a unique chance for trainees to practice surgical skills under the guidance of international experts in both spine and skullbase approaches applying different techniques such as navigation, cadaveric models, virtual reality, and live 3D anatomy.

Finally, European trainees may get additional exposure to neurosimulators by doing an off-site rotation within their country or Europe at large [69].

SESAM Constitution

The name of the society is the "Society in Europe for Simulation Applied to Medicine," known hereafter and registered as "SESAM"(Table 22.2).

The purpose of SESAM is:

- The development and application of simulation in education, research, and quality management in medicine and healthcare

Table 22.2 Society in Europe for Simulation Applied to Medicine (SESAM) Members. Used with permission [70]

Logo	Name of the simulation center
	ADAM – Amsterdam Simulation Centre Amsterdam, Netherlands ADAM – Amsterdam Simulation Centre
	Alpha Medical Concepts (AMC) Linz, Austria AMC is a 300 m2 sim center in Linz, Austria. AMC does 300 high-fidelity trainings per year; 80% of the courses are done in situ and focus on interprofessional, interdisciplinary team trainings. The AMC team consists of physicians, nurses, psychologists, and paramedics. Most of them are licensed hospital managers, executive advisors and of course certified trainers. AMC runs a consulting company besides the sim activities to transfer the issues found during trainings or a system check into a project afterward.
	Antalya Health Directorate – Region Training, Research and Simulation Centre Antalya, Turkey Antalya Health Directorate – Region Training, Research and Simulation Centre
	Application of Science to Simulation Education and Research on Training Centre Cork, Ireland ASSERT aims to decrease medical error and improve patient care by enabling health professionals and trainees to engage in the deliberate practice of skills to predefined proficiency standards in simulated clinical settings
	Arcada Patient Safety and Learning Centre Helsinki, Finland The Arcada Patient Safety and Learning Centre (APSLC) provides educational services to multidisciplinary professionals and students in the healthcare sector. The center's core competencies are patient safety and simulation-based learning
	Association de cardiologie et de réanimation médicale de Zaghouan (ACRMZ) ACRMZ – Association de cardiologie et de réanimation médicale de Zaghouan
	Besta NeuroSim Center Milan, Italy The Besta NeuroSim Center is the first center for training and neurosurgical simulation in Europe dedicated to innovative research in neurosurgical simulation, a means in which neurosurgeons can rehearse surgeries in a superb 3D virtual reality environment. Neurosimulation enables surgeons to plan surgical strategy before performing a real-life operation and reduces medical errors for patients. Our focus is to propose a revolutionary training method for the new generation of neurosurgeons and identify how to achieve performance excellence in surgery
	Biomedical Simulation Center, Faculty of Medicine of University of Porto – CSB The Biomedical Simulation Center of the Faculty of Medicine of U.Porto (CSB-FMUP) opened on December 2003, being a pioneer center in Portugal. Its mission is to create a unique, safe, and sustainable educational environment providing experiential training to students, residents, and healthcare professionals, on technical skills, behavior, decision-making, team work, and clinical communication. Since its opening, BSC-FMUP has trained more than 3500 students and 1200 healthcare professionals, in several clinical areas: physiology, semiology, pharmacology, urology, obstetrics, neonatology, pediatrics, anesthesiology, clinical communication, and crisis resource management, among others. Since 2014 it has accredited training of instructors in clinical simulation

CASE	CASE - Centre of Advanced Simulation and Education Istanbul, Turkey Acibadem University – CASE (Centre of Advanced Simulation and Education) consists of clinical simulation and advanced endoscopic/robotic surgery training departments. With its variety of medical simulation modalities, and technological infrastructure, CASE creates a difference in both undergraduate and postgraduate trainings. Besides its medical simulation labs, CASE has a wet lab with nine stations for laparoscopic surgery, a robotic surgery training center, and a dissection lab for cadaver-based surgical training
ENSOSP	Centre de SIMulation à l'URGence extra-hospitalière de l'ENSOSP Aix-en-Provence – Les Milles, France The ENSOSP trains 25,000 professional firefighter French officers, volunteers, and the health service. The training provided is designed to meet the employers' orders (SDIS) in terms of managerial and operational quality and adaptability and the Civil Security Department (DSC) in normative and prospective terms. Creuset initiatives and partnerships and institutional approaches, supports the training advisers and offers high-level training through specialized master's (risk management, law of civil security, CBRNE)
	Centre de Simulation PRESAGE Lille, France PRESAGE
	Centre Lyonnais d'Enseignement par la Simulation en Santé Lyon, France CLESS (Lyonnais Teaching Centre for Simulation in Healthcare) is located within the Lyon East Faculty of Medicine. It is part of SAMSEI project (Learning Strategies of Health Professionals in Immersive Environment), and their objectives are the training of health professionals in order to improve the quality of care and safety of patients. It also hosts the industrial world of health
	Centro de Simulacao Biomedica, Faculdade de Medicina da Universidade do Porto Porto, Portugal Porto Biomedical Simulation Centre (CSB-FMUP) is an academic center integrated in the Department of Medical Education and Simulation, Faculty of Medicine, at the University of Porto. CSB-FMUP was inaugurated in December 2003, being the first biomedical simulation center in Portugal. Our aim is to create a unique, safe, and sustainable educational environment providing experiential training to students, residents, and healthcare professionals, in the subjects of technical skills, behavior and decision-making, team work, and communication. Research of methods and tools for simulation-based medical education is also part of our action plan, which involves a close working relationship with the simulation industry
CUSIM	Centrul Universitar de Simulare in Instruirea Medicala Chisinau, Republic of Moldova Centrul Universitar de Simulare in Instruirea Medicala
LaC	Clinical Skills Lab of the Faculty of Health Sciences of the University of Beira Interior Covilha, Portugal LaC is the only simulation center located in the countryside of Portugal. It is integrated in a Portuguese public medical school and is focused on undergraduate medical training with simulation. LaC's program accompanies students from their first to their last curricular year, based on peer and near-peer teaching, with excellent feedback and impact on students

(continued)

Table 22.2 (continued)

Logo	Name of the simulation center
	Danish Maritime Authority, Centre of Maritime Health Service The Centre of Maritime Health Service trains Danish and foreign seamen to be in charge of medical care on board ships. The center is part of the Danish Maritime Authority and is situated on Fanoe. The Centre of Maritime Health Service is always ready to answer questions and give guidance concerning health on board Danish ships
	EduSim Therwil, Switzerland EduSim specializes on in situ simulation trainings in the field of both in-hospital and prehospital emergency medicine. EduSim programs cover a broad spectrum from human factors and patient safety to hard skills in emergency medicine. The mutual goal of all EduSim programs is to increase patient safety by the development of individual- and team-oriented knowledge, skills, and competencies
	Emergency Services College – Section of Prehospital Emergency Medical Care Kuopio, Finland Emergency Services College – Section of Prehospital Emergency Medical Care
	Euregional Patient Safety Simulation Liege, Belgium EPaSS Centre
	HELIOS Simulationszentrum Hildesheim Hildesheim, Germany
	Hospital Virtual Valdecilla S L Santander, Spain Hospital Virtual Valdecilla is a center of innovation and high-performance training for health professionals through the use of clinical simulation as a teaching tool. Our training methodology is based on experiential learning and reflection on practice. Each participant is the protagonist of his own process of active training. Participants in our programs have modern facilities and technologies and a wide range of activities specifically designed to meet the needs of any healthcare organization
	iLumens Paris, France Department de Simulation – iLumens
	Institut Toulousain de Simulation en Santé Toulouse, France Institut Toulousain de Simulation en Santé specializes in everyday courses with a very multifunctional platform. They work on standardized patient programs with hospitals, medicine schools, nurse schools, and private health providers
	IrkSTC Irkutsk, Russian Federation IrkSTC is one of the leading medical institutions of the Irkutsk region; it is a clinical base of nine faculties of Irkutsk State Medical University and eight chairs of Irkutsk State Institute of Advanced Medical. The regional hospital has developed and introduced a large number of advanced medical technologies, and the clinic has an important organizational, methodological, and coordinating role in improving the quality of care to the population, transferring lessons learned to other health facilities in the area

	Le SIMU de Nantes Nantes Cedex 1, France Le SiMU de Nantes
	Maudsley Simulation London, England Maudsley Simulation is the UK's first simulation training center focusing on mental health
	Medical Education & Simulation Hub (MESH) – Mid Yorkshire NHS Trust Wakefield, United Kingdom The Mid Yorkshire NHS Trust has a variety of virtual reality simulators, manikins, and simulation models. Their facilities are based in the Trust Headquarters and Education Centre at Pinderfields Hospital, Wakefield, and the Oakwell Centre at Dewsbury Hospital
	Medical Simulation Centre of the Siberian State Medical University Tomsk, Russian Federation MS Center SSMU, Tomsk
	Medical Training & Simulation Center Bilthoven, Netherlands The METS Center develops and facilitates training courses to make healthcare professionals to provide the best and safest patient care.
	MENTOR MEDICUS Moscow, Russian Federation The simulation and assessment center MENTOR MEDICUS was organized by the Sechenov First Moscow State Medical University in 2007, at that time as a center for basic medical skills training. Today this is one of the biggest institutions of this type in Russia, occupying nearly 1,500 square meters – a floor of the Russian Central Medical Scientific Library and services. The simulation center in the "Sechenov First Med" provides annual training for thousands of trainees – medical students and doctors by CME programs. Among the numerous skill labs for different specialties, we facilitate an entire virtual hospital – a complex structure replicating the logistic of universal hospital. It replicates emergency admittance, shock room, diagnostic department, and operation theater with hybrid OR, obstetrics delivery ward, ICU, postop recovery ward, and doctor's offices. A separate room is dedicated for the casualty training by disasters or car accidents – here the numerous realistic emergency scenarios can be represented "in field," and after prehospital aid, the victims are transported by the realistic ambulance to the virtual hospital
	METS Center Bilthoven, Netherlands METS Center is the largest multidisciplinary simulation center in the Netherlands. All simulation instructors in the Netherlands know METS Center because this center provides the EuSim Simulation Instructor Courses (basic/refresher/advanced) in the local language. A lot of foreign instructors followed these courses since we provide international EuSim courses as well
	Royal Free Hospital Simulation Centre London, United Kingdom We provide interprofessional training for both undergraduates and postgraduates. Part of the center is multifunctional, specializing in part-task practical procedural training (often using ultrasound) as well as high-fidelity full immersion simulation and resuscitation training. Other areas are set aside for state-of-the-art virtual reality simulators for training in laparoscopic surgery and endoscopic procedures

(continued)

Table 22.2 (continued)

Logo	Name of the simulation center
	Royal Surrey County Hospital Simulation Centre (UK) Guildford, United Kingdom Medical simulation has been established at Royal Surrey County Hospital and viewed as a center of excellence by the deanery. It has been committed to deliver realistic and immersive simulation with close attention to detail. The service is constantly evolving, driven by a committed team with high standards. We are responsive and reactive to participant feedback. Simulation is delivered on-site within a twin-bedded skills area and periodically at the University of Surrey. Future plans involve using high-fidelity simulators and mobile observation equipment bringing simulation to the multidisciplinary team and allowing real process and systems of work analysis
	School of Nursing, University of Barcelona Barcelona, Spain EUI-EB
	Schweizer Institut fur Rettungsmedizin Nottwil, Switzerland SIRMED
	Scottish Centre for Simulation and Clinical Human Factors The Scottish Centre for Simulation and Clinical Human Factors is a state-of-the-art multi-professional training facility. We run simulation-based courses for hospital healthcare staff – from nursing auxiliaries to anesthetic consultants, as well as industry-based personnel such as offshore gas platform medics. In addition, we facilitate workshops and provide lectures on nontechnical skills and human factors for healthcare personnel, higher education institutions, and businesses.
	SIMNOVA Novara, Italy Centro Interdipartimentale di Didattica Innovativa e di Simulazione in Medicina e Professioni Sanitarie
	Simulatiecentrum Maastricht UMC+ Academie Maastricht, Netherlands The Simulation Center of the Maastricht UMC + Academy is the central facility of the MUMC providing simulation training for healthcare workers from in- and outside the MUMC
	Simulation and Interactive Learning Centre at Guy's and St Thomas' NHS Foundation Hospital London, United Kingdom The Simulation and Interactive Learning Centre at Guy's and St Thomas' NHS Foundation Trust is a state-of-the art training centers dedicated to delivering clinical skills and high-fidelity training for both undergraduate and postgraduate healthcare practitioners. The SaIL Centre at St Thomas' Hospital opened in 2010 and has become one of the most active facilities in London, training over 4000 healthcare students and professionals each year. The center focuses on medical error and human factors/nontechnical skills to improve patient safety. The director, Dr Peter Jaye, is a consultant in emergency medicine and has led the development of simulation within our hospitals and the local community. He has facilitated the development of a national reputation for research into simulation at the St Thomas House SaIL Centre and has also lead the simulation work stream for the South London Health Innovation and Education Cluster
	Simulation Centre of ASL Naples 2 North Naples, Italy MedSimNa2North

	Simulation Training Centre of PFUR Moscow, Russian Federation The Simulation Training Centre of the Peoples' Friendship University of Russia was founded in December of 2013. The center occupies more than 1700 square meters. Our main goal is an acquisition of practical skills in "no stress" conditions, without constant monitoring of the mentor and without risk to the patient. Simulation training courses are part of educational program in our university for students, residents, and fellows. Simulation training programs are held according to following specialties: surgery, endovascular surgery, reanimatology, anesthesiology, obstetrics, gynecology, urology, traumatology, orthopedics, dentistry, nursing, ultrasound diagnostics, endoscopy, pediatrics, neonatology, and ophthalmology
	Simulations & Notfallakademie am HELIOS Klinikum Krefeld – SiNA Krefeld, Lutherplatz 40 47805 Krefeld, Germany
	Simulatorcentrum i vast – Simulation Centre West Gothenburg, Sweden Simulatorcentrum i vast – Simulation Centre West
	SimulHUG Geneva, Switzerland Simulation Centre of the Geneva University Hospital
	Stavanger Acute Medicine Foundation for Education and Research Stavanger, Norway SAFER Simulation Centre
	Swiss Centre for Medical Simulation Basel, Switzerland Swiss Centre for Medical Simulation
	Tbilisi State Medical University Clinical Skills Centre Tbilisi, Georgia TSMUCSC
	The Simulation Center – Gjøvik University College Gjovik, Norway The Simulation Center – Gjøvik University College
	Tupass Centre for Patient Safety and Simulation Tubingen, Germany Tupass Centre for Patient Safety and Simulation
	Unite de Simulation Pedagogique de Strasbourg Strasbourg, France USP-S
	University of Eastern Finland – Taitostudia Kuopio, Finland The simulation center at the University of Eastern Finland is for healthcare students and professionals and specializes in undergraduate students
	West Herts Initiative in Simulation Education and Resuscitation – WISER

(continued)

- Facilitation, exchange, and improvement of the technology and knowledge throughout Europe
- Establishment of combined research facilities

SESAM has its registered office in Göttingen. SESAM is represented by an executive committee and a general assembly. The language used by SESAM is English [71].

Using Simulation for Certification and Board Exams

The Comprehensive Clinical Neurosurgery (CCN) review is becoming one of the most important pre-exam courses in Europe. Its importance comes from using very smart and innovative methods of teaching using simulation to help senior neurosurgery residents and fellows pass their board exams. The course was designed to simulate the oral exam environment by creating what is called "hot seat" sessions where candidates will be sitting on a chair in front of two faculty members of world-class experienced neurosurgeons, and they will be given case scenarios and examined just like if they were in a true final fellowship oral board exam (Fig. 22.6). At the end of each session, the candidates will be marked and will be given immediate feedback about their performance from the faculty members. These sessions are also videotaped so that each candidate accesses these videos and gets a performance feedback from the course director on not only academic knowledge but also on style of delivering information and use of body language [72].

The study which was conducted on candidates attending the CCN review over the past 4 years showed improvement in performance on the hot seat with the use of simulated hot seats provided there is at least moderate knowledge in theory (tested in the study using MCQ exam question style) [73]. In Europe, observed through the British Royal College Fellowship exam (FRCS) and the European Board of Neurological Surgery (EBNS), there was an improvement in candidates' performance after being exposed to this simulation technique, and in fact the top performers in these exams are mainly candidates who took the simulation hot seat review course.

Where Is Simulation Heading in Europe?

Where will simulation go next? A question which was asked and answered by Walsh K. He proposed that a number of different themes will emerge.

- Firstly, simulation will likely become much more closely linked to assessment in the future. The learner of the future will likely spend time in the simulator being continually assessed. The assessment may be by a person

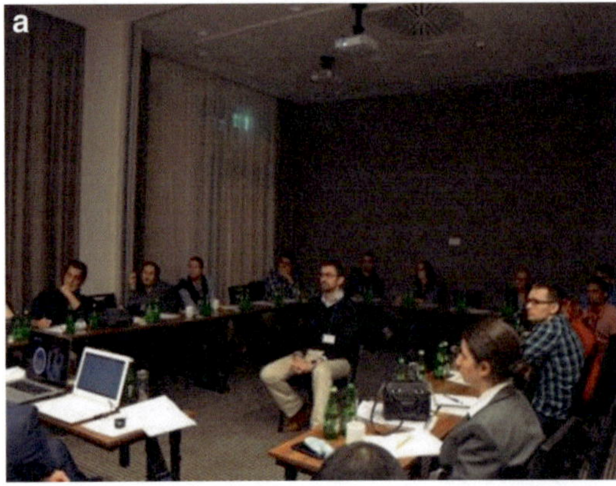
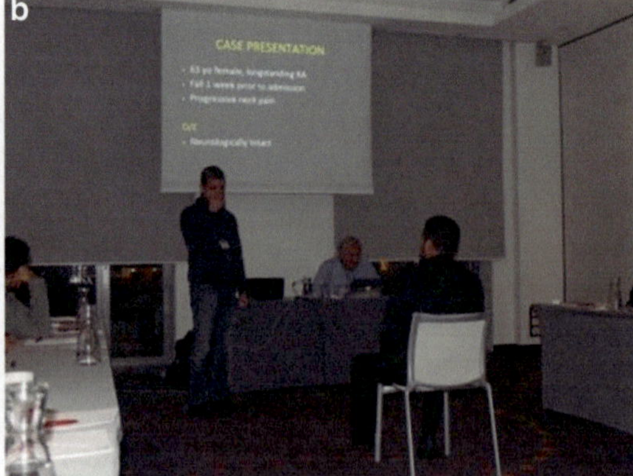

Fig. 22.6 (**a, b**) Hot seat session (board exam simulation) (Courtesy of CCN Review 2014 & 2015 (Krakow, Poland))

or by a machine. Regardless of this, the assessment will be against performance metrics that are important and that can be measured. In keeping with best practice generally in assessment, feedback will be continuous and specific to the task in hand [74].

- Secondly, our vision of what constitutes simulation will change radically in the future. Currently simulation is often seen as a method of learning that can be defined by time and space. So a learner might spend a half-day in the local simulation suite learning a skill. In the future, the concept of simulation will become much more wide so that it captures a range of less well-defined but equally effective activities. For example, mobile simulation suites will enable simulation to happen on the wards or in the outpatient department [75]. Online simulations will enable learners to interact with simulations at a time and place that suits them [76]. Simulation centers themselves will become open access so that a learner can use them as and when they wish to.
- Thirdly, the future of simulation in medical education will follow the same path as the future of healthcare [77].
- Lastly, are we approaching the ultimate dream of simulating human brain? This will be the question to be yet answered.

Obstacles to Implementation of Simulation Training in Europe

Despite obvious benefits of using simulators to teach and assess neurosurgical trainees, there are several large obstacles. Firstly, a relatively high start-up cost [18] may be an important drawback to some European states. Secondly, facilitating an effective training session is a detailed process: a high number of steps involved in designing/planning effective simulation [69]. Thirdly, there may be hesitation of the part of educators to implement simulation training into the residency curriculum. One review [69] emphasized that, to gain full benefits of simulation training, the simulators must become a part of the teaching curriculum. Conversely, some trainees may perceive that

simulation training is somehow less valuable or useful than more operative experience [69]. Finally, there is also a lack of access to the existing simulation facilities [64].

References

1. Ziv A, Wolpe PR, Small SD, Glick S. Simulation-based medical education: an ethical imperative. Acad Med. 2003;78(8):783–8.
2. Jena AB, Seabury S, Lakdawalla D, Chandra A. Malpractice risk according to physician specialty. N Engl J Med. 2011;365(7):629–36.
3. Stone S, Bernstein M. Prospective error recording in surgery: an analysis of 1108 elective neurosurgical cases. Neurosurgery. 2007;60(6):1075–82.
4. Cobb MI, Taekman JM, Zomorodi AR, Gonzalez LF, Turner DA. Simulation in neurosurgery—a brief review and commentary. World Neurosurg. 2016;89:583–6.
5. Marcus H, Vakharia V, Kirkman MA, Murphy M, Nandi D. Practice makes perfect? The role of simulation-based deliberate practice and script-based mental rehearsal in the acquisition and maintenance of operative neurosurgical skills. Neurosurgery. 2013;72:A124–30.
6. Spritz N. Oversight of physicians' conduct by state licensing agencies: lessons from New York's Libby Zion case. Ann Intern Med. 1991;115(3):219–22.
7. McManus IC, Richards P, Winder BC, Sproston KA, Vincent CA. The changing clinical experience of British medical students. Lancet. 1993;341(8850):941–4.
8. Brennum J, van Loon J. Neurosurgical education in Europe. Acta Neurochir. 2016;158:1–2.
9. Smith A, Siassakos D, Crofts J, Draycott T. Simulation: improving patient outcomes. In Seminars in perinatology 2013;37(3):151–156. WB Saunders.
10. Nishisaki A, Keren R, Nadkarni V. Does simulation improve patient safety?: self-efficacy, competence, operational performance, and patient safety. Anesthesiol Clin. 2007;25(2):225–36.
11. Green M, Tariq R, Green P. Improving patient safety through simulation training in anesthesiology: where are we? Anesthesiol Res Pract. 2016;1:2016.
12. Stienen MN, Netuka D, Demetriades AK, Ringel F, Gautschi OP, Gempt J, Kuhlen D, Schaller K. Neurosurgical resident education in Europe—results of a multinational survey. Acta Neurochir. 2016;158(1):3–15.
13. Gladwell M. Outliers: the story of success. New York: Hachette; 2008.
14. Kirkman MA, Ahmed M, Albert AF, Wilson MH, Nandi D, Sevdalis N. The use of simulation in neurosurgical education and training: a systematic review. J Neurosurg. 2014;121(2):228–46.

15. Trojanowski T. Certification of competence in neurosurgery – the European perspective. World Neurosurg. 2010;74(4–5):432–3.

16. Stienen MN, Netuka D, Demetriades AK, Ringel F, Gautschi OP, Gempt J, et al. Working time of neurosurgical residents in Europe – results of a multinational survey. Acta Neurochir. 2016;158(1):17–25.

17. Alshafai N, Falenchuk O, Cusimano MD. International differences in the management of intracranial aneurysms: implications for the education of the next generation of neurosurgeons. Acta Neurochir. 2015;157(9):1467–75.

18. Zanello M, Zerah M, Sainte-Rose C, Di Rocco F. Virtual simulation in neurosurgery: a comparison between pediatric and general neurosurgeons. Acta Neurochir. 2014;156(11):2215–6.

19. Byvaltsev VA, Belykh EG, Konovalov NA. New simulation technologies in neurosurgery. Zh Vopr Neirokhir Im N N Burdenko. 2016;80(2):102–7.

20. Arora S, Darzi A. Introducing technical skills assessment into certification: closing the implementation gap. Ann Surg. 2016;264(1):7–9.

21. Alvand A, Auplish S, Gill H, Rees J. Innate arthroscopic skills in medical students and variation in learning curves. J Bone Joint Surg Am. 2011;93(19):e115.

22. Grantcharov TP, Funch-Jensen P. Can everyone achieve proficiency with the laparoscopic technique? Learning curve patterns in technical skills acquisition. Am J Surg. 2009;197(4):447–9.

23. Sadideen H, Alvand A, Saadeddin M, Kneebone R. Surgical experts: born or made? Int J Surg. 2013;11(9):773–8.

24. Halpenny J. The training of the surgeon. Can Med Assoc J. 1918;8(10):896.

25. Ericsson KA, Krampe RT, Tesch-Römer C. The role of deliberate practice in the acquisition of expert performance. Psychol Rev. 1993;100(3):363.

26. Spiteri A, Aggarwal R, Kersey T, Benjamin L, Darzi A, Bloom P. Phacoemulsification skills training and assessment. Br J Ophthalmol. 2010;94(5):536–41.

27. Okuda Y, Bryson EO, DeMaria S, Jacobson L, Quinones J, Shen B, Levine AI. The utility of simulation in medical education: what is the evidence? Mt Sinai J Med (A Journal of Translational and Personalized Medicine). 2009;76(4):330–43.

28. Weller JM. Simulation in undergraduate medical education: bridging the gap between theory and practice. Med Educ. 2004;38(1):32–8.

29. Limbrick DD Jr, Dacey RG Jr. Simulation in neurosurgery: possibilities and practicalities: foreword. Neurosurgery. 2013;73:S1–3.

30. Cohen AR, Lohani S, Manjila S, Natsupakpong S, Brown N, Cavusoglu MC. Virtual reality simulation: basic concepts and use in endoscopic neurosurgery training. Childs Nerv Syst. 2013;29(8):1235–44.

31. Gélinas-Phaneuf N, Choudhury N, Al-Habib AR, Cabral A, Nadeau E, Mora V, Pazos V, Debergue P, DiRaddo R, Del Maestro RF. Assessing performance in brain tumor resection using a novel virtual reality simulator. Int J Comput Assist Radiol Surg. 2014;9(1):1–9.

32. Harrop J, Rezai AR, Hoh DJ, Ghobrial GM, Sharan A. Neurosurgical training with a novel cervical spine simulator: posterior foraminotomy and laminectomy. Neurosurgery. 2013;73:S94–9.

33. Hassfeld S, Zöller J, Albert FK, Wirtz CR, Knauth M, Mühling J. Preoperative planning and intraoperative navigation in skull base surgery. J Cranio-Maxillofac Surg. 1998;26(4):220–5.

34. Wolfsberger S, Forster MT, Donat M, Neubauer A, Bühler K, Wegenkittl R, Czech T, Hainfellner JA, Knosp E. Virtual endoscopy is a useful device for training and preoperative planning of transsphenoidal endoscopic pituitary surgery. Minim Invasive Neurosurg. 2004;47(4):214–20.

35. Beyer J, Hadwiger M, Wolfsberger S, Bühler K. High-quality multimodal volume rendering for preoperative planning of neurosurgical interventions. IEEE Trans Vis Comput Graph. 2007;13(6):1696–703.

36. Bouyssie JF, Bouyssie S, Sharrock P, Duran D. Stereolithographic models derived from X-ray computed tomography reproduction accuracy. Surg Radiol Anat. 1997;19(3):193–9.

37. Sailer HF, Haers PE, Zollikofer CP, Warnke T, Caris FR, Stucki P. The value of stereolithographic models for preoperative diagnosis of craniofacial deformities and planning of surgical corrections. Int J Oral Maxillofac Surg. 1998;27(5):327–33.

38. Rengier F, Mehndiratta A, von Tengg-Kobligk H, Zechmann CM, Unterhinninghofen R, Kauczor HU, Giesel FL. 3D printing based on imaging data: review of medical applications. Int J Comput Assist Radiol Surg. 2010;5(4):335–41.

39. Rehder R, Abd-El-Barr M, Hooten K, Weinstock P, Madsen JR, Cohen AR. The role of simulation in neurosurgery. Childs Nerv Syst. 2016;32(1):43–54.

40. By Minecraftpsyco – Own work, CC BY-SA 4.0, https://commons.wikimedia.org/w/index.php?curid=47304870.

41. Bradley P. The history of simulation in medical education and possible future directions. Med Educ. 2006;40(3):254–62.

42. Nash R, Sykes R, Majithia A, Arora A, Singh A, Khemani S. Objective assessment of learning curves for the Voxel-Man TempoSurg temporal bone surgery computer simulator. J Laryngol Otol. 2012;126(07):663–9.

43. Kockro RA, Stadie A, Schwandt E, Reisch R, Charalampaki C, Ng I, Yeo TT, Hwang P, Serra L, Perneczky A. A collaborative virtual reality environment for neurosurgical planning and training. Operative Neurosurgery. 2007;61(5):379–91.

44. Amunts K, Ebell C, Muller J, Telefont M, Knoll A, Lippert T. The human brain project: creating a European Research Infrastructure to decode the human brain. Neuron. 2016;92(3):574–81.

45. Huerta MF, Koslow SH, Leshner AI. The human brain project: an international resource. Trends Neurosci. 1993;16(11):436–8.

46. Blue Brain and the Human Brain Project. http://bluebrain.epfl.ch/page-52741-en.html.

47. Human Brain Project from Wikipedia. https://en.wikipedia.org/wiki/Human_Brain_Project.

48. Markram H. The blue brain project. Nat Rev Neurosci. 2006;7(2):153–60.

49. Blue Brain/Project Director. http://bluebrain.epfl.ch/projectdirector.

50. Human Brain Project overview. https://www.human-brainproject.eu/2016-overview.

51. D'Angelo E. The human brain project. Funct Neurol. 2012;27(4):205.

52. Human Brain Project, Framework Partnership Agreement. https://www.humanbrainproject.eu/documents/10180/538356/FPA++Annex+1+Part+B/41c4da2e-0e69-4295-8e98-3484677d661f.

53. Human Brain Project Subproject overview. https://www.humanbrainproject.eu/subprojects-overview.

54. Krichmar JL, Edelman GM. Design principles and constraints underlying the construction of brain-based devices. In International Conference on Neural Information Processing. 2007. Springer Berlin Heidelberg, p. 157–66.

55. Ross T. Machines that think. Health. 1933;243:248.

56. Wikipedia iCub. https://en.wikipedia.org/wiki/ICub.

57. Metta G, Sandini G, Vernon D, Natale L, Nori F. The iCub humanoid robot: an open platform for research in embodied cognition. In: Proceedings of the 8th workshop on performance metrics for intelligent systems; 2008, ACM, p. 50–6.

58. Mizuuchi I, Nakanishi Y, Sodeyama Y, Namiki Y, Nishino T, Muramatsu N, Urata J, Hongo K, Yoshikai T, Inaba M. An advanced musculoskeletal humanoid kojiro. In: Humanoid robots, 2007 7th IEEE-RAS international conference on 2007. IEEE, p. 294–9.

59. Marques HG, Jäntsch M, Wittmeier S, Holland O, Alessandro C, Diamond A, Lungarella M, Knight R. ECCE1: the first of a series of anthropomimetic musculoskeletal upper torsos. In: Humanoid robots (humanoids), 2010 10th IEEE-RAS International Conference on 2010 Dec 6; IEEE, p. 391–6.

60. Health in Europe. Com http://www.healthcare-in-europe.com/en/article/16755-their-parts-are-simply-too-big.html.

61. Olabe J, Olabe J, Sancho V. Human cadaver brain infusion model for neurosurgical training. Surg Neurol. 2009;72(6):700–2.

62. Suslu HT, Tatarli N, Karaaslan A, Demirel N. A practical laboratory study simulating the lumbar microdiscectomy: training model in fresh cadaveric sheep spine. J Neurol Surg A Cent Eur Neurosurg. 2014;75(3):167–9.

63. Tomlinson JE, Yiasemidou M, Watts AL, Roberts DJ, Timothy J. Cadaveric spinal surgery simulation: a comparison of cadaver types. Global. Spine J. 2016;6(4):357–61.

64. Coelho G, Zanon N, Warf B. The role of simulation in neurosurgery. Childs Nerv Syst. 2014;30(12):1997–2000.

65. Alshafai N. European educational survey: results form 38 countries. European Association of Neurosurgical Societies Congress; 2016.

66. NeuroSimulation – Besta Neurosim Center [Internet]. Besta Neurosim Center. 2017 [cited 26 January 2017]. Available from: http://www.bestaneurosim.com/.

67. McGaghie WC, Issenberg SB, Petrusa ER, Scalese RJ. Revisiting 'a critical review of simulation-based medical education research: 2003–2009'. Med Educ. 2016;50(10):986–91.

68. Alshafai N. Cranio Cervical Junction Workshop [Internet]. Craniocervicaljunction.com. 2017 [cited 26 January 2017]. Available from: http://craniocervicaljunction.com/.

69. Stienen MN, Netuka D, Demetriades AK, Ringel F, Gautschi OP, Gempt J, et al. Residency program trainee-satisfaction correlate with results of the European board examination in neurosurgery. Acta Neurochir. 2016;158(10):1823–30.

70. https://www.sesam-web.org/centres/.

71. Society in Europe for Simulation Applied to Medicine SESAM. https://www.sesam-web.org/centres/.

72. Alshafai N. Comprehensive Clinical Neurosurgery Review [Internet]. ccnreview.com. 2017 [cited 26 January 2017]. Available from: http://www.ccnreview.com/.

73. Addressing areas of knowledge gap & oral exam skills deficiencies in Neurosurgical Residents. Al Duais W, Son A, Ulasavets U, Abdulkadir M. The Alshafai lab research day. Krakow, December 3rd; 2016.

74. Walsh K. The future of simulation in medical education. J Biomed Res. 2015;29(3):259.

75. Kneebone R, Arora S, King D, Bello F, Sevdalis N, Kassab E, Aggarwal R, Darzi A, Nestel D. Distributed simulation–accessible immersive training. Med Teach. 2010;32(1):65–70.

76. Walsh K, Dillner L. Launching BMJ learning: online learning resources based on the best available evidence. BMJ. 2003;327(7423):1064.

77. Milburn JA, Khera G, Hornby ST, Malone PS, Fitzgerald JE. Introduction, availability and role of simulation in surgical education and training: review of current evidence and recommendations from the Association of Surgeons in training. Int J Surg. 2012;10(8):393–8.

Part VI

Non-procedural Training

Barbara Stanley

Introduction

In neurosurgery, it is vital that the anaesthetist and surgeon share a mental model of the clinical management goals for perioperative critical incidents. Once bleeding or ischaemia occurs, the brain can become swollen very quickly and blood can obscure the surgical field rapidly making surgical management difficult and leading to acute physiological instability and raised intracranial pressures. The clinical decision-making, physiological manipulation and non-technical skills required for rapid successful management of such incidents can be practised and prepared for using immersive simulation. There is much evidence for the utility of simulation training and its effectiveness in terms of knowledge and practice gains – both in terms of skills acquisition [1], skill demonstration [2] and non-technical skill training [3], to name but a few areas, as well as in terms of participant satisfaction (Table 23.1) which is unsurprising given its foundation in experiential learning theory [4]. This chapter will focus on the techniques and insights from The NeuroSim course – a high-fidelity neuroanaesthesia course mapped to the UK neuroanaesthetic curriculum as set out by the Royal College of Anaesthetists.

B. Stanley (✉)
Department of Anaesthetics, Brighton and Sussex University Hospitals NHS Trust, Brighton, UK

Background and Evidence for Simulation Training

It is likely that the term "simulation training" means different things to different clinicians. In surgery, much of the training undertaken using simulation is of the procedural kind – i.e., cadaver lab work and box training to practice the business of surgery itself – the operative skill. To anaesthetists, "simulation training" most usually occurs in a simulation suite using a mannikin attached to vitals monitoring and involves the diagnosis and management of an acute clinical problem with emphasis on communication, decision-making and situational awareness – the so-called "non-technical" skills. Thus simulation is a hugely versatile platform and offers so many opportunities to practice domain-related knowledge and procedural skills themselves in an environment that is safe for the learner without risking patient safety. Given that in the operating room is a high-risk environment with many distractions, surgeon, anaesthetist and operating room staff need to act effectively as a team – especially in the event of a critical incident occurring. A collegial approach to simulation training in such non-technical skills as communication and situational awareness, as well as the exploration of transactional knowledge and organisational awareness, is arguably long overdue in neurosurgical services, and training together across specialties – rather than in isolation – allows for a

© Springer International Publishing AG, part of Springer Nature 2018
A. Alaraj (ed.), *Comprehensive Healthcare Simulation: Neurosurgery*,
Comprehensive Healthcare Simulation, https://doi.org/10.1007/978-3-319-75583-0_23

Table 23.1 Summary of course feedback for a single NeuroSim course of seven participants. This is a standard representation of the NeuroSim feedback

	Agree	**Disagree**	
I have undertaken my neuroanaesthesia module prior to today	5	2	
The purpose of the scenarios was clear and addressed important and relevant issues	7		
The debriefs clarified how as the anaesthetist I can assist in the resolution of intraoperative events	7		
The debriefs were:	**Too technical**	**Too focused on communication**	**Just right**
			7
The debrief was comprehensive and answered all my questions	7		
The debriefer for my scenario was credible and experienced	7		
My confidence in my neuroanaesthetic knowledge and practice as a result of today has	**Increased**	**Decreased**	
	7		
If there was one thing I could change about today's scenarios or debriefs it would be:			
I would recommend the NeuroSim to my colleagues	7		

shared mental model of the clinical situation and a more robust team approach. Ultimately the simulation scenario provides an "excuse to engage in a good conversation" (P. Weinstock, Boston Sim Peds) about neuroanaesthesia principles in a focused, meaningful and relevant way.

Medicine is a risky industry. Many errors in practice relate to human factors and system failures [5]. There is a mandate from the Institute of Medicine that "(Organizations) should also establish interdisciplinary team training programs—including the use of simulation for trainees and experienced practitioners for personnel in areas such as the emergency department, intensive care unit, and operating room" [6]. Nowhere in medical practice has simulation for multidisciplinary teams been taken up more widely than in anaesthesia. Many courses allow for the teaching and practice of technical skills, but in terms of non-technical skills, anaesthesia has been a pioneer in this field. The practice of non-technical skills – which underpin many of the errors that occur in modern practice [5] – is vital to both patient safety and to quality, and indeed the best courses allow the opportunity to practice and explore both types of skill. The operating suite is a high-risk area where complex technical skills necessarily interplay with the dynamics of team-work, communication, organisational knowledge and situational awareness. Simulation allows the practice of almost any aspect of a clinical situation. High-fidelity simulation submerses the learner into a simulated situation that elicits the emotions, reactions and investment of attention and cognition of a real clinical event. For this reason, it is an excellent tool to refine knowledge structures, for practice and training in complex decision-making under pressure, and for all non-technical skills.

Simulation appears to be highly effective subjectively – in terms of satisfaction and self-assessment of confidence and knowledge outcomes [7] – and moderately effective objectively for knowledge assessment and performance of well-defined tasks or protocols [7] [2]. ,The features of simulation that lead to effective learning have been studied with feedback being the most highly rated [8], and team training, shared mental models, situational awareness and transactional knowledge are all factors shown to produce expert teams in surgery [9]. Thus it can be seen from this brief mention of some of the existing evidence that there is enormous demand for this effective and versatile training modality particularly in high-risk environments such as the operating room.

Neuroanaesthesia Simulation: The NeuroSim

The NeuroSim is one of a group of simulation courses for neuroanaesthesia and neurocritical care. As an entity, these courses cover a broad range of practice relevant to a neurosurgical service. The NeuroSim itself is a high-fidelity simulation suite-based course which allows for team practice of critical incidents within the operating room setting. It is a multidisciplinary course primarily aimed at anaesthesia trainees, but the scenarios can be manipulated to provide vital learning for all clinical practitioners in the neurosurgical setting. NeuroSim is a highly technical course in that the primary aim is to provide participants with a real-time concrete experience upon which to hang their domain-specific knowledge. Moreover, it is a forum in which to share the mental model of the significant and common disease processes such as traumatic brain injury and subarachnoid haemorrhage.

The NeuroSim course was devised from a series of case-based discussions of neuroanaesthetic challenges in 2009. Traditional neuroanaesthesia teaching has revolved around in theatre discussion and lecture-based learning. NeuroSim embraces the tenets of adult learning theory enabling learners to be immersed in a simulated theatre environment, which makes the experience as close to a genuine patient encounter as possible. Each scenario is designed to address different aspects of clinical practice relevant to the domain and allow consolidation of the basic science knowledge that forms the foundation of practice. The standard course scenarios include:

Tight dura + venous sinus bleed	Venous air embolus
TBI in setting of polytrauma	Prone post fossa cardiac arrest
Recovery room deteriorating GCS	
ACOMM or PCOMM aneurysm clip	Unstable C-spine for imaging in a live patient model

These scenarios allow for the inclusion and exploration of all the basic science knowledge relevant to neuroanaesthesia. Multidisciplinary faculty play the roles of surgeon, anaesthetists and scrub/recovery nurse throughout the scenarios which adds validity and buy – into both scenario and debrief – which are so important to the success of a course. The emphasis of NeuroSim is to explore domain-related technical knowledge – i.e. the basic science and anaesthetic management of the patient within the scenario. Human factor exploration comes out as natural consequence of the necessary team interaction within the scenario and is focused on as part of a blended debrief.

Scenario Specifics

The scenarios are designed to be run on any kind of simulation technology that allows for the display and manipulation of vital signs, pupil size and the connection of the mannikin to a ventilator. Currently we use a SimMan 3 g (Laerdal Medical Ltd. UK). The basic structure of the scenario is as follows:

Pre-brief
Participant enters the scenario
Critical incident occurs and gets managed
Debrief

The pre-brief gives the participants the patient story and some basic information. The participant enters the simulation and takes handover from a faculty member. They then act as they would in their own role to diagnose and manage the evolving clinical problem. In other words, they are never expected to be any other clinician than who they are in real life. In this way, the scenario remains realistic, and they are able to use their current knowledge structures and experience to explore the problem before them in real time.

Almost any kind of clinical management dilemma can be simulated. This includes both critical incidents – where the patient deteriorates rapidly and the participant learner is expected to diagnose and treat simultaneously and in real time – but it is also very simple to simulate other aspects of clinical practice, such as a patient consultation. This is a particularly powerful tool to explore communication and information sharing – especially if the consult pertains to a complex clinical issue such as a clinical error, adverse event or taking consent.

The simulation is scripted as to how it is expected to run, and there is a separate sheet with instructions for the simulator technician on parameters for patient vitals and how these are expected to change over the duration of the simulation or in response to participant learner actions. A member of faculty – the person who will lead the debrief for the scenario – sits with the technician in the control booth and observes the scenario as it runs. They advise the technician as to how to change the patient parameters in response to learner actions and liaise with a faculty member inside the scenario via an earpiece. In this way, the scenario can be controlled and manipulated to ensure learning objectives are reached. We will give examples of how these aims are achieved using a traumatic brain injury in polytrauma scenario.

A Sample Scenario: Management of Traumatic Brain Injury in a Polytrauma Patient

The simulation suite and faculty can be seen in Fig. 23.1. The "hot-seat" participant is at the head of the table, and faculty members are playing the roles of surgeons and scrub staff and the anaesthetic nurse is on the telephone. The other participants are observing from outside the room.

The learning objectives for this scenario are as follows:

Briefly review the relevant anatomy and physiology.
Understand the pathophysiology and evolution of TBI as contusions develop.
Understand why hypoxia and hypotension are so detrimental in TBI.
Appreciate the significance of hypotension and the cerebral vascular response.
Manage conflicting requirements of haemorrhage control surgery and TBI.

Develop a shared mental model of the priorities of management and how the seemingly conflicting management goals can be reconciled.

The traumatic brain injury in polytrauma scenario is an immensely rich opportunity to put a great deal of neuroanaesthetic knowledge into practice as well as to explore non-technical skills with an entire operating room team.

The scenario begins with the patient already on the operating table, abdomen open, and surgeon working to stem the ongoing haemorrhage from a ruptured spleen. The participant learner enters the scenario to briefly babysit the patient whilst the anaesthetist leaves the room on some pre-text.

The patient is tachycardic and hypotensive, and the surgeon is struggling to gain control of the bleeding.

Over the next few minutes, the heart rate increases slowly, and the blood pressure falls. The "correct" clinical management of this scenario is for the learner to recognise that blood loss is aggravated by attempts to drive the pressure to protect the cranium. The neurosurgeon calls the theatre and asks how the patient is, thus prompting the participant to notice that the patient has a dilated pupil which is new. There is an expectation of clear communication between surgeon and anaesthetist, and the anaesthetist will ask if haemorrhage control can be achieved through abdominal packing thus allowing the blood pressure to be driven to perfuse the swelling brain. Communication, forward planning and drawing together of domain-related knowledge – as well as situational awareness and team utilisation – all come to the fore in this scenario.

Fidelity

The realism of the simulation, the simulated environment and the reactions the experience elicit are termed fidelity. It is important to realise that fidelity is multifactorial and highly dependent on context. For example, anaesthetists view mannikin simulators as possessing high fidelity when undergoing critical incident

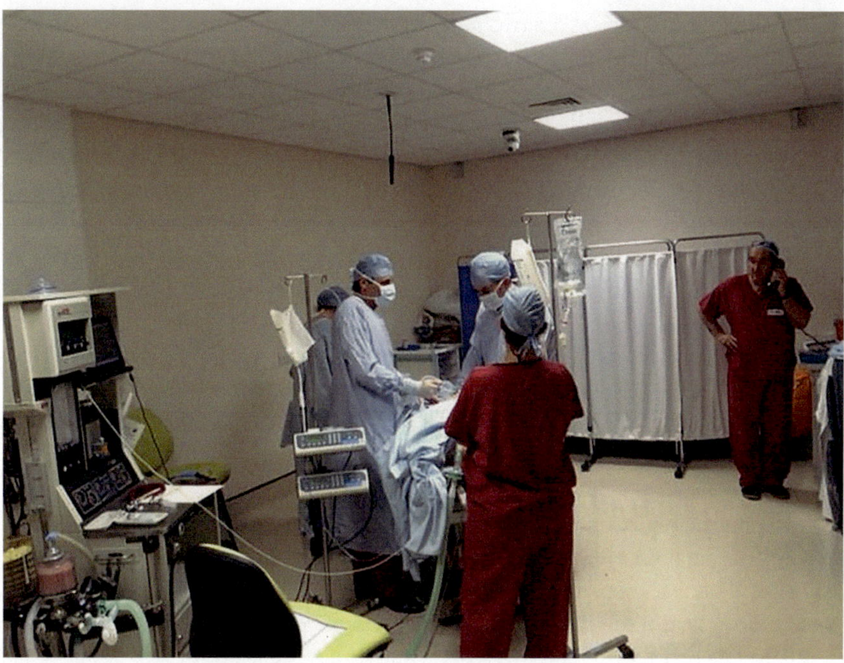

Fig. 23.1   Management of traumatic brain injury in a polytrauma patient

training – because they can see a human-shaped simulator attached to a monitor that has numbers and waveforms resembling a real patient – whereas surgeons regard cadavers and animal models to be of high fidelity when undergoing technique training, because of the tissue and technical fidelity. [10] For the course and scenarios described here, it is functional fidelity (what the simulator does) that matters. The design and the playout of the scenario are far more important to the concrete experience than the look of the simulator per se. If the participant learner gives a bolus of a drug that should increase the patient's blood pressure in reality – if this does not happen in the simulator – the learner will look for reasons why this may have not had the desired effect. If this is not the point of the scenario, then the path the learner takes deviates from that which was intended. Confusion may occur, and the learning objectives may not be reached. Our course focuses on technical management of perioperative critical incidents, so if the participant gets the wrong end of the stick so to speak because the playout of the scenario was incorrect, then

it makes the focus of the debrief change and risks the credibility of the course and buy-in of the participants. It is our belief and view that the physical environment of the simulation should provide adequate fidelity – enabling the learner to buy-in or invest emotionally and cognitively into the experience – but that scenario design and playout need to be of high fidelity to ensure semantic realism and avoid mismatch between the physical reality of the scenario and the meaning that participants will make of it [11]. The other vital ingredient for fidelity for our course is the faculty. They are role players in the scenario, and in this way, they control the timing of events, deal with any problems with equipment that arise during the scenario, act to emphasise certain aspects of the scenario that are of relevance and play the part of the other clinicians, staff or relatives within the scenario. For example, in the venous sinus bleeding scenario, the faculty member playing the surgeon will complain about rapid blood loss, and placed by their foot under the surgical drapes is a chest drain bucket filled with simulated blood that they conveniently move into view at this point in the scenario and which the faculty member playing the anaesthetic assistant comments on at an appropriate moment. In this way the faculty within the scenario control the events and direct the learner's attention appropriately so learning points are achieved. For a course that focuses on technical management of perioperative critical incidents, it is important that the scenario is semantically correct so the scenario is believable.

The Debrief

Of all the factors that make learning successful from high-fidelity simulation, feedback is the most important [8]. Feedback in scenario-based simulation courses is given through the debriefing process. There are many different ways for conducting the debrief and a plethora of published work relevant to the debriefing of simulation. Each debriefing style has advantages, but it is important that a constructive dialogue is entered into and participants are respected and feel safe to engage. Mutual respect for both faculty and participants must be fostered to promote transparency and allow assimilation of new knowledge into existing structures for all participants (including faculty!) and to reflect upon performance.

NeuroSim uses the "debriefing with good Judgement" style [12] which is rooted in Donald Schon's work on reflective practice[13] which aims to engage the participants in a meaningful and relevant conversation whilst keeping them psychologically safe and recognising the debriefers' own stance and values. This style involves not only the "hot-seat" participant but all the participants who watched. Two faculty members conduct the debrief and often involve other faculty on points of practice or experience. The debrief opens with engaging the hot-seat participant by asking them to describe the scenario as they perceived it. This allows them to voice immediately their thoughts and reactions to the scenario and allows the debriefers insight into their perceptions regarding their performance and of their learning needs. The debrief is then conducted through a series of comments regarding observed actions and behaviours which directs the discussion towards the learning objectives. Whilst it is usually straightforward to keep to these objectives, faculty must remain open to the possibility that the scenario may throw up material that doesn't fit with the preconceived objectives, and so the debrief should be allowed a certain natural flow – with faculty steering it to ensure it stays relevant. By allowing this flexibility, the participants reveal their thought processes and mental models or "frames" which explains the actions and decisions they took during the scenario. These may or may not fit with the outlined learning objectives, but identification and reflection upon them lead to learning [12].

Summary

Simulation is a powerful tool to recreate clinical situations which allows clinicians to review, practice and explore their domain-related knowledge and non-technical skills in a real-time immersive environment. It offers a genuine learning experience rooted in adult learning theory and reflective practice – principles at the core of adult education – in a psychologically safe environment. Almost any clinical situation can be simulated to fidelity adequate to elicit genuine actions and responses making learning meaningful and relevant. Simulation training should be both specialty-specific but also undertaken across specialties in a multidisciplinary education experience so as to improve team performance and dynamics as well as patient safety.

References

1. McGaghie WC, Issenberg SB, Cohen ER, Barsuk JH, Wayne DB. Does simulation-based medical education with deliberate practice yield better results than traditional clinical education? A meta-analytic comparative review of the evidence. Acad Med. 2011;86:706–11.
2. Bruppacher HR, et al. Simulation-based training improves physicians' performance in patient care in high-stakes clinical setting of cardiac surgery. Anesthesiology. 2010;112:985–92.
3. Fletcher G, et al. Anaesthetists' non-technical skills (ANTS): evaluation of a behavioural marker system. Br J Anaesth. 2003;90:580–8.
4. Kolb A, Kolb D. The SAGE handbook of management learning, education and development. London: Sage Publications; 2009. p. 42–68.
5. NHS Institute for Innovation and Improvement. Levels of harm in primary care. NHS Inst Innov Improv. 2011.
6. Kohn LT, Corrigan JM, Donaldson MS. To err is human: building a safer health system. Washington, DC: National Academies Press; 1999.
7. Cook DA, et al. Comparative effectiveness of instructional design features in simulation-based education: systematic review and meta-analysis. Med Teac. 2013;35:e867–98.
8. Issenberg SB, McGaghie WC, Petrusa ER, Lee Gordon D, Scalese RJ. BEME: features and uses of high-fidelity medical simulations that lead to effective learning: a BEME systematic review. Med Teach. 2005;27:10–28.
9. Gardner AK, Scott DJ. Concepts for developing expert surgical teams using simulation. Surg Clin North Am. 2015;95:717–28.
10. Hamstra SJ, Brydges R, Hatala R, Zendejas B, Cook DA. Reconsidering fidelity in simulation-based training. Acad Med. 2014;89:387–92.
11. Dieckmann P, Gaba D, Rall M. Deepening the theoretical foundations of patient simulation as social practice. Simul Healthc. 2007;2:183–93.
12. Rudolph JW, Simon R, Dufresne RL, Raemer DB. There's no such thing as 'nonjudgmental' debriefing: a theory and method for debriefing with good judgment. Simul Healthc. 2006;1:49–55.
13. Schön DA. The reflective practitioner. New York: Basic Books; 1983.

Sabine E. M. Kreilinger

Simulation in General Critical Care as a Foundation for Neurocritical Care

Simulation within the specialty of critical care medicine is a rapidly evolving field with the goal to enhance continued education of health professionals and their trainees. Critical care physicians must be proficient in a variety of procedures and algorithms to ensure patient's safety; therefore, excellent hands-on training in technical and non-technical skills is required. Evidence suggests that simulation-based training constitutes an important element in the education of critical care teams, ensuring procedural competence (endotracheal intubation [1–4], central line placement [5–9], point of care ultrasound [10, 11], the complex treatment of disease in a dynamic setting, crisis management [12–18], and cardiac arrest [19–22] (Table 24.1). The use of simulation scenarios is also valuable in teaching communication skills [23–31] both within the multidisciplinary critical care team and with patients and their families (Table 24.2). By creating a learner-focused and nonthreatening educational environment, simulation encourages critical thinking in a realistic fail-safe environment that aids in fostering teamwork and collaboration in a multidisciplinary setting among all levels of providers with the potential for improving patient safety [17, 25, 32–34]. With standardization and repetition of content, trainees are able to solidify their knowledge and increase their confidence levels by interactive learning in a clinical setting without risk of harm to patients.

The Specialty of Neurocritical Care

Neurocritical care is a pioneering subspecialty centering on the unique management and treatment of patients with acute complex neurological disorders, the postoperative medical management of neurosurgical patients, and the management of the neurological manifestations of systemic disease [35, 36]. The seriousness of conditions that affect the nervous system, the rapidity with which these patients can deteriorate, and the profound consequences associated with disease progression necessitate an intense level of observation and management in a critical care setting. There are many publications addressing the benefits of subspecialty trained physicians staffing neurocritical care units, which include decreased hospital mortality and shortened length of stay [37–39]. Specific clinical expertise and specialized neurological monitoring are of paramount importance to care for this subset of patients. Areas of expertise unique to neurocritical care include management of intracranial pressure, hemodynamic augmenta-

S. E. M. Kreilinger (✉)
Department of Anesthesiology (MC 515), University of Illinois Health and Sciences System,
Chicago, IL, USA
e-mail: sabinek@uic.edu

Table 24.1 Technical skills

Airway management and endotracheal intubation
Sedation and pharmacotherapy
Arterial line and central venous line placement
ICP monitor placement, interpretation, and management
Mechanical ventilation
Point-of-care ultrasound
Bronchoscopy
Paracentesis
Thoracentesis
ACLS skills

Table 24.2 Nontechnical skills (cognitive integration skills)

Interdisciplinary team training
Professionalism and communication
Crisis resource management
Clinical decision-making
Transition of patient care and handover of patient care
End-of-life discussion, breaking bad news, and ethical dilemma

tion to optimize cerebral blood flow, and application of advanced neuromonitoring, such as continuous electroencephalography, brain-tissue oxygenation, and microdialysis [40]. Neurointensivists come from a variety of backgrounds including neurosurgery, neurology, anesthesiology, and internal medicine. Their training concentrates on the physiologic interactions between the brain and other organ systems and incorporates all aspects of neurological and medical management into a single care plan [41]. Frequent pathologies encountered in the neuro-critical care unit are ischemic stroke, intracranial hemorrhage, subarachnoid hemorrhage, traumatic brain injury, and status epilepticus.

Why Simulation in Neurocritical Care?

Simulation in neurocritical care is an emerging field that offers an extensive platform for continued research to evaluate potential benefit in medical education, as well as in patient outcomes and safety. This subspecialty provides an exceptional and challenging learning opportunity for providers confronted with high level of acuity and complex patient population. Neurological emergencies can occur in any location starting in the field, in the emergency room, on the ward, in remote locations such as the CT scanner or neurointerventional suite, in the operating room, and in the neurocritical care unit. First responders often have little critical care training and are poorly prepared to diagnose and manage these pathologies given their infrequent exposure to these types of emergencies. Many staff members who are not trained in the subspecialty of neuro-critical care are faced with an unfamiliar situation. They lack confidence and may not appreciate the urgency of these disorders. Among all critical care topics, those involving the nervous system are likely to be the most troublesome and challenging for young physicians to learn and for their educators to teach [42]. Unfortunately, there exists a true risk for misdiagnosing or undertreating the underlying neuropathology which may lead to serious neurological sequelae, increased morbidity, and mortality.

Time is Brain

The chief goal of patient management in the first hours of a neurological emergency is avoiding or reducing secondary neurological injury as this will influence the patient's functional outcome and morbidity and mortality [43, 44]. Therefore, it is of crucial importance to have skilled practitioners provide appropriate and efficient care during the establishment of a diagnosis, the initiation of neurological resuscitation, and the triage process. This will minimize loss of valuable time, decrease medical errors, and increase collaboration in a synergistic multidisciplinary environment with effective and concise communication [45]. The dynamic nature of neurological emergencies and the necessary timely treatment create vast opportunities to implement simulation with the essential goals of reducing secondary injury, improving patient outcomes and communication among care teams and providers.

Most recent endovascular protocols for treatment of ischemic stroke [46–48] have shortened the time course and standardized the associated treatment options for these patients and furthermore require efficient and concise communication among various care teams. The American Heart Association Guidelines address new blood pressure goals and coagulation reversal recommendations in the setting of spontaneous intracerebral hemorrhage [49], which should be targeted and achieved early on in the care of these patients. These concepts can be effectively taught using simulation scenarios.

Simulation-Based Medical Education

Work hour restriction in residency and fellowship training programs has led to decreased practical clinical experience. Multiple medical and surgical specialties have already successfully created simulation programs and incorporated them into their didactic curriculum [50–54]. The importance of attaining adequate neurocritical care exposure and understanding fundamental basic concepts is now recognized and reflected by addition of required milestones in the neurology residency curriculum [54] and in the critical care medicine fellowship curriculum [55]. Critical care trainees require experience in a variety of subspecialties during a very time-constrained training program to ensure clinical competency. Exposure to all pathologies and specifically repetitive exposure is not guaranteed and generates a challenge for critical care educators. Furthermore, exposure to neurological disease may be limited for these general critical care fellows in a setting, where this patient population is mainly cared for by neurointensivists rather than medical or surgical critical care specialists. Because of the complex nature of acute neurological disease with the competing goals of different organ systems and the unfamiliarity of many other specialties when confronted with an acute neurologic crisis, many critical care trainees are uncertain when it comes to manage those patients. Simulation can potentially alleviate these fears, making healthcare providers feel more confident and comfortable with their decision-making process, and help them apply evidence-based management and treatment of these disorders. The management of critically ill patients with neurological pathologies requires special attention to neurophysiological goals to prevent secondary brain injury following the primary insult. This is reflected in hemodynamic management, ventilator strategy, adequate glycemic control, neurosurgical interventions, and hyperosmolar therapy for intracranial hypertension. Simulation-based training is a beneficial tool beyond traditional lectures in educating trainees in these relatively rare occurring scenarios [56].

High-Fidelity Simulation in Neurocritical Care

Simulation in general critical care education has been widely employed. Scenarios are easily created and employed for teaching emergency management [12–22] and interventional procedures [1–11, 57]. Standardized patients, part-task mannequins, and whole-body advanced mannequins with high-fidelity capabilities can be utilized to achieve realistic scenarios. High-fidelity mannequins are capable of running preprogrammed scenarios, which can be manipulated in real time by a proctor. The proctor can use a speaker box and manipulate the mannequin's vital signs including heart rate, blood pressure, respiratory rate, body temperature, end-tidal CO_2, and intracranial pressure (Fig. 24.1). High-fidelity mannequins can also display clinical signs, including palpable pulses, visible respirations, pupil reactivity (Fig. 24.2), as well as seizure activity.

The volume of literature on use of advanced simulation in neurology and specifically in emergency neurology has only recently started to expand. The obvious barriers to simulation in neurocritical care such as the inability of high-fidelity mannequins to emulate neurological deficits (e.g., facial droop) and neurologi-

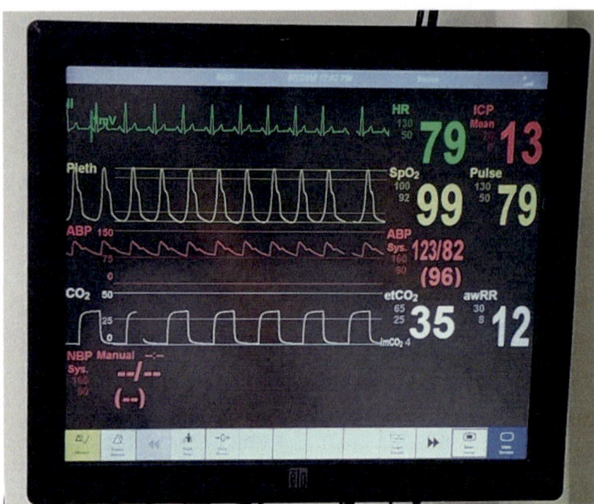

Fig. 24.1 Display of mannequin's vital signs

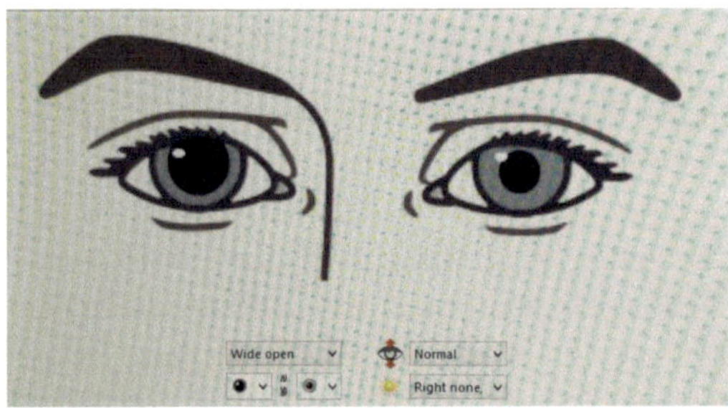

Fig. 24.2 High-fidelity simulation of pupil reactivity

cal signs, which are also difficult to mimic by actors and mannequins, pose a challenge for scenario creation. An advantage of simulation technology is that the data necessary for diagnosis and therapeutic decision-making, such as electroencephalogram (Fig. 24.3), transcranial Doppler, neuroimaging (e.g., CT, MR), and parameters (e.g., intracranial pressure, cerebral perfusion pressure) are easily integrated into simulation [58].

Data and Evidence on Simulation Scenarios in Neurocritical Care

Limited data exists on the effectiveness of simulation in neurocritical care education. What is available is reviewed below by topic.

Acute Cerebral Vasospasm, Closed Head Injury, and Spinal Shock

To date, few studies have been conducted in the neurocritical care setting. Musacchio and colleagues are one of the first groups to investigate and propose a potential benefit of simulation-based educational training in neurological emergencies [59]. These investigators developed successful advanced high-fidelity simulation models for training in the neurocritical care unit that include *acute cerebral vasospasm, closed head injury, and spinal shock.* In these particular scenarios, a high-fidelity mannequin is utilized along with real-time tracings of intracranial pressure and cerebral perfusion pressure. This model is equipped with a speaker box for the proctor to speak for the simulated patient. This group proposed that while traditional lectures can provide a solid knowledge base, simulation, in a protected fail-safe environment, allows for consolidation of knowledge that is necessary to ensure safe and effective interventions.

Lumbar Puncture Skills

This was investigated by Barsuk et al. [60], who focused on a simulation model using part-task mannequins. They demonstrated improvement in *lumbar puncture skills* in neurology residents compared to traditional clinical training, even in those residents who had significant prior clinical experience with the procedure. This reconfirms the potential benefit of simulation as an adjunct to the educational curriculum that increases patient safety and resident confidence.

Brain Code

Papangelou et al. [61] concentrated on the *brain code* scenario associated with herniation with or without intractable intracranial hypertension. This is similar to advanced cardiac life support scenarios. This type of scenario does not demand the presence of a focal neu-

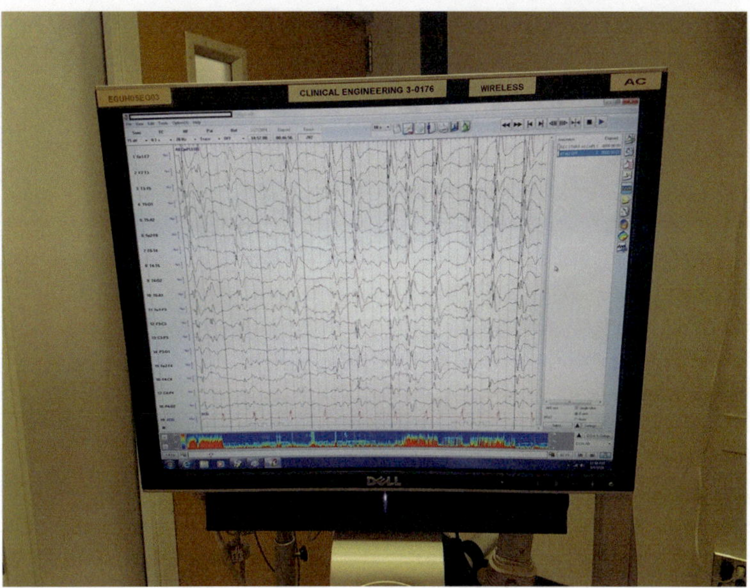

Fig. 24.3 Electrographic seizure activity

rological deficit other than pupillary asymmetry (Fig. 24.1). High-fidelity mannequins are currently capable of displaying both pupil reactivity and seizure functionality. Critical care trainees completed a pretest and then attended a didactic lecture followed by a recorded simulation session and a posttest. After the simulation scenario, a debriefing took place, with the assistance of video replay, and concluded with a satisfaction questionnaire. Performance was assessed with key tasks during the brain code, which included initiating the "ABCs" of basic cardiopulmonary resuscitation, optimizing the patient's position, starting hyperventilation, the use of osmotherapy, ordering neuroimaging, and intracranial pressure monitoring. In addition, the "time to" the intervention was measured as a variable and then compared to performance 3 months later. Papangelou concluded that improvement during the 3-month time interval cannot entirely be attributed to simulation alone, given the ongoing clinical experience and lectures trainees receive. The group suggests that simulation is labor intensive; however, it has the potential for educational benefit and improving patient care and safety.

Acute Ischemic Stroke

Acute ischemic stroke is a neurological emergency and patient outcome is time-sensitive to initial treatment. Garside et al. [62] describe simulation-based interactive scenarios which can be combined with traditional didactic teaching to educate emergency department staff on the recognition and initial management of acute stroke. They successfully integrated video clips of real stroke patients with focal neurological deficits into the simulation scenarios, thereby overcoming the mannequin's inability to mimic such deficits. Learners reported improved self-confidence in the management of acute stroke; however, a long-term change and sustainability in clinical behavior has not yet been investigated.

Status Epilepticus and Acute Stroke

Ermak et al. [58] integrated simulation into the training of third- and fourth-year medical students during their neurology clerkship. Two simulation scenarios were created for the evaluation and treatment *of status epilepticus and acute stroke* using a high-fidelity mannequin programmed with specific vital signs and pupillary responses. A formal neurologic assessment was available when requested by the students. The status epilepticus scenario was supplemented by an actor playing the role of a family member who provided additional pertinent information. Following the simulation, students reviewed their video scenario recording for self-assessment. The simulation facilitator provided additional feedback and encouraged discussion, focusing on key tasks and fundamental knowledge during the debriefing. This allowed for individualized instruction, which addressed knowledge deficits identified during the simulation. The investigators emphasized the importance of the diagnosis and management of a neurological emergency rather than focusing on the recognition of localizing symptoms.

Traumatic Brain Injury

Within the setting of a quality improvement project for the treatment of *traumatic brain-injured* patients in general intensive care units in the United Kingdom, Smith et al. [63] established that simulation-based training improves the intensive care unit staff's knowledge in the management of head injuries. By engaging nurses staffing the general intensive care unit and employing regular and repeated simulation, the investigators were able to demonstrate improvement in skills, knowledge, and confidence levels in caring for these patients. They suggest this may translate into improved patient outcomes at reduced cost [38].

Brain Death

Given the considerable variability in *brain death* determination among institutions in the United States [64–66], as well as the inadequate documentation of brain death in the medical record [67], MacDougall and colleagues [68] sought to implement a program to train physicians from a variety of specialty backgrounds in adherence to the 2010 updated American Academy of Neurology practice parameters [69] with the use

Table 24.3 Determination of brain death in four steps per the American Academy of Neurology Guidelines 2010 [69]

Clinical prerequisites for initiating the determination process
Neurological exam/assessment (including apnea test)
Ancillary testing if deemed necessary
Documentation in the medical record

of didactic and simulation sessions. The American Academy of Neurology suggests a four-step approach (Table 24.3) for providers to declare brain death, which includes clinical prerequisites for initiating the determination process; neurological examination (including apnea test); ancillary testing, if necessary; and proper documentation in the medical record [67]. The investigators used a high-fidelity mannequin and trainees were required to complete a full neurological examination, including performance of the apnea test. Potential cofounders, such as hypothermia, sedating medications, and signs incompatible with brain death, were dispersed throughout the simulator session. Physicians from non-neuroscience background specialties had poor pretest scores, with attendings scoring higher than residents, and neurosurgeons and neurologists significantly outperforming other specialists, demonstrating more familiarity with brain death determination guidelines. This is concerning information, when one considers that most brain death examinations are not performed by neurologists or neurosurgeons in US hospitals [66]. The trainee's performance was evaluated with a checklist based on the American Academy of Neurology guidelines [69]. A neurologist served as a facilitator for the didactic, simulation, and debriefing session. This study showed a 27.9% improvement in mean score from pretest to posttest and uniformly positive feedback. MacDougall et al. concluded that possible limitations to simulation training include a lack of resources and staffing [68]. One suggestion to overcome this lack of resources was partnering with other nearby institutions with simulation centers.

Another group of investigators, [70], tested a new simulation model which put emphasis on accuracy and key pitfalls [71] during brain death determination. This single-center, nonrandomized two-group design study with pre- and post-questionnaires was conducted by two neurointensivists. Neurology and critical care trainees were evaluated with the American Academy of Neurology checklist. Because of the limitations of high-fidelity mannequins in demonstrating neurological exam findings, the group focused mainly on confounders. Confounders such as hypotension, sedating drugs, and autocycling of the ventilator were incorporated into the scenarios. Prebriefing took place 1 week prior to simulation and included literature on common acute neurology topics. Immediately prior to simulation a brief orientation to the simulation center and how to interact with the mannequin took place. 41 trainees completed 71.5% of the prerequisites tasks and 71% of the clinical examination tasks. This study demonstrated improved clinical performance and confidence in critical care and neurology trainees following simulation training. The trainee's confidence in evaluation of brain death and apnea testing improved significantly, demonstrating the value of simulation.

Other reported outcomes of this simulation training include evaluations, trainee's perceptions, and objective improvement in clinical performance on repeat testing. Neurology trainees performed better in neurological examination and obtaining the clinical history, whereas general critical care trainees were more comfortable testing for spontaneous respirations both during mechanical ventilation and apnea testing. Standardized debriefing session included initial reaction to the scenario, discussion of the individual's performance with the help of video playback, as well as a summary of key points [70].

Myasthenia Crisis, Status Epilepticus, and Brain Death Determination

Braksick et al. [72] implemented neurology education for critical care fellows from different specialty backgrounds using a three-scenario high-fidelity simulation course with scenarios of *myasthenia crisis, status epilepticus, and brain death* determination. Fellows were assigned pre-reading material 1 week prior to the simulation. Immediately prior to simulation, they also received a lecture on neurological examination. During simulation, they individually saw three patients with the goal of making a diagnosis and initiating a management plan. Key personnel during the simulation included actors portraying the patient, a nurse, a patient's family member, a respiratory therapist, and the scenario facilitator. Fellows were expected to meet clearly defined individualized scenario objectives. The debriefing session was led by a neurointensivist with the help of video playback in small groups and included discussion of scenario key learning points and common pearls and pitfalls of neurological examination. These structured simulation sessions facilitate interactive debriefing sessions led by experienced physicians were useful in clarifying misconceptions and in delivering immediate feedback to the trainee. These simulation scenarios improved medical knowledge ($p < 0.002$) and confidence ($p < 0.0001$) in managing these neurological conditions. Critical care fellows are able to make diagnosis and treatment decisions in a risk-free environment. Learner satisfaction with this particular course was high. Limitations of Braksick's study were a small sample number of only 16 trainees, and their other clinical obligations may have impacted the trainee's preparation for the simulation session.

Available Training Courses in Neurological Emergencies

The Emergency Neurological Life Support (ENLS) course was developed and first introduced by Wade Smith, a neurologist and intensivist, and Scott Weingart, who specialized in emergency critical care medicine [73]. The certification and training in ENLS is hosted by the Neurocritical Care Society. This course is designed to address basic fundamentals of emergency management of a wide variety of neurological emergencies with simple treatment algorithms to minimize loss of valuable time and enhance communication skills [74]. This course provides a set of protocols, simple checklists, various decision points, and suggested communication to use during patient management. It can be completed as a live or online course. The post course exam focuses on knowledge and skill retention. ENLS recommendations are based on expert opinion due to lack of available data. The audience includes providers from diverse backgrounds, who work in different healthcare settings. Fourteen modules are available in version 2.0 and can serve as guides for development of scenarios in a simulation curriculum [75–88]. This provides a nice framework for simulation education in crises situations that require immediate attention and appropriate treatment.

Another course from the Cleveland Clinic [89] is a web-based approach that encompasses all aspects of brain death determination (brain death exam, relevant legalities, and family discussions) and takes about 1 h to complete. This has great availability; however, there is no hands-on training.

From a live workshop standpoint, the University of Chicago hosts a brain death simulation workshop [90] on a yearly basis. The course offers one full day of simulation stations, lectures, and case studies with the help of expert faculty who provide individualized feedback to the trainee. The advantage of this workshop is extensive practical training though at high cost.

Implementation of Simulation Curriculum

In order to create a meaningful simulation scenario, one must define key educational objectives, clinical pearls of the examination, and potential pitfalls, so that successful knowledge retention ensues. Building teamwork, communication, leadership, situational awareness, and clinical decision-making can benefit not only the patient's care but also communication among the care team members. Potential measurable outcomes include improvement in knowledge, confidence, and time to fulfill key tasks. One can make a simulation scenario more challenging by integrating technical skills (Table 24.1) and nontech-

nical skills (Table 24.2) such as breaking bad news when timely clinical decision-making is necessary. In the intensive care unit, one must adapt quickly to a dynamic environment, especially when working with other team members, other services discussing transfer of care, and family members. Families are often confronted with devastating news and evidence suggests that trainees perform better when having practiced breaking bad news during simulation sessions. Goals of care discussions can be emotionally fueled, and many trainees are not prepared to have these difficult and very complex conversations [29, 91, 92]. Adjuncts to high-fidelity simulation may include a medical history obtained by family member actor or nurse, a neurological exam with the help of videos or actors, as well as laboratory data, neuroimaging, electroencepha-

Table 24.4 Possible neurocritical care simulation scenarios

Traumatic brain injury
Traumatic spine injury and spinal cord compression
Subarachnoid hemorrhage and acute cerebral vasospasm
Intracranial hypertension and herniation (brain code)
Coma
Brain death and organ donor management
Status epilepticus – Convulsive vs nonconvulsive
Acute nontraumatic weakness
Meningitis/encephalitis
Acute ischemic stroke
Intracerebral hemorrhage
Resuscitation in shock states

Table 24.5 What can be simulated in status epilepticus

Medical history	Via *actor (patient, family member, nurse), video, or mannequin*: Seizure history, antiepileptic drug compliance, Onset and length of seizure obtained via family member
Exam	Confusion, inattention, staring Impaired memory of the event Clinical automatisms (e.g., repetitive lip-smacking, fumbling, swallowing movements) Hemiparesis, gaze deviation Subtle nystagmus Prolonged generalized tonic or tonic-clonic seizure Hypotension and cardiac arrhythmias

lography (Fig. 24.3), and transcranial Doppler. Possible scenarios for simulation courses in neurocritical care are listed in Table 24.4. An example of what can potentially be simulated in a scenario of status epilepticus is shown in Table 24.5, and key objectives, actions, and pitfalls are further outlined in Table 24.6 in the form of a checklist based on the evaluation and management guidelines published by the Neurocritical Care Society [93]. Figures 24.4, 24.5, and 24.6 demonstrate a simulation setup with integration of a high-fidelity mannequin.

Table 24.6 Checklist for simulation of status epilepticus (SE) scenario

Objectives	Actions	Pitfalls
ABCs	Evaluate and manage airway and provide supplemental oxygen Monitor vital signs Obtain code status Assess and support ventilation Intubation if necessary Finger stick blood glucose Check or establish vascular access Fluid resuscitation Note time of onset and length of seizure	-Not recognizing need to protect airway with advanced airway -Cervical collar requiring in-line manual stabilization -Failure to obtain IV access -Invasive hemodynamic monitoring if necessary
Control seizures	By 5 min: Emergent initial therapy with benzodiazepine Appropriate choice of medication and dosing Diagnose SE if > 5 min in duration: Urgent control with antiepileptic drug therapy Administer intravenous antiepileptic drugs based on guidelines [93] Diagnose refractory SE: Start continuous infusion, e.g., propofol, pentobarbital, midazolam	-Delay in management and treatment -Incorrect choice of medication -Unawareness of side effects of medications (e.g., hypotension, PR prolongation on EKG, propofol infusion syndrome, arrhythmias, etc.)
Perform seizure workup and determine etiology of seizure	Obtain or review past medical history and perform targeted history (e.g., seizure or alcohol abuse history) Neurological exam Request appropriate labs and imaging studies: Stat labs – Blood glucose, toxicology screening and antiepileptic drug levels, complete blood count, basic metabolic panel, calcium (total and ionized), magnesium CT head, continuous EEG Depending on clinical setting – Request: Blood cultures, urinalysis, cerebrospinal fluid analysis, MRI brain	-Not sending toxicology screen and glucose -Pearl exam: Gold standard for diagnosis is continuous EEG -Failure to obtain imaging -Lumbar puncture only after neuroimaging to rule out potential cerebral herniation
Consider nonconvulsive SE if patient comatose and control electrographic seizure activity	Continuous electroencephalography	-Not recognizing and failing to treat nonconvulsive SE -Not escalating medical management in setting of refractory SE
Management of medication side effects, knowledge of treatment protocol with appropriate intravenous antiepileptic drugs (per current guidelines)	Knowledge of pharmacokinetics and pharmacodynamics Knowledge of SE treatment protocol Recognize and manage antiepileptic medication side effects	-Inappropriate medication selection for treatment -Titrate to goal – Burst suppression on EEG
Communication	Call for help Communicate with primary team Update family in professional manner	-Failure to call for help -Not addressing family's questions and concerns

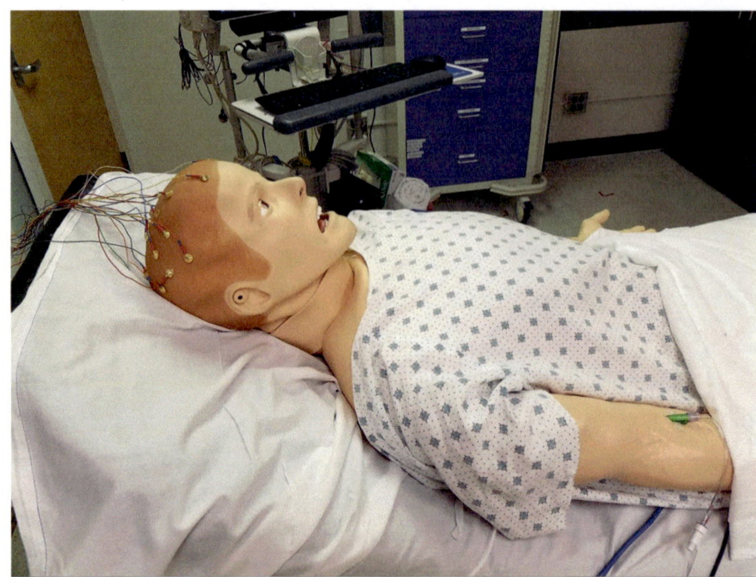

Fig. 24.4 EEG diagnosis of status epilepticus

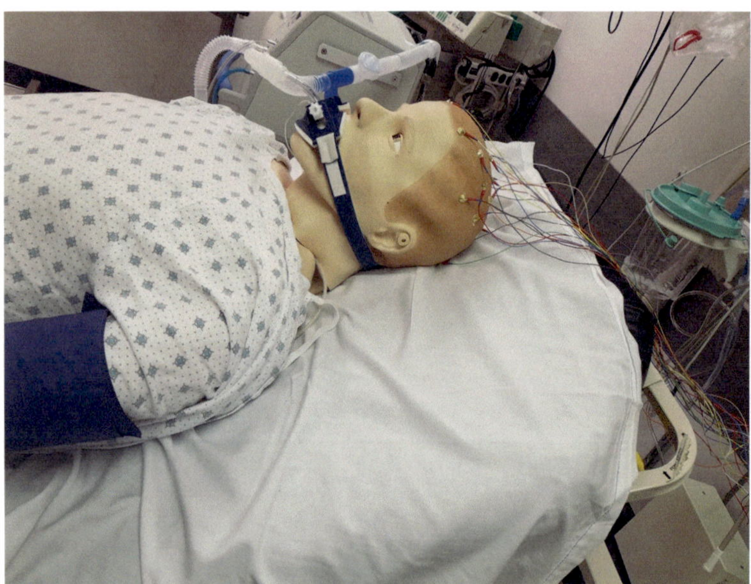

Fig. 24.5 Status post-endotracheal intubation

Conclusion

Neurocritical care or neurological emergency simulation scenarios should target providers across a variety of medical disciplines who have one goal in common – namely the safest, most time-efficient, and effective patient care to avoid secondary neurological injury. Despite the shortcomings of current technology, simulation-based training will not only enhance the trainee's skillset but also improve nontechnical qualities such as confidence levels, knowledge base, and communication skills among critical care team members, interdisciplinary teams, and family members. Specific simulation scenarios to consider implementing are acute ischemic stroke, status epilepticus, traumatic brain injury, and brain death determination. Even

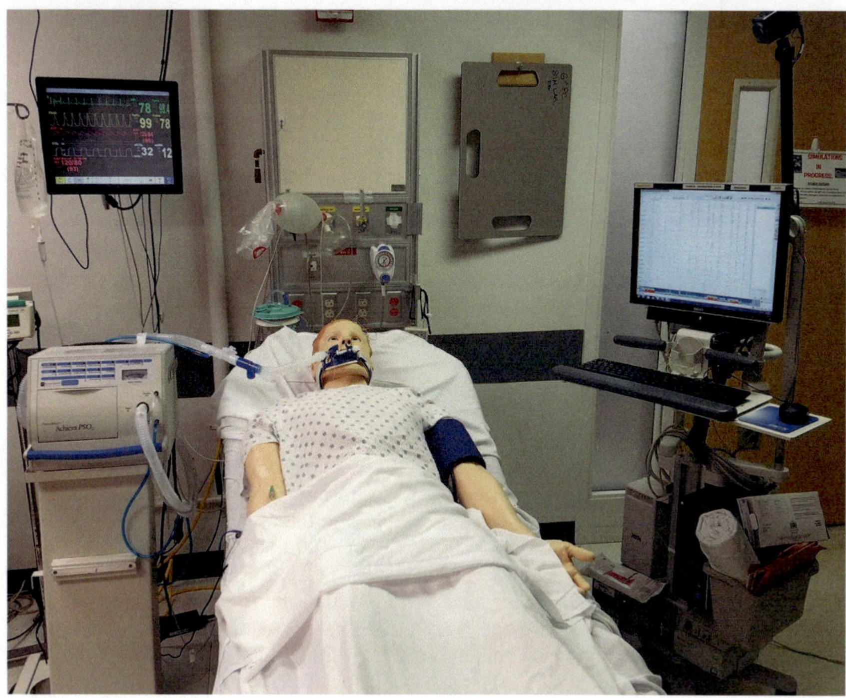

Fig. 24.6 Status epilepticus simulation scenario setup

with limited resources, simulation can be implemented successfully, and collaboration with other facilities may be an option for development of a simulation program. Further outcome measures need to be addressed and continued investigation is necessary to determine the efficacy of scenarios on trainee education and patient outcomes. Given the infancy of simulation in neurocritical care, further studies and great evolution are expected.

References

1. Mayo PH, Hackney JE, Mueck JT, Ribaudo V, Schneider RF. Achieving house staff competence in emergency airway management: results of a teaching program using a computerized patient simulator. Crit Care Med. 2004;32(12):2422–7.
2. Kuduvalli PM, Jervis A, Tighe SQ, Robin NM. Unanticipated difficult airway management in anaesthetised patients: a prospective study of the effect of mannequin training on management strategies and skill retention. Anaesthesia. 2008;63(4):364–9.
3. Rosenthal ME, Adachi M, Ribaudo V, Mueck JT, Schneider RF, Mayo PH. Achieving housestaff competence in emergency airway management using scenario based simulation training: comparison of attending vs housestaff trainers. Chest. 2006;129(6):1453–8.
4. Kory PD, Eisen LA, Adachi M, Ribaudo VA, Rosenthal ME, Mayo PH. Initial airway management skills of senior residents: simulation training compared with traditional training. Chest. 2007;132(6):1927–31.
5. Ma IW, Brindle ME, Ronksley PE, Lorenzetti DL, Sauve RS, Ghali WA. Use of simulation-based education to improve outcomes of central venous catheterization: a systematic review and meta-analysis. Acad Med. 2011;86(9):1137–47.
6. Smith CC, Huang GC, Newman LR, Clardy PF, Feller-Kopman D, Cho M, et al. Simulation training and its effect on long-term resident performance in central venous catheterization. Simul Healthc. 2010;5(3):146–51.
7. Barsuk JH, McGaghie WC, Cohen ER, O'Leary KJ, Wayne DB. Simulation-based mastery learning reduces complications during central venous catheter insertion in a medical intensive care unit. Crit Care Med. 2009;37(10):2697–701.
8. Britt RC, Novosel TJ, Britt LD, Sullivan M. The impact of central line simulation before the ICU experience. Am J Surg. 2009;197(4):533–6.

9. Barsuk JH, Cohen ER, Potts S, Demo H, Gupta S, Feinglass J, et al. Dissemination of a simulation-based mastery learning intervention reduces central line-associated bloodstream infections. BMJ Qual Saf. 2014;23(9):749–56.

10. Sekiguchi H, Bhagra A, Gajic O, Kashani KB. A general critical care ultrasonography workshop: results of a novel web-based learning program combined with simulation-based hands-on training. J Crit Care. 2013;28(2):217.e7–12.

11. Clau-Terre´ F, Sharma V, Cholley B, Gonzalez-Alujas T, Galiñanes M, Evangelista A, et al. Can simulation help to answer the demand for echography education. Anesthesiology. 2014;120:32–41.

12. Shukla A, Kline D, Cherian A, Lescanec A, Rochman A, Plautz C, et al. A simulation course on lifesaving techniques for third-year medical students. Simul Healthc. 2007;2:11–5.

13. Hammond J, Bermann M, Chen B, Kushins L. Incorporation of a computerized human patient simulator in critical care training: a preliminary report. Trauma. 2002;53(6):1064–7.

14. Nishisaki A, Hales R, Biagas K, Cheifetz I, Corriveau C, Garber N, et al. A multi-institutional high-fidelity simulation "boot camp" orientation and training program for first year pediatric critical care fellows. Pediatr Crit Care Med. 2009;10(2):157–62.

15. Freeman J, Dobbie A. Simulation enhances resident confidence in critical care and procedural skills. Fam Med. 2008;40(3):165–7.

16. Hedrick TL, Young JS. The use of "war games" to enhance high-risk clinical decision-making in students and residents. Am J Surg. 2008;195(6):843–9.

17. Steadman RH, Coates WC, Huang YM, Matevosian R, Larmon BR, McCullough L, et al. Simulation-based training is superior to problem-based learning for the acquisition of critical assessment and management skills. Crit Care Med. 2006;34(1):151–7.

18. Holcomb JB, Dumire RD, Crommett JW, Stamateris CE, Fagert MA, Cleveland JA, et al. Evaluation of trauma team performance using an advanced human patient simulator for resuscitation training. J Trauma. 2002;52(6):1078–85. [discussion:1085–6]

19. Wayne DB, Didwania A, Feinglass J, Fudala MJ, Barsuk JH, McGaghie WC. Simulation-based education improves quality of care during cardiac arrest team responses at an academic teaching hospital: a case-control study. Chest. 2008;133(1):56–61.

20. Wayne DB, Butter J, Siddall VJ, Fudala MJ, Wade LD, Feinglass J, et al. Mastery learning of advanced cardiac life support skills by internal medicine residents using simulation technology and deliberate practice. J Gen Intern Med. 2006;21(3):251–6.

21. Wayne DB, Butter J, Siddall VJ, Fudala MJ, Linquist LA, Feinglass J, et al. Simulation-based training of internal medicine residents in advanced cardiac life support protocols: a randomized trial. Teach Learn Med. 2005;17(3):210–6.

22. Andreatta P, Saxton E, Thompson M, Annich G. Simulation-based mock codes significantly correlate with improved pediatric patient cardiopulmonary arrest survival rates. Pediatr Crit Care Med. 2011;12(1):33–8.

23. DeVita MA, Schaefer J, Lutz J, Dongilli T, Wang H. Improving medical crisis team performance. Crit Care Med. 2004;32(Supplement):S61–5.

24. Jankouskas T, Bush MC, Murray B, Rudy S, Henry J, Dyer AM, et al. Crisis resource management: evaluating outcomes of a multidisciplinary team. Simul Healthc. 2007;2(2):96–101.

25. Lighthall GK, Barr J, Howard SK, Gellar E, Sowb Y, Bertacini E, et al. Use of a fully simulated intensive care unit environment for critical event management training for internal medicine residents. Crit Care Med. 2003;31(10):2437–43.

26. Reznek M, Smith-Coggins R, Howard S, Kiran K, Harter P, Sowb Y, et al. Emergency medicine crisis resource management (EMCRM): pilot study of a simulation-based crisis management course for emergency medicine. Acad Emerg Med. 2003;10(4):386–9.

27. Yee B, Naik VN, Joo HS, Savoldelli GL, Chung DY, Houston PL, et al. Nontechnical skills in anesthesia crisis management with repeated exposure to simulation-based education. Anesthesiology. 2005;103(2):241–8.

28. Roberts NK, Williams RG, Schwind CJ, Sutyak JA, McDowell C, Griffen D, et al. The impact of brief team communication, leadership and team behavior training on ad hoc team performance in trauma care settings. Am J Surg. 2014;207(2):170–8.

29. Schmitz CC, Chipman JG, Luxenberg MG, Beilman GJ. Professionalism and communication in the intensive care unit: reliability and validity of a simulated family conference. Simul Healthc. 2008;3(4):224–38.

30. Gisondi MA, Smith-Coggins R, Harter PM, Soltysik RC, Yarnold PR. Assessment of resident professionalism using high-fidelity simulation of ethical dilemmas. Acad Emerg Med. 2004;11(9):931–7.

31. LeBlanc VR, Tabak D, Kneebone R, Nestel D, MacRae H, Moulton CA. Psychometric properties of an integrated assessment of technical and communication skills. Am J Surg. 2009;197(1):96–101.

32. Croley WC, Rothenberg DM. Education of trainees in the intensive care unit. Crit Care Med. 2007;35(2):S117–21.

33. Grenvik A, Schaefer JJ 3rd, DeVita MA, Rogers P. New aspects on critical care medicine training. Curr Opin Crit Care. 2004;10:233–7.

34. Eisold C, Poenicke C, Pfältzer A, Müller MP. Simulation in the intensive care setting. Best Pract Res Clin Anaesthesiol. 2015;29(1):51–60.

35. Rincon F, Mayer SA. Neurocritical care: a distinct discipline? Curr Opin Crit Care. 2007;13(2):115–21.

36. Smith MI. Neurocritical care: has it come of age? Br J Anaesth. 2004;93(6):753–5.

37. Suarez JI. Outcome in neurocritical care: advances in monitoring and treatment and effect of a specialized neurocritical care team. Crit Care Med. 2006;34(9 Suppl):S232–8.

38. Mirski MA, Chang CW, Cowan R. Impact of a neuroscience intensive care unit on neurosurgical patient outcomes and cost of care: evidence-based support for an intensivist-directed specialty ICU model of care. J Neurosurg Anesthesiol. 2001;13:83–92.

39. Diringer MN, Edwards DF. Admission to a neurologic/neurosurgical intensive care unit is associated with reduced mortality rate after intracerebral hemorrhage. Crit Care Med. 2001;29:635–40.

40. Le Roux P, Menon DK, Citerio G, Vespa P, Bader MK, Brophy GM, et al. Consensus summary statement of the international multidisciplinary consensus conference on multimodality monitoring in Neurocritical care: a statement for healthcare professionals from the Neurocritical Care Society and the European Society of Intensive Care Medicine. Neurocrit Care. 2014;21(Suppl 2):S1–26.

41. Goodman DJ, Kumar MA. Evidence-based Neurocritical care. Neurohospitalist. 2014;4(2):102–8.

42. Boulet JR, Murray D, Kras J, Woodhouse J, McAllister J, Ziv A. Reliability and validity of a simulation-based acute care skills assessment for medical students and residents. Anesthesiology. 2003;99(6):1270–80.

43. Saver JL. Time is brain – quantified. Stroke. 2006;37(1):263–6.

44. Schwamm L, Fayad P, Acker JE 3rd, Duncan P, Fonarow GC, Girgus M, et al. Translating evidence into practice: a decade of efforts by the American Heart Association/American Stroke Association to reduce death and disability due to stroke. A presidential advisory from the American Heart Association/American Stroke Association. Stroke. 2010;41(5):1051–65.

45. Herzer G, Illievich U, Voelckel WG, Trimmel H. Current practice in neurocritical care of patients with subarachnoid haemorrhage and severe traumatic brain injury : Results of the Austrian Neurosurvey Study. Wien Klin Wochenschr. 2016 Jul 12.

46. Berkhemer OA, Fransen PS, Beumer D, van den Berg LA, Lingsma HF, Yoo AJ, For the MR CLEAN Investigators, et al. A randomized trial of intraarterial treatment for acute ischemic stroke. N Engl J Med. 2015;372(1):11–20.

47. Goyal M, Demchuk AM, Menon BK, Eesa M, Rempel JL, Thornton J, For the ESCAPE Trial Investigators, et al. Randomized assessment of rapid endovascular treatment of ischemic stroke. N Engl J Med. 2015;372(11):1019–30.

48. Campbell BC, Mitchell PJ, Yan B, Parsons MW, Christensen S, Churilov L, for the EXTEND-IA Investigators, et al. A multicenter, randomized, controlled study to investigate extending the time for thrombolysis in emergency neurological deficits with intra-arterial therapy (EXTEND-IA). Int J Stroke. 2014;9(1):126–32.

49. Hemphill JC 3rd, Greenberg SM, Anderson CS, Becker K, Bendok BR, Cushman M, et al. Guidelines for the management of spontaneous intracerebral hemorrhage: a guideline for healthcare professionals from the American heart association/American stroke association. Stroke. 2015;46:2032–60.

50. Dagnone JD, McGraw R, Howes D, Messenger D, Bruder E, Hall A, et al. How we developed a comprehensive resuscitation-based simulation curriculum in emergency medicine. Med Teach. 2014;38:1–6.

51. Laack TA, Dong Y, Goyal DG, Sadosty AT, Suri HS, Dunn WF. Short-term and long-term impact of the central line workshop on resident clinical performance during simulated central line placement. Simul Healthc. 2014;9:228–33.

52. Miyasaka KW, Martin ND, Pascual JL, Buchholz J, Aggarwal R. A simulation curriculum for management of trauma and surgical critical care patients. J Surg Educ. 2015;72:803–10.

53. Murray DJ. Progress in simulation education: developing an anesthesia curriculum. Curr Opin Anaesthesiol. 2014;27:610–5.

54. Lewis SL, Józefowicz RF, Kilgore S, Dhand A, Edgar L. Introducing the neurology milestones. J Grad Med Educ. 2014;6(1 Suppl 1):102–4.

55. Fessler HE, Addrizzo-Harris D, Beck JM, Buckley JD, Pastores SM, Piquette CA, et al. Entrustable professional activities and curricular milestones for fellowship training in pulmonary and critical care medicine: executive summary from the Multi-Society Working Group. Crit Care Med. 2014;42(10):2290–1.

56. McGaghie WC, Issenberg SB, Cohen ER, Barsuk JH, Wayne DB. Does simulation-based medical education with deliberate practice yield better results than traditional clinical education? A meta-analytic comparative review of the evidence. Acad Med. 2011;86(6):706–11.

57. Cooke JM, Larsen J, Hamstra SJ, Andreatta PB. Simulation enhances resident confidence in critical care and procedural skills. Fam Med. 2008;40(3):165–7.

58. Ermak DM, Bower DW, Wood J, Sinz EH, Kothari MJ. Incorporating simulation technology into a neurology clerkship. J Am Osteopath Assoc. 2013;113(8):628–35.

59. Musacchio MJ Jr, Smith AP, McNeal CA, Munoz L, Rothenberg DM, von Roenn KA, et al. Neuro-critical care skills training using a human patient simulator. Neurocrit Care. 2010;13(2):169–75.

60. Barsuk JH, Cohen ER, Caprio T, McGaghie WC, Simuni T, Wayne DB. Simulation-based education with mastery learning improves residents' lumbar puncture skills. Neurology. 2012;79(2):132–7.

61. Papangelou A, Ziai W. The birth of neuro-simulation. Neurocrit Care. 2010;13(2):167–8.

62. Garside MJ, Rudd MP, Price CI. Stroke and TIA assessment training: a new simulation-based approach to teaching acute stroke assessment. Simul Healthc. 2012;7(2):117–22.

63. Smith M, Jankowski S. Simulation-based training improves ITU staff knowledge in the management of head injuries. BMJ Qual Improv Rep. 2014;3(1): pii: u201041–w972.

64. Greer DM, Varelas PN, Haque S, Wijdicks EF. Variability of brain death determination guidelines

in leading US neurologic institutions. Neurology. 2008;70:284–9.

65. Shappell CN, Frank JI, Husari K, Sanchez M, Goldenberg F, Ardelt A. Practice variability in brain death determination: a call to action. Neurology. 2013;81:2009–14.

66. Greer DM, Wang HH, Robinson JD, Varelas PN, Henderson GV, Wijdicks EF. Variability of brain death policies in the United States. JAMA Neurol. 2016;73(2):213–8.

67. Wang M, Wallace P, Gruen JP. Brain death documentation: analysis and issues. Neurosurgery. 2002;51:731–6.

68. MacDougall BJ, Robinson JD, Kappus L, Sudikoff SN, Greer DM. Simulation-based training in brain death determination. Neurocrit Care. 2014;21:383–91.

69. Wijdicks EF, Varelas PN, Gronseth GS, Greer DM. Evidence based guideline update: determining brain death in adults: report of the quality standards subcommittee of the American Academy of Neurology. Neurology. 2010;74:1911–8.

70. Hocker S, Schumacher D, Mandrekar J, Wijdicks EF. Testing confounders in brain death determination: a new simulation model. Neurocrit Care. 2015;23:401–8.

71. Wijdicks EF. Pitfalls and slip-ups in brain death determination. Neurol Res. 2013;35(2):169–73.

72. Braksick SA, Kashani K, Hocker S. Neurology Education for Critical Care Fellows Using High-Fidelity Simulation. Neurocrit Care. 2017;26(1):96–102.

73. Smith WS, Weingart S. Emergency Neurological Life Support (ENLS): what to do in the first hour of a neurological emergency. Neurocrit Care. 2012;17(Suppl1):S1–3.

74. Miller CM, Pineda J, Corry M, Brophy G, Smith WS. Emergency Neurologic Life Support (ENLS): evolution of management in the first hour of a neurological emergency. Neurocrit Care. 2015;23(Suppl 2):S1–4.

75. Stein DM, Pineda JA, Roddy V, Knight WA 4th. Emergency neurological life support: traumatic spine injury. Neurocrit Care. 2015;23(Suppl 2):S155–64.

76. Garvin R, Venkatasubramanian C, Lumba-Brown A, Miller CM. Emergency neurological life support: traumatic brain injury. Neurocrit Care. 2015;23(Suppl 2):S143–54.

77. Edlow JA, Figaji A, Samuels O. Emergency neurological life support: subarachnoid hemorrhage. Neurocrit Care. 2015;23(Suppl 2):S103–9.

78. Claassen J, Riviello JJ Jr, Silbergleit R. Emergency neurological life support: status epilepticus. Neurocrit Care. 2015;23(Suppl 2):S136–42.

79. O'Phalen KH, Bunney EB, Kuluz JW. Emergency neurologic life support: spinal cord compression. Neurocrit Care. 2015;23(Suppl 2):S129–35.

80. Rittenberger JC, Friess S, Polderman KH. Emergency neurological life support: resuscitation following cardiac arrest. Neurocrit Care. 2015;23(Suppl 2):S119–28.

81. Flower O, Wainwright MS, Caulfield AF. Emergency neurological life support: acute non-traumatic weakness. Neurocrit Care. 2015;23(Suppl 2):S23–47.

82. Stevens RD, Cadena RS, Pineda J. Emergency neurological life support: approach to the patient with coma. Neurocrit Care. 2015;23(Suppl 2):S69–75.

83. Jauch EC, Pineda JA, Hemphill JC. Emergency neurological life support: intracerebral hemorrhage. Neurocrit Care. 2015;23(Suppl 2):S83–93.

84. Stevens RD, Shoykhet M, Cadena R. Emergency neurological life support: intracranial hypertension and herniation. Neurocrit Care. 2015;23(Suppl 2):S76–82.

85. Gross H, Guilliams KP, Sung G. Emergency neurological life support: acute ischemic stroke. Neurocrit Care. 2015;23(Suppl 2):S94–102.

86. Gaieski DF, Nathan BR, O'Brien NF. Emergency neurologic life support: meningitis and encephalitis. Neurocrit Care. 2015;23(Suppl 2):S110–8.

87. Brophy GM, Human T, Shutter L. Emergency neurological life support: pharmacotherapy. Neurocrit Care. 2015;23(Suppl 2):S48–68.

88. Seder DB, Jagoda A, Riggs B. Emergency neurological life support: airway, ventilation, and sedation. Neurocrit Care. 2015;23(Suppl 2):S5–22.

89. The Cleveland Clinic Death by Neurologic Criteria course website: https://www.cchs.net/onlinelearning/cometvs10/dncPortal/default.htm.

90. University of Chicago International Brain Death Simulation Workshop website: http://events.uchicago.edu/cal/event/showEventMore.rdo;jsessionid=C50E5D92211CB65C99BED86509B148FB.

91. Efstathiou N, Walker WM. Interprofessional, simulation-based training in end of life care communication: a pilot study. J Interprof Care. 2014;28(1):68–70.

92. Schmitz CC, Braman JP, Turner N, Heller S, Radosevich DM, Yan Y, et al. Learning by (video) example: a randomized study of communication skills training for end-of-life and error disclosure family care conferences. Am J Surg. 2016;212:996–1004.

93. Brophy GM, Bell R, Claassen J, Alldredge B, Bleck TP, Glauser T, et al. Neurocritical care society status epilepticus guideline writing committee. Guidelines for the evaluation and management of status epilepticus. Neurocrit Care. 2012;17(1):3–23.

Index

© Springer International Publishing AG, part of Springer Nature 2018
A. Alaraj (ed.), *Comprehensive Healthcare Simulation: Neurosurgery*,
Comprehensive Healthcare Simulation, https://doi.org/10.1007/978-3-319-75583-0

Isaacs, R.E., 127
Ismail, R., 185–190, 192–195, 197, 265–277
Isolated brain, 114, 116

J
Jerry, Y., 128
Ju, C., 199–209
Jung, Y., 125
Junhui, 128

K
Kahol, K., 18
Kawashima, M., 69
Keen's point, 17
Keens, W.W., 17
Kessler, J., 127
Keyhole approach, 174
Kim, T.E., 79–86
Kimura, T., 49
Kinesthesia, 144
Kinesthetic receptors, 144
Kirkman, M.A., 18
Kocher, T., 18
Kocher's point, 18, 19
Kockro, R.A., 159–163, 165–169, 171, 172, 174–177, 179, 181, 296
Kondo, K., 55
Kreilinger, S.E.M., 323
Krishna, C., 65–71, 73, 74
Krisht, A., 103–105, 107–116
Kshettry, V.R., 120, 245
Kuhlen, T., 150
Kwasnicki, A., 185–190, 192–195, 197, 265–277

L
Lan, Q., 50
Lanier, J., 11
Laparoscopic surgery, 79
Large vessel occlusion, 34
Laser ablation amygdalo-hippocampectomy
    AC and PC localization, 260
    Brainlab software, 261
    image fusion, 260
    iPlan® Stereotaxy, 258
    laser cooling catheter and stylets, 261
    mesial temporal lobe epilepsy, 260
    MRI thermography, 262
    Visualase laser fiber, 260
Laser sintering technique, 54
Lawton, M., 285–288, 290
Lærdal, Å., 5, 8
Le Cat, C.-N., 17
Learning curve, 120–122, 125
    cadavers
        advantages and disadvantages, 120, 122
        CNS, 120
        lack of experience, 120

minimally invasive spinal procedures, 120
    residents, 120, 121
    TS, 125
    LS, 125–126
Learning theory, 317, 320
Lee, J.T., 80
Left ventricle every cardiac cycle, 31
Lemole, G.M., 21
Leonardo's physiological sketch, human brain and skull, 4, 6
Li, C., 60
Li, Z., 61
Libby Zion, 65
Lieber, B.B., 29–33, 35, 37–39
Limitations, neurocritical care, 328, 329
Link, E., 10
Liquid investment molding, 35
Liquid polymers, 35
Live and nonlive laboratory animals, 94
Live cadaver, 104–111
    aneurysm model, 116
    artificial tumor resection, 113–114, 116
    cisternal and vascular dissection, 112–114
    connections and settings, 104
    craniotomy, 112, 113
    development, 117
    embalming techniques, 116
    endoscopic procedures, 111–112
    health hazard, 116
    model evaluation
        questionnaire, 111
        trainees to practice aneurysmal clip placement, 111
    preparation
        head specimen, 104–105
        pseudoaneurysms, 106–108
    technical skills training, 114
    thrombectomy, 113, 115
    training exercises
        aneurysm clipping exercises, 106–109
        aneurysmal clipping and management of rupture, 106, 108
        management of intraoperative rupture, 109–110
    vascular surgery, 114
    vascular suturing and anastomosis, 113, 115
Live cadaver model, 289, 290
Living cadavers, 286
Living human cerebral vasculature, 104
Lobel, D.A., 201
Low back pain, 131
Luciano, C., 57
Luciano, C.J., 141–143, 145–150
Ludwig, C.S., 127
Lumbar cadaveric spine
    complications, 126, 127
    decompression and stabilization procedures, 126
    diagnosis, 126
    operations, 126
Lumbar disc herniation, 126